Natural Compounds as Inducers of Cell Death

Marc Diederich • Karoline Noworyta
Editors

Natural Compounds as Inducers of Cell Death

Volume 1

Springer

Editors
Marc Diederich
Laboratoire de Biologie
Moléculaire et Cellulaire du Cancer
Hôpotal Kirchberg
Steichen, Luxembourg

Karoline Noworyta
Laboratoire de Biologie
Moléculaire et Cellulaire du Cancer
Hôpotal Kirchberg
Steichen, Luxembourg

ISBN 978-94-007-4574-2 ISBN 978-94-007-4575-9 (eBook)
DOI 10.1007/978-94-007-4575-9
Springer Dordrecht Heidelberg New York London

Library of Congress Control Number: 2012947412

Printed on acid-free paper

Springer is part of Springer Science+Business Media (www.springer.com)

Editorial

Natural Products Research in the Greater Saar-Lor-Lux Region: Corena

This book was edited under the patronage of CORENA, a network aiming to create an internationally competitive cluster within the Greater Region (Saarland, Lorraine, Luxembourg, Wallonia, Rhineland-Palatinate). CORENA is co-funded by European Regional development fund within the INTERREG IVA Greater Region program. The European Union invests in your future.

Since its official foundation in April 2009, the CORENA Network has brought together existing researchers and research structures from various scientific and institutional backgrounds throughout the greater Saar-Lor-Lux region to join forces in the field of natural product research. Since then, the Network has been a catalyst to initiate and deepen cross-border research and development – and has resulted in a crystallization point for natural product research involving various universities, research institutes, and companies in the Greater Region.

The CORENA network is the combination of research, development, and applications. The aim of the project is to create an internationally competitive cluster that links the particular research institutions and companies within the Greater Region (Saarland, Lorraine, Luxembourg, Wallonia, Rhineland-Palatinate). Scientifically, the Network aims at the promotion of the use of natural products in medicine and agriculture. In biomedical research, natural ingredients, such as antioxidants and chemopreventive agents, have recently come back into focus. Here, ageing Societies provide an impetus to (re-)consider nutri-therapeutics, from simple vitamins to highly promising, natural product based nutri-epigenetic substances. At the same time, the CORENA Network supports the idea of green, eco-friendly pesticides extracted from natural substances such as plants or fungi. Within this context, the focus has been no substances derived from edible plants, which promise low or now toxicity to animals and humans, yet may be effective against common agricultural pests.

The CORENA Network established in the Saar-Lor-Lux region is a highly successful network of major research institutions, companies, producers and users.

During the last three years, existing expertise in the field of natural products within the greater Saar-Lor-Lux area has been bundled, thereby increasing the scientific potential and industrial competitiveness of the whole region. As part of the network, closer cross-border cooperation between industry and research in the field of natural products is now easily possible. Thus, small and medium enterprises (SMEs) have gained access to the latest research, while the researchers in exchange have benefited from new ideas and stimuli provided by the companies. This mutually beneficial exchange has contributed significantly to the innovation potential of the Greater Region in this area of Science. The CORENA Network will certainly grow and deepen further in the years to come, attracting researchers and companies from throughout the Region and beyond.

Marc Diederich and Karoline Noworyta
(Recherchhes Scientifiques Luxembourg asbl), editors
Claus Jacob
(Universität des Saarlandes, Germany)
Gilbert Kirsch
(Université de Metz, France)

Contents

Part I
Phytochemicals as Inducers of Cell Death Mechanisms

Chapter 1
Phytochemicals and Amino Acids: Inducers or Inhibitors of Cell Death?

Asser Ghoneim

Abstract Phytochemicals and amino acids have long been considered as important inducers of cell death. However, many of these natural compounds have been demonstrating dual action effects on cell death through inhibition as well as induction. Clinical applications may require dosage adjustment and determination of selectively vulnerable cells, either normal or cancer cells. Indeed, the opposing actions and controversial uses as cytoprotective and/or cytotoxic agents, in different tissues and diseases, need further scrutiny. The potential usefulness of these natural compounds as combined chemoprotectants for cancer chemotherapy should also be taken into consideration. Special emphasis will be placed on curcumin and *Astragalus* constituents as potential phytochemicals. Relevant amino acids include the excitatory and branched-chain ones, as well as glycine and cysteine.

1.1 Phytochemicals

1.1.1 Terminology, Definition and Classification

The word part "*phyto-*" is a root derived from a Greek origin meaning "plant". Hence, *phyto*chemicals, also known as plant secondary metabolites, represent a diverse group of bioactive natural organic chemical products. They can be generally classified as phenolics, terpenoids, glycosides, and alkaloids (Barrett 2004; Liu 2004). Phenolics are compounds possessing one or more hydroxyl groups attached to an

A. Ghoneim, Ph.D. (✉)
Department of Pharmacology and Toxicology, Faculty of Pharmacy,
Damanhour University (formerly Alexandria University, Damanhour Branch),
El Gomhouria street, Damanhour 22514, Egypt
e-mail: asser.ghoneim@alexpharmacy.edu.eg; asserg2001@yahoo.com

M. Diederich and K. Noworyta (eds.), *Natural Compounds as Inducers of Cell Death: Volume 1*, DOI 10.1007/978-94-007-4575-9_1,

aromatic ring system. Among the most commonly consumed green and yellow fruits and vegetables that possess the highest phenolic content we can mention cranberry, apple, broccoli, and spinach. The terpenoids, sometimes called isoprenoids, are naturally-occurring organic chemicals similar to terpenes, derived from five-carbon isoprene units (hydrocarbons containing two unsaturated bonds). The most common plant sources of terpenoids are carrots and tomatoes. Alkaloids are organic substances having a nitrogen atom and exhibiting alkaline properties and physiologic actions. They are particularly common in certain families such as Fabaceae, Solanaceae and Papaveraceae. Alkaloids affecting cell death comprise taxol from *Taxus* and swainsonine from *Astragalus*. Glycosides are molecules containing sugar bound to non-carbohydrate moiety. Some glycosides can be found in nature as sugars bound to flavonoids (polyphenolics). Glycosides are widespread throughout the plant kingdom with some toxic members especially the cyanogenic and the cardiac glycosides (Liu 2004; Molyneux et al. 2007; Pengelly 2004).

1.1.2 Phytochemicals as Cancer Chemopreventive Agents

Chemoprevention refers to the use of non-toxic chemical substances to prevent carcinogenesis. Epidemiologic studies indicate that the regular consumption of phytochemicals, can reduce the risk of certain cancers. Besides, the current cancer control approach involves a shift from chemotherapy to chemoprevention. Selected chemopreventive phytochemicals include curcumin (Cur) and resveratrol (Kundu and Surh 2009).

1.1.2.1 Mechanisms of Cancer Prevention by Phytochemicals

Most chemopreventive phytochemicals are defined as either blocking agents, which act immediately before or during the initiation of chemical carcinogenesis, or suppressing agents, which act thereafter during the stages of promotion and progression (Duvoix et al. 2005; Johnson 2007). Chemoprevention can be achieved mechanistically by enhancing cellular antioxidant activity, promoting carcinogen detoxificating enzymes, blocking carcinogen activating enzymes, suppressing abnormally activated pro-inflammatory signals, inhibition of metastasis, immunostimulation, antiangiogenesis, and induction of cell death (Fig. 1.1). In brief, the major actions involve almost the whole spectrum of cellular basic machinery, from cell membrane to signaling cytoplasmic molecules and to the major nuclear components (Kampa et al. 2007; Kundu and Surh 2009; Liu 2004).

1.1.2.2 Phytochemicals as Inducers of Cell Death

Phytochemicals may induce cell death by stimulation of apoptosis and/or necrosis, modulation of oxidative stress, inhibition of cell proliferation, tumor suppressor gene expression, inhibition of oncogene expression, induction of cell-cycle arrest,

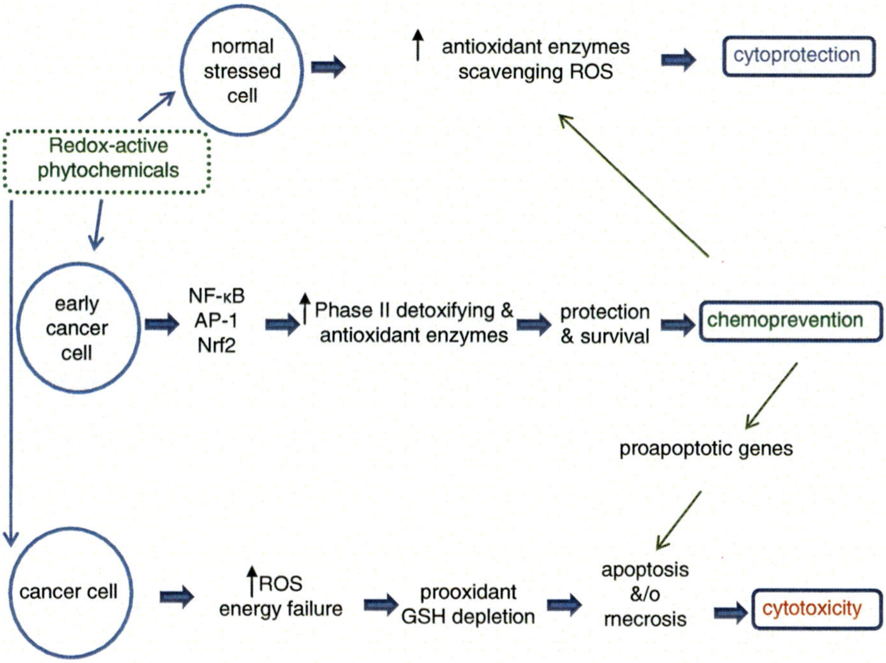

Fig. 1.1 Redox-active phytochemicals as cytoprotective, cytotoxic and/or chemopreventive agents

and inhibition of signal transduction pathways (Kundu and Surh 2009; Liu 2004; Tosetti et al. 2009). The apoptosis signaling pathways have profound effect on the progression of cancer. Induction of apoptosis is, hence, an important goal of treatment strategies for cancer (Hu et al. 2009; Lowe and Lin 2000). Indeed, polyphenols have been found to affect cancer cell growth by inducing apoptosis in many cell lines, both in vitro and in vivo. In many cases, apoptosis induced by polyphenols was caspase 3-dependent (Hu et al. 2009; Kampa et al. 2007). Examples of phytochemical inducers of cell death include quercetin, kaempferol, apigenin, resveratrol, EGCG, catechins, Cur, etc. The types of cells responding to these phytochemicals by undergoing cell death include both normal and tumor cells. For example, different cells exist such as rat primary hepatocytes, the hepatocellular carcinoma HepG2, the colon CaCo-2, the prostate DU145, the breast MCF7, the melanoma SK-MEL-1, the Molt 4B leukemia cells, etc (Ghoneim 2009; Kampa et al. 2007).

1.1.2.3 Phytochemicals as Inhibitors of Cell Death

On the other hand, an antiapoptotic effect based on the ability of polyphenols to scavenge free radicals, has also been observed. For example, resveratrol prevents apoptosis by inhibiting lipoxygenase and cyclooxygenase activity in K562 cells.

A similar effect of cell death inhibition was also observed in PC12 cells with tea catechins as well as, Cur and different crude plant extracts in liver cells (Badr et al. 2009; Ghoneim 2009; Ghoneim and Eldahshan 2012; (Kampa et al. 2007). In addition, silymarin (16 mg/kg/day) has proven effective in preventing apoptotic and necrotic cell death in mice liver (Patel et al. 2010).

1.1.2.4 Phytochemicals as Redox Active Compounds with Dual Effects

Redox-sensitive transcription factors might also be potential targets for chemoprevention by phytochemicals (Kundu and Surh 2009). Their key molecular targets include the nuclear transcription factor NF-κB, AP-1, hypoxia-inducible transcription factor and AKT, which are redox-sensitive molecules. Numerous phytochemicals such as curcumin (Cur) target the transcription factor Nrf2 (nuclear factor (erythroid-derived 2)-related factor). Nrf2 activates an antioxidant defense response by ARE antioxidant response element-mediated induction of Phase II detoxifying and antioxidant enzymes (Tosetti et al. 2009). For example, Cur supplementation in mice results in increased expression of detoxification enzymes glutathione-s-transferases, glutathione reductase, and catalase in the liver, small intestine and kidney tissues. Besides, Cur induces Nrf2/ARE pathway in human monocytes and rat kidney epithelial cells and HepG2 cells (Gopalakrishnan and Tony Kong 2008; Kundu and Surh 2009). Furthermore, opposing redox effects of several phytochemicals in different pathophysiological situations have been reported including Cur and resveratrol. For example, resveratrol can be both antioxidant or prooxidant in different conditions and tumor cell types (Holme and Pervaiz 2007). Cur, also, can produce a dose-dependent prooxidant state inside tumor cells. This effect is exerted by promoting either reactive oxygen species (ROS) generation by mitochondria or NADPH oxidases. Another mechanism may be through induction of redox imbalance through glutathione (GSH) depletion or impairment of its biosynthesis (Hail and Lotan 2009). Conversely, several phytochemicals act as antioxidants by scavenging ROS directly or by enhancing antioxidant enzymes activity (Tosetti et al. 2009).

1.1.3 Cytotoxic Phytochemicals Are Cytoprotective to Normal Cells

Many redox-active phytochemicals are apparently able to induce cytoprotection and cell survival in normal cells by improving cell defense systems. However, they can act as cytotoxic agents in tumor cells whose survival depends on energetic resources mainly occupied to maintain an unstable redox equilibrium. The control of energy balance at the cellular level may explain these apparently opposite effects. This might comprise the pathophysiological contexts regarding ROS production and the functionality of the antioxidant defense systems. One should also consider the dose used and duration of the drug use, along with tissue-specific effects on redox balance (Hail and Lotan 2009; Tosetti et al. 2009). Redox perturbation, in both a prooxidant or antioxidant direction, shows homeostatic responses by phytochemicals. These apparently produce an overall balancing effect through preconditioning, to protect against a severe stress, by reinforcing normal cell defenses (Mattson 2008). Concerning mild redox stress, the antioxidant defense response seems to be cytoprotective for normal and untransformed cells, probably because it counteracts genotoxic damage and detoxifies excessive ROS. This might explain the hepato-, neuro- and cardioprotective effects of phytochemicals such as Cur and resveratrol in corresponding normal cells (Ghoneim 2009; Tosetti et al. 2009). Meanwhile, the same signals can become intolerable for tumor cells, where elevated ROS and impaired antioxidant systems, fueled by enhanced glucose metabolism, are unsuitable to maintain viability and proliferation (Nair et al. 2007; Tosetti et al. 2009). Moreover, by activating Nrf2, phytochemicals can enhance the detoxification of carcinogens and thus block tumor initiation in non-neo-plastic cells. Alternatively, abnormal cancer cells constitutively express amplified signaling pathways of cell proliferation and suppressed apoptosis. By modulating transcription factors such as NFκB and AP-1, the same phytochemicals may inhibit these signaling pathways leading to apoptosis. Both Cur and resveratrol suppress NF-κB activity, resulting in increased apoptosis in human breast cancer cells, mantle cell lymphoma and multiple myeloma cells. Furthermore, both phenolics attenuate AP-1 activity in human cervical cancer (HeLa) and HaCaT cells. However, in human colon cancer HT-29 cells resveratrol has been shown to increase lipopolysaccharide-induced AP-1 activity (Gopalakrishnan and Tony Kong 2008; Kundu and Surh 2009). For a better description of the meanings of terms "chemopreventive", "cytotoxic", and "cytoprotective", refer to (Fig. 1.1).

1.1.4 Toxic Phytochemicals as Chemoprotective Agents

Phytochemicals investigated initially for their toxic properties in normal cells in poisoning animals may eventually prove to have benefits to humans as therapeutics. For example, swainsonine alkaloid, identified in species of Astragalus and Oxytropis, was historically associated with locoweed poisoning as a toxic phytochemical to normal cells. Besides, swainsonine, as a cytotoxic phytochemical to tumor cells, is used for treatment of cancer by inhibition of glycoprotein-processing pathways, and enhancement of natural killer cell activity (Bowlin et al. 1989). Swainsonine has also been shown to protect from cytotoxicity of cyclophosphamide without interfering with its chemotherapeutic activity. Thus, it may be considered as a chemoprotective phytochemical against chemotherapy-induced toxicity in normal cells. Swainsonine has also important immunomodulation, increasing colony forming unit capacity, indicating a potential to overcome the bone marrow suppressive effects of chemotherapy (Molyneux et al. 2007).

1.1.5 Curcumin

Curcumin (Cur), among phenolic phytochemicals, is made of two ferulic acids linked by a methylene in a diketone structure (Liu 2004). Cur is regarded as the most active constituent of turmeric preparations. Cur has been the subject of many articles studying its antioxidant, antiinflammatory, cytoprotective, and chemotherapeutic properties (Ghoneim 2009; Ravindran et al. 2009; Salvioli et al. 2007; Sharma et al. 2005)

1.1.5.1 Mechanisms of Anti-cancer Activity

The molecular targets of anti-cancer activity of Cur may originate from its antioxidant activity and induction of phase II detoxifying enzymes (Iqbal et al. 2003). Other Cur activities with potential anticancer effects include down-regulation of transcription factors such as NF-kB and AP-1; down-regulation of the expression of enzymes such as cyclooxygenase, nitric oxide synthase, matrix metalloproteinase; down-regulation of tumor necrosis factor, chemokines, and growth factor receptors; and inhibition of the activity of c-Jun N-terminal kinase and other protein kinases. Additionally, Cur has an anti-angiogenic activity (Maheshwari et al. 2006) and it induces both types of cell death, apoptosis and necrosis, in many types of cancer and normal cells (Aggarwal et al. 2003; Duvoix et al. 2005; Ravindran et al. 2009; Salvioli et al. 2007), see Fig. 1.2 (Ghoneim 2009). Cur ability to induce apoptosis in preclinical models supports its potential utility in cancer chemotherapy (Sharma et al. 2005).

1.1.5.2 Mechanisms of Apoptosis Induction

Cur can induce the intracellular mitochondrial apoptotic pathway as well as the extracellular one (Anto et al. 2002; Rashmi et al. 2005). The induction of apoptosis pathways involves mitochondrial activation and DNA fragmentation (Ravindran et al. 2009). Cur-induced apoptosis is either p53-dependent or independent (Salvioli et al. 2007). The role of ROS in Cur-induced apoptosis is controversial, since Cur can exert both pro- and anti-oxidant effects (Ahsan et al. 1999). The sensitivity of many tumor cells to Cur correlates with generation of ROS (Mishra et al. 2005) and many antioxidants prevent Cur-induced apoptosis. Besides, Cur inhibits apoptosis via a GSH-independent pathway in normal cells (Jaruga et al. 1998). However, Cur is a potent scavenger of ROS and increases the level of GSH (Salvioli et al. 2007). This pleiotropic activity of Cur can be explained by its activity on gene transcription regulation. Cur inhibits AP-1 and NF-kB transcription factors, which are involved in cell proliferation and apoptotic pathways (Salvioli et al. 2007; Sharma et al. 2005; Sikora et al. 1997). Cur can overcome resistance to many apoptosis-inducing factors

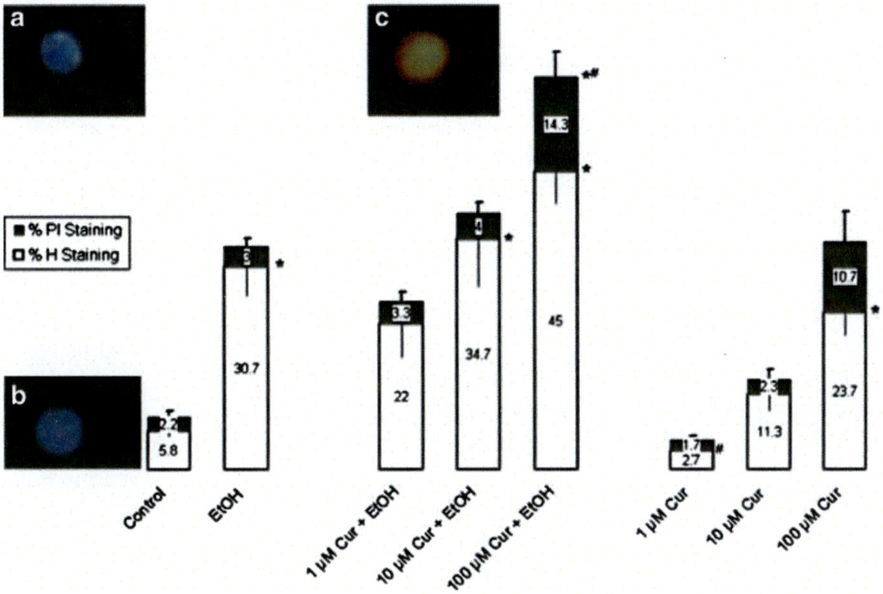

Fig. 1.2 Effects of curcumin (*Cur*) on ethanol (*EtOH*)-induced apoptosis and/or necrosis in hepatocyte monolayers. Hepatocytes were preincubated with increasing concentrations (1–100 µM) of Cur for 30 min before addition of 0.1 M EtOH where indicated together. Fluorescence microscopy was used for monitoring nuclear alterations and membrane dysfunction after an additional 4 h of monolayer culture (37°C, 5% CO2). Apoptotic cells, as represented by the hepatocyte shown in panel a, exhibiting chromatin condensation, fragmentation, and margination, are counted for percent Hoechst 33258 (H) staining of the total number of cells in *panel A* plus normal viable hepatocytes as that shown in *panel B*. Changing filters allows for monitoring of necrotic cells, as represented by the hepatocyte shown in *panel C*, counted for percent propidium iodide (*PI*)-stained cells of the total number of cells in *panels A* and *B*. Data shown are representatives of the means ± standard error of mean (*SEM*) of three to five experiments. Statistically significant difference among groups is indicated as $^*p<0.05$ vs. corresponding control group and $\#p<0.05$ vs. corresponding EtOH group. Statistical analysis was done using analysis of variance (*ANOVA*) followed by Tukey-Kramer as post hoc test for multiple comparisons (Ghoneim 2009). The data herein indicated that 100 µM Cur provoked apoptosis. In addition, this relatively high Cur concentration added to EtOH showed progressive necrosis in hepatocyte monolayers. Technically, necrosis and apoptosis can occur simultaneously depending on insult intensity reiterating the importance of the new terminology "necrapoptosis," describing the implication of both forms of cell death clearly using the H/PI double staining for hepatocytotoxicity by curcumin (Ghoneim 2009)

by affecting multiple signaling pathways and by affecting survivin, thus potentiating the effect of chemotherapy (Aggarwal and Shishodia 2006; Ravindran et al. 2009). Cur can also induce cell death in many types of normal cells, such as rat thymocytes and hepatocytes leading to undesirable side effects (Donatus et al. 1990; Ghoneim 2009; Ravindran et al. 2009).

1.1.5.3 Curcumin Protects Against Cell Death

Concomitantly, with Cur as a cytotoxic agents that may enhance the cytotoxicity of chemotherapeutic agents (Chan et al. 2003), there are many reports showing that Cur treatment is not associated with programmed cell death (Mehta et al. 1997; Raza et al. 2008; Syng-Ai et al. 2004). In addition, Cur has been shown to protect normal and cancer cells against apoptosis (Jaruga et al. 1998; Piwocka et al. 2001; Sikora et al. 1997; Somasundaram et al. 2002; Zhu et al. 2004). Indeed, Cur administration has been shown to be hepatoprotective in liver injury caused by many hepatotoxins (Donatus et al. 1990; Park et al. 2000; Shapiro et al. 2006). Moreover, Cur, as a neuroprotectant, exerts a protective effect against neurodegeneration and stroke (Bala et al. 2006; Ghoneim et al. 2002). Possible mechanisms of neuroprotection exerted by Cur include inhibition of excytotoxicity, antioxidant activity, and induction of chaperone proteins (Bala et al. 2006; Yazawa et al. 2006). It is obvious, therefore, that the effects of Cur may be tissue specific and that it may target proliferating cells more efficiently than differentiated ones (Ghoneim 2009; Sharma et al. 2005; Syng-Ai et al. 2004). Possible explanations might include the higher cellular uptake of Cur is in tumor cells than in normal cells (Kunwar et al. 2008). Second, lower GSH levels exist in tumor cells compared to normal cells (Syng-Ai et al. 2004). Third, most tumor cells, but not normal cells, express constitutively active NF-κB that is suppressed by Cur (Ravindran et al. 2009; Shishodia et al. 2005). In addition, Cur has been demonstrated to inhibit both cell growth and cell death. The capacity of Cur to inhibit both cell growth and death implies that these two biological processes may share common pathways (Sikora et al. 1997). Furthermore, this contradiction can be explained by the pleiotropic activity of Cur, which has many molecular targets inside the cell. Moreover, many of the studies are based on the assumption that apoptosis is detected by oligonucleosomal DNA degradation. This can be a misleading concept, since Cur can induce cell death despite a simultaneous inhibition on endonuclease activity (Sikora et al. 2006). Besides, the methods used for lipid peroxidation (LP) are relatively blunt tools in vivo where alterations may be too circumscribed to show up in whole tissue analysis, and because products accumulated may be metabolized (Agardh et al. 1991). Moreover, a direct causal relationship between LP, as a hallmark of oxidative stress, and cell death is still disputed (Ghoneim 2009; Plaa 2000). Another suggested reason for this divergence relies on the capability of Cur to exert a biphasic effect, depending on its concentration. For example, Cur at different concentrations elicits a biphasic effect on apoptosis in keratinocytes (Jana et al. 2004) and hepatocytes (Ghoneim 2009). The biphasic effect of Cur can also impose on the type of cell death; either apoptosis or necrosis depending on ROS generation and ATP levels (Chan et al. 2006). Indeed, Cur has been shown to exhibit concentration-dependent antilipid peroxidant cytoprotectant as well as GSH-depleting cytotoxic effects in isolated hepatocytes. Besides, Cur may have important pharmacological applications as a potential concentration-dependent modulator of cytochrome c release-induced apoptosis (Ghoneim 2009). Furthermore, a temporal biphasic activity is given by the effect of Cur on NF-κB levels (Notarbartolo et al. 2005).

1.1.6 *Astragalus*

1.1.6.1 History and Origin

Astragalus L. (Fabaçeae, Papillinoideae) is a widely distributed genus throughout the temperate regions of the world, with about 2,000 species described (Boulos 1999). The plant was given its traditional names, Astragalus and milk vetch; from the belief that the genus vetch 'Vicia' of the bean family increases the milk 'gala' yield of livestock, besides, its legumes have a star-shape 'astr' (Asaad 1977).

1.1.6.2 Chemistry

The genus Astragalus appears highly uniform from chemical point of view, with three main pharmacologically active principles and three kinds of toxic compounds (e.g., swainsonine). The major pharmacologically active constituents of Astragalus belong to cycloartane- and oleanane-type saponins, flavonoids and polysaccharides (Rios and Waterman 1997; Pistelli 2002; Sinclair 1998).

1.1.6.3 Pharmacology

The most interesting pharmacological activities include: cytotoxic, cytoprotective, immunomodulator, antimicrobial, anti–inflammatory and cardiovascular effects (Rios and Waterman 1997; Sinclair 1998; Mills and Bone 2000; Pistelli 2002).

Protective Effects of Astragalus

Pretreatment with Astragalus mongholicus isoflavonoids has increased the activities of antioxidant enzymes and prevented the release of LDH in glutamate-injured cells (Yu et al. 2005). The Astragalus membranaceous root extracts have been widely studied for hepatoprotective properties (Li et al. 2003). Zhang et al. (1992) reported the hepatoprotective effect of the saponins isolated from Astragalus membranaceous and Astragalus sieversianus against the chemically induced liver injury in mice. Besides, the saponins were evaluated in cultured rat hepatocytes and indicated that hepatoprotection may be attributable to antioxidant action, enhanced protein synthesis and immunoregulatory effect. Moreover, an Astragalus polysaccharide isolated from Astragalus mongholicus exhibited a dose-dependent decrease in MDA, increase in GSH and ATP and increase of survival rate in mouse liver damage (Rios and Waterman 1997). In addition, a triterpenoidal glucuronide and a flavonoid, both obtained from Astragalus complanatus, showed hepatoprotective action on immunological liver injury in cultured hepatocytes and anti-fibrotic action in rat liver, respectively (Kinjo et al. 1999; Liu et al. 2005). Astragalus normalized elevated SGPT levels in chronic viral hepatitis patients (Mills and Bone 2000). Furthermore, several Astragalus species exhibited promising protective effects against programmed cell death. For example, Astragalus membranaceous inhibits free radical production, inhibits LDH release, and decreases apoptosis of cardiomyocytes (Luo et al. 2009). In addition, it inhibits apoptosis of human peritoneal mesothelial cells (Na et al. 2009). Also, Astragalus reduces spermatogenic cell apoptosis, decreases the level of LP and protects GSH in the torsional testis (Zhen et al. 2008). Besides, Astragalus lowers plasma levels of apoptosis-related factors improving cardiac function (Zhang et al. 2005).

Cytotoxic Activities of Astragalus

On the other hand, the roots of Astragalus spp. are known to be rich in polysaccharides and saponins that are reported to possess anticancer and immunostimulating effects (Rios and Waterman 1997; Bedir et al. 2000; Yesilada et al. 2005). Apoptosis was induced in HEL cells by Astragalus membranaceus. Upregulation of Apaf-1, casp-3 and acetylcholinesterase may have played a crucial role in the process of apoptosis. The prospect of inducing apoptosis selectively in cancer cells is obviously attractive from a therapeutic point of view (Cheng et al. 2004). Indeed, Astragalus is reported to treat various types of cancers (Yesilada et al. 2005). It has also shown to potentiate the activity of chemotherapeutic agents, reduce their adverse toxicities, inhibit recurrences and to prolong survival time (Zee-Cheng 1992; Sinclair 1998). In parallel, Astragalus-based Chinese herbal medicine have been shown to increase effectiveness of platinum-based chemotherapy (McCulloch et al. 2006). Recently, flavonoids from Astragalus complanatus induced apoptosis in human hepatocarcinoma cells via mitochondria-dependent and death receptor-dependent apoptotic pathways (Hu et al. 2009). Besides, Astragalus mongholicus induced apoptosis and inhibited proliferation in different tumor cell lines (Yan et al. 2009; Zhou et al. 2009). Moreover, Astragalus saponins induced growth inhibition and apoptosis via an ERK-independent NF-kappaB signaling pathway in HepG2 cell line and colon cancer cells (Auyeung et al. 2009; Tin et al. 2007). Furthermore, the volatile fractions from Astragalus corniculatus Bieb. were found to be cytotoxic by induction of necrotic cell death, which could mainly be ascribed to the high content of hydrocarbons and squalene (Krasteva et al. 2008).

1.1.6.4 Egyptian Astragalus Species

Pharmacology

Astragalus L., the largest genus in the family Fabaçeae (Leguminoseae), is represented by 32 species in Egypt (Laurent-Täckholm 1974; Boulos 1999). Some species of this genus have been reported as having immunostimulant, cytotoxic and antiviral activities (Verotta and El-Sebakhy 2001). For example, Astragaloside II, isolated from A. spinosus has shown good activity against human cancer cell lines; particularly, the colon and the leukemia cell lines. It also exhibited a 100% protective effect on T–lymphocytes against human immunodeficiency virus (Abdallah et al. 1993). Moreover, Astragalus kahiricus initial extract has reproducible cytotoxicity against ovarian cancer cell line (Radwan et al. 2004).

Chemistry

Previous phytochemical studies performed on some Egyptian Astragalus spp. have resulted in the isolation of large series of cycloartane- and oleanane-type saponins (Asaad 2000; Radwan et al. 2004), as well as flavonoids (Asaad 1983; Radwan 2004).

Selected Example of Egyptian Astragalus

Two Astragalus extracts were screened for modulatory effect on hepatocyte necrosis. It was found that A. spinosus extract didn't protect hepatocytes in suspension culture, but it showed a slight cytotoxic trend over the whole range of concentrations tested (Ghoneim 2006). This might be further screened for probable activity against hepatic carcinoma, in the light of the anticancer activity of one of the triterpene saponins of this species (Abdallah et al. 1993), and the presence of Astragaloside IV; a strong scavenger for superoxide and hydroxyl radicals (Luo et al. 2004).

On the other hand, the extract of A. boeticus conferred significant protection against both EtOH- and spontaneously- induced hepatocyte death. A. boeticus seemed safe over all tested concentrations (Ghoneim 2006). The marked difference between the two species might be attributable to a difference in the amount of pharmacologically active constituents that are concentrated in the polar n-butanolic extract. An important preliminary TLC screening revealed a remarkable increase in the flavonoids in the case of the A. boeticus whole herb much more than the roots of A. spinosus that contains mainly cycloartane saponins. See Fig. 1.3 (Ghoneim 2006). The flavonoids, that are normally prevalent in the flowers and leaves of the whole herbs, are well reputed for their antioxidant, radical scavenging, an hepatoprotective activities through their chemical structure that gives them their characteristic beautiful colors (Mills and Bone 2000; Liu et al. 2005). Generally, the flavonoids represent the main active constituents of the standard and most studied hepatoprotective and membrane stabilizer plant extract; silymarin (Badr et al. 2009; Luper 1998; Liu et al. 2005). Also, the saponin glycosides are documented in several Astragalus spp. to have potential hepatoprotective and anti-oxidant activities (Zhang et al. 1992; Luo et al. 2004).

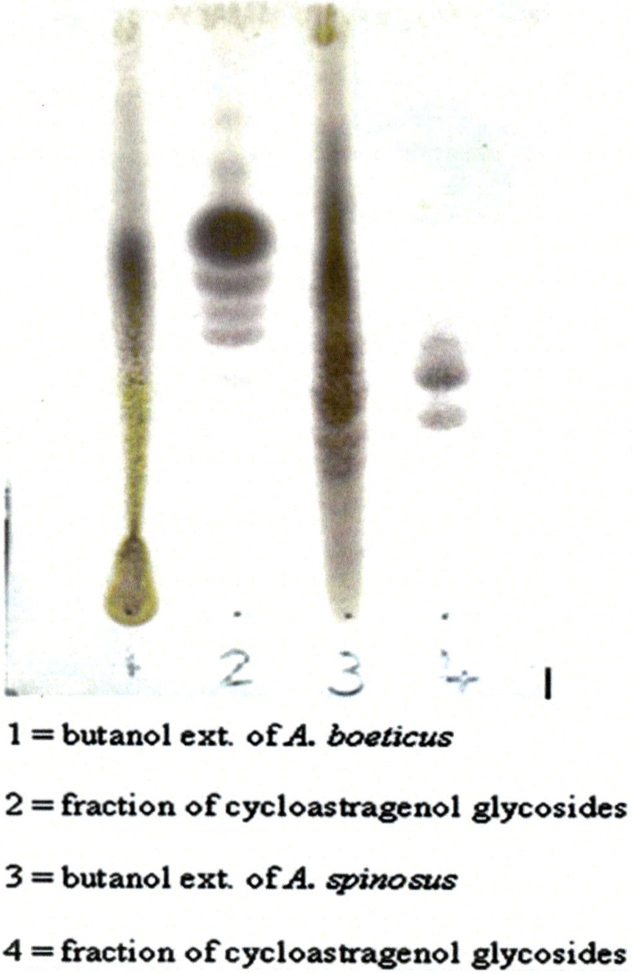

Fig. 1.3 TLC plate of the n-butanolic extracts of *A. boeticus* L. and *A. spinosus* Forssk. Spray Reagent: Modified Anisaldehyde/sulfuric, then heated at 120°C for 2 min. The *yellowish spots* are flavonoids in nature. The *violet spots* are tetracyclic cycloartane saponins in nature (Stahl 1969; Asaad 1983; Radwan 2004). The plant extraction and the TLC were performed by Prof. Dr. Aya Asaad (Faculty of Pharmacy, Alexandria University) (Ghoneim 2006)

1.2 Amino Acids

1.2.1 Introduction

Proteins are essential components of all cells. They help maintain the cell's structure, transport certain substances in and out of cells, and act as enzymes that mediate almost all biochemical reactions occurring in the cells; including the antioxidant enzymes. Proteins are composed of approximately 20 different building blocks called amino acids. Some of the amino acids have free radical scavenging activity. Amino acids for clinical purposes should not be viewed simply as building blocks for protein synthesis, but as important modulators of cell functions and as drugs (Battezzati and Riso 2002; Fang et al. 2002; Ghoneim 2006).

1.2.2 Amino Acids as Inducers of Cell Death

Varying reports can be found on the application and effect of amino acids to tumor bearing animals, probably due to nature of tumors, experimental animals and amino acid concentrations (Grossie et al. 1992; Ma et al. 1996). Amino acids that are able to potentiate starvation-induced apoptosis (e.g., L-norleucine and arginine) deserve further attention as possible candidates for novel anti-tumor agents (Franek et al. 2002).

1.2.2.1 Excitatory Amino Acids and Cell Death

A prolonged or excessive activation of excitatory amino acid receptors leads to irreversible cell death. Anti-excitotoxic drugs include N-methyl-D-aspartate (NMDA) receptor antagonists and glycine site antagonists (Doble 1999). Various mechanisms have been proposed to explain the excitotoxic cell death characteristic of neurodegenerative diseases, including elevation of intracellular calcium, oxidative stress, and activation of apoptosis (Dong et al. 2009).

Excitotoxicity and Apoptosis

Apoptosis is the programmed cell death that contrasts with classical necrosis (Thompson 1995). Excitotoxicity was considered to be mainly caused by necrosis with swelling and cell lysis. However, more recent findings suggest that these two modes are complementary and interchangeable (Doble 1999). The stimulation of ionotropic glutamate receptors in neurons results in a p53-dependent apoptosis (Uberti et al. 1998).

Glycine as an Excitatory Co-transmitter

Glycine (Gly) is an essential co-agonist at an NMDA receptor site different from that of glutamate (Johnson and Ascher 1987). Exogenous Gly also potentiates the synaptic effects of glutamate (Doble 1999). Indeed, the administration of high dose Gly resulted in convulsions and death of injected rats (unpublished observation). In connection, homocysteine, an excitatory amino acid homolog of cysteine, induces neuronal cell death via stimulation of NMDA receptors. In the whole animal studies, homocysteine administered also at very high dosages induced seizures in rats (Moore et al. 2001).

Excitatory Amino Acids as Inhibitors of Cell Death

Alternatively, Glutamate may be either trophic or toxic for neurons (Balazs et al. 1988). The chronic treatment with NMDA prevents the excitotoxic response produced by a later "acute" administration of glutamate receptor agonists. Early activation of NMDA receptors inhibits apoptosis by receptor downregulation (Lladó et al. 1999).

1.2.2.2 Branched-Chain Amino Acids and Cell Death

Branched-chain amino acids (BCAAs) diminish neoplastic cell proliferation at supraphysiological concentrations. The use of high concentrations of arginine may disturb cancer proliferation. In addition to defects in protein synthesis, caspase-mediated and mitochondrial dysfunction apoptosis occur with both arginine and leucine (Wakshlag et al. 2006). Generally speaking, tumors may be more sensitive to amino acid depletion than host tissues (Baracos and Mackenzie 2006). Additionally, valine, leucine and isoleucine are neurotoxic at concentrations found in plasma and tissues of maple syrup urine disease patients, with necrosis as the presumed mode of cell death (Funchal et al. 2005). Meanwhile, studies on alcoholic cirrhosis patients have shown that these BCAAs supplementing can enhance protein synthesis in liver and muscle cells, help restore liver function, and prevent chronic encephalopathy (Chalasani and Gitlin 1996).

1.2.3 Cytoprotective Effects of Amino Acids

Among more than 45 amino acids and analogs examined by Weinberg et al. (1990), only Gly, L-alanine, D-alanine, β-alanine and a neuronal Gly-binding site agonist have been active in protecting kidney tubular cells against hypoxic injury. The protective effect could not be explained by either amino acid metabolism or concentration or turnover of ATP in cells. These data indicate that a highly specific configuration is responsible for activity and that a comparison of structure activity relationships with neuronal Gly receptors is relevant. Scavenging of ROS by the amino acids is unlikely to be critical for protection. Also, taurine was an effective scavenger of HOCl as evidenced by its cytoprotective actions in PC12 cells (Kearns and Dawson 2000).

1.2.3.1 Amino Acids as Anti-apoptotic Agents

Apoptosis-preventing amino acids include Gly, L-alanine, L-serine, L-threonine, L-proline, L-asparagine, L-glutamine, L-histidine. The apoptosis-preventing amino acids act as signal molecules of survival factor, rather than critical nutritive substrates of metabolism (Franěk and Srámková 1996). Besides, Serine and Gly were found to improve viability of rat neurons (Yang et al. 2000). Moreover, Hybridoma cells could be rescued from apoptotic death by Gly, L-alanine, L-serine, L-threonine, L-proline, L-asparagine, L-glutamine, L-histidine, D-serine, β-alanine, or taurine (Franek et al. 2002). Furthermore, Gly-Pro-Arg three amino acid peptide can rescue cultured rat hippocampal neurons from cell death by inhibiting caspase-3/p53-dependent apoptosis (Ioudina and Uemura 2003). In particular, taurine decreases apoptosis induced by different factors in several cell types (Pasantes-Morales 2007). However, taurine addition show either inhibition of cell proliferation as in hepatic stellate cells (Chen et al. 2004) or increasing proliferation as in fetal pancreatic cells (Boujendar et al. 2002). In parallel, L-carnitine has important dual functions in apoptosis that differ in normal cells from cancer cells (Fan et al. 2009). L-carnitine could prevent apoptosis of skeletal and cardiac muscle cells (Vescovo et al. 2002). Also, L-carnitine can protect cardiomyocytes from doxorubicin-induced apoptosis through PPARα activation and PGI2 (Chao et al. 2009). Alternatively, L-carnitine induces apoptosis in cancer leukemic cells (Wenzel et al. 2005) and inhibits hepatocarcinogenesis in vivo (Chang et al. 2005). L-carnitine induces death in mouse liver cancer cells, not in normal ones. This may be due to the different metabolic changes between cancer cells and normal cells. Some cancer cells have been shown to have lower levels of free L-carnitine than normal cells (Peluso et al. 2000b), with a cancer-associated metabolic dysfunction related to carnitine (Fan et al. 2009).

1.2.3.2 Amino Acids as Osmolytes

A decrease in cell volume has been always recognized as a hallmark of apoptosis. Cell shrinkage normally precedes apoptotic events such as cytochrome c release, caspase 3 activation, nuclear condensation, and DNA fragmentation (Maeno et al. 2000). The mechanisms of cell shrinkage during apoptosis include K and Cl loss through activated K and Cl channels. Indeed, the role for amino acids as osmolytes in volume regulation, particularly those being synaptically inhibitory or inert is of significance. Especially, taurine decreases apoptosis induced by different factors in several cell types (Pasantes-Morales 2007). Also, carnitine is an example of active osmolytes that exert metabolic functions (Peluso et al. 2000a). In particular, Gly is an osmoprotectant against stresses such as salinity, high temperature, desiccation and urea-concentrating environments (Hall 1998). It is believed that such amino acids stabilize enzymes, nucleic acids, membrane-associated proteins and intracellular organelles (Buche et al. 1993). In addition, solutions of hypotonic Gly are used to irrigate the bladder in patients undergoing transurethral resection of the prostate (TURP) with underlying pathophysiology including more than just direct osmotic effects (Stalberg et al. 1993).

1.2.3.3 Amino Acids as Chemoprotective Inhibitors of Cell Death

The narrow selectivity of anticancer drugs led to the evolution of the concept of cytoprotection with the use of leucovorin as a cytoprotectant against methotrexate toxicity (Klein and Muggia 1999). Positive or negative modulation of thiol levels, particularly GSH, may provide means to enhance chemotherapy activity at the tumor site and to protect against toxicity in normal cells. The elevated intracellular GSH is associated with opposition to chemotherapeutic agents such as cisplatin and melphalan in tumor cells (Zhang et al. 1998). On the other hand, it may be possible to reduce the toxicities of anti-cancer agents by using sulfur-containing chemoprotective agents (Links and Lewis 1999). Clinically relevant amino acids that may provide chemoprotection include N-acetylcysteine, D-methionine, and GSH ethyl ester. The interactions of chemoprotectants with chemotherapy efficacy may be prevented by separating treatments in time or space (Muldoon et al. 2001).

1.2.4 N-Acetylcysteine and Cysteine

N-acetylcysteine (NAC) is a derivative of cysteine (Cys) and an intermediary in the conversion of Cys to GSH (Parcell 2002). Made endogenously and found in foods, NAC and Cys both have sulfhydryl groups that can scavenge free radicals. Cys's protective mechanisms could relate to its antioxidant properties, its promotion of GSH or even, to some ability to participate in DNA repair (MECo. 1999). NAC is a reducing agent and has antioxidant activity. It is also a mucolytic and a hepatoprotectant, and it may have anti-apoptotic and antiviral activities (Parcell 2002). Moreover, NAC is gaining use as a chemoprotective agent against cisplatin-induced toxicities, such as ototoxicity and nephrotoxicity (Dickey et al. 2008). Although, Cys and NAC have been documented as hepatoprotectives by increasing level of the antioxidant GSH (MECo. 1999), other studies failed to demonstrate their cytoprotection (Ghoneim 2006; Vina et al. 1980; Weinberg et al. 1990). Furthermore, Cys severely damages isolated hepatocytes by killing more than half of the population (Ghoneim 2006), in accordance with its hepatotoxic potential as formerly reported by Viña et al. (1983). Additionally, Cys, at concentrations as low as 0.2 mM, caused a GSH depletion in isolated hepatocytes (Vina et al. 1978). That's why; this amino acid should be used with great caution even at minute concentrations. Furthermore, it is known that relatively low doses of Cys can be toxic to rats in vivo (Birnbaum et al. 1957), and to cultured cells (Nishiuch et al. 1976). It has been documented that the critical event leading to Cys cytotoxicity is its rapid autoxidation to cystine with the production of H_2O_2 and then of hydroxyl radicals' oxidative stress leading to hepatocytes destruction (Saez et al. 1982; Vina et al. 1983):

$$2\,\text{Cys} + O_2 \rightarrow \text{cystine} + H_2O_2$$

The reason underlying many conflicting results may be the unwanted consequences of standard cell isolation procedures and/or viability assessment. Besides, freshly isolated hepatocytes are under enormous oxidative stress which increases GSH consumption and turnover (Dalhoff and Poulsen 1992). Also, extremely high doses (more than 7 g) of Cys should be avoided because it may be toxic to human cells and may even lead to death (MECo. 1999). In addition, large doses of Cys are neuroexcitotoxic in several species (Kidd 1997). Moreover, several researchers have reported a depletion of GSH by both NAC (Vina et al. 1980) and Cys (Vina et al. 1980, 1983). Indeed, Cys is unstable in the blood because the ambient oxygen is high enough to oxidize it, yet its availability limits GSH synthesis (Kidd 1997). Regarding NAC, similar results to ours (Ghoneim 2006) were obtained by its pretreatment of hepatocytes; failing to mitigate the EtOH-induced insult (Lee and Shukla 2005), and indicating oxidative stress-independent toxicity (Higuchi et al. 2001). Furthermore, other preliminary experiments have indicated that NAC failed to adequately raise GSH levels, and more impor tantly, it stimulated hepatocyte LP (Gumpricht et al. 2000). Nevertheless, as NAC has already proved to be a good acetaminophen antagonist, then, the hepatoprotective role of liver GSH has been suggested to be reconsidered. A feasible explanation was through NAC deacetylation to Cys in the liver (USP DI 1999) that is oxidized to cystine which is not a good GSH precursor. Thus, the NAC anti-oxidative protective effect could have been counteracted by its conversion to the pro-oxidant Cys (Ghoneim 2006).

1.2.5 Glycine

1.2.5.1 The Receptors

There exists strychnine (str)-sensitive as well as str-insensitive Gly binding sites. The str-sensitive Gly receptor forms a chloride (Cl^-)-selective transmembrane channel, which is predominantly expressed in the spinal cord and brain stem. In these regions, Gly acts as an inhibitory neurotransmitter (Hall 1998). Alternatively, the str-insensitive Gly-binding site is located on the NMDA receptor complex. This GlyB site is necessary for NMDA receptor activation as a co-agonist. Preclinical evidence suggests that GlyB antagonists are most likely used as neuroprotectants (Danysz and Parsons 1998).

1.2.5.2 Anti-cancer Activity

Animal studies demonstrate that Gly may have anti-cancer properties. The proposed pathophysiologic mechanism may be based on the fact that Gly prevents activation of Kupffer cells and, hence, TNF-α release, which has a mitogenic effect (Roth et al. 2003). In another study (Rose et al. 1999), dietary Gly inhibited B16 melanoma tumors in mice through inhibition of angiogenesis.

1.2.5.3 Protective Effects

Gly protects in a variety of disease states and experimental models such as ischemia/reperfusion (I/R) injury, shock, transplantation, alcoholic hepatitis, hepatic fibrosis, liver transplantation, gastric ulcer, arthritis, tumor and drug toxicity, regardless of controversies on mechanisms (Roth et al. 2003; Zhong et al. 2003). Briefly, Gly exerts several protective effects, including antiinflammatory, immunomodulatory and direct cytoprotective actions (Ghoneim 2006; Roth et al. 2003; Zhong et al. 2003). Indeed, Gly has been found to exert a cytoprotective effect against hypoxic injury to in vitro renal tubules (Weinberg et al. 1987) and endothelial cells (Weinberg et al. 1992). Besides, Gly has protected rat hepatocytes against anoxic injury (Marsh et al. 1993) and against I/R injury of the whole liver (Zhong et al. 1996). Gly has also been shown to antagonize the toxic effects of valproate and paracetamol (Vance et al. 1994). Moreover, a potential therapeutic benefit of Gly treatment of hepatocytes cultured at high density in a bioartificial liver has been identified (Nyberg et al. 2000). Furthermore, Gly has been shown to protect against in vivo and in vitro ethanol-induced liver injury (Ghoneim et al. 2005; Iimuro et al. 1996; Senthilkumar et al. 2004). Therefore, Gly can prevent cell death induced by anoxia, oxidative stress and various toxic agents at the cell, organ and whole body levels in a variety of species (Deters et al. 1998; Ghoneim 2006; Roth et al. 2003; Zhong et al. 2003).

1.2.5.4 Protective Mechanisms

The mechanisms by which Gly protects remain incompletely understood, and it may be through multiple mechanisms with additive or synergistic effects (Zhong et al. 2003). Proposed mechanisms include suppression of Ca^{2+} signaling, inhibition of inflammatory cell activation, decreased formation of free radicals and other toxic mediators, and blockage of plasma membrane permeabilization preceding oncotic necrosis. Gly has also been shown to inhibit nonlysosomal Ca^{2+}-dependent degradative proteolysis (Carini et al. 1997). Besides, Schilling et al. (1991) found that Gly stabilized cell membrane by inhibition of phospholipase A_2.

Gly and Cell Death

Gly has been demonstrated to possess significant anti-apoptotic effects (Ghoneim 2006; Ghoneim et al. 2005; Zhang et al. 2000; Franek et al. 2002; Jacob et al. 2003). Interestingly, the antiapoptotic effect of Gly in hepatic SECs was antagonized in part by str. It is postulated, therefore, that SECs most likely contain a Gly receptor, through which antiapoptotic effects are elicited. Moreover, Gly prevented the induced decrease in Bcl-2 protein levels (Zhang et al. 2000). In addition, immunohistochemical studies on small bowel specimens have revealed significantly increased expression of the pro-apoptotic mediators; Bax, CPP-32 and Fas that were saline-treated as compared with Gly-treated segments. There has also been a strong expression of Bcl-2 in the Gly-treated specimens (Jacob et al. 2003). Besides, cytoprotection by Gly was not dependent on blockade of mitochondrial depolarization in case of necrapoptosis. Reperfusion with Gly alone was poorly effective at restoring ATP and did not promote apoptosis, although Gly prevented necrotic cell death (Kim et al. 2003). Moreover, Gly's effects are most likely linked to cellular regeneration potential and reduced both apoptotic and necrotic cell death (Rentsch et al. 2005). Furthermore, Gly significantly protects against EtOH-induced casp-3 activation in both suspended and monolayered hepatocytes (Ghoneim 2006; Ghoneim et al. 2005). Very low doses have also been shown efficacious in preventing hepatocyte DNA fragmentation (Neuman et al. 1999). Nonetheless, Nyberg et al. (2000) and Kim et al (2003) denied an anti-casp-3 activity of Gly. The protection might hence be attributable to the Gly's membrane and protein stabilization, as well as, anti-proteolytic activity (Hall 1998; Zhong et al. 2003). Moreover, Gly (10 mM) showed a potential protective effect against both apoptosis and necrosis inferred by EtOH (Ghoneim 2006; Ghoneim et al. 2005). Gly's downregulation of PARP (Jacob et al. 2003) as well as DNA stabilization (Buche et al. 1993) could explain its marked prevention of apoptotic chromatin fragmentation and condensation. Gly might have been more effective at later stages of apoptosis that culminate into secondary necrosis. Kim et al. (2003) showed a potential anti-necrotic effect for Gly against I/R-induced hepatocyte death. The authors mentioned neither a pro- nor an anti-apoptotic potential for Gly. Concerning necrosis, Gly has been shown to be very active in preventing cell death in a variety of cell types (Carini et al. 1997).

Gly and Ion Channels

Gly has been reported to be protective against hypoxia, ischemia and various cytotoxic substances in renal proximal tubules via Gly-gated Cl^- channels (Miller et al. 1994). Besides, studies have demonstrated that dietary Gly prevents polysaccharide-induced arthritis in the rat by reducing cytokine release from macrophages via Gly-gated Cl^- channel (Li et al. 2001). In another study (Qu et al. 2002) on isolated rat hepatocytes, the effect of Gly was specific and the inhibitory effect of Gly on increases in $[Ca^{2+}]_i$ in hepatocytes occurs via Gly receptors, as in neurons. One possibility is that this receptor/Cl^- channel increases the Cl^- influx, thereby preventing the shrinkage of cells during the apoptotic process. Alternatively, Gly, at high concentrations, is known to desensitize and block Cl^- channels in many cell types. Gly inhibition of Cl^- conductance protects against hepatocyte killing by interfering with intracellular Na^+ accumulation triggered by ATP depletion (Carini et al. 1997). In addition, it has been hypothesized that Gly-sensitive Cl^- anion channel opening causes rapid cell swelling and stretching of the plasma membrane bilayer that lead secondarily to porous defects. Gly, which slows anion entry, also decreases the rate of bleb formation and cell swelling (Nishimura and Lemasters 2001). Besides, a postulated pro-apoptotic mitochondrial Cl^- channel (Fernández-Salas et al. 2002) might have been partially blocked by Gly, as well as Bax, (Barros et al. 2002) both affecting cyt c release through postulated anion channels. Furthermore, Gly blocks the opening of relatively non-specific anion and cation pores in the plasma membrane that occurs as the penultimate event leading to necrotic cell death (Frank et al. 2000; Zhong et al. 2003). Gly is, therefore, documented to inhibit opening of both the non-specific cationic pores and/or the anion/death channels (Frank et al. 2000; Nishimura and Lemasters 2001; Zhong et al. 2003). Moreover, in apoptotic cell death, cyt c release, casp-3 activation and DNA laddering were all blocked by a Cl^- channel blocker in different cell types (Maeno et al. 2000; Okada et al. 2001). Furthermore, in Jurkat T-cells, stimulated with anti-Fas antibodies, sustained plasma membrane depolarization, attributable to increased intracellular Na^+ but reduced K^+ uptake, was observed prior to cell shrinkage (Bortner et al. 2001). Therefore, Gly, through postulated Cl^- and/or Na^+ channels inhibition, could prevent Na^+-induced apoptotic cell death, as well as, necrotic one.

Gly and GSH

Gly has been demonstrated to enhance GSH synthesis in hepatocytes (Neuman et al. 1999; Nishida et al. 1997). Nevertheless, protection of isolated tubules appears to be mediated by Gly produced from GSH metabolism, and the cytoprotective to be due to Gly directly and not one of its metabolites (Weinberg et al. 1987; Deters et al. 1998). In parallel, Ozaki et al. (1994) demonstrated that Gly could protect liver from reperfusion injury by reducing LP, an effect that was not due to alteration of GSH. GSH also informs about cell viability as a universal parameter. In connection with the above-listed findings, the Gly-induced GSH replenishment, if not due to an enhanced synthesis, it could rather be a consequence of the Gly's general cytoprotective mechanism.

Gly and Lipid Peroxidation

The level of LP is an index for oxidative stress and cell injury. However, several researchers could not find anti-LP by their demonstrated anti-necrotic agents, and vice versa (Donatus et al. 1990; Cobreros et al. 1997; Ghoneim 2006; Ghoneim et al. 2005). Indeed, Gly cytoprotection might be independent of its antioxidative potential under many experimental conditions. Undeniably, a direct causal relationship between LP and cell death is still disputed (Berry et al. 1991; Plaa 2000). The technique most commonly used is the measurement of malondialdehyde accumulation, but frequently non-physiological conditions are required to detect this accumulation, and artifacts are encountered. Accordingly, there is some degree of agreement that it is not a reliable measure of LP (Berry et al. 1991; Dianzani 1985).

Gly as a Membrane Stabilizer

Gly might have two opposite effects on cell swelling and blebbing, as an estimate for membrane stabilization. The anti-swelling one is based on the hypothesis that death channel opening initiates entry of anions, swelling, bleb formation and porous defects in the plasma membrane (Nishimura and Lemasters 2001). This death channel is presumably identical to the Gly-sensitive Cl^- channel postulated earlier to be blocked by Gly (Miller et al. 1994; Carini et al. 1997). The opposite effect is a Gly-induced membrane swelling and/or blebbing; perhaps due to extensive urea production, and osmotic swelling secondary to Gly transport (Vincent et al. 1992). This might also lead to anti-apoptotic effect through inhibition of shrinkage through a proposed increased Cl^{-}/water influx (Zhang et al. 2000). Another logic hypothesis postulated in 2005 by Del Monte depends on the assumption that an increase of non-perturbing solutes maintains the physiological intracellular osmotic pressure leading to osmoprotection.

1.3 Concluding Remarks

Phytochemicals and amino acids have long been considered as important inducers of cell death. However, many of these natural compounds have been demonstrating dual action effects on cell death through inhibition as well as induction. The cellular energy balance seems to be an explanation for the opposing redox effects of several phytochemicals that apparently show either antioxidant or prooxidant effects. Homeostatic responses by phytochemicals can also have a profound influence on the direction of signaling between cell survival in normal cells and cell death in cancer cells. Important considerations include the dose used and the duration of use, along with tissue-specific effects on redox balance and on gene transcription regulation, which are involved in apoptosis.

Cur, like other phytochemicals, shows multiple signaling pathways and targets, that it might counteract rather than potentiate the effect of anti-cancer agents. Accordingly, any possible drug interaction must be checked before concomitant clinical use. In addition, Cur exerts biphasic effects, depending on its concentration and temporal administration. The effects of Cur may be tissue specific and it may target cancer cells more efficiently than normal ones. Possible explanations might include the higher cellular uptake of Cur in tumor cells having a lower GSH level and a higher NF-κB expression. Moreover, many of the studies are based on probably misleading methodological models regarding cell death detection and its association with estimated oxidative stress parameters. Furthermore, future research is warranted to investigate the risk-to-benefit ratio vis-à-vis the controversial use of Cur as a liver cytoprotectant antioxidant and/or cytotoxic chemotherapeutic agent with hepatotoxic side effects.

Several Astragalus plant extracts demonstrate remarkable protective effects against both types of cell death. Conversely, Astragalus as an inducer of cell death, is reported to treat various types of cancers. Besides, it has been shown to potentiate the activity of chemotherapeutic agents, and reduce their toxicities. The marked difference between the different species might be attributable to a difference in the type and amount of pharmacologically active constituents that are concentrated in the different extract fractions. Based on the recommendations of several researchers (Liu 2004; Temple 2002; van Breda et al. 2008), phytochemicals may need to act in combination with rest of extract constituents, rather than a single magically active substance. Taken alone, the individual phytochemicals do not appear to have consistent disease-preventive effects. The isolated pure phytochemical compound may not behave the same way as in the whole mixture. More emphasis may be placed on simple unbiased research of epidemiologic studies and clinical trials. The information of practical value should also receive bulk of resources and attention as complex mechanistic reductionistic research is receiving.

Concerning amino acids, they should not be viewed simply as building blocks for protein synthesis, but as important modulators of cell function and as drugs used for different clinical purposes. Particularly, several amino acids deserve further attention as possible candidates for novel apoptosis-inducing anti-tumor agents. Amino acids including the excitatory, branched-chain, taurine and carnitine may be considered as either inducers or inhibitors of cell death depending on the dose used, its duration, and the type of cells, either normal or cancer. Alternatively, the apoptosis-preventing amino acids act as signal molecules of survival factor. In addition, the role for amino acids as osmolytes in volume regulation, particularly Gly, taurine and carnitine is of importance to the program of cell death.

Sulfur-containing chemoprotective amino acids may provide efficacy when separated in time or space (route) from chemotherapy. However, Cys should be used with great caution even at low doses due to its cytotoxicity and autoxidation. Besides, the NAC anti-oxidative protective effect could be counteracted by its deacetylation in the liver to the pro-oxidant Cys. Since Cys and NAC are used as therapeutic agents, it should be reiterated that being a documented antioxidant amino acid is obviously not sufficient to confer cytoprotection.

Gly exerts general cytoprotection in a variety of experimental models regardless of controversies on mechanisms. Gly cytoprotection might be independent of its antioxidative potential. Gly, dose-dependently, and through postulated modulation of anion and/or cation channels and pores, could prevent apoptotic and necrotic cell death. Gly-gated channels could, hence, represent a potential therapeutic target to control both forms of death in different cell types. In addition to its benefits in case of cancer, Gly could be very effective clinically to ameliorate different injuries because it prevents both forms of cell death that is a fundamental feature of many diseases, including the viral-induced. Thus, research for new cytoprotective preparations is strongly recommended. These preparations may include Gly and phytochemical extracts and may share a degree of similarity with another ones (Milliman et al. 2000) that help prevent liver cancer in hepatitis C patients. In conclusion, the opposing actions and controversial uses of phytochemicals and amino acids, as cytoprotective and/or cytotoxic agents, in different tissues and diseases, are still in need of much further scrutiny. The pharmacogenomic screening of these natural compounds for their dual actions on cell death should also be taken into consideration. This technology of "personalized medicine" may provide a tool to answer the title question: Are they inducers or inhibitors of cell death? At which concentration? In which tissue? and of which "person"? …

Acknowledgment The author is greatly indebted to Dr. Aya Asaad, Professor of Pharmacognosy, Faculty of Pharmacy, Alexandria University, for reading and commenting on the manuscript.

References

Abdallah RM, Ghazy NM, El-Sebakhy NA, Pirillo A, Verotta L (1993) Astragalosides from Egyptian Astragalus spinosus vahl. Pharmazie 48:452–454

Acamovic T, Brooker J (2005) Biochemistry of plant secondary metabolites and their effects in animals. Proc Nutr Soc 64:403–412

Agardh C, Zhang H, Smith M, Siesjö B (1991) Free radical production and ischemic brain damage: influence of postischemic oxygen tension. Int J Dev Neurosci 9:127–138

Aggarwal B, Shishodia S (2006) Molecular targets of dietary agents for prevention and therapy of cancer. Biochem Pharmacol 71:1397–1421

Aggarwal B, Kumar A, Bharti A (2003) Anticancer potential of curcumin: preclinical and clinical studies. Anticancer Res 23:363–398

Ahsan H, Parveen N, Khan N, Hadi S (1999) Pro-oxidant, anti-oxidant and cleavage activities on DNA of curcumin and its derivatives demethoxycurcumin and bisdemethoxycurcumin. Chem Biol Interact 121:161–175

Anto R, Mukhopadhyay A, Denning K, Aggarwal B (2002) Curcumin (diferuloylmethane) induces apoptosis through activation of caspase-8, BID cleavage and cytochrome c release: its suppression by ectopic expression of Bcl-2 and Bcl-xl. Carcinogenesis 23:143–150

Asaad AM (1977) M.Sc. Pharm. thesis, Faculty of Pharmacy, Alexandria University, Egypt

Asaad AM (1983) Ph.D. Pharm. thesis, Faculty of Pharmacy, Alexandria University, Egypt

Asaad AM (2000) A minor cycloartane saponin from Astragalus boeticus L. Alex J Pharm Sci 14(2):105–108

Auyeung K, Law P, Ko J (2009) Astragalus saponins induce apoptosis via an ERK-independent NF-kappaB signaling pathway in the human hepatocellular HepG2 cell line. Int J Mol Med 23:189–196

Badr AM, El-Demerdash E, Khalifa AE, Ghoneim AI, Ayoub NA and Abdel-Naim AB (2009) Rubus sanctus protects against carbon tetrachloride-induced toxicity in rat isolated hepatocytes: isolation and characterization of its galloylated flavonoids. J Pharm Pharmacol 61:1511–1520

Bala K, Tripathy B, Sharma D (2006) Neuroprotective and anti-ageing effects of curcumin in aged rat brain regions. Biogerontology 7:81–89

Balazs R, Hack N, Jørgensen OS (1988) N-methyl-D-aspartate promotes the survival of cerebellar granule cells in culture. Neuroscience 27:437–451

Baracos V, Mackenzie M (2006) Investigations of branched-chain amino acids and their metabolites in animal models of cancer. J Nutr 136:237S–242S

Barrett, M. (2004) The handbook of clinically tested herbal remedies. Haworth Herbal Press, New York

Barros LF, Castro J, Bittner CX (2002) Ion movements in cell death: from protection to execution. Biol Res 35:209–214

Battezzati A, Riso P (2002) Amino acids: fuel, building blocks for proteins, and signals. Nutrition 18:773–774

Bedir E, Pugh N, Calis I, Pasco DS, Khan IA (2000) Immunostimulatory effects of cycloartane-type triterpene glycosides from astragalus species. Biol Pharm Bull 23:834–837

Berry MN, Edwards AM, Barritt GJ, Grivell MB (1991) Isolated hepatocytes: preparation, properties and applications. Elsevier, Amsterdam

Birnbaum SM, Winitz M, Greenstein JP (1957) Quantitative nutritional studies with water-soluble, chemically defined diets. III. Individual amino acids as sources of non-essential nitrogen. Arch Biochem Biophys 72:428–436

Bortner CD, Gomez-Angelats M, Cidlowski JA (2001) Plasma membrane depolarization without repolarization is an early molecular event in anti-Fas-induced apoptosis. J Biol Chem 276:4304–4314

Boujendar S, Reusens B, Merezak S, Ahn M, Arany E, Hill D, Remacle C (2002) Taurine supplementation to a low protein diet during foetal and early postnatal life restores a normal proliferation and apoptosis of rat pancreatic islets. Diabetologia 45:856–866

Boulos L (1999) Flora of Egypt, vol 1, 1st edn. Alhadara Publishing, Egypt, pp 320–336
Bowlin T, McKown B, Kang M, Sunkara P (1989) Potentiation of human lymphokine-activated killer cell activity by swainsonine, an inhibitor of glycoprotein processing. Cancer Res 49:4109–4113
Buche A, Colson P, Houssier C (1993) Effect of organic effectors on chromatin solubility, DNA-histone H1 interactions, DNA and histone H1 structures. J Biomol Struct Dyn 11:95–119
Carini R, Bellomo G, Grazia De Cesaris M, Albano E (1997) Glycine protects against hepatocyte killing by KCN or hypoxia by preventing intracellular Na+ overload in the rat. Hepatology 26:107–112
Chalasani N, Gitlin N (1996) Severe recurrent hepatic encephalopathy that responded to oral branched chain amino acids. Am J Gastroenterol 91:1266–1268
Chan M, Fong D, Soprano K, Holmes W, Heverling H (2003) Inhibition of growth and sensitization to cisplatin-mediated killing of ovarian cancer cells by polyphenolic chemopreventive agents. J Cell Physiol 194:63–70
Chan W, Wu H, Chang W (2006) Dosage effects of curcumin on cell death types in a human osteoblast cell line. Food Chem Toxicol 44:1362–1371
Chang B, Nishikawa M, Nishiguchi S, Inoue M (2005) L-carnitine inhibits hepatocarcinogenesis via protection of mitochondria. Int J Cancer 113:719–729
Chao H, Liu J, Hong H, Lin J, Chen C, Cheng T (2009) L-carnitine reduces doxorubicin-induced apoptosis through a prostacyclin-mediated pathway in neonatal rat cardiomyocytes. Int J Cardiol 15(3):532–537
Chen Y, Zhang X, Xie W, Li S (2004) Effects of taurine on proliferation and apoptosis of hepatic stellate cells in vitro. Hepatobiliary Pancreat Dis Int 3:106–109
Cheng XD, Hou CH, Zhang XJ, Xie HY, Zhou WY, Yang L, Zhang SB, Qian RL (2004) Effects of Huangqi (Hex) on inducing cell differentiation and cell death in K562 and HEL cells. Acta Biochim Biophys Sin (Shanghai) 36:211–217
Cobreros A, Sainz L, Lasheras B, Cenarruzabeitia E (1997) Hepatotoxicity of ethanol: protective effect of calcium channel blockers in isolated hepatocytes. Liver 17:76–82
Dalhoff K, Poulsen HE (1992) Effects of cysteine and acetaminophen on the syntheses of glutathione and adenosine 3′-phosphate 5′-phosphosulfate in isolated rat hepatocytes. Biochem Pharmacol 44:447–454
Danysz W, Parsons AC (1998) Glycine and N-methyl-D-aspartate receptors: physiological significance and possible therapeutic applications. Pharmacol Rev 50:597–664
Deters M, Siegers CP, Strubelt O (1998) Influence of glycine on the damage induced in isolated perfused rat liver by five hepatotoxic agents. Toxicology 128:63–72
Dianzani MU (1985) Lipid peroxidation in ethanol poisoning: a critical reconsideration. Alcohol Alcohol 20:161–173
Dickey D, Muldoon L, Doolittle N, Peterson D, Kraemer D, Neuwelt E (2008) Effect of N-acetylcysteine route of administration on chemoprotection against cisplatin-induced toxicity in rat models. Cancer Chemother Pharmacol 62:235–241
Doble A (1999) The role of excitotoxicity in neurodegenerative disease: implications for therapy. Pharmacol Ther 81:163–221
Donatus I, Sardjoko VN, Vermeulen N (1990) Cytotoxic and cytoprotective activities of curcumin. Effects on paracetamol-induced cytotoxicity, lipid peroxidation and glutathione depletion in rat hepatocytes. Biochem Pharmacol 39:1869–1875
Dong X, Wang Y, Qin Z (2009) Molecular mechanisms of excitotoxicity and their relevance to pathogenesis of neurodegenerative diseases. Acta Pharmacol Sin 30:379–387
Duvoix A, Blasius R, Delhalle S, Schnekenburger M, Morceau F, Henry E, Dicato M, Diederich M (2005) Chemopreventive and therapeutic effects of curcumin. Cancer Lett 223:181–190
Fan JP, Kim HS, Han GD (2009) Induction of apoptosis by L-carnitine through regulation of two main pathways in Hepa1c1c 7 cells. Amino Acids 36:365–372
Fang YZ, Yang S, Wu G (2002) Free radicals, antioxidants, and nutrition. Nutrition 18:872–879
Fernández-Salas E, Suh KS, Speransky VV, Bowers WL, Levy JM, Adams T, Pathak KR, Edwards LE, Hayes DD, Cheng C, Steven AC, Weinberg WC, Yuspa SH (2002) mtCLIC/CLIC4, an

organellular chloride channel protein, is increased by DNA damage and participates in the apoptotic response to p53. Mol Cell Biol 22:3610–3620
Franěk F, Srámková K (1996) Protection of B lymphocyte hybridoma against starvation-induced apoptosis: survival-signal role of some amino acids. Immunol Lett 52:139–144
Franek F, Fismolova I, Eckschlager T (2002) Antiapoptotic and proapoptotic action of various amino acids and analogs in starving MOLT-4 cells. Arch Biochem Biophys 398:141–146
Frank A, Rauen U, de Groot H (2000) Protection by glycine against hypoxic injury of rat hepatocytes: inhibition of ion fluxes through nonspecific leaks. J Hepatol 32:58–66
Funchal C, Gottfried C, de Almeida L, dos Santos A, Wajner M, Pessoa-Pureur R (2005) Morphological alterations and cell death provoked by the branched-chain alpha-amino acids accumulating in maple syrup urine disease in astrocytes from rat cerebral cortex. Cell Mol Neurobiol 25:851–867
Ghoneim AI (2006) Ph.D. Pharm. thesis, Faculty of Pharmacy, Ain Shams University, Egypt
Ghoneim A (2009) Effects of curcumin on ethanol-induced hepatocyte necrosis and apoptosis: implication of lipid peroxidation and cytochrome c. Naunyn Schmiedebergs Arch Pharmacol 379:47–60
Ghoneim A, Abdel-Naim A, Khalifa A, El-Denshary E (2002) Protective effects of curcumin against ischaemia/reperfusion insult in rat forebrain. Pharmacol Res 46:273–279
Ghoneim AI, Eldahshan OA (2012) Anti-apoptotic effects of tamarind leaves against ethanol-induced rat liver injury. J Pharm Pharmacol 64:430–438
Ghoneim AI, Khalifa AE, El-Demerdash E, Abdel-Naim AB (2005) Hepatoprotective effects of glycine and Astragalus boeticus against ethanol-induced hepatocyte death. In: Forty-seventh annual conference of the Egyptian Society of Pharmacology & Experimental Therapeutics:17 [abstract], Dec 1st, Helwan University, Egypt
Gopalakrishnan A, Tony Kong A (2008) Anticarcinogenesis by dietary phytochemicals: cytoprotection by Nrf2 in normal cells and cytotoxicity by modulation of transcription factors NF-kappa B and AP-1 in abnormal cancer cells. Food Chem Toxicol 46:1257–1270
Grossie VB, Nishioka K, Ajani JA, Ote DM (1992) Substituting ornithine for arginine in total parenteral nutrition eliminates enhanced tumor growth. J Surg Oncol 50:161–167
Gumpricht E, Devereaux MW, Dahl RH, Sokol RJ (2000) Glutathione status of isolated rat hepatocytes affects bile acid-induced cellular necrosis but not apoptosis. Toxicol Appl Pharmacol 164:102–111
Hail NJ, Lotan R (2009) Cancer chemoprevention and mitochondria: targeting apoptosis in transformed cells via the disruption of mitochondrial bioenergetics/redox state. Mol Nutr Food Res 53:49–67
Hall JC (1998) Glycine. JPEN J Parenter Enteral Nutr 22:393–398
Higuchi H, Adachi M, Miura S, Gores GJ, Ishii H (2001) The mitochondrial permeability transition contributes to acute ethanol-induced apoptosis in rat hepatocytes. Hepatology 34:320–328
Holme A, Pervaiz S (2007) Resveratrol in cell fate decisions. J Bioenerg Biomembr 39:59–63
Hu Y, Liu C, Du C, Zhang J, Wu W, Gu Z (2009) Induction of apoptosis in human hepatocarcinoma SMMC-7721 cells in vitro by flavonoids from Astragalus complanatus. J Ethnopharmacol 123:293–301
Iimuro Y, Bradford BU, Forman DT, Thurman RG (1996) Glycine prevents alcohol-induced liver injury by decreasing alcohol in the rat stomach. Gastroenterology 110:1536–1542
Ioudina M, Uemura E (2003) A three amino acid peptide, Gly-Pro-Arg, protects and rescues cell death induced by amyloid beta-peptide. Exp Neurol 184:923–929
Iqbal M, Sharma S, Okazaki Y, Fujisawa M, Okada S (2003) Dietary supplementation of curcumin enhances antioxidant and phase II metabolizing enzymes in ddY male mice: possible role in protection against chemical carcinogenesis and toxicity. Pharmacol Toxicol 92:33–38
Jacob T, Ascher E, Hingorani A, Kallakuri S (2003) Glycine prevents the induction of apoptosis attributed to mesenteric ischemia/reperfusion injury in a rat model. Surgery 134:457–466
Jana N, Dikshit P, Goswami A, Nukina N (2004) Inhibition of proteasomal function by curcumin induces apoptosis through mitochondrial pathway. J Biol Chem 279:11680–11685

Jaruga E, Bielak-Zmijewska A, Sikora E, Skierski J, Radziszewska E, Piwocka K, Bartosz G (1998) Glutathione-independent mechanism of apoptosis inhibition by curcumin in rat thymocytes. Biochem Pharmacol 56:961–965

Johnson I (2007) Phytochemicals and cancer. Proc Nutr Soc 66:207–215

Johnson J, Ascher P (1987) Glycine potentiates the NMDA response in cultured mouse brain neurons. Nature 325:529–531

Kampa M, Nifli A, Notas G, Castanas E (2007) Polyphenols and cancer cell growth. Rev Physiol Biochem Pharmacol 159:79–113

Kearns S, Dawson RJ (2000) Cytoprotective effect of taurine against hypochlorous acid toxicity to PC12 cells. Adv Exp Med Biol 483:563–570

Kidd PM (1997) Glutathione: systemic protectant against oxidative and free radical damage. Altern Med Rev 2(3):155–176

Kim JS, Qian T, Lemasters JJ (2003) Mitochondrial permeability transition in the switch from necrotic to apoptotic cell death in ischemic rat hepatocytes. Gastroenterology 124:494–503

Kinjo J, Udayama M, Okawa M, Nohara T (1999) Study of structure–hepatoprotective relationships of oleanene-type triterpenoidal glucuronides obtained from several fabaceous plants on rat primary hepatocyte cultures. Biol Pharm Bull 22:203–206

Klein P, Muggia F (1999) Cytoprotection: shelter from the storm. Oncologist 4:112–121

Krasteva I, Platikanov S, Momekov G, Konstantinov S, Nikolov S (2008) Phytochemical analysis and in vitro cytotoxic activity of volatiles from Astragalus corniculatus. Nat Prod Res 22:969–974

Kundu JK, Surh YJ (2009) Molecular basis of chemoprevention with dietary phytochemicals: redox-regulated transcription factors as relevant targets. Phytochem Rev 8:333–347

Kunwar A, Barik A, Mishra B, Rathinasamy K, Pandey R, Priyadarsini K (2008) Quantitative cellular uptake, localization and cytotoxicity of curcumin in normal and tumor cells. Biochim Biophys Acta 1780:673–679

Laurent-Täckholm V (1974) Students's Flora of Egypt. Cairo University, Beirut

Lee YJ, Shukla SD (2005) Pro- and anti-apoptotic roles of c-Jun N-terminal kinase (JNK) in ethanol and acetaldehyde exposed rat hepatocytes. Eur J Pharmacol 508:31–45

Li X, Bradford BU, Wheeler MD, Stimpson SA, Pink HM, Brodie TA, Schwab JH, Thurman RG (2001) Dietary glycine prevents peptidoglycan polysaccharide-induced reactive arthritis in the rat: role for glycine-gated chloride channel. Infect Immun 69:5883–5891

Li C, Luo J, Li L, Cheng M, Huang N, Liu J, Waalkes MP (2003) The collagenolytic effects of the traditional Chinese medicine preparation, Han-Dan-Gan-Le, contribute to reversal of chemical-induced liver fibrosis in rats. Life Sci 72:1563–1571

Links M, Lewis C (1999) Chemoprotectants. A review of their clinical pharmacology and therapeutic efficacy. Drugs 57:293–308

Liu R (2004) Potential synergy of phytochemicals in cancer prevention: mechanism of action. J Nutr 134:3479S–3485S

Liu CY, Gu ZL, Zhou WX, Guo CY (2005) Effect of Astragalus complanatus flavonoid on anti-liver fibrosis in rats. World J Gastroenterol 11:5782–5786

Lladó J, Calderó J, Ribera J, Tarabal O, Oppenheim R, Esquerda J (1999) Opposing effects of excitatory amino acids on chick embryo spinal cord motoneurons: excitotoxic degeneration or prevention of programmed cell death. J Neurosci 19:10803–10812

Lowe S, Lin A (2000) Apoptosis in cancer. Carcinogenesis 21:485–495

Luo Y, Qin Z, Hong Z, Zhang X, Ding D, Fu JH, Zhang WD, Chen J (2004) Astragaloside IV protects against ischemic brain injury in a murine model of transient focal ischemia. Neurosci Lett 363:218–223

Luo Z, Zhong L, Han X, Wang H, Zhong J, Xuan Z (2009) Astragalus membranaceus prevents daunorubicin-induced apoptosis of cultured neonatal cardiomyocytes: role of free radical effect of Astragalus membranaceus on daunorubicin cardiotoxicity. Phyther Res 23:761–767

Luper S (1998) A review of plants used in the treatment of liver disease: part 1. Altern Med Rev 3:410–421

Ma Q, Hoper M, Anderson M, Rowlends BJ (1996) Effect of supplemental L-arginine in chemically induced model of colorectal cancer. World J Surg 20:1087–1091

Maeno E, Ishizaki Y, Kanaseki T, Hazama A, Okada Y (2000) Normotonic cell shrinkage because of disordered volume regulation is an early prerequisite to apoptosis. Proc Natl Acad Sci USA 97:9487–9492

Maheshwari R, Singh A, Gaddipati J, Srimal R (2006) Multiple biological activities of curcumin: a short review. Life Sci 78:2081–2087

Marsh DC, Vreugdenhil PK, Mack VE, Belzer FO, Southard JH (1993) Glycine protects hepatocytes from injury caused by anoxia, cold ischemia and mitochondrial inhibitors, but not injury caused by calcium ionophores or oxidative stress. Hepatology 17:91–98

Mattson M (2008) Hormesis defined. Ageing Res Rev 7:1–7

McCulloch M, See C, Shu X, Broffman M, Kramer A, Fan W, Gao J, Lieb W, Shieh K, Colford JJ (2006) Astragalus-based Chinese herbs and platinum-based chemotherapy for advanced non-small-cell lung cancer: meta-analysis of randomized trials. J Clin Oncol 24:419–430

Medical Economics Company: MECo. (1999) Physicans' Desk reference for nonprescription drugs and dietary supplements. Medical Economics Co., Montvale

Mehta K, Pantazis P, McQueen T, Aggarwal B (1997) Antiproliferative effect of curcumin (diferuloylmethane) against human breast tumor cell lines. Anticancer Drugs 8:470–481

Miller GW, Lock EA, Schnellmann RG (1994) Strychnine and glycine protect renal proximal tubules from various nephrotoxicants and act in the late phase of necrotic cell injury. Toxicol Appl Pharmacol 125:192–197

Milliman WB, Lamson DW, Brignall MS (2000) Hepatitis C; a retrospective study, literature review, and naturopathic protocol. Altern Med Rev 5:355–371

Mills S, Bone K (2000) Principles and practice of phytotherapy: modern herbal medicine. Churchill Livingstone, Edinburgh/Toronto

Mishra S, Kapoor N, Mubarak Ali A, Pardhasaradhi B, Kumari A, Khar A, Misra K (2005) Differential apoptotic and redox regulatory activities of curcumin and its derivatives. Free Radic Biol Med 38:1353–1360

Molyneux R, Lee S, Gardner D, Panter K, James L (2007) Phytochemicals: the good, the bad and the ugly? Phytochemistry 68:2973–2985

Moore P, El-sherbeny A, Roon P, Schoenlein P, Ganapathy V, Smith S (2001) Apoptotic cell death in the mouse retinal ganglion cell layer is induced in vivo by the excitatory amino acid homocysteine. Exp Eye Res 73:45–57

Muldoon LL, Walker-Rosenfeld SL, Hale C, Purcell SE, Bennett LC, Neuwelt EA (2001) Rescue from enhanced alkylator-induced cell death with low molecular weight sulfur-containing chemoprotectants. J Pharmacol Exp Ther 296:797–805

Na D, Liu F, Miao Z, Du Z, Xu H (2009) Astragalus extract inhibits destruction of gastric cancer cells to mesothelial cells by anti-apoptosis. World J Gastroenterol 15:570–577

Nair S, Li W, Kong A (2007) Natural dietary anti-cancer chemopreventive compounds: redox-mediated differential signaling mechanisms in cytoprotection of normal cells versus cytotoxicity in tumor cells. Acta Pharmacol Sin 28:459–472

Neuman MG, Shear NH, Cameron RG, Katz G, Tiribelli C (1999) Ethanol-induced apoptosis in vitro. Clin Biochem 32:547–555

Nishida K, Ohta Y, Ishiguro I (1997) Glycine facilitates gamma-glutamylcysteinylethyl ester-mediated increase in liver glutathione level. Eur J Pharmacol 333:289–292

Nishimura Y, Lemasters JJ (2001) Glycine blocks opening of a death channel in cultured hepatic sinusoidal endothelial cells during chemical hypoxia. Cell Death Differ 8:850–858

Nishiuch Y, Sasaki M, Nakayasu M, Oikawa A (1976) Cytotoxicity of cysteine in culture media. In Vitro 12:635–638

Notarbartolo M, Poma P, Perri D, Dusonchet L, Cervello M, D'Alessandro N (2005) Antitumor effects of curcumin, alone or in combination with cisplatin or doxorubicin, on human hepatic cancer cells. Analysis of their possible relationship to changes in NF-kB activation levels and in IAP gene expression. Cancer Lett 224:53–65

Nyberg SL, Hardin JA, Matos LE, Rivera DJ, Misra SP, Gores GJ (2000) Cytoprotective influence of ZVAD-fmk and glycine on gel-entrapped rat hepatocytes in a bioartificial liver. Surgery 127:447–455

Okada Y, Maeno E, Shimizu T, Dezaki K, Wang J, Morishima S (2001) Receptor-mediated control of regulatory volume decrease (RVD) and apoptotic volume decrease (AVD). J Physiol 532:3–16
Ozaki M, Ozasa H, Fuchinoue S, Teraoka S, Ota K (1994) Protective effects of glycine and esterified gamma-glutamylcysteine on ischemia/reoxygenation injury of rat liver. Transplantation 58:753–755
Parcell S (2002) Sulfur in human nutrition and applications in medicine. Altern Med Rev 7:22–44
Park E, Jeon C, Ko G, Kim J, Sohn D (2000) Protective effect of curcumin in rat liver injury induced by carbon tetrachloride. J Pharm Pharmacol 52:437–440
Pasantes-Morales H (2007) Amino acids and brain volume regulation: contribution and mechanisms. In: Lajtha A (ed) Handbook of neurochemistry and molecular neurobiology. Amino acids and peptides in the nervous system, 3rd edn. Springer-Verlag Berlin Heidelberg, pp 225–248
Peluso G, Barbarisi A, Savica V, Reda E, Nicolai R, Benatti P, Calvani M (2000a) Carnitine: an osmolyte that plays a metabolic role. J Cell Biochem 80:1–10
Peluso G, Nicolai R, Reda E, Benatti P, Barbarisi A, Calvani M (2000b) Cancer and anticancer therapy-induced modifications on metabolism mediated by carnitine system. J Cell Physiol 182:339–350
Pengelly A (2004) Constituents of medicinal plants: an introduction to the chemistry and therapeutics of herbal medicine. CABI Pub., Wallingford, Oxon, UK ; Cambridge, MA
Pistelli L (2002) Secondary metabolites of genus Astragalus; Structure and biological activity. In: Atta-Ur-Rhaman (ed) Studies in natural products chemistry, vol 27 (part H), 1st edn. Elsevier Science Publishers, Amsterdam, pp 443–545
Piwocka K, Jaruga E, Skierski J, Gradzka I, Sikora E (2001) Effect of glutathione depletion on caspase-3 independent apoptosis pathway induced by curcumin in Jurkat cells. Free Radic Biol Med 31:670–678
Plaa G (2000) Chlorinated methanes and liver injury: highlights of the past 50 years. Annu Rev Pharmacol Toxicol 40:42–65
Qu W, Ikejima K, Zhong Z, Waalkes MP, Thurman RG (2002) Glycine blocks the increase in intracellular free Ca^{2+} due to vasoactive mediators in hepatic parenchymal cells. Am J Physiol Gastrointest Liver Physiol 283:G1249–1256
Radwan MM (2004) Ph.D. Pharm. thesis, Faculty of Pharmacy, Alexandria University, Egypt
Radwan MM, El-Sebakhy NA, Asaad AM, Toaima SM, Kingston DG (2004) Kahiricosides II-V, cycloartane glycosides from an Egyptian collection of Astragalus kahiricus. Phytochemistry 65:2909–2913
Rashmi R, Kumar S, Karunagaran D (2005) Human colon cancer cells lacking Bax resist curcumin-induced apoptosis and Bax requirement is dispensable with ectopic expression of Smac or downregulation of Bcl-XL. Carcinogenesis 26:713–723
Ravindran J, Prasad S, Aggarwal B (2009) Curcumin and cancer cells: how many ways can curry kill tumor cells selectively? AAPS J 11:495–510
Raza H, John A, Brown E, Benedict S, Kambal A (2008) Alterations in mitochondrial respiratory functions, redox metabolism and apoptosis by oxidant 4-hydroxynonenal and antioxidants curcumin and melatonin in PC12 cells. Toxicol Appl Pharmacol 226:161–168
Rentsch M, Puellmann K, Sirek S, Iesalnieks I, Kienle K, Mueller T, Bolder U, Geissler E, Jauch K, Beham A (2005) Benefit of Kupffer cell modulation with glycine versus Kupffer cell depletion after liver transplantation in the rat: effects on postischemic reperfusion injury, apoptotic cell death graft regeneration and survival. Transpl Int 18:1079–1089
Rios JL, Waterman PG (1997) A review of the pharmacology and toxicology of Astragalus. Phytochem Res 11:411–418
Rose ML, Madren J, Bunzendahl H, Thurman RG (1999) Dietary glycine inhibits the growth of B16 melanoma tumors in mice. Carcinogenesis 20:793–798
Roth E, Zellner M, Wessner B, Strasser E, Manhart N, Oehler R, Spittler A (2003) Glycine–an inert amino acid comes alive. Nutrition 19:817–818
Saez G, Thornalley PJ, Hill HA, Hems R, Bannister JV (1982) The production of free radicals during the autoxidation of cysteine and their effect on isolated rat hepatocytes. Biochim Biophys Acta 719:24–31

Salvioli S, Sikora E, Cooper E, Franceschi C (2007) Curcumin in cell death processes: a challenge for CAM of age-related pathologies. Evid Based Complement Altern Med 4:181–190
Schilling MK, den Butter G, Saunder A, Lindell S, Belzer FO, Southard JH (1991) Membrane stabilizing effects of glycine during kidney cold storage and reperfusion. Transplant Proc 23:2387–2389
Senthilkumar R, Viswanathan P, Nalini N (2004) Effect of glycine on oxidative stress in rats with alcohol induced liver injury. Pharmazie 59:55–60
Shapiro H, Ashkenazi M, Weizman N, Shahmurov M, Aeed H, Bruck R (2006) Curcumin ameliorates acute thioacetamide-induced hepatotoxicity. J Gastroenterol Hepatol 21:358–366
Sharma R, Gescher A, Steward W (2005) Curcumin: the story so far. Eur J Cancer 41:1955–1968
Shishodia S, Amin H, Lai R, Aggarwal B (2005) Curcumin (diferuloylmethane) inhibits constitutive NF-kappaB activation, induces G1/S arrest, suppresses proliferation, and induces apoptosis in mantle cell lymphoma. Biochem Pharmacol 70:700–713
Sikora E, Bielak-Zmijewska A, Piwocka K, Skierski J, Radziszewska E (1997) Inhibition of proliferation and apoptosis of human and rat T lymphocytes by curcumin, a curry pigment. Biochem Pharmacol 54:899–907
Sikora E, Bielak-Zmijewska A, Magalska A, Piwocka K, Mosieniak G, Kalinowska M, Widlak P, Cymerman I, Bujnicki J (2006) Curcumin induces caspase-3-dependent apoptotic pathway but inhibits DNA fragmentation factor 40/caspase-activated DNase endonuclease in human Jurkat cells. Mol Cancer Ther 5:927–934
Sinclair S (1998) Chinese herbs: a clinical review of Astragalus, Ligusticum, and Schizandrae. Altern Med Rev 3:338–344
Somasundaram S, Edmund N, Moore D, Small G, Shi Y, Orlowski R (2002) Dietary curcumin inhibits chemotherapy-induced apoptosis in models of human breast cancer. Cancer Res 62:3868–3875
Stahl E (1969) Thin-layer chromatography. A laboratory handbook. Springer, Berlin/Heidelberg/New York, p 857
Stalberg HP, Hahn RG, Hjelmqvist H, Ullman J, Rundgren M (1993) Haemodynamics and fluid balance after intravenous infusion of 1.5% glycine in sheep. Acta Anaesthesiol Scand 37:281–287
Syng-Ai C, Kumari A, Khar A (2004) Effect of curcumin on normal and tumor cells: role of glutathione and bcl-2. Mol Cancer Ther 3:1101–1108
Temple N (2002) Nutrition and disease: challenges of research design. Nutrition 18:343–347
Thompson C (1995) Apoptosis in the pathogenesis and treatment of disease. Science 267:1456–1462
Tin M, Cho C, Chan K, James A, Ko J (2007) Astragalus saponins induce growth inhibition and apoptosis in human colon cancer cells and tumor xenograft. Carcinogenesis 28:1347–1355
Tosetti F, Noonan D, Albini A (2009) Metabolic regulation and redox activity as mechanisms for angioprevention by dietary phytochemicals. Int J Cancer 125:1997–2003
Uberti D, Belloni M, Grilli M, Spano P, Memo M (1998) Induction of tumour-suppressor phosphoprotein p53 in the apoptosis of cultured rat cerebellar neurones triggered by excitatory amino acids. Eur J Neurosci 10:246–254
United States Pharmacopeial Convention (1999) United States pharmacopeia dispensing information: USP DI, 19th edn. United States Pharmacopeial Convention, Rockville
van Breda S, de Kok T, van Delft J (2008) Mechanisms of colorectal and lung cancer prevention by vegetables: a genomic approach. J Nutr Biochem 19:139–157
Vance MA, Gray PD, Tolman KG (1994) Effect of glycine on valproate toxicity in rat hepatocytes. Epilepsia 35:1016–1022
Verotta L, El-Sebakhy NA (2001) Cycloartane and oleanane saponins from Astragalus. In: Atta-Ur-Rhaman (ed) Studies in natural products chemistry, vol 25 (part F), 1st edn. Elsevier Science Publishers, Amsterdam, pp 179–234
Vescovo G, Ravara B, Gobbo V, Sandri M, Angelini A, Della Barbera M, Dona M, Peluso G, Calvani M, Mosconi L, Dalla Libera L (2002) L-Carnitine: a potential treatment for blocking apoptosis and preventing skeletal muscle myopathy in heart failure. Am J Physiol Cell Physiol 283:C802–C810

Vina J, Hems R, Krebs HA (1978) Maintenance of glutathione content is isolated hepatocyctes. Biochem J 170:627–630
Vina J, Romero FJ, Estrela JM, Vina JR (1980) Effect of acetaminophen (paracetamol) and its antagonists on glutathione (GSH) content in rat liver. Biochem Pharmacol 29:1968–1970
Vina J, Saez GT, Wiggins D, Roberts AF, Hems R, Krebs HA (1983) The effect of cysteine oxidation on isolated hepatocytes. Biochem J 212:39–44
Vincent N, Martin G, Baverel G (1992) Glycine, a new regulator of glutamine metabolism in isolated rat-liver cells. Biochim Biophys Acta 1175:13–20
Wakshlag J, Kallfelz F, Wakshlag R, Davenport G (2006) The effects of branched-chain amino acids on canine neoplastic cell proliferation and death. J Nutr 136:2007S–2010S
Weinberg JM, Davis JA, Abarzua M, Rajan T (1987) Cytoprotective effects of glycine and glutathione against hypoxic injury to renal tubules. J Clin Invest 80:1446–1454
Weinberg JM, Venkatachalam MA, Garzo-Quintero R, Roeser NF, Davis JA (1990) Structural requirements for protection by small amino acids against hypoxic injury in kidney proximal tubules. FASEB J 4:3347–3354
Weinberg JM, Varani J, Johnson KJ, Roeser NF, Dame MK, Davis JA, Venkatachalam MA (1992) Protection of human umbilical vein endothelial cells by glycine and structurally similar amino acids against calcium and hydrogen peroxide-induced lethal cell injury. Am J Pathol 140:457–471
Wenzel U, Nickel A, Daniel H (2005) Increased carnitine-dependent fatty acid uptake into mitochondria of human colon cancer cells induces apoptosis. J Nutr 135:1510–1514
Yan Q, Li Y, Jiang Z, Sun Y, Zhu L, Ding Z (2009) Antiproliferation and apoptosis of human tumor cell lines by a lectin (AMML) of Astragalus mongholicus. Phytomedicine 16:586–593
Yang L, Zhang B, Toku K, Maeda N, Sakanaka M, Tanaka J (2000) Improvement of the viability of cultured rat neurons by the non-essential amino acids L-serine and glycine that upregulates expression of the anti-apoptotic gene product Bcl-w. Neurosci Lett 295:97–100
Yazawa K, Kihara T, Shen H, Shimmyo Y, Niidome T, Sugimoto H (2006) Distinct mechanisms underlie distinct polyphenol-induced neuroprotection. FEBS Lett 580:6623–6628
Yesilada E, Bedir E, Calis I, Takaishi Y, Ohmoto Y (2005) Effects of triterpene saponins from Astragalus species on in vitro cytokine release. J Ethnopharmacol 96:71–77
Yu D, Duan Y, Bao Y, Wei C, An L (2005) Isoflavonoids from Astragalus mongholicus protect PC12 cells from toxicity induced by L-glutamate. J Ethnopharmacol 98:89–94
Zee-Cheng RK (1992) Shi-quan-da-bu-tang (ten significant tonic decoction), SQT. A potent Chinese biological response modifier in cancer immunotherapy, potentiation and detoxification of anticancer drugs. Methods Find Exp Clin Pharmacol 14:725–736
Zhang YD, Shen JP, Zhu SH, Huang DK, Ding Y, Zhang XL (1992) Effects of Astragalus (ASI, SK) on experimental liver injury. Yao Xue Xue Bao 27:401–406
Zhang K, Mack P, Wong KP (1998) Glutathione-related mechanisms in cellular resistance to anticancer drugs. Int J Oncol 12:871–882
Zhang Y, Ikejima K, Honda H, Kitamura T, Takei Y, Sato N (2000) Glycine prevents apoptosis of rat sinusoidal endothelial cells caused by deprivation of vascular endothelial growth factor. Hepatology 32:542–546
Zhang J, Yang N, He H, Wei G, Gao D, Wang X, Wang X, Song G (2005) Effect of Astragalus injection on plasma levels of apoptosis-related factors in aged patients with chronic heart failure. Chin J Integr Med 11:187–190
Zhen J, Li W, Zuo Y, Xu Y, Wang Y (2008) Astragalus protects the testis following testicular torsion/detorsion in rats. Zhonghua Nan Ke Xue 14:951–953
Zhong Z, Jones S, Thurman RG (1996) Glycine minimizes reperfusion injury in a low-flow, reflow liver perfusion model in the rat. Am J Physiol 270:G332–G338
Zhong Z, Wheeler MD, Li X, Froh M, Schemmer P, Yin M, Bunzendaul H, Bradford B, Lemasters JJ (2003) L-Glycine: a novel antiinflammatory, immunomodulatory, and cytoprotective agent. Curr Opin Clin Nutr Metab Care 6:229–240
Zhou R, Liu P, Tan M (2009) Effect of Astragalus mongholicus injection on proliferation and apoptosis of hormone sensitive (MCF-7) breast cancer cell lines with physiological dose E2. Zhong Yao Cai 32:744–747
Zhu Y, Chen X, Chen Z, Zeng Y, Shi G, Su Y, Peng X (2004) Curcumin protects mitochondria from oxidative damage and attenuates apoptosis in cortical neurons. Acta Pharmacol Sin 25:1606–1612

Chapter 2
Pomegranate-Derived Constituents as Inducers of Cell Death: Implications in Cancer Prevention and Therapy

Anupam Bishayee and Altaf S. Darvesh

Abstract Cancer chemoprevention, the process of administrating agents which inhibit, delay or reverse the process of carcinogenesis, represents one of the most novel and promising approaches in cancer research. Significant epidemiological evidence suggests an association between increased consumption of fruits, vegetables and spices with a reduced risk of cancer. Bioactive components present in fruits and vegetables, especially polyphenolic flavonoids such as anthocyanins and catechins, show antioxidant, anti-inflammatory and pro-apoptotic effects which afford chemopreventive properties. Pomegranate, obtained from the tree *Punica granatum* has been suggested as an excellent chemopreventive dietary agent. The pomegranate tree, especially the fruit has been a part of medical and religious folklore for centuries. Pomegranates are an extremely rich source of several complex polyphenolic flavonoids such as anthocyanins, hydrolyzable tannins such as punicalin and ellagic acid as well as fatty acids such as punicic acid. Pomegranate phytochemicals have been shown to demonstrate potent anti-tumor promoting effects due to its antioxidant, anti-inflammatory and apoptosis-inducing properties. Apoptosis, programmed cell death, is one of the most important cancer arresting mechanisms and an important target for chemopreventive strategy. Several studies provide evidence highlighting the pro-apoptotic effects of both the polyphenolic and non-polyphenolic bioactive components of pomegranate. This chapter reviews, in detail, the pro-apoptotic and anti-tumor effects of pomegranate-derived constituents in both *in vivo* as well as *in vitro* studies in pre-clinical models of breast, colon, hematological, skin and prostate cancer. The role of synergy, highlighting the importance of poly-constituent

A. Bishayee, Ph.D., M.Pharm. (✉)
Department of Pharmaceutical Sciences, American University of Health Sciences, 1600 East Hill Street, Signal Hill, CA 90755, USA
e-mail: abishayee@auhs.edu

A.S. Darvesh
Department of Pharmaceutical Sciences, College of Pharmacy, Northeast Ohio Medical University, 4209 State Route 44, Rootstown, OH 44272, USA

M. Diederich and K. Noworyta (eds.), *Natural Compounds as Inducers of Cell Death: Volume 1*, DOI 10.1007/978-94-007-4575-9_2,

pomegranate extracts, bioavailability studies as well as the critical need for clinical studies are discussed.

Keywords Apoptosis • Chemoprevention • Chemotherapy • Pomegranate • Polyphenols

2.1 Introduction

Phytochemicals, obtained from both dietary and non-dietary sources, have recently gained prominence in their role as chemopreventive, prophylactic and therapeutic agents for several age-related chronic illnesses, such as cardiovascular and neurodegenerative diseases as well as cancer (Lee et al. 2004; Aggarwal and Shishodia 2006; Ullah and Khan 2008; Khan et al. 2008; Moiseeva and Manson 2009; Bishayee and Darvesh 2010). Dietary phytoconstituents, such as polyphenolic compounds, present in a plethora of fruits and vegetables have demonstrated anti-cancer effects in pre-clinical models and a potential ability to thwart the appearance of cancer in high-risk populations (Johnson 2007; Russo 2007; Khan et al. 2008; Stan et al. 2008). Chemoprevention, using dietary measures, remains the most prominent and promising strategy in cancer research. Polyphenols, obtained from dietary sources, such as anthocyanins from berries and pomegranate, catechins obtained from green and oolong tea leaves, ellagic acid from pomegranate, lycopene present in tomatoes and pink guavas, resveratrol in grapes and red wine as well as several others have gained recent prominence as potential preventive and therapeutic agents in breast, colon, lung, liver, skin as well as prostate cancer. Polyphenolic compounds owe their anti-cancer effects to their ability to modulate a multitude of diverse signaling mechanisms implicated in carcinogenesis as well as their potent antioxidant, anti-inflammatory and anti-apoptotic effects (Galati et al. 2000; Surh 2003; Manach et al. 2004; Rahman et al. 2005; Lee and Lee 2006; Ullah and Khan 2008; Khan et al. 2010).

The pro-apoptotic properties of dietary phytochemicals, polyphenols in particular, have been a subject of considerable investigation over the past decade. The contribution of phytochemical-induced apoptosis in their anti-cancer effects has been elucidated in several pre-clinical models of breast, colon, skin as well as prostate cancer (Galati et al. 2000; Fan et al. 2008; Meeran and Katiyar 2008; Khan et al. 2010). Phytochemicals such as antocyanidins, curcuminoids, ellagitannins, green tea catechins and resveratrol have demonstrated their ability to modulate cell cycle mechanisms including activation of apoptotic pathways (Khan et al. 2006; Meeran and Katiyar 2008; Gupta et al. 2010; Keijer et al. 2011). In this chapter, we examine the apoptotic properties of pomegranate constituents and their contribution to the therapeutic and chemopreventive effects of pomegranate.

2.2 Apoptosis

Programmed cell death mechanisms are deemed essential for the development, homeostasis and elimination of damaged and unwanted cells from multicellular organisms (Sinha and El-Bayoumy 2004). Ever since Kerr and colleagues (1972)

conceptualized the phenomenon of apoptosis, it has been implicated in the pathogenesis of a multitude of illnesses. Apoptosis, a highly conserved mechanism of programmed cell death, ensures maintenance of cell numbers and positioning within varied cell tissue (Fadeel and Orrenius 2005). Apoptosis is defined by distinct morphological changes with characteristic features, such as cell shrinkage, membrane blebbling, chromatin condensation, and DNA ladder formation with final engulfment by macrophages which prevent inflammation in surrounding tissue. Apoptotic events are mediated by a family of cystenine proteases called caspases, activated following an apoptotic stimulus (Thompson 1995; Savill and Fadok 2000). Apoptotic mechanisms involve an extrinsic death receptor-mediated pathway and an intrinsic mitochondria-mediated pathway.

The extrinsic pathway is initiated due to the ligation of transmembrane death receptors which results in activation of membrane-proximal caspases. The caspase signaling cascade ultimately results in the initiation of cell degradation and inevitable apoptosis. The intrinsic pathway is activated due to the loss of growth factor signals in response to detrimental stimuli, such as hypoxia, oxidative damage, toxins as well as chemotherapeutic agents. Pro- and anti-apoptotic members of the Bcl-2 family regulate mitochondrial membrane permeabilization and thus control the release of apoptotic factors from the mitochondrial intermembrane space. Cytochorme *c* (cyt. *c*) release causes downstream start of the caspase cascade which results in the start of apoptotic events (Adams and Cory 1998; Green 2000; Wang 2001; Iannolo et al. 2008).

Disruption of the complex equilibrium between cell growth, cell proliferation and apoptotic mechanisms has been strongly implicated in carcinogenesis. The over-expression of factors implicated in cell survival and the accompanying uncontrolled proliferation with a concurrent loss of apoptotic signals is key to the progression of tumorigenesis and cancer. Disruption of the intrinsic pathway has been shown to play a major role in the growth of cancer cells. The activation of pro-apoptotic mechanisms has been the cornerstone in the development of chemopreventive and therapeutic strategies against cancer (Johnstone et al. 2002). Galati and colleagues (2000) have reviewed the mechanisms, such as mitochondrial cytotoxicity, DNA topoisomerase inhibition as well as signal transduction events which are involved in the apoptotic effects of dietary phytochemicals, including flavonoids and polyphenolic compounds.

2.3 Pomegranate

2.3.1 The Tree and the Fruit

The pomegranate, *Punica granatum* L., is a highly prized fruit and the predominant member of Punicaceae family which consists of only two species. The pomegranate has been mentioned since ancient times in the Bible, the Torah and the Babylonian Talmud as a sacred fruit. The fruit also features in ancient Egyptian ceremonies and Greek mythology as well as the prominent religions of the world, such as Buddhism, Christianity, Judaism, Islam and Zoroastrianism. Lansky and

Newman (2007) have written an enchanting review about the history of this mythical fruit. The pomegranate, of which over a thousand cultivars exist, originated in the Middle East and is now spread throughout the Mediterranean, China, India as well as the American Southwest (Arizona, California and Texas) and Mexico (Levin 1994; Langley 2000).

The pomegranate tree, typically 12–16 ft tall, can live over 200 years. It has glossy lance shaped leaves with the bark turning grey with age. The tree bears large red, white, or variegated flowers which eventually become the fruit. The pomegranate fruit, growing upto 5 in. in diameter, is grenade shaped with a crown shaped calyx. The skin is deep red and leathery and the fruit contains arils (seeds) surrounded by a sac filled with tart, red juice and separated by white membranous pericarp providing a lattice-like network from which the arils are suspended. The seeds constitute about 3% of fruit weight and the juice about 30% of the fruit weight (Lansky and Newman 2007; Syed et al. 2007; Jurenka 2008).

Pomegranates, recently termed "*super fruit*" have long been a symbol of life, longevity, and health (Mahdihassan 1984). The pomegranate fruit as well as other plant parts such as leaves, bark and roots has been considered to be a "*pharmacy unto itself*" and has found a multitude of uses in Ayurvedic and Unani medicine (Izhar 1989; Naovi et al. 1991). Pomegranates have found use in cardiovascular ailments such as atherosclerosis, hyperlipidemia and hypertension, diabetes, bacterial infections, oral hygiene, neurodegenerative diseases, for example Alzheimer's disease as well as cancers of several organ systems, such as breast, colon and the prostate (Burton 2003; Longtin 2003; Basu and Penugonda 2008; Heber 2008; Jurenka 2008; Khan 2009; Sturgeon and Ronnenberg 2009).

2.3.2 *Chemical Constituents*

The pomegranate tree and fruit are a rich source of polyphenolic compounds, such as anthocyanins, catechins and other complex flavonoids along with hydrolysable tannins, such as punicalin, punicalagin and ellagic acid as well as polyunsaturated fatty acids (Artik 1998; Halvorsen et al. 2002; Afaq et al. 2005; Lansky and Newman 2007).

Pomegranate seed oil, which consists of 20% seed weight, contains unsaturated fatty acids, such as linoleic acid and punicic acid as well as minor constituents, such as sterols. Pomegranate juice owes its brilliant red color to a group of potent antioxidant flavonoid compounds known as anthocyanins. Flavonoid glycosides of cyanidin, delphinidin and pelargonidin have been characterized in pomegranate juice along with several minerals (Hernandez et al. 1999; Halvorsen et al. 2002). Hydrolyzable ellagitannins, such as punicalin, pedunculagin and punicalagin as well as gallagic and ellagic acid esters of glucose are found present in the pericarp (peel, rind, and hull) and tree bark. Unique tannins as well as other distinctive compounds are found present in the leaves and flowers of the pomegranate tree. The chemical constituents present in the various different parts of the pomegranate tree have been systematically reviewed by Lansky and Newman (2007).

2.3.3 Pomegranate and Cancer

In recent years, a multitude of studies have examined the anti-cancer potential of pomegranate constituents both in pre-clinical *in vivo* and *in vitro* research as well as in clinical paradigms. The various pomegranate constituents owe their anticancer potential to their ability or modulate apoptotic and inflammatory pathways, affect signal transduction mechanisms as well as their potent antioxidant properties. Pomegranate constituents have been studied and have shown growth inhibition in pre-clinical models of breast, colon, lung, skin and prostate cancers (Bernis et al. 2006; Khan et al. 2009; Lansky and Newman 2007; Syed et al. 2007; Adhami et al. 2009). Recently, for the very first time, we have demonstrated a striking chemopreventive effect of a novel pomegranate formulation in the chemically-induced rodent hepatocarcinogenesis model. The aforementioned effect was achieved through modulation of hepatic nuclear factor E2-related factor 2-mediated antioxidant signaling pathways (Bishayee et al. 2011). Significant progress has been made in evaluating the chemopreventive and therapeutic potential of pomegranate-derived phytochemicals in prostate cancer with an initial phase II clinical trial reporting significant prolongation of prostate specific antigen doubling time in patients with prostate cancer (Adhami and Mukhtar 2006, 2007; Bell and Hawthorne 2008; Siddiqui et al. 2008; Syed et al. 2008; Trottier et al. 2010).

2.3.4 Bioavailability, Toxicity and Synergy of Pomegranate Constituents

The bioavailability and the pharmacokinetic profile of pomegranate phytoconstituents has not yet been completely characterized. Perez-Vicente et al. (2002) elucidated the metabolism of anthocyanins found present in pomegranate juice in an *in vitro* digestion study. A few clinical studies have examined the metabolic profile of certain pomegranate-derived phytochemicals, such as ellagic acid. Healthy human subjects who consumed 180 ml of pomegranate juice concentrate showed presence of ellagic acid metabolites in the plasma as well as urine, both in conjugated as well as free forms. Dimethylellagic acid glucuronide, detected in human plasma and urine samples after consumption of the fruit juice concentrate, has been proposed as a reliable biomarker of pomegranate intake (Seeram et al. 2006). In general, the metabolites found present in human samples after consumption of pomegranate juice coincides with those found in rats administered pomegranate extracts (Cerda et al. 2003). Syed and colleagues (2007) have summarized the bioavailability and pharmacokinetic studies of pomegranate constituents.

Pomegranates have been widely consumed through several millennia across cultures largely without any untoward effects and are deemed safe. However, several investigators have reported toxic events after intake of pomegranate products (Lansky and Newman 2007). One of the earliest reports was published by Squillaci and Di Maggio (1946) who described the acute gastric inflammation followed by death due to consumption of pomegranate tree bark decoction. Allergic reactions after pomegranate fruit consumption have also been reported (Hedge et al. 2002).

Dietary phytochemicals do not exist in isolation in nature but in combination. This adage is best illustrated by the examples of a group of catechins present in green tea and curcuminoids in turmeric (de Kok et al. 2008; Korkina et al. 2009). Pomegranate, both the fruit and the tree, with its varied constituents, such as anthocyanins, ellagitannins, unsaturated fatty acids and many other classes of compounds represents the perfect example of a dietary agent containing a multitude of diverse and important phytoconstituents. The role of synergy, especially in the chemopreventive and therapeutic properties of pomegranate has been a subject of recent investigation (Lansky 2006). It has been shown that although ellagic acid, an important pomegranate phytochemical with potent antioxidant and anti-inflammatory properties, showed inhibitory effects against cell growth and proliferation and promoted apoptosis the effects were more pronounced in combination with flavonoids and other polyphenolics, such as resveratrol (Mertens-Talcott and Percival 2005). Lansky and colleagues (2005a, b) have demonstrated that the anti-invasive effects of combination of extracts obtained from pomegranate peel, seed oil and fermented fruit juice was much greater that any one alone in prostate cancer cells. Similar results have been obtained with the combination of pure constituents, such as ellagic acid and punicic acid. The aforementioned studies thus provide substantial evidence in the relevance of synergy in the effects of varied pomegranate constituents.

2.4 Pomegranate-Mediated Apoptotic and Anti-cancer Effects

2.4.1 In Vitro and In Vivo Studies

Several investigators, over the past decade, have investigated the potential apoptotic effects of pomegranate constituents in pre-clinical cancer models of various organ systems. In this section we review these studies which have been highlighted in Table 2.1.

2.4.1.1 Breast Cancer

In one of the earliest studies investigating the effects of pomegranate, Kim and co-workers (2002) demonstrated that pomegranate seed oil-mediated inhibition of both invasion and proliferation of estrogen-dependent MCF-7 human breast cancer cells was accompanied by apoptosis. Similar anti-invasive and pro-apoptotic effects were also obtained with total pomegranate extract (Jeune et al. 2005). Several studies,

Table 2.1 Pomegranate-mediated apoptotic and anti-cancer effects: *in vitro* and *in vivo* studies

Pomegranate constituents	Biological effects	Apoptotic mechanisms	Concentration	Reference
Breast cancer				
Seed oil	Inhibited proliferation and invasion, and induced apoptosis in estrogen-dependent MCF-7 human breast cancer cells	–	25, 50, 100 μg/ml	Kim et al. (2002)
Total extract	Suppressed growth and invasion, as well as induced apoptosis in MCF-7 cells	–	12, 28, 40, 60, 80 μg/ml	Jeune et al. (2005)
Fermented juice extract	Inhibited growth, proliferation and invasion, and stimulated apoptosis in MDA-231 and SUM 149 breast cancer cells	–	100, 200 μg/ml	Khan et al. (2009)
Standardized fruit extract	Decreased viability, inhibited proliferation, and induced apoptosis in WA4 mouse mammary cancer cells	↑caspase-3 activity	25, 50, 100, 150 μg/ml	Dai et al. (2010)
Punicic acid	Suppressed proliferation and induced apoptosis in both estrogen sensitive (MDA-ERα7) and estrogen insensitive (MDA-MB-231) cells	↓ΔΨm	2.5, 5, 10, 20, 40 μM	Grossmann et al. (2010)
Colon cancer				
Juice, ellagic acid, punicalagin, and total tannin extract	Inhibited proliferation and induced apoptosis in H29 and HCT116 colon tumor cells	–	100 μg/ml	Seeram et al. (2005)
Ellagic acid, and punicalagin	Initiated apoptosis via the mitochondrial intrinsic pathway in human colon adenocarcinoma Caco-2 cells	↑cyt. *c*, ↓bcl-X_L, ↑procaspase-3,-9	1, 10, 30, 100 μM	Larrosa et al. (2006)
Ellagitannins, and urolithins	Inhibited colony formation and induced apoptosis in colon carcinoma HT-29 cells	↑caspase-3 activity	12.5, 25, 50, 100 μM	Kasimsetty et al. (2010)
Hematological cancer				
Peel extract	Produced apoptosis in Raji and P3HR-1 human Burkitt's lymphoma cells	–	1.3, 1.9, 2.5 μl/ml	Settheetham and Ishida (1995)

(continued)

Table 2.1 (continued)

Pomegranate constituents	Biological effects	Apoptotic mechanisms	Concentration	Reference
Skin cancer				
Fruit juice extract	Induced cell cycle arrest and apoptosis in normal human epidermal keratinocytes subjected to UVA radiation	↑bax, ↑bad, ↓bcl-X_L	60, 80, 100 μg/ml	Syed et al. (2006)
Delphinidin	Protected against UVB-induced apoptosis in normal human epidermal keratinocytes	↓PARP, ↓bax, ↑bcl-X_L, ↓procaspase-3,-8,-9	10 μM	Afaq et al. (2006)
Standardized extract	Prevented apoptosis in SKU-1064 human skin fibroblast cells after UV irradiation	↓caspase-3	5, 10, 20 μg/ml	Pacheco-Palencia et al. (2008)
Prostate cancer				
Pericarp extract, juice extract, and seed oil	Suppressed proliferation and induced apoptosis in PC-3 and DU-145 human prostate cancer cells	↑caspase-3	50, 100 μg/ml	Albrecht et al. (2004)
Fruit extract	Inhibited proliferation and induced apoptosis in PC3 human prostate cancer cells	↑bax, ↑bak, ↓bcl-2, ↓bcl-X_L	10, 20, 40, 60, 80, 100 μg/ml	Malik et al. (2005)
Juice extract and skin extract	Decreased cell viability and induced apoptosis in DU-145 cells	–	Dilution factor: 1,000, 2,000, 3,000	Rettig et al. (2008)
Juice extract and skin extract	Prevented proliferation, induced apoptosis and delayed the emergence of LAPC4 xenograft in mice		1.0 ml/kg p.o.	Rettig et al. (2008)
Punicalagin, ellagic acid, extract, and fruit juice	Down-regulated androgen synthesizing gene expression and induced apoptosis in LNCaP, LNCaP-AR and DU-145 human prostate cancer cells	–	50, 100 μg/ml	Hong et al. (2008)
Aril and skin extract	Inhibited cell proliferation and induced apoptosis in LAPC4 prostate cancer cells	–	10 μg/ml	Koyoma et al. (2010)

Abbreviations: *cyt. c* cytochrome *c*, $\Delta\Psi m$ mitochondrial membrane potential, *PARP* poly(ADP-ribose) polymerase, *p.o. per os*, *UVA* ultraviolet A, *UVB* ultraviolet B conduced in recent years, have also demonstrated the involvement of apoptotic mechanisms in the anti-cancer effects of pomegranate constituents. The fermented juice extract of the pomegranate fruit showed anti-invasive, anti-proliferative and apoptotic effects in both MDA-231 as well as SUM 149 breast cancer cells (Khan et al. 2009). Dai and colleagues (2010) showed that the standardized extract of the pomegranate fruit decreased cell viability, inhibited the proliferative effects and induced apoptosis in WA4 mouse mammary cancer cells as evidenced by an increase in caspase-3 activity. Punicic acid, a conjugated fatty acid present in pomegranate seed oil, showed anti-proliferative effects and induced apoptosis with an accompanying lowering of the mitochondrial membrane potential in both estrogen sensitive (MDA-ERα7) as well as estrogen insensitive (MDA-MB-231) breast cancer cells (Grossmann et al. 2010).

2.4.1.2 Colon Cancer

Several pomegranate constituents have been a subject of relatively recent investigation for their potential anticancer and apoptotic effects in pre-clinical models of colon cancer. Seeram and co-workers (2005) showed that both isolated constituents, such as ellagic acid and punicalagin as well as pomegranate juice and total tannic extract inhibited the proliferative effects and promoted apoptosis in H29 and HCT116 colon cancer cells. Mechanistic studies by Larrosa et al. (2006) showed that both ellagic acid as well as punicalagin initiated apoptosis in the human colon adenocarcinoma Caco-2 cells as evidenced by an increase in cyt. *c* release, decreased bcl-X_L and increased procaspase-3 and -9 expression. A recent study by Kasimesetty et al. (2010) showed that both ellagitannins and urolithins produced apoptotic effects in colon carcinoma HT-29 cells as demonstrated by increased caspase-3 activity.

2.4.1.3 Hematological Cancer

In the only study of its kind, Settheetham and Ishida (1995) demonstrated the apoptotic properties of pomegranate peel extract in both Raji and P3HR-1 human Burkitt's lymphoma cells.

2.4.1.4 Skin Cancer

A few studies have investigated the potential apoptotic properties of pomegranate constituents in models of skin cancer. Pomegranate fruit juice extract caused cell cycle arrest and produced apoptosis as evidenced by an increased bax/bcl-X_L ratio in human epidermal keratinocytes (Syed et al. 2006). However, two studies have demonstrated the anti-apoptotic activities of pomegranate constituents. Delphinidin, a prominent anthocyanin found present in pomegranate, as well as standardized pomegranate extract prevented the ultraviolet radiation-induced apoptosis in both human epidermal keratinocytes and SKU-1064 human skin fibroblast cells with accompanying decrease in bax/bcl-X_L ratio and caspase activity (Afaq et al. 2006; Pacheco-Palencia et al. 2008).

2.4.1.5 Prostate Cancer

The apoptotic properties of pomegranate components have been studied extensively in pre-clinical models of prostate cancer. Albrecht and colleagues (2004) demonstrated the anti-proliferative and accompanying apoptotic effects of pericarp extract, juice extract as well as pomegranate seed oil in PC-3 and DU-145 human prostate cancer cells as evidenced by elevated caspase-3 expression. Pomegranate fruit extract showed similar results in PC-3 cells with simultaneous increase in bax/bcl-X_L ratio in PC-3 cells (Malik et al. 2005). Rettig and co-workers (2008) demonstrated that both pomegranate juice extract and skin extract reduced cell viability and induced apoptosis in DU-145 cells. Besides the aforementioned *in vitro* study, Rettig et al. (2008) also showed that the pomegranate juice extract and skin extract also produced anti-proliferative and apoptotic effects with the accompanying delay in the emergence of LAPC4 xenografted tumor in mice. Punicalagin, ellagic acid, pomegranate extract as well as fruit juice produced apoptosis in LNCaP, LNCaP-AR and DU-145 human prostate cancer cells (Hong et al. 2008). In a recent study, Koyoma and colleagues (2010) showed the anti-proliferative and apoptotic effects of pomegranate aril and skin extract in LAPC4 prostate cancer cells.

2.4.1.6 Liver Cancer

Recently, pomegranate phytoconstituents showed significant chemoprevention against diethylnitrosamine (DENA)-initiated and phenobarbital (PB)-promoted rat liver tumorigenesis (Bishayee et al. 2011). Pomegranate-mediated chemoprevention was achieved through substantial induction of apoptosis in the liver tissues of carcinogen-exposed animals (Fig. 2.1, unpublished observations).

2.5 Conclusion and Future Directions

The scientific rationale for the potential usefulness of pomegranate-derived phytoconstituents as chemopreventive and therapeutic agents in cancer is based on their proven antioxidant, anti-inflammatory and pro-apoptotic properties as well as its demonstrated ability to modulate a multitude of signaling pathways implicated in the process of carcinogenesis. In this chapter, we have reviewed the contribution of the apoptotic properties of pomegranate constituents in its anti-cancer effects. It is clearly evident that the use of pomegranate-derived phytochemicals holds tremendous promise as chemopreventive and therapeutic agents in cancer. Nevertheless,

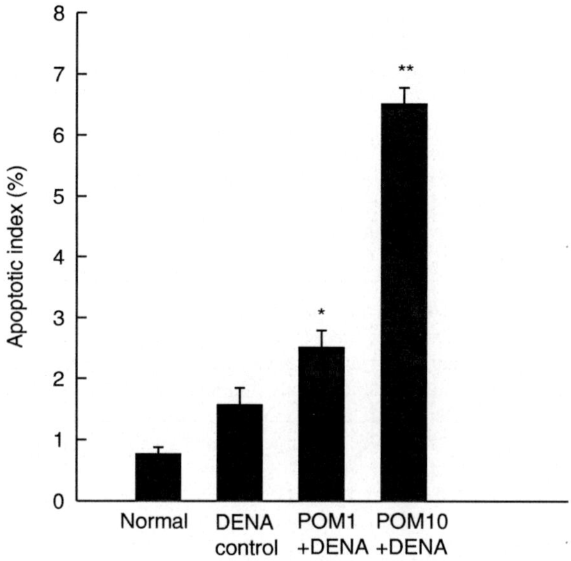

Fig. 2.1 Immunohistochemical analysis of DNA fragmentation in apoptotic cells in hepatic tissues during experimental hepatocarcinogenesis in rats in the presence or absence of pomegranate treatment. Rat liver tumorigenesis was initiated with DENA (200 mg/kg; i.p.) and subsequently promoted by PB (0.05% in drinking water). Oral administration of pomegranate emulsion (1 or 10 g/kg; three times a week) was initiated 4 weeks prior to the initiation and continued for 22 weeks. All rats were sacrificed 18 weeks following DENA exposure and liver sections were subjected to immunohistochemical analysis. The apoptotic index was expressed as the number of positively stained cells per 100 hepatocytes based on a count of 1,000 cells per animal. Each bar represents the mean ± SE ($n=4$ animals). $^{*}P<0.05$ and $^{**}P<0.001$ as compared to DENA control

a significant amount of effort would be required to ensure successful use of pomegranate constituents. The pro-apoptotic properties of pomegranate need further elucidation in pre-clinical *in vivo* cancer models of several organ systems, such as breast, colon, lung, liver and prostate. Translational research, carried out using well designed clinical trials, is critical to the development of pomegranate constituents as anti-cancer agents. Systematic epidemiological evolution in world regions where pomegranates form an integral part of the diet would provide valuable clues in its anti-cancer potential. A systematic multi-dose "*head-to-head*" comparison, in both pre-clinical and clinical studies, of important pomegranate phytochemicals, namely delphinidin and ellagic acid with pomegranate extract with various pomegranate constituents, such as fruit juice, seed oil, bark extract, peel and leaf extract would provide valuable insight into the synergistic potential of pomegranate. Clinical bioavailability, dosing and safety studies also have paramount importance in advancing the use of pomegranate for wide spread therapeutic use. Another major challenge remains the development of commercially available pomegranate formulation with stable shelf life which would contain all the goodness of the pomegranate constituents and be easily available and acceptable for consumption.

References

Adams JM, Cory S (1998) The Bcl-2 protein family: arbiters of cell survival. Science 281:1322–1326

Adhami VM, Mukhtar H (2006) Polyphenols from green tea and pomegranate for prevention of prostate cancer. Free Radic Res 40:1095–1104

Adhami VM, Mukhtar H (2007) Antioxidants from green tea and pomegranate for chemoprevention of prostate cancer. Mol Biotechnol 37:52–57

Adhami VM, Khan N, Mukhtar H (2009) Cancer chemoprevention by pomegranate: laboratory and clinical evidence. Nutr Cancer 61:811–815

Afaq F, Saleem M, Krueger CG, Reed JD, Mukhtar H (2005) Anthocyanin- and hydrolyzable tannin-rich pomegranate fruit extracts modulates MAPK and NF-kappaB pathways and inhibits skin tumorigenesis in CD-1 mice. Int J Cancer 113:423–433

Afaq F, Syed DN, Malik A, Hadi N, Sarfaraz S, Kweon MH et al (2006) Delphinidin, an anthocyanidin in pigmented fruits and vegetables, protects human HaCaT keratinocytes and mouse skin against UVB-mediated oxidative stress and apoptosis. J Invest Dermatol 127:222–232

Aggarwal BB, Shishodia S (2006) Molecular targets of dietary agents for prevention and therapy of cancer. Biochem Pharmacol 71:1379–1421

Albrecht M, Jiang W, Kumi-Diaka J, Lansky EP, Gommersall LM, Patel A et al (2004) Pomegranate extracts potently suppress proliferation, xenograft growth, and invasion of human prostate cancer cells. J Med Food 7:274–283

Artik N (1998) Determination of phenolic compounds in pomegranate juice by using HPLC. Fruit Process 8:492–499

Basu A, Penugonda K (2008) Pomegranate juice: a heart-healthy fruit juice. Nutr Rev 67:49–56

Bell C, Hawthorne S (2008) Ellagic acid, pomegranate and prostate cancer – a mini review. J Pharm Pharmacol 60:139–144

Bernis DL, Katz AE, Buttyan R (2006) Clinical trials of natural products as chemopreventive agents for prostate cancer. Expert Opin Invest Drugs 15:1191–1200

Bishayee A, Darvesh AS (2010) Oxidative stress in cancer and neurodegenerative diseases: prevention and treatment by dietary antioxidants. In: Kozyrev D, Slutsky V (eds) Free radicals: formation, types and effects. Nova Science Publishers, Inc, Hauppauge, pp 1–55

Bishayee A, Bhatia D, Thoppil RJ, Darvesh AS, Eviatar N, Lansky EP (2011) Pomegranate-mediated chemoprevention of experimental hepatocarcinogenesis involves Nrf2-regulated antioxidant mechanisms. Carcinogenesis 32:888–896

Burton A (2003) Chemoprevention: eat ginger, rub on pomegranate. Lancet 4:715

Cerda B, Llorach R, Ceron JJ, Espin JC, Tomar-Barberan FA (2003) Evaluation of the bioavailability and metabolism in the rat of punicalagin, an antioxidant polyphenol from pomegranate juice. Eur J Nutr 42:18–28

Dai Z, Nair V, Khan M, Ciolino HP (2010) Pomegranate extract inhibits the proliferation and viability of MMTV-Wnt-1 mouse mammary cancer stem cells *in vitro*. Int J Oncol 24:1087–1091

de Kok TM, van Breda SG, Manson MM (2008) Mechanisms of combined action of different chemopreventive dietary compounds. Eur J Nutr 47:51–59

Fadeel B, Orrenius S (2005) Apoptosis: a basic biological phenomenon with wide-ranging implications in human disease. J Int Med 258:479–517

Fan E, Jiang S, Zhang L, Bai Y (2008) Molecular mechanism of apoptosis induction by resveratrol, a natural cancer chemopreventive agent. Int J Vitam Nutr Res 78:3–8

Galati G, Teng S, Moridani MY, Chan TS, O'Brien PJ (2000) Cancer chemoprevention and apoptosis mechanisms by dietary polyphenolics. Drug Metabol Interact 17:311–349

Green DR (2000) Apoptotic pathways: paper wraps stone blunts scissors. Cell 102:1–4

Grossmann ME, Mizuno NK, Schuster T, Cleary MP (2010) Punicic acid is an ω-5 fatty acid capable of inhibiting breast cancer proliferation. Int J Oncol 36:421–426

Gupta SC, Kim JH, Prasad S, Aggarwal BB (2010) Regulation of survival, proliferation, invasion, angiogenesis, and metastasis of tumor cells through modulation of inflammatory pathways by nutraceuticals. Cancer Metastasis Rev 29:405–434

Halvorsen BL, Holte K, Myhrstad MC, Barikmo I, Hvattum E, Remberg SF et al (2002) A systematic screening of total antioxidants in dietary plants. J Nutr 132:461–471

Heber D (2008) Multitargeted therapy of cancer by ellagitannins. Cancer Lett 269:262–268

Hegde VL, Mahesh PA, Venkatesh YP (2002) Anaphylaxis caused by mannitol in pomegranate (*Punica granatum*). Allergy Clin Immunol Int 14:37–39

Hernandez F, Melgarejo P, Tomas-Barberan FA, Artes F (1999) Evolution of juice anthocyanins during ripening of new selected pomegranate (*Punica granatum*) clones. Eur Food Res Technol 210:39–42

Hong MY, Seeram NP, Heber D (2008) Pomegranate polyphenols down-regulate expression of androgen-synthesizing genes in human prostate cancer cells overexpressing the androgen receptor. J Nutr Biochem 19:848–855

Iannolo G, Conticello C, Memeo L, De Maria R (2008) Apoptosis in normal and cancer stem cells. Crit Rev Oncol Hematol 66:42–51

Izhar N (1989) The Unani traditional medical system in India: a case study in health behavior. Geogr Med 19:163–185

Jeune MA, Diaka-Kumi J, Brown J (2005) Anticancer activities of pomegranate extracts and genistein in human breast cancer cells. J Med Food 8:469–475

Johnson IT (2007) Phytochemicals and cancer. Proc Nutr Soc 6:207–215

Johnstone RW, Ruefli AA, Lowe SW (2002) Apoptosis: a link between cancer genetics and chemotherapy. Cell 108:152–164

Jurenka J (2008) Therapeutic applications of pomegranate (*Punica granatum* L.): a review. Altern Med Rev 13:128–144

Kasimsetty SG, Bialonska D, Reddy MK, Ma G, Khan SI, Ferreira D (2010) Colon cancer chemopreventive activities of pomegranate ellagitannins and urolithins. J Agric Food Chem 58:2180–2187

Keijer J, Bekkenkamp-Grovenstein M, Venema D, Dommels YEM (2011) Bioactive food components, cancer cell growth limitation and reversal of glycolytic metabolism. Biochim Biophys Acta 1807:697–706

Kerr JF, Wyllie AH, Currie AR (1972) Apoptosis: a basic biological phenomenon with wide-ranging implications in tissue kinetics. Br J Cancer 26:239–257

Khan SA (2009) The role of pomegranate (*Punica Granatum* L.) in colon cancer. Pak J Pharm Sci 22:346–348

Khan N, Afaq F, Saleem M, Ahmad N, Mukhtar H (2006) Targeting multiple signaling pathways by green tea polyphenol (−)-epigallocetechin-3-galate. Cancer Res 66:2500–2505

Khan N, Afaq F, Mukhtar H (2008) Cancer chemoprevention through dietary antioxidants: progress and promise. Antioxid Redox Signal 10:475–510

Khan GN, Gorin MA, Rosenthal D, Pan Q, Bao LW, Wu ZF et al (2009) Pomegranate fruit extract impairs invasion and motility in human breast cancer. Integr Cancer Ther 8:242–253

Khan N, Adhami VM, Mukhtar H (2010) Apoptosis by dietary agents for prevention and treatment of prostate cancer. Endocr Relat Cancer 17:R39–R52

Kim ND, Mehta R, Yu W, Neeman I, Livney T, Amichay A et al (2002) Chemopreventive and adjuvant therapeutic potential of pomegranate (*Punica granatum*) for human breast cancer. Breast Cancer Res Treat 71:203–217

Korkina LG, de Luca C, Kostyuk VA, Pastore S (2009) Plant polyphenols and tumors: from mechanisms to therapies, prevention and protection against toxicity of anti-cancer treatments. Curr Med Chem 16:3943–3965

Koyoma S, Cobb LJ, Mehta HH, Seeram NP, Heber D, Pantuck AJ et al (2010) Pomegranate extract induces apoptosis in human prostate cancer cells by modulation of the IGF-IGFBP axis. Growth Horm IGF Res 20:55–62

Langley P (2000) Why a pomegranate? Br Med J 321:1153–1154

Lansky EP (2006) Beware of pomegranates bearing 40% ellagic acid. J Med Food 9:119–122

Lansky EP, Newman RA (2007) *Punica granatum* (pomegranate) and its potential for prevention and treatment of inflammation and cancer. J Ethnopharmacol 109:177–206

Lansky EP, Harrison G, Froom P, Jiang WG (2005a) Pomegranate (*Punica granatum*) pure chemical show possible synergistic inhibition of human PC-3 prostate cancer cell invasion across Matrigel™. Invest New Drugs 23:121–122

Lansky EP, Jiang W, Mo H, Bravo L, Froom P, Yu W et al (2005b) Possible synergistic prostate cancer suppression by anatomically discreet pomegranate fractions. Invest New Drugs 22:11–20

Larrosa M, Tomás-Barberán FA, Espín JC (2006) The dietary hydrolysable tannin punicalagin releases ellagic acid that induces apoptosis in human colon adenocarcinoma Caco-2 cells by using the mitochondrial pathway. J Nutr Biochem 17:611–625

Lee KW, Lee HJ (2006) The roles of polyphenols in cancer chemoprevention. Biofactors 26:105–121

Lee KW, Lee HJ, Lee CY (2004) Vitamins, phytochemicals, diet, and their implementation in cancer chemoprevention. Crit Rev Food Sci Nutr 44:437–452

Levin GM (1994) Pomegranate (*Punica granatum*) plant genetic resources in Turkmenistan. Plant Genetic Res Newslett 97:31–37

Longtin R (2003) The pomegranate: nature's power fruit? J Natl Cancer Inst 95:346–348

Mahdihassan S (1984) Outline of the beginnings of alchemy and its antecedents. Am J Chin Med 12:32–42

Malik A, Afaq F, Sarfaraz S, Adhami VM, Syed DN, Mukhtar H (2005) Pomegranate fruit juice for chemoprevention and chemotherapy of prostate cancer. Proc Natl Acad Sci USA 102:14813–14818

Manach C, Scalbert A, Morand C, Remesy C, Jimenes L (2004) Polyphenols: food sources and bioavailability. Am J Clin Nutr 79:727–747

Meeran SM, Katiyar SK (2008) Cell cycle control as a basis for cancer chemoprevention through dietary agents. Front Biosci 13:2191–2202

Mertens-Talcott SU, Percival SS (2005) Ellagic acid and quercetin interact synergistically with resveratrol in the induction of apoptosis and cause transient cell cycle arrest in human leukemia cells. Cancer Lett 218:141–151

Moiseeva EP, Manson MM (2009) Dietary chemopreventive phytochemicals: too little or too much. Cancer Prev Res 2:611–616

Naovi SAH, Khan MSY, Vohora SB (1991) Antibacterial, anti-fungal and anthelmintic investigations on Indian medicinal plants. Fitoterapia 62:221–228

Pacheco-Palencia LA, Noratto G, Hingorani L, Talcott ST, Mertens-Talcott SU (2008) Protective effects of standardized pomegranate (*Punica granatum* L.) polyphenolic extract in ultraviolet-irradiated human skin fibroblasts. J Agric Food Chem 56:8434–8441

Perez-Vicente A, Gil-Izquierdo A, Garcia-Viguera C (2002) In vitro gastrointestinal digestion study of pomegranate juice phenolic compounds, anthocyanins, and vitamin C. J Agric Food Chem 50:2308–2312

Rahman I, Biswas SK, Kirkham PA (2005) Regulation of inflammation and redox signaling by dietary polyphenols. Biochem Pharmacol 72:1439–1452

Rettig MB, Heber D, An J, Seeram NP, Rao JY, Liu H et al (2008) Pomegranate extract inhibits androgen-independent prostate cancer growth through nuclear factor-κB-dependent mechanism. Mol Cancer Ther 7:2662–2671

Russo GL (2007) Ins and outs of dietary phytochemicals in cancer chemoprevention. Biochem Pharmacol 74:533–544

Savill J, Fadok V (2000) Corpse clearance defines the meaning of cell death. Nature 407:784–788

Seeram NP, Adams LS, Henning SM, Niu Y, Zhang Y, Nair MG et al (2005) In vitro antiproliferative, apoptotic and antioxidant activities of punicalagin, ellagic acid and a total pomegranate tannin extract are enhanced in combination with other polyphenols as found in pomegranate juice. J Nutr Biochem 16:360–367

Seeram NP, Henning SM, Zhang Y, Suchard M, Li Z, Heber D (2006) Pomegranate juice ellagitannin metabolites are present in human plasma and some persist in urine for up to 48 h. J Nutr 136:2481–2485

Settheetham W, Ishida T (1995) Study of genotoxic effects of antidiarrheal medicinal herbs on human cells in vitro. Southeast Asian J Trop Med Public Health 26:306–310

Siddiqui IA, Afaq F, Adhami VM, Mukhtar H (2008) Prevention of prostate cancer through custom tailoring of chemopreventive regimen. Chem Biol Interact 171:122–132

Sinha R, El-Bayoumy K (2004) Apoptosis is a critical cellular event in cancer chemoprevention and chemotherapy by selenium compounds. Curr Cancer Drug Targets 4:13–28

Squillaci G, Di Maggio G (1946) Acute morbidity and mortality from decoctions of the bark of *Punica granatum*. Bollettino Soc Ital Biol 1946:1095–1096

Stan SD, Kar S, Stoner GD, Singh SV (2008) Bioactive food components and cancer risk reduction. J Cell Biochem 104:339–356

Sturgeon SR, Ronnenberg (2009) Pomegranate and breast cancer: possible mechanisms of prevention. Nutr Revs 68:122–128

Surh YJ (2003) Cancer chemoprevention with dietary phytochemicals. Nat Rev Cancer 3:768–780

Syed DN, Malik A, Hadi N, Sarfaraz S, Afaq F, Mukhtar H (2006) Photochemopreventive effect of pomegranate fruit extract on UVA-mediated activation of cellular pathways in normal human epidermal ketatinocytes. Photochem Photobiol 82:398–405

Syed DN, Afaq F, Mukhtar H (2007) Pomegranate derived products for cancer chemoprevention 2007. Semin Cancer Biol 17:377–385

Syed DN, Suh Y, Afaq F, Mukhtar H (2008) Dietary agents for chemoprevention of prostate cancer. Cancer Lett 265:167–176

Thompson CB (1995) Apoptosis in pathogenesis and treatment disease. Science 267:1456–1462

Trottier G, Boström PJ, Lawrentschuk N, Fleshner NE (2010) Nutraceuticals and prostate cancer prevention: a current review. Nat Rev Urol 7:21–30

Ullah MF, Khan MW (2008) Potential therapeutic tendencies of plant derived polyphenolic compounds. Asian Pacific J Cancer Prev 9:187–196

Wang X (2001) The expanding role of mitochondria in apoptosis. Genes Dev 15:2922–2933

Chapter 3
Antitumor Effects of Anthocyanins: Focus on Apoptosis

Carmela Fimognari

Abstract Aberrantly regulated apoptosis is involved in the pathogenesis of several diseases and defective apoptosis leads to uncontrolled cell proliferation and tumorigenesis. Cancer, one of the major causes of death across the world, is a pathologic condition characterized by a dysfunction of the normal mechanisms of cell-cycle regulation either by excessive cell proliferation, inhibited/suppressed apoptosis or both. Conceivably, the carcinogenetic process can be targeted and interrupted along different stages through the induction of apoptosis. Many naturally occurring dietary compounds from our daily consumption of fruits and vegetables have been shown to possess cancer preventive and/or therapeutic effects. Anthocyanins are serious candidates since they are responsible for the cancer protective properties of a diet rich in vegetables and fruit. Numerous anthocyanins indeed show antiproliferative and cytotoxic effects, and more specifically pro-apoptotic activities, in several cancer cell lines and animal tumour models. The aim of the present chapter is to analyze and summarize the most recent advances related to the molecular mechanisms of apoptosis induced by anthocyanins and to delineate the involvement of apoptosis in the activity of anthocyanins at all different stages of the carcinogenetic process.

Abbreviations

ADPRTL1	ADP-ribosyltransferase (NAD+poly (ADP-ribose) polymerase)-like 1
BIRC3	baculoviral IAP repeat-containing 3″
CYP1A1	cytochrome P450 1A1
EGFR	epidermal growth factor receptor

C. Fimognari (✉)
Department of Pharmacology, Alma Mater Studiorum - Università di Bologna, via Irnerio 48, 40126 Bologna, Italy
e-mail: carmela.fimognari@unibo.it

M. Diederich and K. Noworyta (eds.), *Natural Compounds as Inducers of Cell Death: Volume 1*, DOI 10.1007/978-94-007-4575-9_3,

FasL Fas ligand
IAP inhibitor of apoptosis protein
JNK Jun N-terminal Kinase
MEK MAP kinase or ERK kinase
ROS reactive oxygen species

3.1 Introduction

The longstanding dogma of multistage carcinogenesis divides the development of malignancies into three temporally ordered and mechanistically distinct stages of initiation, promotion and progression (Hursting et al. 1999). Initiation, the first stage, is an early mutagenic event that produces a cell with the genetic code for a benign tumor phenotype. The second stage, tumor promotion, is a slow and reversible, epigenetically controlled clonal expansion of the initiated cell that produces a benign tumor. Tumor progression is the irreversible conversion of the benign tumor to a malignant phenotype (Hursting et al. 1999).

Anthocyanins occur ubiquitously in the plant kingdom and confer the bright red, blue and purple colors to fruits and vegetables such as berries, grapes, apples, purple cabbage and corn. Of potential importance to human health is the relatively high concentration of anthocyanins in the diet. The daily intake of anthocyanins in the U.S. diet is estimated to be about 200 mg or about ninefold higher than that of other dietary flavonoids. For example, the intake of genistein, quercetin and apigenin is only 20–25 mg/day (Hertog et al. 1993). Epidemiologic studies suggest that the consumption of anthocyanins lowers the risk of different chronic-degenerative diseases, such as cancer (Prior and Wu 2006). They have indeed multiple effects that inhibit carcinogenesis at each discrete stage and involve interactions between anthocyanins and several targets.

The present chapter focuses on the modulation of apoptosis as a fundamental mechanism by which anthocyanins exert anticancer activity. The most recent results from *in vitro* cell culture and *in vivo* animal model tumor systems will be highlighted.

3.2 Chemistry of Anthocyanins

Anthocyanins belong to a wider class of phenolic compounds. They are glycosides, having glucose, galactose, rhamnose, xylose or arabinose attached to a polyhydroxy and polymethoxy derivatives of 2-phenylbenzopyrylium or flavylium salts (Mazza 1995; Harborne and Grayer 1988). In contrast to other flavonoids, the anthocyanins have a positive charge in acidic solution (Mazza 1995). Their color depends upon pH and the presence of chelating metal ions: many anthocyanins are red at acidic conditions

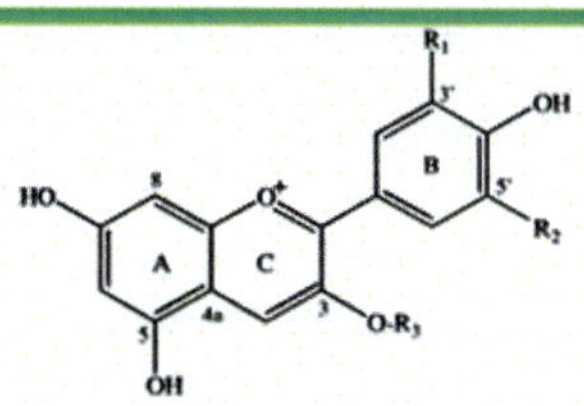

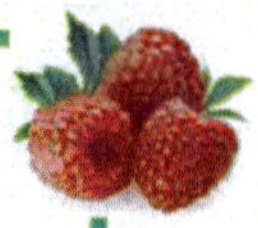

Percentage abundance	
Delphinidin	50%
Cyanidin	12%
Petunidin	12%
Pelargonidin	12%
Peonidin	7%
Malvidin	7%

Anthocyanidins & Anthocyanins	R_1	R_2	R_3
Pelargonidin	H	H	H
Cyanidin	OH	H	H
Delphinidin	OH	OH	H
Peonidin	OMe	OH	H
Malvidin	OMe	OMe	H
Pelargonidin-3-galactoside	H	H	galactose
Cyanidin-3-galactoside	OH	H	galactose
Cyanidin-3-rutinoside	OH	OH	rutinose
Cyanidin-3-glucosylrutinoside	OH	OH	glucose-rutinose
Delphinidin-3-galactoside	OH	OH	galactose

Fig. 3.1 Chemical structures and percentage abundance of anthocyanins

and turn blue at less acid conditions. The aglycone forms of anthocyanins are known as anthocyanidins. The six most common anthocyanidin skeletons are cyanidin, delphinidin, petunidin, peonidin, malvidin, pelargonidin (Fig. 3.1). The sugar components of anthocyanins are usually conjugated to the anthocyanidin skeleton via the C-ring C-3 hydroxyl group. Several hundred anthocyanins are known varying in the basic anthocyanidin skeleton, the number of hydroxyl groups, the nature and number of sugars attached to the molecule, the position of this attachment and the nature and number of aliphatic or aromatic acids attached to the sugars in the molecule (Harborne and Grayer 1988).

3.3 Modulation of Apoptosis by Anthocyanins

Apoptosis, or programmed cell death, plays a key role in the development and growth regulation of normal cells, and is often dysregulated in cancer cells. Some of the most effective chemopreventive agents are strong inducers of apoptosis in premalignant and malignant cells. Anthocyanin-rich extracts from berries and grapes, and several pure anthocyanins and anthocyanidins, exhibit pro-apoptotic effects in multiple experimental systems. In some instances (e.g. UVB-induced damage), the chemopreventive potential of anthocyanins is linked to their ability to inhibit apoptosis induced by toxic agents. Of note, the modulation of apoptotic pathways is widely involved in the inhibitory effects of anthocyanins at all different stages of the carcinogenetic process.

3.3.1 *In Vitro Studies*

3.3.1.1 Induction of Apoptosis

The anti-mutagenic properties elicited by natural dietary components have a range of possible applications in human health care. They can potentially protect against electrophilic (e.g., free radical) attack on DNA and its possible outcomes, such as ageing and cancer. One of the possible mechanisms of their antimutagenic action could be an increase in the apoptotic elimination of heavily-damaged cells from a culture. The antimutagenic activity of anthocyanins was established in a battery of short-term cytogenetic tests in lymphocyte cultures exposed to genotoxic agents: hydrogen peroxide, benzo[a]pyrene, ethyl methanesulfonate, mitomycin C, and colchicine. By microscopic examination, it was assessed that the frequencies of cells exhibiting morphological features of apoptosis considerably increased in the cultures containing anthocyanins. However, the enhancement of apoptosis can explain a major part of their activity against the genotoxicity of hydrogen peroxide, ethyl methanesulfonate, and colchicine, whereas other mechanisms of antimutagenic action should be sought for the other genotoxic compounds (Fimognari et al. 2001; Gasiorowski et al. 2001).

Several studies demonstrated the ability of anthocyanins to modulate further events involved in cancer development through the induction of apoptosis on already transformed or tumor cells.

The effects of anthocyanins on apoptosis induction were described in several cell models. Table 3.1 reports all the transformed and cancer cell lines where apoptosis induction by anthocyanins was recorded together with the range of concentrations tested. For example, many studies reported that exposure of different human breast cancer cells (breast adenocarcinoma cells; human epidermal growth factor receptor (EGFR) 2-positive cells; estrogen-dependent/aromatase-positive cells; estrogen-independent cells; estrogen-, progesterone- and human EGFR 2-negative cells) to anthocyanin-containing extracts and isolated anthocyanidins caused the cells to become apoptotic (Afaq et al. 2008; Chen et al. 2005; Hakimuddin et al. 2004; Kuo et al. 2004; Li and Jiang 2007; Li et al. 2009; Nguyen et al. 2010). An anthocyanin-containing extract obtained by litchi fruit pericarp affected the gene expression profile of breast cancer cells by up-regulation of 41 genes (1.22%) and down-regulation of 129 genes (3.84%), involved in various biological functions including apoptosis. Furthermore, the expressions of ADPRTL1 [ADP-ribosyltransferase (NAD+; poly (ADP-ribose) polymerase)-like 1] and CYP1A1 (cytochrome P450 1A1) increased and the expression of BIRC3 (baculoviral IAP repeat-containing 3″) decreased significantly, suggesting that the extract inhibited proliferation and induced apoptosis of breast cancer cells mainly through up-regulation of CYP1A1 and ADPRTL1, and down-regulation of BIRC genes (Li and Jiang 2007).

The proapoptotic effect of anthocyanins was widely investigated also in human leukemia cells. Most of the studies were performed on a human promyelocytic

Table 3.1 Apoptosis induction by anthocyanins in different transformed and cancer cell models

Cell line	Substance	Concentrations	Apoptosis biomarker and mechanism	References
Colon cancer cells				
Human adenocarcinoma Caco-2 cells	Cabernet Sauvignon anthocyanin extract	140 μM	Caspase-3 activity	Forester and Waterhouse (2010)
Human adenocarcinoma Caco-2 cells	Grape extract, anthocyanin fraction from grape extract	50–1,600 μg/ml	DNA fragmentation	Yi et al. (2005a)
Human adenocarcinoma Caco-2 cells	Anthocyanin fraction from blueberry extract	0–350 μg/ml	DNA fragmentation	Yi et al. (2005b)
Human HCT-116 cells	Delphinidin	30–240 μM	DNA fragmentation, procaspase-3, 8 and 9 cleavage, poly(ADP-ribose) polymerase cleavage, Bcl-2 and Bax expression, NFκB signaling	Yun et al. (2009)
Human adenocarcinoma HT-29 cells	Anthocyanin fraction from Georgia-grown blueberries	50–150 μg/ml	DNA fragmentation, caspase-3 activity	Srivastava et al. (2007)
Human adenocarcinoma HT-29 cells	Berry phenolic extracts	10–60 mg/ml	DNA fragmentation, Bax expression	Wu et al. (2007)
Human adenocarcinoma HT-29 cells	Strawberry extract, black raspberry extract	200 μg/ml	DNA fragmentation	Seeram et al. (2006)
Human adenocarcinoma HT-29 cells	Grape extract, anthocyanin fraction from grape extract	10–1,200 μg/ml	DNA fragmentation	Yi et al. (2005a)
Human adenocarcinoma HT-29 cells	Anthocyanin fraction from blueberry extract	0–900 μg/ml	DNA fragmentation	Yi et al. (2005b)
Gastric cancer cells				
Human adenocarcinoma AGS cells	Malvidin	50–200 μM	DNA content, cell morphology, caspase-3 activity, mitochondrial membrane potential, poly (ADP-ribose) polymerase cleavage, p38 mitogen-activated protein kinase expression, extracellular signal-regulated kinase expression	Shih et al. (2005)

(continued)

Table 3.1 (continued)

Cell line	Substance	Concentrations	Apoptosis biomarker and mechanism	References
Esophageal cancer cells				
Rat highly tumorigenic RE-149 DHD cells	Freeze-dried black raspberries	100 μg/ml	Caspase-3 and caspase-7 activity	Zikri et al. (2009)
Rat highly tumorigenic RE-149 DHD cells	Cyanidin-3-O-rutinoside	50 μg/ml	Caspase-3 and caspase-7 activity	Zikri et al. (2009)
Hepatic cancer cells				
Human hepatocellular carcinoma PLC/PRF/5 cells	Anthocyanins from the berries of *Pistacia lentiscus*	0.1–0.8 mg/ml	DNA fragmentation, Bcl-2 expression, Bax translocation, caspase-3 activity, cytochrome *c* release	Longo et al. (2008)
Human HepG2 cells	Extracts from *Graptopetalum paraguayense*	62.5–500 μg/ml	DNA content	Chen et al. (2008)
Human HepG2 cells	Cyanidin, delphinidin, malvidin	100 μM	DNA fragmentation, caspase-3 activity, c-Jun expression, c-Jun NH2-terminal kinase activation	Yeh and Yen (2005)
Leukemia cells				
Human promyelocytic HL-60 cells	Cyanidin-3-rutinoside	60 μM	Condensed or fragmented nuclei	Feng et al. (2010)
Human promyelocytic HL-60 cells	Delphinidin	20 μM	Condensed or fragmented nuclei	Feng et al. (2010)
Human promyelocytic HL-60 cells	Cyanidin-3-rutinoside	20, 40 and 80 μM	DNA fragmentation, caspase-3 and caspase-9 activity, cytochrome *c* and Smac release, activation of p38 mitogen-activated protein kinase and c-Jun NH2-terminal kinase, Bax and Bak expression, Bim_{EL} migration	Feng et al. (2007)
Human promyelocytic HL-60 cells	Isolated anthocyanins from *Euterpe oleracea* Mart.	0.17–10.7 μM	Caspase-3 activity	Del Pozo-Insfran et al. (2006)
Human promyelocytic HL-60 cells	Cyanidin 3-O-β-glucopyranoside	50–200 μg/ml	Phosphatydilserine exposure, Bcl-2 and c-Myc expression	Fimognari et al. (2004)

Human promyelocytic HL-60 cells	Delphinidin 3-sambubioside	75 and 100 μM	DNA fragmentation; caspase-3, caspase-8 and caspase-9 activity; mitochondrial membrane potential, cytochrome *c* release, Bid truncation	Hou et al. (2005)
Human promyelocytic HL-60 cells	Anthocyanins from *Hibiscus sabdariffa* extract	2 and 3 mg/ml	DNA fragmentation, DNA content, activation of p38 and c-Jun kinases, Das and FasL expression, caspase-3 and caspase-8 activity, Bid activation, cytochrome *c* release	Chang et al. (2005)
Human promyelocytic HL-60 cells	Bilberry extract, malvidin, delphinidin, cyanidin	4 mg/ml (bilberry extract), 200 μM (malvidin, delphinidin, cyanidin)	DNA fragmentation	Katsube et al. (2003)
Human acute leukemia T MOLT-4 cells	Cyanidin-3-rutinoside	20, 40 and 80 μM	DNA fragmentation	Feng et al. (2007)
Human acute leukemia T MOLT-4 cells	Delphinidin 3-*O*-β-D-glucoside, petunidin 3-*O*-β-D-glucoside, malvidin 3-*O*-β-D-glucoside, cyanidin 3-*O*-β-D-glucoside	0.2, 0.4, 0.8, 1 mM	DNA fragmentation, cell morphology	Katsuzaki et al. (2003)
Human Burkitt lymphoma Daudi cells	Cyanidin-3-rutinoside	20, 40 and 80 μM	DNA fragmentation	Feng et al. (2007)
Human T leukemia CCRF-CEM cells	Cyanidin-3-rutinoside	20, 40 and 80 μM	DNA fragmentation	Feng et al. (2007)
Human U937 cells	Anthocyanins isolated from *Vitis coignetiae*	5–55 μg/ml	Chromatin condensation; apoptotic bodies; DNA fragmentation; mitochondrial membrane potential; Bcl-2 and Bax expression; caspase-3, caspase-8 and caspase-9 activity; inhibitor of apoptosis protein (IAP) activity; poly(ADP-ribose) polymerase cleavage; truncated Bid translocation	Lee et al. (2009)

(continued)

Table 3.1 (continued)

Cell line	Substance	Concentrations	Apoptosis biomarker and mechanism	References
Human U937 cells	Cyanidin, malvidin	60 μM (cyanidin), 40 μM (malvidin)	DNA fragmentation, DNA content	Hyun and Chung (2004)
Human acute leukemia T Jurkat cells	Cyanidin 3-O-β-glucopyranoside	12.5–200 μg/ml	Phosphatydilserine exposure; p53, Bcl-2 and c-Myc expression	Fimognari et al. (2004)
Mammary cancer cells				
Hormone-responsive human MCF-7 cells	Bilberry extract	0.125, 0.25, 0.50 mg/ml	DNA fragmentation	Nguyen et al. (2010)
Rat mammary carcinoma cells from dimethylbenz[a]anthracene-induced tumors in female c-Ha-*ras* transgenic rats	Cyanidin 3-*O*-β-D-glucoside	0.25, 0.5 and 5 mM	DNA fragmentation, caspase-3 cleavage	Fukamachi et al. (2008)
Human estrogen dependent/aromatase positive MCF-7aro cells	Freeze-dried Jamun (*Eugenia jambolana*) fruit extract	100 and 200 μg/ml	DNA fragmentation	Li et al. (2009)
Human estrogen independent/aromatase positive MDA-MB-231 cells	Freeze-dried Jamun (*Eugenia jambolana*) fruit extract	100 and 200 μg/ml	DNA fragmentation	Li et al. (2009)
Human EGFR positive AU-565 cells	Delphinidin	5–40 μM	DNA fragmentation, phosphatydilserine exposure, poly(ADP-ribose) polymerase cleavage, Bax and Bcl-2 expression, caspase-3 activity	Afaq et al. (2008)
Human HS578T cells	Cyanidin 3-glucoside, peonidin 3-glucoside	10 and 30 μM (cyanidin 3-glucoside), 30 and 50 μM (peonidin 3-glucoside)	Cell morphology, caspase-3 activity, poly(ADP-ribose) polymerase cleavage, DNA content	Chen et al. (2005)

Prostate cancer cells				
Androgen refractory human PCa 22Rnu1 cells	Delphinidin	30, 60 and 90 μM	Poly(ADP-ribose) polymerase cleavage; Bax and Bcl-2 expression; caspase-3 and caspase-9 activity, NFκB signaling	Hafeez et al. (2008b)
Human PC3 cells	Delphinidin	60, 120 and 180 μM	Phosphatydilserine exposure, poly(ADP-ribose) polymerase cleavage, Bax and Bcl-2 expression, caspase-3 and caspase-9 activity, NFκB signaling	Hafeez et al. (2008a)
Human androgen-dependent LNCaP cells	Anthocyanin fraction from potatoes	5 and 10 μg/ml	DNA fragmentation, poly(ADP-ribose) polymerase cleavage, cleaved caspase-3 and cleaved caspase-9 proteins, Bax expression, nuclear apoptosis-inducing factor and endonuclease G protein levels, activation of kinases and endoplasmic reticulum stress	Reddivari et al. (2007)
Human androgen-independent PC-3 cells	Anthocyanin fraction from potatoes	5 and 10 μg/ml	DNA fragmentation, Bax expression, nuclear apoptosis-inducing factor and endonuclease G protein levels, activation of kinases and endoplasmic reticulum stress	Reddivari et al. (2007)
Uterus cancer cells				
Human HeLa S3 cells	Delphinidin	100, 150 and 200 μM	Cell morphology, DNA fragmentation, phosphatydilserine exposure, mitochondrial membrane potential, poly(ADP-ribose) polymerase cleavage	Lazzè et al. (2004)

leukemia cell line (HL-60), where different anthocyanins or anthocyanidins and anthocyanin-containing extracts were tested for their proapoptotic potential (Chang et al. 2005; Del Pozo-Insfran et al. 2006; Fimognari et al. 2004; Hou et al. 2003, 2005; Katsube et al. 2003; Yi et al. 2005a). HL-60 is a tumorigenic promyelocytic cell line that consists predominantly of promyelocytes and can be induced to terminally differentiate toward granulocytes and/or macrophages. Differentiated cells contain amounts of survival-maintaining molecules lower than their immature progenitors, whose great immaturity is likely to account for their resistance to apoptosis (Pae et al. 2001). For cyanidin 3-*O*-β-glucopyranoside (the main anthocyanin present in the juice of pigmented oranges), the induction of apoptosis represented an event only partly dependent on cytodifferentiation. In fact, after 8 h of exposure (a time-point where no cytodifferentiation was recorded) to cyanidin 3-*O*-β-glucopyranoside, an increase in the apoptotic cell fraction was observed (Fimognari et al. 2004). Of note, HL-60 cells harbor defective p53 (Iwamoto et al. 1996). This suggests a p53-independent effect of cyanidin 3-*O*-β-glucopyranoside in this cell system. However, the analysis of p53 protein level in another leukemia cell line (Jurkat, a T lymphoblastoid cell line) showed that the induction of apoptosis by cyanidin 3-*O*-β-glucopyranoside was associated with a significant change in p53 levels. An alteration in the levels of p53 protein can be directly responsible for the death signal delivered by cyanidin 3-*O*-β-glucopyranoside and explain the less sensitivity of HL-60 cells to the effects of cyanidin 3-*O*-β-glucopyranoside than Jurkat cells (Fimognari et al. 2004).

Other molecular mechanisms were demonstrated to be involved in the proapoptotic activity of anthocyanins on HL-60 cells. Anthocyanins extracted from *Hibiscus sabdariffa* Linn. markedly increased phosphorylation in p38 and c-Jun, cytochrome c release, and expression of tBid, Fas, and FasL (Fas ligand). The use of different inhibitors [SB203580 as p38 inhibitor, PD98059 as MEK (MAP kinase or ERK kinase) inhibitor, SP600125 as JNK (Jun N-terminal Kinase) inhibitor, and wortmannin as phosphatidylinositol 3-kinase inhibitor] showed that only SB203580 had strong potential in inhibiting HL-60 cell apoptosis and related protein expression and phosphorylation. The apoptosis induced by hibiscus anthocyanins is therefore mediated via the p38-FasL and Bid pathway (Chang et al. 2005).

Human glyoxalase I was identified as a new target involved in the proapoptotic activity of delphinidin (a major anthocyanidin present in many pigmented fruits and vegetables) in HL-60 cells (Takasawa et al. 2010). Glyoxalase I is the rate-limiting enzyme for detoxification of methylglyoxal, one of the side-product of glycolysis. Methylglyoxal is highly reactive with DNA and proteins, and thereby induces apoptosis (Thornalley et al. 1996). Delphinidin possessed strong inhibitory activity of the human glyoxalase I activity and suppressed the growth of HL-60 cells in a dose- and time-dependent manner. In contrast, cyanidin and pelargonidin that had less inhibitory effects on the enzyme had little suppressive effects on the cell growth. Furthermore, delphinidin induced apoptosis. The kinetics of delphinidin-induced apoptosis was slow. This can suggest that the onset of apoptosis by delphinidin treatment was the consequence of the accumulation of methylglyoxal by glyoxalase I inhibition. However, further studies should be performed to investigate whether delphinidin actually enters the cells, inhibits glyoxalase and induces the accumulation of methylglyoxal cells (Takasawa et al. 2010).

Finally, different berry extracts and two cyanidins (delphinidin and cyanidin) were able to induce apoptosit on colon cancer cell lines (Katsube et al. 2003; Lazzè et al. 2004; Seeram et al. 2006; Shin et al. 2009; Srivastava et al. 2007; Wu et al. 2007; Yi et al. 2005a, b; Yun et al. 2009). Considering the increasing evidence suggesting an association between cancer and COX-2 (Marnett and Dubois 2002), a COX-2 expressing colon cancer cell line (HT-29) was also used. Black raspberry and strawberry extracts showed the most significant pro-apoptotic effects against this cell line (Seeram et al. 2006). The pro-apoptotit marker Bax was increased 1.3-fold in cloudberry- and bilberry-treated cells, whereas the prosurvival marker Bcl-2 was detected only in untreated cells (Wu et al. 2007).

Taken together, these results show that anthocyanins induce apoptosis through the modulation of both intrinsic (mitochondrial) and extrinsic (FAS) pathways (Chang et al. 2005; Kuo et al. 2004; Reddivari et al. 2007). Treatment of cancer cells with anthocyanins resulted in a loss of mitochondrial membrane potential, cytochrome *c* release and modulation of caspase-dependent anti- and pro-apoptotic proteins, such as downregulation of Bcl-2 and increased expression of Bax (Afaq et al. 2008). In the extrinsic pathway, anthocyanins modulated the expression of FAS and FasL (Chang et al. 2005).

The role of reactive oxygen species (ROS) in the induction of apoptosis by anthocyanins is still controversial. Two studies reported that treatment of cancer cells, but not normal cells, with extracted and purified anthocyanins leads to an accumulation of ROS and subsequent apoptosis. Treatment with antioxidants such as N-acetyl-L-cysteine and catalase effectively blocked anthocyanin-induced ROS generation, caspase-3 activity, and DNA fragmentation, suggesting that the ROS-mediated mitochondrial-dependent pathway is important for anthocyanin-induced apoptosis (Feng et al. 2007; Hou et al. 2005).

However, numerous studies reported a positive correlation between fruit or vegetable pigment content and antioxidant capacities (Abuja et al. 1998; Moyer et al. 2002; Wang and Jiao 2000). For example, purified anthocyanin extracts from crude blackberry suppressed peroxyil radical-initiated Caco-2 intracellular oxidation in a concentration-dependent manner and prior exposure of Caco-2 cells to anthocyanin extract suppressed the peroxydil radical-induced apoptosis (Elisia and Kitts 2008). Structural variations in anthocyanins seem to influence antioxidant activities (Stintzing et al. 2002; Wang et al. 1997). Furthermore, the bioactivities of anthocyanins are pH-dependent. This is due to different ratios of flavylium cation, hemiketal and quinoidal bases at different pH values (Stintzing and Carle 2004). This means that variations in the pH value of cell culture medium could modify the biological activity of anthocyanins.

Another possibility could be related to the phenolic nature of anthocyanins. Isolated anthocyanins are prone to oxidation/decomposition when purified and taken out of the matrix of the whole fruit/juice. More research is needed in order to completely elucidate whether prooxidant action or antioxidant action mediate the anticancer and apoptosis-inducing properties of anthocyanins.

Some studies suggested a potential selective effect of anthocyanins towards tumor cells. Although cyanidin 3-*O*-β-glucopyranoside induced apoptosis in both transformed (Jurkat cells) and non-transformed (human lymphocytes) T cells, normal T cells were much less sensitive to this effect than transformed cells. A significant induction of apoptosis was detected in Jurkat cells even at the concentration 12.5 μg/ml of cyanidin 3-*O*-β-glucopyranoside. In normal T cells, 100 μg/ml of anthocyanin were required to trigger a significant increase in apoptosis. Moreover, the highest amount of apoptosis induced in Jurkat cells was substantially greater than that recorded in normal lymphocytes (4.4- vs. 1.7-fold increases vs. controls). The behavior of cyanidin 3-*O*-β-glucopyranoside on transformed and non-transformed T cells is, therefore, quantitatively different (Fimognari et al. 2005).

More recent studies demonstrated selective effects of extracts containing anthocyanins and isolated anthocyanins on human hepatoma cells, breast and esophageal cancer cells (Li et al. 2009; Shin et al. 2009; Yeh and Yen 2005; Zikri et al. 2009). A standardized *Eugenia jambolana* Lam. fruit extract exhibited pro-apoptotic effects against estrogen-dependent/aromatase positive (MCF-7aro) breast cancer cells and estrogen-independent (MDA-MB-231) breast cancer cells, but not toward the normal/non-tumorigenic (MCF-10A) breast cells (Li et al. 2009). Furthermore, an ethanol extract of freeze-dried black raspberries and two component anthocyanins (cyanidin-3-O-glucoside and cyanidin-3-O-rutinoside) selectively caused significant induction of apoptosis in a highly tumorigenic rat esophageal epithelial cell line (RE-149 DHD) but not in a weakly tumorigenic rat esophageal epithelial cell line (RE-149). The uptake of anthocyanins into RE-149 DHD cells far exceeded their uptake into RE-149 cells, which may have accounted for their selective effects on apoptosis of RE-149 DHD cells (Zikri et al. 2009).

As above reported, anthocyanidins are able to induce apoptosis through the inhibition of human glyoxalase I (Takasawa et al. 2010), an enzyme known to be highly expressed in the most tumor cells and little in normal cells. Abnormal expression or higher activity of glyoxalase I was reported in many human tumors including colon, prostate and lung (Davidson et al. 1999; Ranganathan and Tew 1993). This mechanism could further support a selective activity of anthocyanins for cancer cell.

Of note, gut metabolites of anthocyanins, such as gallic acid, 3-O-methylgallic acid and 2,4,6-trihydroxybenzaldehyde, exhibited cytotoxic effects at a wide range of concentrations in colon cancer cells. The results from these treatments were compared with results from a Cabernet Sauvignon anthocyanin grape extract. It is notable that these compounds were more effective than the anthocyanin extract. This evidence supports the hypothesis that metabolites are responsible for the biological activities of anthocyanin consumption (Forester and Waterhouse 2010).

In addition, these same metabolites degraded quickly in growth media (Forester and Waterhouse 2010). A reduction in cell population may be associated with oxidative reactions caused by treatment compounds, resulting in a cytotoxic effect by hydrogen peroxide production and subsequent hydroxyl radical formation. The instability of gallic acid in growth media was shown and linked to the production of hydrogen peroxide (Kern et al. 2007).

3.3.1.2 Inhibition of Apoptosis

UVB radiation proves to be one of the most important etiological factors in premature skin aging and especially skin photocarcinogenesis. Increased production of ROS and oxidative stress condition are known to play a central role in initiating and driving the signaling events that lead to cellular response following UV irradiation (Halliday 2005). Anthocyanins from black soybean [Glycine max (L.) Merr] seed coats reduced UVB-induced ROS levels and inhibited UVB-induced apoptotic cell death through the prevention of caspase-3 pathway activation and reduction of proapoptotic Bax protein levels (Tsoyi et al. 2008). A photoprotective activity was also recorded for a standardized extract from red orange, obtained from three red orange varieties. In human keratinocytes, the red orange extract efficiently counteracted some events implicated in UVB-induced inflammation and apoptosis such as NF-kB and AP-1 translocation and procaspase-3 cleavage (Cimino et al. 2007).

Also isolated anthocyanins and anthocyanidins are endowed with a photochemopreventive activity. Pretreatment of human keratinocytes with delphinidin or cyanidin-3-O-glucoside protected against UVB-mediated decrease in cell viability and induction of apoptosis and inhibited in poly(ADP-ribose) polymerase cleavage, activation of caspases, Bax increase, upregulation of Bid and Bak, and downregulation of Bcl-xL (Afaq et al. 2007; Cimino et al. 2006).

3.3.2 *In Vivo Studies on Animals*

3.3.2.1 Induction of Apoptosis

The induction of apoptosis by anthocyanins was confirmed in different *in vivo* preclinical setting. The effects of anthocyanins on apoptosis induction on animal models are reported in Table 3.2. Some berry extracts prevented esophageal tumors in rats. Rats were divided in three groups, consuming diets containing (1) 5% whole black raspberries; (2) an anthocyanin-rich fraction; (3) an organic solvent-soluble extract. Each treatment contained approximately 3.8 μmol anthocyanins/g diet. Animals were fed diets 2 weeks before treatment with N-nitrosomethylbenzylamine and throughout the study. N-nitrosomethylbenzylamine is one of the most potent organ-specific carcinogens routinely used in rat esophageal tumorigenesis. Animals were killed at week 30, and esophageal tumors were enumerated. The anthocyanin treatments were about equally effective in reducing N-nitrosomethylbenzylamine tumorigenesis in the esophagus. Diet groups 1 and 2 both induced apoptosis in both preneoplastic and papillomatous esophageal tissues (Wang et al. 2009).

A single anthocyanidin, delphinidin, significantly inhibited tumor growth in a xenograft mouse model originated by implanting of human prostate cancer PC3 cells in athymic nude mice. PC3 cells were selected as a model system because of

Table 3.2 Apoptosis induction by anthocyanins in different animal models

Animal model	Substance	Doses	Apoptosis biomarker and mechanism	References
Breast, 7,12-dimethylbenz[a] anthracene-treated rats	Purple corn seed extract	0.01, 0.1 and 1 (% diet)	DNA fragmentation, caspase-3 cleavage	Fukamachi et al. (2008)
Eesophagus, N-nitrosomethylbenzylamine-treated rats	Freeze-dried black raspberry powder/extract	Not reported	DNA fragmentation	Wang et al. (2009)
Skin, UVB-treated mice	Delphinidin	1 mg topical	DNA fragmentation	Afaq et al. (2007)
Xenograft, PC3 human prostate carcinoma cells in mice	Delphinidin	2 mg intraperitoneal, three times/week	Bcl-2 and Bax expression	Hafeez et al. (2008a)

their highly aggressive proliferative nature. The primary mode of delphinidin-mediated inhibition of tumor growth was through the induction of apoptosis, governed primarily by the activation of caspases. The analysis of the expression levels of Bax and Bcl-2 in tumors excised from both delphinidin-treated and untreated groups of animals demonstrated a decrease in the expression level of Bcl-2 protein. Inversely, a significant increase in the expression level of Bax was observed in tumor tissues of animals treated with delphinidin (Hafeez et al. 2008a). These observations suggest the involvement of an intrinsic apoptotic pathway by which delphinidin inhibits tumor growth in athymic nude mice.

An anthocyanin containing extract of purple corn seeds was studied for its ability to modulate 7,12-dimethylbenz[*a*]anthracene-induced mammary carcinogenesis in human c-Ha-*ras* proto-oncogene transgenic (Hras128) rats and in their non-transgenic counterpart's rats. The extract inhibited 7,12-dimethylbenz[*a*]anthracene-induced mammary carcinogenesis in both animal models. It significantly decreased the incidence of middle-sized (0.5–2.0 g) mammary tumors in transgenic rats and induced a not statistically significant decrease in the number of large-sized (>2.0 g) mammary tumors. On the other hand, the number and incidence of smaller-sized (<0.5 g) mammary tumors were not suppressed by the extract. This indicates that the extract was not able to inhibit the emergence of mammary tumors in transgenic rats. At the molecular level, the extract treatment resulted in a preferential activation of caspase-3 and reduction of Ras protein levels in tumor cells (Fukamachi et al. 2008).

3.3.2.2 Inhibition of Apoptosis

UVB irradiation-induced apoptotic cell death was inhibited by topical application of both anthocyanins and anthocyanidins. In hairless mice, UVB increased the fraction of apoptotic cells in the epidermis, which was inhibited by topical application of anthocyanins from black soybean seed coats or delphinidin (Afaq et al. 2007; Tsoyi et al. 2008). Cleaved caspase-3 and Bax proapoptotic protein levels were increased in UVB-treated mice skin, which were decreased by treatment of anthocyanins. UVB-mediated decrease of Bcl-2 antiapoptotic protein level was also recovered (Tsoyi et al. 2008).

3.4 Conclusions

Anthocyanins and anthocyanidins, predominantly in the form of mixtures, have been shown to exhibit anti-carcinogenic activity against multiple cancer cell types *in vitro* and tumor types *in vivo* through the induction of apoptosis. Anthocyanins have been shown to stimulate apoptosis and modulate different oncogenic signaling events *in vitro* in the 5–240 μM (Prior and Wu 2006) concentration range. These amounts far exceed the amounts observed in human plasma *in vivo*. The apparent bioavailability of anthocyanins is indeed consistently very low across animal species including humans with often less than 0.1% of the ingested dose appearing in the urine (Thomasset et al. 2009).

For example, Frank and coworkers (2003) compared pharmacokinetic parameters and bioavailability of several dietary anthocyanins following consumption of red grape juice in nine healthy volunteers. They were given a single oral dose of 283.5 mg total anthocyanins and the relative bioavailability of cyanidine-3-glucoside was calculated to be 65.7%. Moreover, it was demonstrated that, after the ingestion of 153 mg of anthocyanins, only 0.020–0.050% of the oral doses was excreted in the urine (Netzel et al. 2001). However, more recent studies indicated that the C_{max} in plasma of anthocyanins following a meal is in the range of 1 nM to <1 μM (Prior and Wu 2006). Thus, it is unclear whether the concentrations *in vivo* are sufficient to elicit anti-carcinogenic effects in humans.

Furthermore, much of the detail is missing about how anthocyanins are absorbed, how the variation of molecular structures consumed in food and the forms generated *in vivo* contribute to the health benefits. Anthocyanidins released locally from their glycosides could mediate, at least in part, the efficacy of anthocyanins. Formation of anthocyanidins from anthocyanins has indeed been demonstrated in the biomatrix *in vivo*, even if at miniscule concentrations (Thomasset et al. 2009). Therefore, it is possible, but not likely, that the anthocyanidins mediate the pharmacological effects of their parent glycosides.

It is also important to note that many studies have used the aglycone of the anthocyanin. However, anthocyanidins are chemical instable. In cell culture medium, delphinidin and cyanidin break down with half-lives of less than 30 min; the half-lives of pelargonidin and peonidin is approximately an hour (Kern et al. 2007). Furthermore, anthocyanidins generate hydrogen peroxide in cellular incubations. This indicates that their proapoptotic activity *in vitro* may well be the combined effect of a complicated mixture. The stability of anthocyanidins in plasma and tissues has not been clearly defined, except that they break down rapidly in the presence of intestinal microflora (Fleschhut et al. 2006).

Anthocyanins are chemically more stable than anthocyanidins, as demonstrated under conditions of neutral pH (Fleschhut et al. 2006). The sugar moiety indeed prevents or delays their degradation. In human plasma cyanidin- and delphinidin-3-glucosides are stable for 4 h at room temperature (Giordano et al. 2007).

Thus, interpretation and extrapolation of results from studies using relatively high concentrations and the aglycone form of anthocyanins need to be carefully interpreted.

In conclusion, anthocyanins may play an important role in health promotion in terms of anti-cancer effects. They modulate different events, involved in both the initiation and the late stages of carcinogenetic process. However, although experimental studies have clearly demonstrated the anti-cancer activity of anthocyanins, epidemiological studies have not revealed protective effects of anthocyanin consumption on cancer risk in humans (Wang and Stoner 2008). Much remains to be done with *in vivo* studies in animal models and human clinical trials for a thorough understanding of their overall biological effects and their optimal use in the chemoprevention of human cancer.

References

Abuja PM, Murkovic M, Pfannhauser W (1998) Antioxidant and prooxidant activities of elderberry (Sambucus nigra) extract in low-density lipoprotein oxidation. J Agric Food Chem 46:4091–4096

Afaq F, Syed DN, Malik A, Hadi N, Sarfaraz S, Kweon MH, Khan N, Zaid MA, Mukhtar H (2007) Delphinidin, an anthocyanidin in pigmented fruits and vegetables, protects human HaCaT keratinocytes and mouse skin against UVB-mediated oxidative stress and apoptosis. J Invest Dermatol 127:222–232

Afaq F, Zaman N, Khan N, Syed DN, Sarfaraz S, Zaid MA, Mukhtar H (2008) Inhibition of epidermal growth factor receptor signaling pathway by delphinidin, an anthocyanidin in pigmented fruits and vegetables. Int J Cancer 123:1508–1515

Chang YC, Huang HP, Hsu JD, Yang SF, Wang CJ (2005) Hibiscus anthocyanins rich extract-induced apoptotic cell death in human promyelocytic leukemia cells. Toxicol Appl Pharmacol 205:201–212

Chen PN, Chu SC, Chiou HL, Chiang CL, Yang SF, Hsieh YS (2005) Cyanidin 3-glucoside and peonidin 3-glucoside inhibit tumor cell growth and induce apoptosis in vitro and suppress tumor growth in vivo. Nutr Cancer 53:232–243

Chen SJ, Chung JG, Chung YC, Chou ST (2008) In vitro antioxidant and antiproliferative activity of the stem extracts from Graptopetalum paraguayense. Am J Chin Med 36:369–383

Cimino F, Ambra R, Canali R, Saija A, Virgili F (2006) Effect of cyanidin-3-O-glucoside on UVB-induced response in human keratinocytes. J Agric Food Chem 54:4041–4047

Cimino F, Cristiani M, Saija A, Bonina FP, Virgili F (2007) Protective effects of a red orange extract on UVB-induced damage in human keratinocytes. Biofactors 30:129–138

Davidson SD, Cherry JP, Choudhury MS, Tazaki H, Mallouh C, Konno S (1999) Glyoxalase I activity in human prostate cancer: a potential marker and importance in chemotherapy. J Urol 161:690–691

Del Pozo-Insfran D, Percival SS, Talcott ST (2006) Açai (Euterpe oleracea Mart.) polyphenolics in their glycoside and aglycone forms induce apoptosis of HL-60 leukemia cells. J Agric Food Chem 54:1222–1229

Elisia I, Kitts DD (2008) Anthocyanins inhibit peroxyl radical-induced apoptosis in Caco-2 cells. Mol Cell Biochem 312:139–145

Feng R, Ni HM, Wang SY, Tourkova IL, Shurin MR, Harada H, Yin XM (2007) Cyanidin-3-rutinoside, a natural polyphenol antioxidant, selectively kills leukemic cells by induction of oxidative stress. J Biol Chem 282:13468–13476

Feng R, Wang SY, Shi YH, Fan J, Yin XM (2010) Delphinidin induces necrosis in hepatocellular carcinoma cells in the presence of 3-methyladenine, an autophagy inhibitor. J Agric Food Chem 58:3957–3964

Fimognari C, Berti F, Cantelli-Forti G, Hrelia P (2001) Effect of cyanidin 3-*O*-β-glucopyranoside on micronucleus induction in cultured human lymphocytes by four different mutagens. Environ Mol Mutagen 43:45–52

Fimognari C, Berti F, Nüsse M, Cantelli-Forti G, Hrelia P (2004) Induction of apoptosis in two human leukemia cell lines as well as differentiation in human promyelocytic cells by cyanidin-3-O-beta-glucopyranoside. Biochem Pharmacol 67:2047–2056

Fimognari C, Berti F, Nüsse M, Cantelli-Forti G, Hrelia P (2005) In vitro antitumor activity of cyanidin-3-*O*-β-glucopyranoside. Chemotherapy 51:332–335

Fleschhut JKF, Rechkemmer G, Kulling SE (2006) Stability and biotransformation of various dietary anthocyanins in vitro. Eur J Nutr 45:7–18

Forester SC, Waterhouse AL (2010) Gut metabolites of anthocyanins, gallic acid, 3-O-methylgallic acid, and 2,4,6-trihydroxybenzaldehyde, inhibit cell proliferation of Caco-2 cells. J Agric Food Chem 58:5320–5327

Frank T, Netzel M, Strass G, Bitsch R, Bitsch I (2003) Bioavailability of anthocyanidin-3-glucosides following consumption of red wine and red grape juice. Can J Physiol Pharmacol 81:423–435

Fukamachi K, Imada T, Ohshima Y, Xu J, Tsuda H (2008) Purple corn color suppresses Ras protein level and inhibits 7,12-dimethylbenz[a]anthracene-induced mammary carcinogenesis in the rat. Cancer Sci 99:1841–1846

Gasiorowski K, Brokos B, Kulma A, Ogorzałek A, Skórkowska K (2001) Impact of four antimutagens on apoptosis in genotoxically damaged lymphocytes in vitro. Cell Mol Biol Lett 6:649–675

Giordano LCW, Rapisarda P, Donati MB, Rotilio D (2007) Development and validation of an LC-MS/MS analysis for simultaneous determination of delphinidin-3-glucoside, cyanidin-3-glucoside and cyanidin-3-(6-malonylglucoside) in human plasma and urine after blood orange juice administration. J Sep Sci 30:3127–3136

Hafeez BB, Siddiqui IA, Asim M, Malik A, Afaq F, Adhami VM, Saleem M, Din M, Mukhtar H (2008a) A dietary anthocyanidin delphinidin induces apoptosis of human prostate cancer PC3 cells in vitro and in vivo: involvement of nuclear factor-kappaB signaling. Cancer Res 68:8564–8572

Hafeez BB, Asim M, Siddiqui IA, Adhami VM, Murtaza I, Mukhtar H (2008b) Delphinidin, a dietary anthocyanidin in pigmented fruits and vegetables: a new weapon to blunt prostate cancer growth. Cell Cycle 7:3320–3326

Hakimuddin F, Paliyath G, Meckling K (2004) Selective cytotoxicity of a red grape wine flavonoid fraction against MCF-7 cells. Breast Cancer Res Treat 85:65–79

Halliday GM (2005) Inflammation, gene mutation and photoimmunosuppression in response to UVR-induced oxidative damage contributes to photocarcinogenesis. Mutat Res 571:107–120

Harborne JB, Grayer RJ (1988) The anthocyanins. In: Harborne JB (ed) The flavonoids. Chapman and Hall, London

Hertog MG, Hollman PC, Katan MB, Kromhout D (1993) Intake of potentially anticarcinogenic flavonoids and their determinants in adults in the Netherlands. Nutr Cancer 20:21–29

Hou DX, Ose T, Lin S, Harazoro K, Imamura I, Kubo M, Uto T, Terahara N, Yoshimoto M, Fujii M (2003) Anthocyanidins induce apoptosis in human promyelocytic leukemia cells: structure-activity relationship and mechanisms involved. Int J Oncol 23:705–712

Hou DX, Tong X, Terahara N, Luo D, Fujii M (2005) Delphinidin 3-sambubioside, a Hibiscus anthocyanin, induces apoptosis in human leukemia cells through reactive oxygen species-mediated mitochondrial pathway. Arch Biochem Biophys 440:101–109

Hursting SD, Slaga TJ, Fischer SM, Di Giovanni J, Phang JM (1999) Mechanism-based cancer prevention approaches: targets, examples, and the use of transgenic mice. J Natl Cancer Inst 91:215–225

Hyun JW, Chung HS (2004) Cyanidin and Malvidin from Oryza sativa cv. Heugjinjubyeo mediate cytotoxicity against human monocytic leukemia cells by arrest of G(2)/M phase and induction of apoptosis. J Agric Food Chem 52:2213–2217

Iwamoto KS, Mizuno T, Ito T, Tsuyama N, Kyoizumi S, Seyama T (1996) Gain-of-function p53 mutations enhance alteration of the T-cell receptor following X-irradiation, independently of the cell cycle and cell survival. Cancer Res 56:3862–3865

Katsube N, Iwashita K, Tsushida T, Yamaki K, Kobori M (2003) Induction of apoptosis in cancer cells by Bilberry (Vaccinium myrtillus) and the anthocyanins. J Agric Food Chem 51:68–75

Katsuzaki H, Hibasami H, Ohwaki S, Ishikawa K, Imai K, Date K, Kimura Y, Komiya T (2003) Cyanidin 3-O-beta-D-glucoside isolated from skin of black Glycine max and other anthocyanins isolated from skin of red grape induce apoptosis in human lymphoid leukemia Molt 4B cells. Oncol Rep 10:297–300

Kern M, Fridrich D, Reichert J, Skrbek S, Nussher A, Hofem S (2007) Limited stability in cell culture medium and hydrogen peroxide formation affect the growth inhibitory properties of delphinidin and its degradation product gallic acid. Mol Nutr Food Res 51:1163–1172

Kuo PL, Hsu YL, Lin TC, Lin LT, Lin CC (2004) Induction of apoptosis in human breast adenocarcinoma MCF-7 cells by prodelphinidin B-2 3,3′-di-O-gallate from Myrica rubra via Fas-mediated pathway. J Pharm Pharmacol 56:1399–1406

Lazzè MC, Savio M, Pizzala R, Cazzalini O, Perucca P, Scovassi AI, Stivala LA, Bianchi L (2004) Anthocyanins induce cell cycle perturbations and apoptosis in different human cell lines. Carcinogenesis 25:1427–1433

Lee SH, Park SM, Park SM, Park JH, Shin DY, Kim GY, Ryu CH, Shin SC, Jung JM, Kang HS, Lee WS, Choi YH (2009) Induction of apoptosis in human leukemia U937 cells by anthocyanins through down-regulation of Bcl-2 and activation of caspases. Int J Oncol 34:1077–1083

Li J, Jiang Y (2007) Litchi flavonoids: isolation, identification and biological activity. Molecules 12:745–758

Li L, Adams LS, Chen S, Killian C, Ahmed A, Seeram NP (2009) Eugenia jambolana Lam. berry extract inhibits growth and induces apoptosis of human breast cancer but not non-tumorigenic breast cells. J Agric Food Chem 57:826–831

Longo L, Platini F, Scardino A, Alabiso O, Vasapollo G, Tessitore L (2008) Autophagy inhibition enhances anthocyanin-induced apoptosis in hepatocellular carcinoma. Mol Cancer Ther 7:2476–2485

Marnett LJ, Dubois RN (2002) COX-2: a target for colon cancer prevention. Annu Rev Pharmacol Toxicol 42:55–80

Mazza G (1995) Anthocyanins in grapes and grape products. Crit Rev Food Sci Nutr 35:341–371

Moyer RA, Hummer KE, Finn CE, Frei B, Wrolstad RE (2002) Anthocyanins, phenolics, and antioxidant capacity in diverse small fruits: vaccinium, rubus, and ribes. J Agric Food Chem 50:519–525

Netzel M, Strass G, Janssen M, Bitsch I, Bitsch R (2001) Bioactive anthocyanins detected in human urine after ingestion of blackcurrant juice. J Environ Pathol Toxicol Oncol 20:89–95

Nguyen V, Tang J, Oroudjev E, Lee CJ, Marasigan C, Wilson L, Ayoub G (2010) Cytotoxic effects of bilberry extract on MCF7-GFP-tubulin breast cancer cells. J Med Food 13:278–285

Pae HO, Seo WG, Kim NY, Oh GS, Kim GE, Kim YH, Kwak HJ, Yun YG, Jun CD, Chung HT (2001) Induction of granulocytic differentiation in acute promyelocytic leukemia cells (HL-60) by water-soluble chitosan oligomer. Leuk Res 25:339–346

Prior RL, Wu X (2006) Anthocyanins: structural characteristics that result in unique metabolic patterns and biological activities. Free Radic Res 40:1014–1028

Ranganathan S, Tew KD (1993) Analysis of glyoxalase-I from normal and tumor tissue. Biochim Biophys Acta 1182:311–316

Reddivari L, Vanamala J, Chintharlapalli S, Safe SH, Miller JC Jr (2007) Anthocyanin fraction from potato extracts is cytotoxic to prostate cancer cells through activation of caspase-dependent and caspase-independent pathways. Carcinogenesis 28:2227–2235

Seeram NP, Adams LS, Zhang Y, Lee R, Sand D, Scheuller HS, Heber D (2006) Blackberry, black raspberry, blueberry, cranberry, red raspberry, and strawberry extracts inhibit growth and stimulate apoptosis of human cancer cells in vitro. J Agric Food Chem 54:9329–9339

Shih PH, Yeh CT, Yen GC (2005) Effects of anthocyanidin on the inhibition of proliferation and induction of apoptosis in human gastric adenocarcinoma cells. Food Chem Toxicol 43:1557–1566

Shin DY, Ryu CH, Lee WS, Kim DC, Kim SH, Hah YS, Lee SJ, Shin SC, Kang HS, Choi YH (2009) Induction of apoptosis and inhibition of invasion in human hepatoma cells by anthocyanins from meoru. Ann N Y Acad Sci 1171:137–148

Srivastava A, Akoh CC, Fischer J, Krewer G (2007) Effect of anthocyanin fractions from selected cultivars of Georgia-grown blueberries on apoptosis and phase II enzymes. J Agric Food Chem 55:3180–3185

Stintzing FC, Carle R (2004) Functional properties of anthocyanins and betalains in plants, food, and in human nutrition. Trends Food Sci Technol 15:19–38

Stintzing FC, Stintzing AS, Carle R, Frei B, Wrolstad RE (2002) Color and antioxidant properties of cyanidin-based anthocyanin pigments. J Agric Food Chem 50:6172–6181

Takasawa R, Saeki K, Tao A, Yoshimori A, Uchiro H, Fujiwara M, Tanuma SI (2010) Delphinidin, a dietary anthocyanidin in berry fruits, inhibits human glyoxalase I. Bioorg Med Chem 18:7029–7033

Thomasset S, Teller N, Cai H, Marko D, Berry DP, Steward WP, Gescher AJ (2009) Do anthocyanins and anthocyanidins, cancer chemopreventive pigments in the diet, merit development as potential drugs? Cancer Chemother Pharmacol 64:201–211

Thornalley PJ, Edwards LG, Kang Y, Wyatt C, Davies N, Ladan MJ, Double J (1996) Antitumour activity of S-p-bromobenzylglutathione cyclopentyl diester *in vitro* and *in vivo*: inhibition of glyoxalase I and induction of apoptosis. Biochem Pharmacol 51:1365–1372

Tsoyi K, Park HB, Kim YM, Chung JI, Shin SC, Shim HJ, Lee WS, Seo HG, Lee JH, Chang KC, Kim HJ (2008) Protective effect of anthocyanins from black soybean seed coats on UVB-induced apoptotic cell death in vitro and in vivo. J Agric Food Chem 56:10600–10605

Wang SY, Jiao H (2000) Scavenging capacity of berry crops on superoxide radicals, hydrogen peroxide, hydroxyl radicals, and singlet oxygen. J Agric Food Chem 48:5677–5684

Wang LS, Stoner GD (2008) Anthocyanins and their role in cancer prevention. Cancer Lett 269:281–290

Wang H, Cao G, Prior RL (1997) Oxygen radical absorbing capacity of anthocyanins. J Agric Food Chem 45:304–309

Wang LS, Hecht SS, Carmella SG, Yu N, Larue B, Henry C, McIntyre C, Rocha C, Lechner JF, Stoner GD (2009) Anthocyanins in black raspberries prevent esophageal tumors in rats. Cancer Prev Res (Phila Pa) 2:84–93

Wu QK, Koponen JM, Mykkänen HM, Törrönen AR (2007) Berry phenolic extracts modulate the expression of p21(WAF1) and Bax but not Bcl-2 in HT-29 colon cancer cells. J Agric Food Chem 55:1156–1163

Yeh CT, Yen GC (2005) Induction of apoptosis by the Anthocyanidins through regulation of Bcl-2 gene and activation of c-Jun N-terminal kinase cascade in hepatoma cells. J Agric Food Chem 53:1740–1749

Yi W, Fischer J, Akoh CC (2005a) Study of anticancer activities of muscadine grape phenolics in vitro. J Agric Food Chem 53:8804–8812

Yi W, Fischer J, Krewer G, Akoh CC (2005b) Phenolic compounds from blueberries can inhibit colon cancer cell proliferation and induce apoptosis. J Agric Food Chem 53:7320–7329

Yun JM, Afaq F, Khan N, Mukhtar H (2009) Delphinidin, an anthocyanidin in pigmented fruits and vegetables, induces apoptosis and cell cycle arrest in human colon cancer HCT116 cells. Mol Carcinog 48:260–270

Zikri NN, Riedl KM, Wang LS, Lechner J, Schwartz SJ, Stoner GD (2009) Black raspberry components inhibit proliferation, induce apoptosis, and modulate gene expression in rat esophageal epithelial cells. Nutr Cancer 61:816–826

Chapter 4
Anti-proliferative and Apoptosis-Inducing Properties of Xanthohumol, a Prenylated Chalcone from Hops (*Humulus lupulus* L.)

Julia Strathmann and Clarissa Gerhauser

Abstract Xanthohumol (XN) is a prenylated chalcone found at high concentrations in hop cones (*Humulus lupulus* L.). XN has been characterized as a promising cancer chemopreventive lead structure that acts *via* a broad spectrum of bioactivities. This chapter summarizes the anti-proliferative and apoptosis-inducing potential of XN and gives a detailed overview of underlying mechanisms and pathways targeted by XN to induced programmed cell death. XN is a potent inhibitor of NF-κB and inhibits activation of the death-receptor pathway by tumor necrosis factor (TNF). In various cell lines, XN treatment results in an immediate transient increase in mitochondria-derived reactive oxygen species (ROS) that is considered as the initial trigger of apoptosis induction *via* the intrinsic pathway by breakdown of the mitochondrial membrane potential, release of cytochrome *c* and activation of the caspase cascade. Oxidative stress may also contribute to the activation of endoplasmatic reticulum (ER) stress and unfolded protein response recently identified as a novel mechanisms underlying XN-mediated apoptosis induction.

Abbreviations

AML	acute myelocytic leukemia
A-SMase	acid sphingomyelinase
ATF	activating transcription factor

J. Strathmann
Division Epigenomics and Cancer Risk Factors, German Cancer Research Center, Heidelberg, Germany

Current address: German Center for Neurodegenerative Diseases (DZNE), Munich

Department of Biochemistry, Adolf-Butenandt-Institute, Munich, Germany

C. Gerhauser (✉)
Division Epigenomics and Cancer Risk Factors, German Cancer Research Center, Heidelberg, Germany
e-mail: c.gerhauser@dkfz.de

M. Diederich and K. Noworyta (eds.), *Natural Compounds as Inducers of Cell Death: Volume 1*, DOI 10.1007/978-94-007-4575-9_4,

ATP	adenosine triphosphate
BiP	immunoglobulin-heavy-chain binding protein
BPH	benign prostate hyperplasia
CHOP	CAAT/enhancer-binding protein (C/EBP) homologous protein
CLL	chronic lymphocytic leukemia
Cox	cyclooxygenase
CYP	cytochrome P450
DC	dendritic cells
DCF-DA	dichlorofluorescein-diacetate
DHE	dihydroethidium
DISC	death-inducing signaling complex
DMBA	dimethylbenz-*[a]*-anthracene
DMSO	dimethylsulfoxide
DR	death receptor
ER	endoplasmatic reticulum
FADD	Fas-associated death domain
FITC	fluorescein isothiocyanate
Gadd153	growth arrest and DNA damage 153
GRP78	glucose-regulated protein 78
GSH	glutathione
H_2O_2	hydrogen peroxide
HUVEC	human umbilical vein endothelial cells
IC_{50}	half-maximal inhibitory concentration
IKK	I-κB kinase
IL	interleukin
Ire1α	inositol-requiring 1α
LDH	lactate dehydrogenase
MMP	matrix metalloprotease
MnTMPyP	manganese(III) tetrakis(1-methyl-4-pyridyl)porphyrin
MTT	3-(4,5-dimethyl thiazol-2-yl)-2,5-diphenyl tetrazoliumbromide
NAC	N-acetyl cysteine
NAD(P)H	nicotinamide adenine dinucleotide phosphate
NF-κB	nuclear factor κB
$O_2^{-\bullet}$	superoxide anion radicals
$OH^{\bullet}$	hydroxyl radicals
PARP	poly(ADP-ribose)polymerase
PERK	double stranded RNA-dependent protein kinase (PKR)-like ER kinase
RIP	receptor interacting kinase
ROS	reactive oxygen species
SCID	severe combined immuno-deficient
SM	sphingomyelin
SOD	superoxide dismutase
SRB	sulforhodamine B

TNF	tumor necrosis factor
TNF-R1	TNF-receptor 1
TRAF	TNF receptor-associated factor
TRAIL	TNF-related apoptosis-inducing ligand
Trb3	Tribble homolog 3
TUNEL	TdT-mediated dUTP-biotin nick end labeling
UPR	unfolded protein response
XBP1	X-box-binding protein 1
XN	Xanthohumol
Ψ_m	mitochondrial membrane potential
ρ^0	rho zero

4.1 Introduction

Evading apoptosis has been recognized as one of the hallmarks of cancer cells (Hanahan and Weinberg 2000). Consequently, the induction of apoptosis by cancer chemotherapeutic or chemopreventive agents is one of the key mechanisms to effectively kill cancer cells and thus prevent or inhibit tumor growth. Anti-proliferative action has been demonstrated for a large number of natural compounds in human cancer cell lines as well as in *in vivo* models of carcinogenesis. One of these natural compounds is xanthohumol (XN, 2′,4,4′-trihydroxy-3′-prenyl-6′-methoxychalcone, Fig. 4.1), a prenylated chalcone found in hops (*Humulus lupulus* L.).

Prenylated hop flavonoids are secreted together with bitter acids and essential oils by lupulin glands of the female hops inflorescences (hop cones). Since lupulin glands do not express the enzyme necessary for the conversion of chalcones to flavanones, they exclusively produce chalcone type flavonoids with XN as the most abundant one (82–89% of the total amount of prenylated flavonoids in European hop varieties) (Stevens et al. 1997).

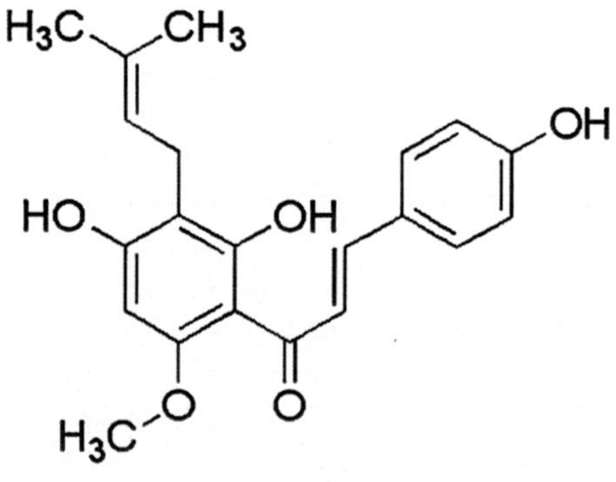

Fig. 4.1 Chemical structure of xanthohumol (2′,4,4′-trihydroxy-3′-prenyl-6′-methoxychalcone)

4.2 Xanthohumol as a Cancer Chemopreventive Lead Structure

Interest in the cancer chemopreventive potential of hops components started in the late 1990s, when prenylated flavonoids from hops were first described to modulate carcinogen metabolism *in vitro* (Henderson et al. 2000; Miranda et al. 2000a) and to possess antioxidant (Miranda et al. 2000b), anti-proliferative and cytotoxic activity (Miranda et al. 1999). Subsequently, we identified XN as a broad spectrum cancer chemopreventive agent able to interfere with the initiation, promotion and progression phase of carcinogenesis (Gerhauser et al. 2002). Several recent reviews have comprehensively summarized the cancer preventive and health promoting activities of XN and other hops components (Gerhauser et al. 2002; Stevens and Page 2004; Gerhauser 2005; Zanoli and Zavatti 2008; Magalhaes et al. 2009; Chadwick et al. 2006; Strathmann et al. 2009; Botta et al. 2005). Therefore, we will present here only a short overview of XN-mediated chemopreventive activities to emphasize that anti-proliferative and apoptosis-inducing properties, although the focus of this chapter, are not the sole or most important biological activities of this interesting lead structure.

During the initiation step of carcinogenesis, XN modulates xenobiotic metabolism by inhibiting the phase I enzyme cytochrome P450 (CYP) 1A and monofunctionally inducing phase II enzymes, such as NAD(P)H: quinone oxidoreductase and intracellular glutathione levels (GSH), leading to reduced metabolic activation and increased detoxification of xenobiotics and carcinogens (Henderson et al. 2000; Gerhauser et al. 2002). Antioxidant and radical scavenging properties can also contribute to the inhibition of tumor initiation by XN (Gerhauser et al. 2002; reviewed in Gerhauser 2005; Strathmann et al. 2009). XN inhibits cyclooxygenases (Cox)-1 and -2 activities as well as the production of nitric oxide (Gerhauser et al. 2002). These anti-inflammatory properties may contribute to the inhibition of tumor promotion. XN also acts as an anti-inflammatory agent by inhibition of nuclear factor κB (NF-κB) signaling and subsequent downregulation of pro-inflammatory key factors (Albini et al. 2006; Colgate et al. 2007; Dell'Eva et al. 2007; Harikumar et al. 2009). Estrogen-mediated tumor promotion may be prevented by anti-estrogenic effects of XN that were demonstrated *in vitro* by the inhibition of estrogen-mediated alkaline phosphatase activation in human endometrial cancer cells (Gerhauser et al. 2002; Guerreiro et al. 2007). XN also inhibits the enzyme aromatase (CYP19), which plays a crucial role in the conversion of testosterone to estrogen (Strathmann et al. 2009; Monteiro et al. 2006). In the progression phase, XN affects cell proliferation by induction of cell differentiation (Gerhauser et al. 2002) and apoptosis (as outlined below). In addition, XN may inhibit tumor progression by inhibition of angiogenesis. This was demonstrated in a human *in vitro* anti-angiogenesis model using fragments of human placenta, by downregulation of pro-angiogenic signaling, and by inhibition of endothelia cell migration and vessel formation using human microendothelial cells (Gerhauser 2005). *In vivo*, inhibition of angiogenesis was demonstrated in human breast cancer xenografts in a skinfold chamber model (Klenke 2008), and with a matrigel sponge angiogenesis assay as described by Albini et al. (2006). These activities contribute to the inhibitory effects of XN during malignant progression of tumorigenesis. Breast cancer chemopreventive potential of XN was first indicated by inhibition of 7,12-dimethylbenz-*[a]*-anthracene (DMBA)-induced preneoplastic lesions in a mammary mouse organ culture model at low nM concentrations (Gerhauser et al. 2002). Recently, we have demonstrated that XN also possess breast cancer preventive efficacy in the DMBA-induced rat mammary carcinogenesis model. Application of XN at a dose of 100 mg/kg bodyweight/day significantly inhibited tumor latency, tumor multiplicity ($p<0.05$) and tumor weight ($p=0.07$) when applied during the initiation and promotion phase of carcinogenesis (Strathmann et al. in preparation).

4.3 Cell-Growth Inhibitory Potential of Xanthohumol

The first indication of anti-proliferative potential of XN was reported by Miranda et al. (1999). Since then, more than 25 studies have investigated XN in anti-proliferation and cytotoxicity assays using ovarian, breast, endometrial, cervical, prostate, colon, liver, and lung cancer, as well as leukemia, myeloma, sarcoma and melanoma cell lines, macrophages, adipocytes, dendritic cells and T-cells (summary in Table 1 in the Annex). Early studies investigated anti-proliferative activity based on [^{3}H]-thymidine incorporation, sulforhodamin B (SRB) or crystal violet staining, lactate dehydrogenase (LDH) release, MTT (3-(4,5-dimethyl thiazol-2-yl)-2, 5-diphenyl tetrazoliumbromide) reduction, calcein hydrolysis, trypan blue exclusion and cell counting, and determined halfmaximal inhibitory concentrations (IC_{50} values) of cell viability in the range of 0.5–25 μM, depending on cell line and incubation times. Cell growth inhibition by XN is apparently not cancer site or organ specific, at least not in *in vitro* studies. Interestingly however, XN more potently reduced cell growth of HT-1080 sarcoma cell under hypoxic conditions than under normoxic conditions (Goto et al. 2005). Also, data by Monteiro et al. suggest that XN-mediated inhibition of breast cancer cell growth may be partly related to a reduction of estrogen levels by aromatase inhibition (Monteiro et al. 2007). Importantly, primary hepatocytes were more resistant to the anti-proliferative effects of XN than liver cancer cells (Ho et al. 2008; Dorn et al. 2010a, b).

4.4 Mechanisms of Apoptosis Induction by Xanthohumol

Generally, apoptosis can be induced by two major pathways: the extrinsic, death receptor-mediated and the intrinsic, mitochondria-mediated pathway (Jin and El-Deiry 2005). In addition, apoptosis can be triggered by endoplasmatic reticulum (ER) stress and unfolded protein response (Faitova et al. 2006; Heath-Engel et al. 2008). There is accumulating evidence that XN targets all three pathways.

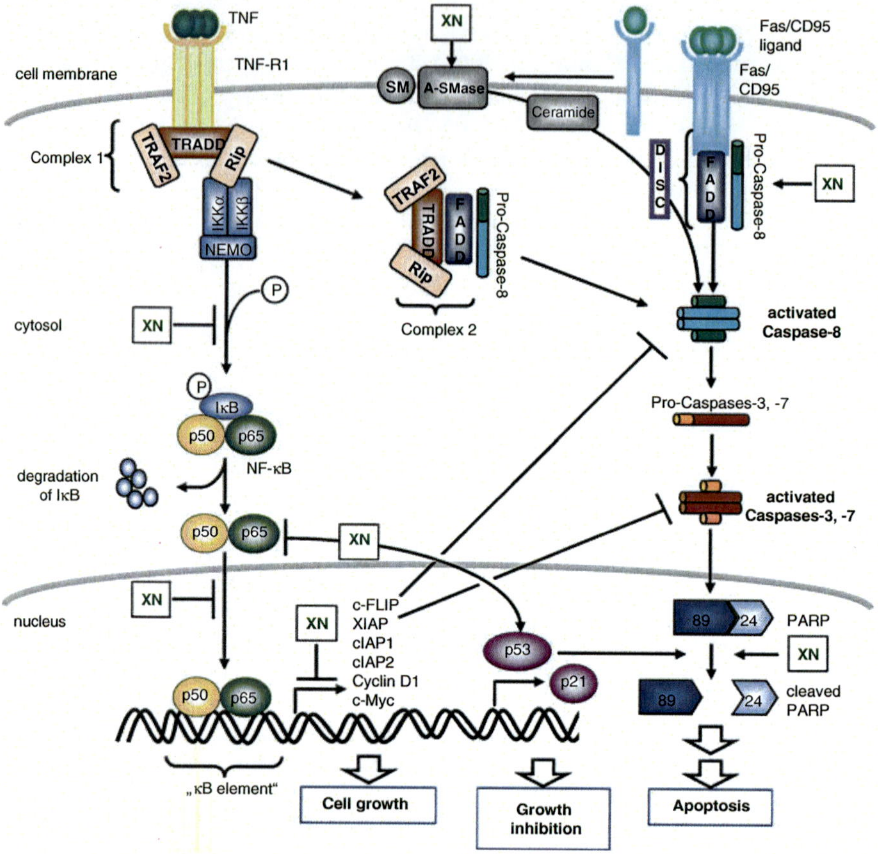

Fig. 4.2 Induction of apoptosis via the death receptor pathway, and the influence of XN on these mechanisms (see text for description)

4.4.1 *Death Receptor Pathway, TNF and NF-κB*

Death receptors of the TNF (tumor-necrosis factor) receptor superfamily such as TNF receptor 1 (TNF-R1), CD95 (APO-1/Fas), and TNF-related apoptosis-inducing ligand (TRAIL) receptors DR4 and DR5 play an important role in the extrinsic pathway of apoptosis induction. As an example, activation of the CD95/Fas by the CD95/Fas ligand results in receptor aggregation and recruitment of the adaptor molecule FADD (Fas-Associated Death Domain) and initiator caspase-8 (Fig. 4.2, right). Consequently, caspase-8 becomes activated and initiates apoptosis by cleavage of downstream effector caspases. Caspases are synthesized as inactive pro-caspases and act in a caspase cascade to initiate apoptosis. Initiator caspases are characterized by longer pro-domains that mediate the assembly of activating complexes, such as the death-inducing signalling complex (DISC), resulting in the transduction of death signals. The major effector caspases-3, -6 and -7 execute apoptosis by cleavage of key cellular proteins that cause the typical morphological changes observed in cells undergoing apoptosis, including apoptotic and structural proteins, cell cycle proteins and proteins belonging to the cellular DNA repair machinery (summary in Jin and El-Deiry 2005). Cleavage of the DNA repair-associated enzyme poly(ADP-ribose)polymerase (PARP) is accepted as a prominent marker of apoptosis.

Activation of sphingomyelinases such as the acid sphingomyelinase (A-SMase) results in the formation of ceramide from sphingomyelin (SM). Ceramide is acting as a second messenger involved in regulating various cellular functions including proliferation and apoptosis (Carpinteiro et al. 2008). Activation of death receptors has been shown to activate A-SMase, enhancing ceramide production, which in turn facilitates death receptor clustering, DISC formation and caspase-8 activation (Grassme et al. 2003).

TNF is a multifunctional pro-inflammatory protein that activates the NF-κB pathway through binding to TNF-receptors (Fig. 4.2, left). After TNF-binding, the adaptor protein TRADD is recruited to the activated TNF-R1 and serves as a platform for binding of TNF receptor-associated factor (TRAF) 2 and the receptor interacting kinase (RIP), forming complex 1. TNF activates NF-κB through phosphorylation and subsequent ubiquitin-mediated degradation of its inhibitor I-κB by I-κB kinase (IKK), which is recruited to the TNF-R1 complex through TRAF2 and stabilized by RIP. Degradation of I-κB liberates NF-κB and allows nuclear translocation, where it interacts with the κB element. In a second step after formation of the TNF-R1 complex 1, TRAF2 and RIP interact with FADD and pro-caspase 8, forming complex 2 that results in activation of caspase-8 and the caspase cascade.

Different from Fas and TRAIL signalling, TNF does not induce apoptosis spontaneously, since activation of NF-κB mediates a strong pro-survival mechanism. NF-κB is involved in the regulation of gene expression of about 200 genes involved in inflammation, development, cell growth, and inhibition of apoptosis (Ak and Levine 2010). Consequently, the cell-death inducing capacity of TNF is only apparent when NF-κB activation is blocked. Ak and Levine have recently postulated that NF-κB and p53 have mutually exclusive functions: inactivation of NF-κB enhances the stability of p53, which then contributes to cell growth inhibition and apoptosis induction (Ak and Levine 2010).

In 2005, we were first to describe that XN induced apoptosis in the HCT-116 derived colon cancer cell line 40–16 *via* the extrinsic apoptotic pathway (Pan et al. 2005). XN treatment led to cleavage and activation of the initiator caspase-8 in a dose-and time-dependent manner. Consequently, XN also activated downstream effector caspases-3 and -7 and PARP cleavage as a marker of apoptosis induction. Several other groups subsequently demonstrated similar activation of the caspase cascade, PARP cleavage and apoptosis induction by XN in breast cancer cell lines and patient-derived B-cell lymphocytic leukemia (B-CLL) cells (Vanhoecke et al. 2005; Lust et al. 2005) (Table 1 in the Annex). Interestingly, Xuan et al. recently identified a role of A-SMase-derived ceramide in XN-mediated apoptosis induction in dendritic cells (DC) (Xuan et al. 2010).

Unlike in DC from wildtype mice, in DC from A-SMase knockout mice, XN was unable to activate caspase-8 and -3 and to stimulate PARP cleavage and DNA fragmentation, underlining the importance of A-SMase activity for XN-mediated apoptosis induction in DC.

An influence of XN on NF-κB signaling was first described by Albini et al. in 2006. The authors investigated anti-angiogenic modes of action of XN. Treatment of human umbilical vein endothelial cells (HUVEC) with TNF for 15 min resulted in nuclear translocation of NF-κB, which was completely blocked by pretreatment with 10 μM XN. This was attributed to the inhibition I-κB phosphorylation by XN. In addition to blocking TNF-induced NF-κB activation, XN inhibited the constitutive activity of NF-κB in BPH-1 prostate epithelial cells, but not in the PC-3 prostate cancer cell line. Effects in BPH-1 cells were not associated with inhibition of NF-κB nuclear translocation. Still, caspases were activated, and XN treatment resulted in cell growth inhibition and cell death (Colgate et al. 2007). In MM6 and U937 leukemia cells stimulated with TNF, inhibition of NF-κB activation by XN led to downregulation of matrix metalloproteases (MMP) expression and reduced invasive potential. Also, XN reduced proliferation of MM6 and U937 leukemia cells and primary samples from acute myelocytic leukemia (AML) patients (Dell'Eva et al. 2007). Anti-leukemic efficacy of XN was further confirmed in the myeloid leukemia cell line K562 positive for the tyrosine kinase Bcr-Abl. Bcr-Abl activates several signaling pathways including Akt and NF-κB. XN treatment reduced cell viability and led to apoptosis induction. Also, cell invasion was reduced. Both effects were attributed to suppression of NF-κB activation as well as IκB and IKK expression. Levels of the anti-apoptotic protein survivin, which is induced by Bcr-Abl, and of Bcr-Abl itself were reduced by XN, whereas expression of p53 and its effector p21 were elevated (Monteghirfo et al. 2008). Most of these XN-mediated effects on cell proliferation, apoptosis induction, Bcr-Abl expression, and NF-κB activation were mediated by increased oxidative stress after XN treatment, and were prevented by pretreatment with the antioxidant N-acetyl cysteine (NAC)(see also below). In a more mechanistic study in leukemia cell lines, Harikumar et al. confirmed that XN induced apoptosis by affecting NF-κB signaling. XN treatment blocked constitutive NF-κB activity and NF-κB activation by TNF, prevented nuclear translocation of the NF-κB p65 subunit to the nucleus, suppressed NF-κB-regulated proliferative (cyclin D1, c-Myc) as well as anti-apoptotic gene products (Bcl-xL, XIAP, cIAP1, cIAP2), thus promoting apoptosis. The authors postulate that XN may directly interact with cysteine residues of IκB kinase (IKK) and the p65 subunit of NF-κB through its unsaturated ketone moiety (Harikumar et al. 2009). Inhibition of NF-κB activation by XN and increased caspases 3 activity was also involved in apoptosis induction in hepatic stellate cells and Huh7 human liver cancer cells (Dorn et al. 2010a, b). In a recent study, Szliszka et al. demonstrated that combined treatment with TRAIL and XN or a series of other chalcones enhanced the apoptosis inducing capacity of TRAIL in prostate cancer cells (Szliszka et al. 2010).

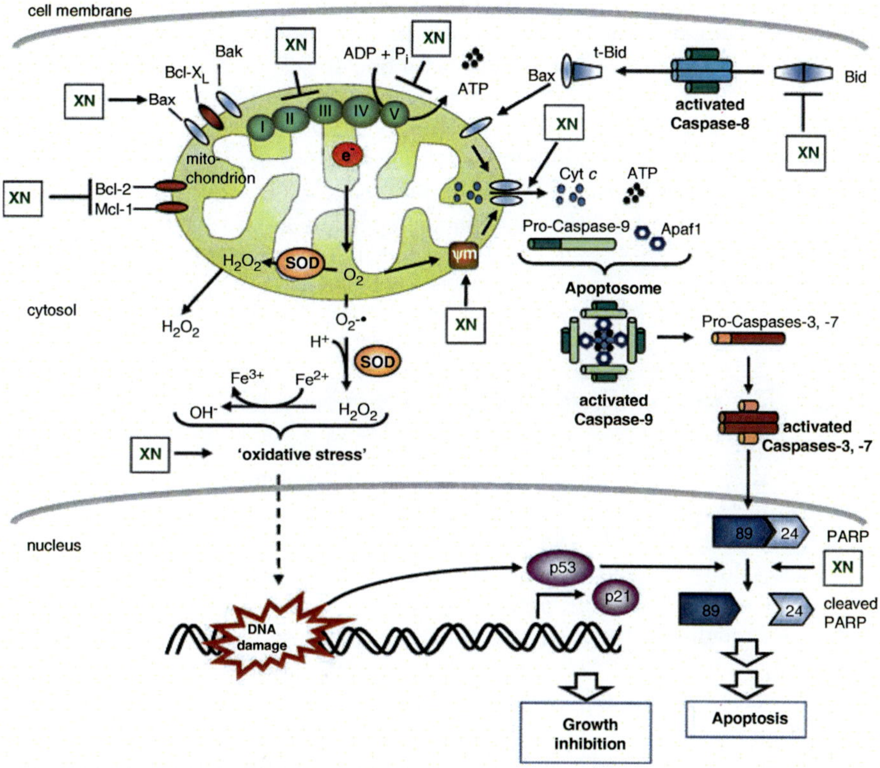

Fig. 4.3 Induction of apoptosis via the mitochondrial pathway, including the role of reactive oxygen species (*ROS*). Mechanisms targeted by XN are indicated (see text for description)

4.4.2 Mitochondria-Mediated Apoptosis Induction

The intrinsic mitochondrial pathway of apoptosis induction is initiated by Bcl-2 family proteins, which regulate the passage of small molecules like cytochrome *c* through the mitochondrial permeability transition pore (Fig. 4.3). The Bcl-2 protein family includes anti-apoptotic (e.g. Bcl-2, Bcl-xL, Bcl-w, Mcl-1) and pro-apoptotic proteins (e.g. Bax, Bak, Bad). The small BH3 domain-only protein Bid activates pro-apoptotic Bax after cleavage by caspase-8 and thus interconnects the death receptor- and the mitochondrial pathway. Intracellular stress signals trigger the translocation of Bax from the cytosol to the mitochondria, where it homodimerizes and contributes to the permeabilization of the mitochondrial membrane. Release of cytochrome *c* then activates assembly of the multiprotein complex Apoptosome, resulting in activation of pro-caspase-9 and the downstream effector caspase cascade (Jin and El-Deiry 2005).

Our study with 40–16 colon cancer cells indicated that XN not only activates the death receptor pathway, but also the intrinsic apoptosis pathway (Pan et al. 2005). XN decreased the expression of anti-apoptotic Bcl-2, leading to cleavage and subsequent activation of pro-caspase-9 and downstream effector caspases. Further, XN treatment induced p53 and pro-apoptotic Bax expression in BPH-1 prostate epithelial cells, whereas anti-apoptotic Bcl-2 was downregulated (Colgate et al. 2007). Lust et al. demonstrated induction of apoptosis by XN *via* the mitochondrial pathway in human chronic lymphocytic leukemia (CLL) cells. XN reduced the expression of Bcl-2, Mcl-1 and Bid, and induced caspase-9 and -3 activity (Lust et al. 2009).

4.4.3 The Role of Reactive Oxygen Species (ROS)

Recently, ROS have been identified as key redox regulators of cellular signaling cascades, metabolic processes and transcription factors. Numerous cellular pathways generate ROS, with hydrogen peroxide (H_2O_2), superoxide anion radicals ($O_2^{-\bullet}$) and hydroxyl radicals ($OH^{\bullet}$) being the most abundant ones (Kamata and Hirata 1999). In aerobic cells, mitochondria are believed to be the major source of ROS, since roughly 1–2% of all transported electrons escape oxidative phosphorylation and reduce O_2 to $O_2^{-\bullet}$ (Boveris and Chance 1973; Boveris and Cadenas 1975; Fruehauf and Meyskens 2007; Pani et al. 2009).

Acute high levels of ROS oxidize intracellular proteins, inactivate iron-sulfur complex-containing enzymes and damage cellular compartments, which ultimately trigger cells into apoptosis. For example, mitochondrial dysfunction has been shown to play a key role in the induction of apoptosis (Green and Reed 1998; Desagher and Martinou 2000). Impaired mitochondrial functions suppress mitochondrial metabolism, imbalance the mitochondrial membrane potential, block respiration and oxidative phosphorylation (Orrenius et al. 2007), finally leading to apoptosis induction (Simon et al. 2000). Interestingly, cells with an imbalanced redox homeostasis are apparently more susceptible to oxidative stress-induced apoptosis than normal cells. Therefore, induction of ROS might be very effective in eliminating cancer cells by disrupting mitochondrial functions and inducing apoptosis (Trachootham et al. 2009).

Despite its antioxidant activity (Gerhauser et al. 2002), several recent reports suggest that induction of apoptosis by XN is linked to the induction of ROS (Fig. 4.3). As a first indication, Yang et al. reported in 2007 that XN inhibited adipocyte differentiation and subsequently induced apoptosis in human preadipocytes *via* a ROS-mediated mechanism. Incubation of preadipocytes with XN resulted in a transient increase in 'oxidative stress', detected by dichlorofluorescein (DCF) fluorescence. This was accompanied by a rapid breakdown of the mitochondrial membrane potential and release of cytochrome *c* from the mitochondria to the cytosol, activation of caspase-3 and -7, PARP cleavage and apoptosis induction indicated by single stranded DNA. The role of ROS induction was confirmed by pre-treatment

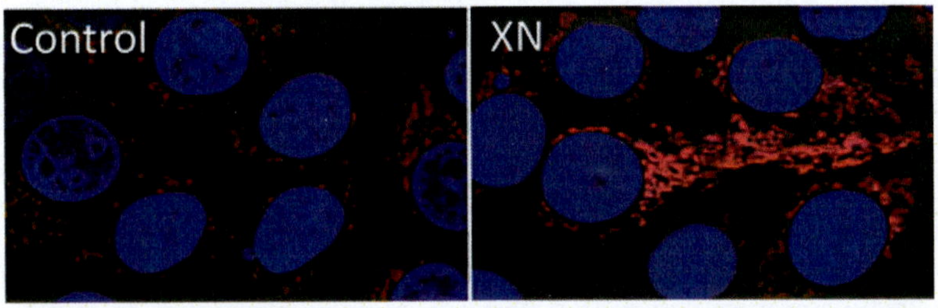

Fig. 4.4 Mitochondria are the source of XN-induced $O_2^{-\bullet}$. MCF-7 cells were loaded with MitoSOX Red and then incubated with 50 μM XN for 25 min. *Red* fluorescent staining of mitochondria indicates $O_2^{-\bullet}$ formation, blue staining depicts the position of nuclei. Pictures were acquired by confocal microscopy

with the antioxidants ascorbic acid and β-mercaptoethanol, which efficiently prevented XN-mediated apoptosis induction (Yang et al. 2007). As mentioned above, data by Monteghirfo et al. also suggested that apoptosis induction by XN in K562 leukemia cells was related to the induction of 'oxidative stress' detected with the fluorescent dye DCF diacetate (DA). XN-mediated effects, *i.e.* inhibition of NF-κB activation, reduced Bcr-Abl expression, inhibition of cell proliferation, and apoptosis induction were inhibited by co-exposure with the antioxidant NAC. The authors speculated that increased ROS levels might lead to DNA damage, which could activate p53 to establish an amplification loop (Monteghirfo et al. 2008).

Only recently, we could provide detailed information on the nature and source of ROS induced after XN treatment, and their link to apoptosis induction (Strathmann et al. 2010). We confirmed a rapid time- and dose-dependent increase in intracellular ROS formation detected by DCF-DA fluorescence in BPH-1 prostate epithelial cells by XN. DCF-DA is considered as a sensor for unspecific 'oxidative stress' rather than for a particular ROS (Halliwell and Whiteman 2004). By using the dye dihydroethidium (DHE), which is specifically oxidized by $O_2^{-\bullet}$ (Zhao et al. 2005), we could demonstrate that XN treatment resulted in enhanced $O_2^{-\bullet}$-generation. $O_2^{-\bullet}$ induction by XN was transient and significantly scavenged by co-treatment with the antioxidants ascorbic acid and NAC, as well as by pre-treatment with the superoxide dismutase (SOD) mimetic MnTMPyP (manganese(III) tetrakis(1-methyl-4-pyridyl) porphyrin). In BPH-1 cells loaded with MitoSOX Red specific for mitochondrial $O_2^{-\bullet}$, XN treatment caused a rapid increase in red fluorescent staining of mitochondria, suggesting that mitochondria are targeted by XN, leading to $O_2^{-\bullet}$-formation (Fig. 4.4). In contrast, XN treatment of BPH-1 ρ^0 (rho zero) cells (characterized by non-functional mitochondria) in the presence of DHE resulted in significantly lower DHE oxidation than in intact BPH-1 cells, further confirming the important role of mitochondria in $O_2^{-\bullet}$-generation induced by XN.

Blocking of mitochondrial respiration is believed to be one of the major sources of mitochondrial $O_2^{-\bullet}$ formation. When oxygen consumption was measured in isolated mouse liver mitochondria, XN treatment was as potent in blocking mitochondrial respiration as Antimycin A, a prominent inhibitor of Complex III of the respiratory chain. A more detailed analysis of XN-mediated effects on complexes of the respiratory chain indicated that XN nonspecifically inhibited Complexes I to III at high concentrations, blocked the electron flux from Complex I to Complexes II and III and caused a rapid depletion of ATP. These data supported the hypothesis that XN inhibits mitochondrial respiration. Consistently, XN caused a rapid breakdown of the mitochondrial membrane potential (Ψ_m), followed by the release of cytochrome *c* to the cytosol and induction of PARP cleavage in a time- and dose-dependent manner. Importantly, anti-proliferative as well as apoptosis-inducing effects of XN were significantly reduced by co-treatment with the SOD mimetic MnTMPyP. Overall, these data strongly suggest that XN-mediated $O_2^{-\bullet}$ formation is the initial trigger of XN-induced apoptosis (Strathmann et al. 2010).

4.4.4 ER Stress and Unfolded Protein Response

Besides the death receptor- and the mitochondria-mediated pathway of apoptosis induction, endoplasmatic reticulum (ER) stress and unfolded protein response (UPR) is another cellular program activating apoptosis cascades. Interestingly, ER stress is closely linked to oxidative stress. Protein folding itself is an oxidizing process that leads to the generation of ROS during oxidizing protein folding and the formation of disulfide bonds (Malhotra and Kaufman 2007). ROS can target ER-based calcium channels, stimulating the release of Ca^{2+} ions to the cytosol, which then accumulate in the inner matrix of mitochondria, disrupt the electron transport chain and stimulate the production of more ROS. Excessive ROS production and changes in cellular redox status then directly or indirectly affect protein folding and aggravate ER stress (Fig. 4.5).

The ER is the cellular site of protein biosynthesis, folding, assembly and modifications. It is composed of protein chaperones, proteins that catalyze folding and sensors for the detection of mis- or unfolded proteins. Also, it is a major calcium store and functions as a sensor to signals mediated by growth factors, hormones, changes in energy levels, nutrient availability and redox status (Zhang and Kaufman 2008). Alterations in cellular homeostasis that cause accumulation of unfolded proteins in the ER lumen by an imbalance between protein folding demand and protein folding capacity (referred to as ER stress) activate the unfolded protein response (UPR).

The UPR signaling cascades are activated by three ER membrane-localized sensor proteins: ATF6 (activating transcription factor 6), Ire1α (inositol-requiring 1α) and PERK (double stranded RNA-dependent protein kinase (PKR)-like ER kinase). Under non-stressed conditions, they are maintained in an inactive state through interaction of their luminal unfolded protein-sensing domain with the abundant ER chaperone BiP (immunoglobulin-heavy-chain binding protein, also known as glucose-regulated protein GRP78). ER stress causes release of BiP and activates PERK through homodimerization and *trans*-autophosphorylation.

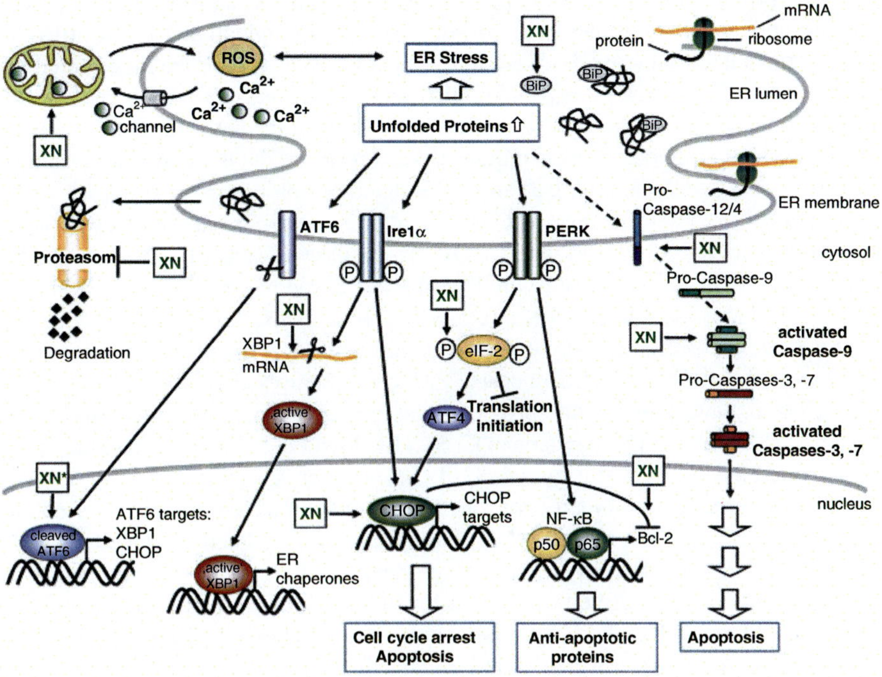

Fig. 4.5 Link between ER stress and unfolded protein response (*UPR*) and induction of apoptosis (Adapted from Faitova et al. 2006; Zhang and Kaufman 2008). Mechanisms targeted by XN in CLL cells are indicated (From Lust et al. 2009, *only in T47D cells used as control)

Activated PERK then phosphorylates the translation initiation factor eIF2α, thereby reducing the general frequency of mRNA translation initiation. On the other hand, specific mRNAs such as the basic leucine zipper domain (bZIP)-containing transcription factor ATF4 are preferentially translated and activate the transcription of UPR target genes involved in amino acid biosynthesis, antioxidative stress response and ER stress-induced apoptosis. PERK is also required for NF-κB activation which mainly up-regulates anti-apoptotic proteins (see above) and thus contributes to the balance between survival and cell death. In addition to PERK, ER stress activates autophosphorylation of Ire1α, which has protein kinase and site-specific endoribonuclease (RNase) activity. It initiates the removal of a 26 base intron from the mRNA of XBP1 (X-box-binding protein 1), resulting in the translation of 'active' XBP1 with potent transcription factor activity (Zhang and Kaufman 2008). As a third important factor, ER stress initiates the processing of ATF6 to release a functional fragment ('cleaved' ATF6) that acts as a transcription factor with similar functions as 'active' XBP1. These transcription factors stimulate the transcription of UPR target genes including ER chaperones and enzymes that promote protein folding, maturation, secretion and ER-associated protein degradation (Zhang and Kaufman 2008).

If the protein-folding defect is persisting and cannot be resolved, the UPR will initiate apoptosis to remove stressed cells. Apoptosis induction *via* ER-stress is mainly mediated by the bZIP transcription factor CHOP (CAAT/enhancer-binding protein (C/EBP) homologous protein, also known as Gadd153 (growth arrest and DNA damage 153). For maximal induction of CHOP, activation of all three ER-stress signalling pathways is required. Activation of CHOP target genes such as Gadd34, Trb3 (tribble homolog 3) and DR5 (death receptor 5) induces growth arrest and apoptosis. CHOP has also been implicated in repressing the transcription of anti-apoptotic Bcl-2. In addition to CHOP, pro-caspase-12 (probably represented by pro-caspase-4 in humans) associated with the ER membrane is involved in the induction of apoptosis during ER stress. The mechanisms of caspase 12 activation by ER stress are presently not clear. However, it activates processing and activation of caspase-9 and the downstream caspase cascade (Faitova et al. 2006).

Lust et al. have only recently provided first indication that XN induces apoptosis *via* an UPR-mediated mechanisms in CLL cells (Lust et al. 2009). The authors first demonstrated activation of caspases-3, -4, and -9 after XN treatment of CLL cells for 12 h and more prominently for 24 h. Next, they detected upregulation of the chaperone BiP (GRP78) at the mRNA and protein level. XN activated the ER stress sensor IRE1α, indicated by detection of the processed, shorter XBP1 mRNA. However, active XBP1 protein was not detectable by Western blotting. The authors concluded that either CLL cells do not translate the processed XPB1 transcript, or that levels were too low for detection by Western blotting. Cleaved ATF6 was also not unambiguously detectable by Western blotting in CLL cells, whereas XN treatment clearly induced the processing of ATF6 in T47D breast cancer cells used as a positive control. PERK activation was demonstrated by eIF2α phosphorylation, which was strongly enhanced by XN treatment already after 3 h of treatment. Also, CHOP protein levels were strongly induced by XN treatment for 12 and 24 h. The authors detected ROS by DCF-DA fluorescence microscopy. However, since the influence of co-treatment with antioxidants was not tested, it is unclear whether ROS induction is a cause or consequence of UPR. XN also inhibited protein degradation *via* the proteasome and caused an accumulation of ubiquitinated proteins. These data provide an interesting new insight into the apoptosis inducing capacity of XN in CLL cells. Further studies have to demonstrate whether these observation are also relevant for other cell types and *in vivo*.

4.5 Inhibition of Tumor Growth *In Vivo*

Only few studies so far have investigated the anti-proliferative and tumor growth inhibiting potential of XN in animal models. In the course of a study by our group (Gerhauser 2005; Klenke 2008), intravital microscopy was used to investigate the effect of XN on tumor angiogenesis and tumor growth *in vivo*. Human MX-1 breast tumor xenografts were implanted in dorsal skinfold chamber preparations in female

Severe Combined Immuno-Deficient (SCID) mice. Starting from day 15 after tumor implantation, animals were treated with XN applied subcutaneously at a dose of 1,000 mg/kg body weight per day or DMSO as solvent control, respectively, for 7 and 14 days. To assess tumor growth, the two-dimensional tumor surface was documented with digital photography using bright field microscopy. Functional vessel density was quantified by intravital fluorescence video microscopy after injection of FITC-labelled dextran. Application of XN for 7 and 14 days inhibited the growth of the breast tumor xenografts by 46% and 83%, respectively, in comparison with the solvent-treated control group, and reduced the size of established tumors by 30% and 56%, respectively. Concomitantly, XN-treatment for 14 days reduced tumor-induced neovascularization by 33% (Gerhauser 2005; Klenke 2008).

Albini et al. tested the effect of XN applied orally at a dose of 20 μM in drinking water on the growth of Karposi's sarcoma xenografts (Albini et al. 2006). KS-IMM cells mixed with matrigel were injected on the flanks of 7 week old *nu/nu* (CD-1) BR mice. XN application was started 4 days before cell injection. Twenty-four days after injection, the average tumor volume was significantly reduced by 70% by XN intervention. The average tumor weight was also significantly inhibited by about 45%. Inhibition of tumor growth was accompanied by a reduction of vascularisation and extensive areas of necrosis and fibrosis in comparison with control tumors (Albini et al. 2006).

In a third investigation, Monteiro et al. tested the effect of orally applied XN on the growth of MCF-7 breast cancer xenografts in male nude mice. XN was applied at a dose of 100 μM in 0.1% ethanol as drinking source for 60 days. In comparison with the solvent control, XN treatment non-significantly reduced average tumor weights. Morphologically, tumors from XN-treated animals showed large areas of necrosis, a decrease in the number of infiltrating inflammatory cells, and decreased NF-κB, phosphorylated IκB, and cytokine IL1β staining. XN treatment also reduced cell proliferation assessed by Ki67 staining from a diffuse pattern in control tumors to focal areas of proliferating cells, and doubled the number of TUNEL-positive cells as an indication of apoptosis induction. Consistent with previous studies, tumors of XN-treated animals presented significantly lower microvessel density than tumors of control mice. Also, expression of factor VIII as an endothelial marker was significantly reduced.

4.6 Summary and Conclusion

As outlined above, XN is a natural product with a broad spectrum of biological activities. There is consistent evidence from in vitro studies that XN inhibits cell proliferation by inhibition of DNA synthesis, induction of cell cycle arrest and induction of apoptosis. Apoptosis induction is observed in a wide panel of cell types and in cancer cells derived from a large spectrum of tumor sites. Primary cells appear to be less sensitive to the anti-proliferative activity of XN than transformed cells.

XN induces apoptosis by activation of the death receptor-mediated extrinsic as well as the mitochondria-mediated intrinsic pathway. Inhibition of TNF-mediated activation of NF-κB by XN has been associated with induction of apoptosis *via* the extrinsic pathway in various studies. In cell culture, XN treatment results in an immediate transient increase in $O_2^{-\bullet}$ generation by inhibition of the mitochondrial respiratory chain. This increase in oxidative stress is considered as the trigger of apoptosis induction. Recent evidence indicates that XN induces ER stress as an additional mechanism of apoptosis induction, which might also be activated by ROS production.

Only few studies so far have addressed the question of whether XN reduces tumor growth *in vivo*. Inhibition of mammary cancer and Karposi's sarcoma xenograft growth by XN has consistently been related to the inhibition of angiogenesis. There is limited evidence that induction of apoptosis also contributes to tumor growth inhibition. The mechanisms of apoptosis induction *in vivo* may involve prevention of TNF-induced NF-κB activity.

Annex

Table 1 Anti-proliferative and apoptosis-inducing potential of XN *in vitro*

Organ	Cell lines	Xanthohumol concentration	Treatment time	Effect	Reference
Ovary	A-2780	0.1–100 μM	48, 96 h	↓ proliferation	Miranda et al. (1999)
Ovary	SK-OV-3	not stated	48 h	↓ proliferation	Lee et al. (2007)
Breast	MCF7	0. 1–100 μM	48, 96 h	↓ proliferation	Miranda et al. (1999)
		0.01–100 μM	8, 24, 48 h	Cytotoxicity at 100 μM	
		0.1–100 μM	24–96 h	↓ DNA synthesis	
		10, 40, 100 μM	8, 24 h	↔ induction of apoptosis	
Breast	MDA-MB-435	3–50 μM	72 h	↓ proliferation	Gerhauser et al. (2002)
		3–50 μM	72 h	↓ DNA synthesis	
		5–50 μM	24 h	S-phase cell cycle arrest	
Breast	MCF-7; T47D	1–20 μM	8 days	↓ proliferation	Vanhoecke et al. (2005)
	MCF-7	10 μM	96 h	↑ nuclear condensation	
	T47D	5–25 μM	48 h	↑ PARP cleavage	
Breast	Sk-Br-3	0.005–25 μM	72 h	↓ proliferation	Monteiro et al. (2007)
		0.005–25 μM	72 h	↓ DNA synthesis	
		5 μM	24 h	↓ proliferation	
		5 μM	24 h	↑ apoptosis	
Breast	MCF-7	10 μM	24 h	↓ viable cells	Guerreiro et al. (2007)
		10 μM	24 h	↓ proliferation	
		10 μM	24 h	↓ apoptosis	
Breast	MCF7	0.1–100 μM	24, 72 h	↓ viable cells; ↑ cytotoxicity	Monteiro et al. (2008)
		0.1–100 μM	24, 72 h	↓ DNA synthesis	
		10 μM	24 h	↓ proliferation	
Endometrium	Ishikawa	1.6–50 μM	72 h	↓ proliferation	Gerhauser et al. (2002)
Cervix	HeLa	not stated	72 h	↓ proliferation	Vogel and Heilmann (2008) and Vogel et al. (2008, 2010)

(contiuned)

Table 1 (continued)

Organ	Cell lines	Xanthohumol concentration	Treatment time	Effect	Reference
Prostate	BPH-1[a]/PC-3	2.5–20 μM	48 h	↓ proliferation	Colgate et al. (2007)
		10, 20 μM	48 h	↑ cell death	
		10, 20 μM	48 h	↑ caspase activity	
	BPH-1	10, 20 μM	48 h	S-phase cell cycle arrest	
		10, 20 μM	48 h	↓ NF-κB activity	
				↑ p65 nuclear translocation	
		10, 20 μM	48 h	↑ expression of Bax, p53	
				↓ Bcl-2 expression	
Prostate	PC-3, DU145	100, 200 μM	2 h	↓ cell viability	Delmulle et al. (2008)
		200 μM	up to 2 h	↔ caspase 3 activation	
Prostate	LNCaP	20–50 μM + TRAIL	48 h	↑ cytotoxicity in combination with TRAIL	Szliszka et al. (2010)
		20, 50 μM + TRAIL		synergistic ↑ apoptosis no necrotic cell death	
Prostate	BPH-1	1.6–50 μM	72 h	↓ proliferation	Strathmann et al. (2010)
		1.6–50 μM	5–45 min	↑ ROS production	
		3.1–50 μM	10–30 min	↓ Ψ_m	
		6.3–50 μM	30 min-24 h	↑ cytochrome *c* release	
		10–40 μM	48 h	↑ PARP cleavage	
		10–40 μM	72 h	↑ apoptosis (sub-G_1 fraction)	
Colon	HT-29	0.01–100 μM	48, 96 h	Cytotoxicity at 100 μM	Miranda et al. (1999)
Colon	HCT116 cl. 40-16	0.5–10 μM 5-15 μM	72 h 24-72 h	↓ proliferation ↑ PARP cleavage	Pan et al. (2005)
		5–15 μM	24–72 h	↑ caspase-3, -7, -8, -9 cleavage	
		5–15 μM	24–72 h	↓ Bcl-2 expression	
Colon	HCT15	not stated	48 h	↓ proliferation	Lee et al. (2007)
Liver	Primary rat hepatocytes	0.1–100 μM	24 h	Cytotoxicity at 100 μM	Miranda et al. (1999)
Liver	Hepa1c1c7	0.4–25 μM	48 h	↓ proliferation	Gerhauser et al. (2002)

Liver	AML12[a]; HA22T/VGH; HEP3B	10–225 µM	24 h	↓ proliferation	Ho et al. (2008)
	HA22T/VGH; HEP3B	90, 135 µM	4 h	↑ apoptosis	
		90 µM	24 h	↑ nuclear condensation	
		45, 90, 135 µM	24 h	↑ DNA fragmentation	
Liver	HSC[b]	0–40 µM	6 h	↑ caspase-3 activity	Dorn et al. (2010a)
		5, 10, 20 µM	24 h	↑ apoptosis/necrosis	
		5–40 µM	24 h	↓ vitality	
		5 µM	2 h	↓ basal and TNF-induced NF-κB activity	
	PHH[a]	25, 50 µM	24 h	↔ vitality	
		25, 50 µM	24 h	↔ apoptosis/necrosis	
		25, 50 µM	24 h	↓ basal and palmitate-induced pro-inflammatory IL-8 mRNA expression	
Liver	HepG2, Huh7	10–100 µM	24 h	↓ proliferation	Dorn et al. (2010b)
		25 µM		↑ caspase-3 activity	
	Huh7	2.5 µM	3 h preinc.	↓ TNF-induced NF-κB activity and IL-8 mRNA expression	
	PHH	10–100 µM	24 h	no inhibition of cell viability	
Lung	A549	not stated	48 h	↓ proliferation	Lee et al. (2007)
Leukemia	HL-60	0.5–10 µM	72 h	↓ proliferation	Gerhauser et al. (2002)
Leukemia	Primary B-CLL cells	10, 25 µM	24, 48 h	↑ cell death/apoptosis	Lust et al. (2005)
		25 µM	24, 48 h	↑ PARP cleavage	
Leukemia	MM6, U937	2.5–10 µM	24–72 h	↓ proliferation	Dell'Eva et al. (2007)
	primary AML and CLL cells	2.5–10 µM	24–72 h	↑ cell death	
		5 µM	6 h	↓ TNF-induced NF-κB signaling	
Leukemia	K562	2.5–10 µM	24–72 h	↓ proliferation	Monteghirfo et al. (2008)

(continued)

Table 1 (continued)

Organ	Cell lines	Xanthohumol concentration	Treatment time	Effect	Reference
	Primary CML cells	5 μM	24 h	↑ apoptosis	
		5 μM	6 h	↑ ROS, ↓ TNF-induced NF-κB signalling, ↑ p21, p53 mRNA and protein expression	
		5 μM	16, 24 h	↓ survivin mRNA and protein expression	
Leukemia	Primary CLL cells	25 μM	12, 24 h	↑ caspase-3, -4, -9 cleavage	Lust et al. (2009)
		25 μM	3–24 h	↓ Bid, Mcl-1 expression	
		25 μM	24 h	↓ Bcl-2 expression	
		25 μM	12, 24 h	↑ ER-stress, ↑ UPR	
		25 μM	12 h	↑ ROS	
		25–100 μM		↓ S20 proteasomal activity	
		25 μM	12 h	↑ ubiquitinated proteins	
Leukemia	KBM-5 (CML)	50 μM	4 h	↑ TNF-induced apoptosis	Harikumar et al. (2009)
		50 μM	12, 24 h	↑ TNF-induced PARP cleavage	
		50 μM	4 h + 0–12 h	↓ expression of TNF-induced proliferative and anti-apoptotic proteins	
		50 μM/5–50 μM	1–12 h/4 h	↓ TNF-induced activation of NF-κB, IκBα kinase activity	
Myeloma	U266	50 μM	4 h	↑ TNF-induced apoptosis	Harikumar et al. (2009)
Sarcoma	HT-1080	3 μM	72 h	↓ proliferation under hypoxia	Goto et al. (2005)
Sarcoma	KS-IMM	2.5–25 μM	48–72 h	↓ proliferation	Albini et al. (2006)
Melanoma	SK-Mel2	not stated	48 h	↓ proliferation	Lee et al. (2007)
Macrophages	Raw264.7	0.4–50 μM	24 h	↔ proliferation	Gerhauser et al. (2002)
Endothelial cells	HUVEC	2.5–25 μM	48–72 h	↓ proliferation (10–15 μM); ↑ cell death (25 μM)	Albini et al. (2006)
		10 μM	3 h pre-treatment	↓ TNF-induced NF-κB nuclear translocation, ↓ IκBα phosphorylation	

Endothelial cells cells	HUVEC	2.5-10 μM	24-72 h	↓ proliferation	Dell'Eva et al. (2007)
Adipocytes	From 3 T3-L1	25–100 μM	24, 48 h	↓ proliferation	Yang et al. (2007; 2008); Rayalam et al. (2009)
		25–100 μM	24, 48 h	↑ apoptosis	
		75 μM	0–3 h	↑ ROS production	
		75 μM	0–1.5 h	↓ mitochondrial membrane potential	
		75 μM	6–48 h	↑ cytochrome *c* release	
		75, 100 μM	3–12 h	↑ caspase3/7 activity	
		75 μM	6–24 h	↑ PARP cleavage	
Adipocytes	From 3 T3-L1	0.1–50 μM	24–72 h	↓ proliferation	Mendes et al. (2008)
		5 μM	24 h	↓ proliferation	
		5 μM	24 h	↑ apoptosis	
Dendritic cells	From bone marrow	2–50 μM	24 h	↑ caspase-3, -8 activity	Xuan et al. (2010)
		20 μM	24 h	↑ caspase-3, -8 cleavage	
		2–50 μM	24 h	↑ apoptosis (sub-G_1 fraction)	
T-cells	Murine T-lymphocytes	1.25–40 μM	72, 96 h	↓ Con A or IL-2-induced proliferation	(Gao et al. 2009)
		1.25–40 μM	72 h	↓ cell viability at high, ↑ cell counts at low concentrations	

[a]Non-cancerous cell lines: *AML12* normal murine hepatocyte cell line, *PHH* primary human hepatocytes, *BPH-1* benign prostatic hyperplasia (prostate epithelial cells)
[b]*HSC* hepatic stellate cells

References

Ak P, Levine AJ (2010) p53 and NF-kappaB: different strategies for responding to stress lead to a functional antagonism. FASEB J 24(10):3643–3652. doi:fj.10-160549 [pii] 10.1096/fj.10-160549

Albini A, Dell'Eva R, Vene R, Ferrari N, Buhler DR, Noonan DM, Fassina G (2006) Mechanisms of the antiangiogenic activity by the hop flavonoid xanthohumol: NF-kappaB and Akt as targets. FASEB J 20(3):527–529

Botta B, Vitali A, Menendez P, Misiti D, Delle MG (2005) Prenylated flavonoids: pharmacology and biotechnology. Curr Med Chem 12(6):717–739

Boveris A, Cadenas E (1975) Mitochondrial production of superoxide anions and its relationship to the antimycin insensitive respiration. FEBS Lett 54(3):311–314

Boveris A, Chance B (1973) The mitochondrial generation of hydrogen peroxide. General properties and effect of hyperbaric oxygen. Biochem J 134(3):707–716

Carpinteiro A, Dumitru C, Schenck M, Gulbins E (2008) Ceramide-induced cell death in malignant cells. Cancer Lett 264(1):1–10. doi:S0304-3835(08)00082-7 [pii] 10.1016/j.canlet.2008.02.020

Chadwick LR, Pauli GF, Farnsworth NR (2006) The pharmacognosy of Humulus lupulus L. (hops) with an emphasis on estrogenic properties. Phytomedicine 13(1-2):119–131

Colgate EC, Miranda CL, Stevens JF, Bray TM, Ho E (2007) Xanthohumol, a prenylflavonoid derived from hops induces apoptosis and inhibits NF-kappaB activation in prostate epithelial cells. Cancer Lett 246(1–2):201–209

Dell'Eva R, Ambrosini C, Vannini N, Piaggio G, Albini A, Ferrari N (2007) AKT/NF-kappaB inhibitor xanthohumol targets cell growth and angiogenesis in hematologic malignancies. Cancer 110(9):2007–2011

Delmulle L, Vanden Berghe T, Keukeleire DD, Vandenabeele P (2008) Treatment of PC-3 and DU145 prostate cancer cells by prenylflavonoids from hop (Humulus lupulus L.) induces a caspase-independent form of cell death. Phytother Res 22(2):197–203. doi:10.1002/ptr.2286

Desagher S, Martinou JC (2000) Mitochondria as the central control point of apoptosis. Trends Cell Biol 10(9):369–377

Dorn C, Kraus B, Motyl M, Weiss TS, Gehrig M, Scholmerich J, Heilmann J, Hellerbrand C (2010a) Xanthohumol, a chalcon derived from hops, inhibits hepatic inflammation and fibrosis. Mol Nutr Food Res 54(Suppl 2):S205–213. doi:10.1002/mnfr.200900314

Dorn C, Weiss TS, Heilmann J, Hellerbrand C (2010b) Xanthohumol, a prenylated chalcone derived from hops, inhibits proliferation, migration and interleukin-8 expression of hepatocellular carcinoma cells. Int J Oncol 36(2):435–441

Faitova J, Krekac D, Hrstka R, Vojtesek B (2006) Endoplasmic reticulum stress and apoptosis. Cell Mol Biol Lett 11(4):488–505. doi:10.2478/s11658-006-0040-4

Fruehauf JP, Meyskens FL Jr (2007) Reactive oxygen species: a breath of life or death? Clin Cancer Res 13(3):789–794

Gao X, Deeb D, Liu Y, Gautam S, Dulchavsky SA, Gautam SC (2009) Immunomodulatory activity of xanthohumol: inhibition of T cell proliferation, cell-mediated cytotoxicity and Th1 cytokine production through suppression of NF-kappaB. Immunopharmacol Immunotoxicol 31(3):477–484. doi:10.1080/08923970902798132

Gerhauser C (2005) Beer constituents as potential cancer chemopreventive agents. Eur J Cancer 41(13):1941–1954

Gerhauser C, Alt A, Heiss E, Gamal-Eldeen A, Klimo K, Knauft J, Neumann I, Scherf HR, Frank N, Bartsch H, Becker H (2002) Cancer chemopreventive activity of Xanthohumol, a natural product derived from hop. Mol Cancer Ther 1(11):959–969

Goto K, Asai T, Hara S, Namatame I, Tomoda H, Ikemoto M, Oku N (2005) Enhanced antitumor activity of xanthohumol, a diacylglycerol acyltransferase inhibitor, under hypoxia. Cancer Lett 219(2):215–222. doi:S0304-3835(04)00577-4 [pii] 10.1016/j.canlet.2004.07.034

Grassme H, Cremesti A, Kolesnick R, Gulbins E (2003) Ceramide-mediated clustering is required for CD95-DISC formation. Oncogene 22(35):5457–5470. doi:10.1038/sj.onc.1206540 1206540 [pii]

Green DR, Reed JC (1998) Mitochondria and apoptosis. Science 281(5381):1309–1312
Guerreiro S, Monteiro R, Martins MJ, Calhau C, Azevedo I, Soares R (2007) Distinct modulation of alkaline phosphatase isoenzymes by 17beta-estradiol and xanthohumol in breast cancer MCF-7 cells. Clin Biochem 40(3–4):268–273
Halliwell B, Whiteman M (2004) Measuring reactive species and oxidative damage in vivo and in cell culture: how should you do it and what do the results mean? Br J Pharmacol 142(2):231–255
Hanahan D, Weinberg RA (2000) The hallmarks of cancer. Cell 100(1):57–70
Harikumar KB, Kunnumakkara AB, Ahn KS, Anand P, Krishnan S, Guha S, Aggarwal BB (2009) Modification of the cysteine residues in IkappaBalpha kinase and NF-kappaB (p65) by xanthohumol leads to suppression of NF-kappaB-regulated gene products and potentiation of apoptosis in leukemia cells. Blood 113(9):2003–2013
Heath-Engel HM, Chang NC, Shore GC (2008) The endoplasmic reticulum in apoptosis and autophagy: role of the BCL-2 protein family. Oncogene 27(50):6419–6433. doi:onc2008309 [pii] 10.1038/onc.2008.309
Henderson MC, Miranda CL, Stevens JF, Deinzer ML, Buhler DR (2000) In vitro inhibition of human P450 enzymes by prenylated flavonoids from hops, Humulus lupulus. Xenobiotica 30(3):235–251
Ho YC, Liu CH, Chen CN, Duan KJ, Lin MT (2008) Inhibitory effects of xanthohumol from hops (Humulus lupulus L.) on human hepatocellular carcinoma cell lines. Phytother Res 22(11):1465–1468. doi:10.1002/ptr.2481
Jin Z, El-Deiry WS (2005) Overview of cell death signaling pathways. Cancer Biol Ther 4(2):139–163. doi:1508 [pii]
Kamata H, Hirata H (1999) Redox regulation of cellular signalling. Cell Signal 11(1):1–14
Klenke E (2008) Inhibition of angiogenesis by potential chemopreventive agents, vol 1. Vdm Verlag Dr Müller, Saarbrücken
Lee SH, Kim HJ, Lee JS, Lee IS, Kang BY (2007) Inhibition of topoisomerase I activity and efflux drug transporters' expression by xanthohumol. from hops. Arch Pharm Res 30(11):1435–1439
Lust S, Vanhoecke B, Janssens A, Philippe J, Bracke M, Offner F (2005) Xanthohumol kills B-chronic lymphocytic leukemia cells by an apoptotic mechanism. Mol Nutr Food Res 49(9):844–850. doi:10.1002/mnfr.200500045
Lust S, Vanhoecke B, Van GM, Boelens J, Van MH, Kaileh M, Vanden Berghe W, Haegeman G, Philippe J, Bracke M, Offner F (2009) Xanthohumol activates the proapoptotic arm of the unfolded protein response in chronic lymphocytic leukemia. Anticancer Res 29(10):3797–3805
Magalhaes PJ, Carvalho DO, Cruz JM, Guido LF, Barros AA (2009) Fundamentals and health benefits of xanthohumol, a natural product derived from hops and beer. Nat Prod Commun 4(5):591–610
Malhotra JD, Kaufman RJ (2007) Endoplasmic reticulum stress and oxidative stress: a vicious cycle or a double-edged sword? Antioxid Redox Signal 9(12):2277–2293. doi:10.1089/ars.2007.1782
Mendes V, Monteiro R, Pestana D, Teixeira D, Calhau C, Azevedo I (2008) Xanthohumol influences preadipocyte differentiation: implication of antiproliferative and apoptotic effects. J Agric Food Chem 56(24):11631–11637. doi:10.1021/jf802233q10.1021/jf802233q [pii]
Miranda CL, Stevens JF, Helmrich A, Henderson MC, Rodriguez RJ, Yang YH, Deinzer ML, Barnes DW, Buhler DR (1999) Antiproliferative and cytotoxic effects of prenylated flavonoids from hops (Humulus lupulus) in human cancer cell lines. Food Chem Toxicol 37(4):271–285. doi:S0278691599000198 [pii]
Miranda CL, Aponso GL, Stevens JF, Deinzer ML, Buhler DR (2000a) Prenylated chalcones and flavanones as inducers of quinone reductase in mouse Hepa 1c1c7 cells. Cancer Lett 149(1–2):21–29
Miranda CL, Stevens JF, Ivanov V, McCall M, Frei B, Deinzer ML, Buhler DR (2000b) Antioxidant and prooxidant actions of prenylated and nonprenylated chalcones and flavanones in vitro. J Agric Food Chem 48(9):3876–3884. doi:10.1021/Jf0002995
Monteghirfo S, Tosetti F, Ambrosini C, Stigliani S, Pozzi S, Frassoni F, Fassina G, Soverini S, Albini A, Ferrari N (2008) Antileukemia effects of xanthohumol in Bcr/Abl-transformed cells involve nuclear factor-kappaB and p53 modulation. Mol Cancer Ther 7(9):2692–2702

Monteiro R, Becker H, Azevedo I, Calhau C (2006) Effect of hop (Humulus lupulus L.) flavonoids on aromatase (estrogen synthase) activity. J Agric Food Chem 54(8):2938–2943

Monteiro R, Faria A, Azevedo I, Calhau C (2007) Modulation of breast cancer cell survival by aromatase inhibiting hop (Humulus lupulus L.) flavonoids. J Steroid Biochem Mol Biol 105(1–5):124–130. doi:S0960-0760(07)00105-7 [pii] 10.1016/j.jsbmb.2006.11.026

Monteiro R, Calhau C, Silva AO, Pinheiro-Silva S, Guerreiro S, Gartner F, Azevedo I, Soares R (2008) Xanthohumol inhibits inflammatory factor production and angiogenesis in breast cancer xenografts. J Cell Biochem 104(5):1699–1707

Orrenius S, Gogvadze V, Zhivotovsky B (2007) Mitochondrial oxidative stress: implications for cell death. Annu Rev Pharmacol Toxicol 47:143–183

Pan L, Becker H, Gerhauser C (2005) Xanthohumol induces apoptosis in cultured 40–16 human colon cancer cells by activation of the death receptor- and mitochondrial pathway. Mol Nutr Food Res 49(9):837–843

Pani G, Koch OR, Galeotti T (2009) The p53-p66shc-Manganese Superoxide Dismutase (MnSOD) network: a mitochondrial intrigue to generate reactive oxygen species. Int J Biochem Cell Biol 41(5):1002–1005

Rayalam S, Yang JY, Della-Fera MA, Park HJ, Ambati S, Baile CA (2009) Anti-obesity effects of xanthohumol plus guggulsterone in 3T3-L1 adipocytes. J Med Food 12(4):846–853. doi:10.1089/jmf.2008.0158

Simon HU, Haj-Yehia A, Levi-Schaffer F (2000) Role of reactive oxygen species (ROS) in apoptosis induction. Apoptosis 5(5):415–418

Stevens JF, Page JE (2004) Xanthohumol and related prenylflavonoids from hops and beer: to your good health! Phytochemistry 65(10):1317–1330

Stevens JF, Ivancic M, Hsu VL, Deinzer ML (1997) Prenylflavonoids from Humulus lupulus. Phytochemistry 44(8):1575–1585

Strathmann J, Klimo K, Steinle R, Hussong R, Frank N, Gerhauser C (2009) Xanthohumol from Hops Prevents Hormone-dependent Tumorigenesis in vitro and in vivo. Acta Hortic. Proceedings of the second international humulus symposium 848:179–190

Strathmann J, Klimo K, Sauer SW, Okun JG, Prehn JHM, Gerhauser C (2010) Xanthohumol-induced transient superoxide anion radical formation triggers cancer cells into apoptosis via a mitochondria-mediated mechanism. FASEB J 24(8):2938–2950. doi:10.1096/fj.10-155846

Szliszka E, Czuba ZP, Mazur B, Paradysz A, Krol W (2010) Chalcones and dihydrochalcones augment TRAIL-mediated apoptosis in prostate cancer cells. Molecules 15(8):5336–5353. doi:molecules15085336 [pii] 10.3390/molecules15085336

Trachootham D, Alexandre J, Huang P (2009) Targeting cancer cells by ROS-mediated mechanisms: a radical therapeutic approach? Nat Rev Drug Discov 8(7):579–591

Vanhoecke B, Derycke L, Van Marck V, Depypere H, De Keukeleire D, Bracke M (2005) Antiinvasive effect of xanthohumol, a prenylated chalcone present in hops (Humulus lupulus L.) and beer. Int J Cancer 117(6):889–895. doi:10.1002/ijc.21249

Vogel S, Heilmann J (2008) Synthesis, cytotoxicity, and antioxidative activity of minor prenylated chalcones from Humulus lupulus. J Nat Prod 71(7):1237–1241. doi:10.1021/np800188b

Vogel S, Ohmayer S, Brunner G, Heilmann J (2008) Natural and non-natural prenylated chalcones: synthesis, cytotoxicity and anti-oxidative activity. Bioorg Med Chem 16(8):4286–4293. doi:S0968-0896(08)00198-3 [pii] 10.1016/j.bmc.2008.02.079

Vogel S, Barbic M, Jurgenliemk G, Heilmann J (2010) Synthesis, cytotoxicity, anti-oxidative and anti-inflammatory activity of chalcones and influence of A-ring modifications on the pharmacological effect. Eur J Med Chem 45(6):2206–2213. doi:S0223-5234(10)00105-4 [pii] 10.1016/j.ejmech.2010.01.060

Xuan NT, Shumilina E, Gulbins E, Gu S, Götz F, Lang F (2010) Triggering of dendritic cell apoptosis by xanthohumol. Mol Nutr Food Res 54(S2):S214–S224. doi:10.1002/mnfr.200900324

Yang JY, la-Fera MA, Rayalam S, Baile CA (2007) Effect of xanthohumol and isoxanthohumol on 3T3-L1 cell apoptosis and adipogenesis. Apoptosis 12(11):1953–1963

Yang JY, Della-Fera MA, Rayalam S, Baile CA (2008) Enhanced effects of xanthohumol plus honokiol on apoptosis in 3T3-L1 adipocytes. Obesity (Silver Spring) 16(6):1232–1238. doi:oby200866 [pii] 10.1038/oby.2008.66

Zanoli P, Zavatti M (2008) Pharmacognostic and pharmacological profile of Humulus lupulus L. J Ethnopharmacol 116(3):383–396
Zhang K, Kaufman RJ (2008) From endoplasmic-reticulum stress to the inflammatory response. Nature 454(7203):455–462. doi:nature07203 [pii] 10.1038/nature07203
Zhao H, Joseph J, Fales HM, Sokoloski EA, Levine RL, Vasquez-Vivar J, Kalyanaraman B (2005) Detection and characterization of the product of hydroethidine and intracellular superoxide by HPLC and limitations of fluorescence. Proc Natl Acad Sci USA 102(16):5727–5732

Chapter 5
Bioavailability and Metabolism of Curcuminoids

Wolfgang W. Quitschke

Abstract Curcuminoids are biologically active polyphenols present in the spice and coloring agent turmeric. Dietary intake of curcuminoids has been associated a wide range of medicinal properties, including possible beneficial effects in the prevention of many forms of cancer. Studies carried out *in vitro* on cultured cells show that curcuminoids reduce the rate of cell division and induce apoptosis by affecting signal transduction pathways. However, there is a discrepancy between the curcuminoid dosage required for these *in vitro* effects and the most optimistic estimates on curcuminoid bioavailability following oral uptake. Therefore, the mechanism by which curcuminoids exert their biological effects through dietary intake remains incompletely understood. Curcuminoid bioavailability is dependent on several factors. These include solubility, chemical stability, efficiency of digestive uptake, metabolic processing, and excretion. This review attempts to illuminate the current state of knowledge on the effect of these factors on curcuminoid bioavailability. In addition, efforts to augment curcuminoid bioavailability through chemical modifications, improved solubilization, increased stability, or alternative routes of administration are addressed.

5.1 Introduction

Curcuminoids are polyphenols extracted from the root of *Curcuma longa* (Braga et al. 2003; Verghese 1993). They impart the yellow color to the spice turmeric, where they occur in amounts of 2–8% (Hiserodt et al. 1996; Jayaprakasha et al. 2002; Tayyem et al. 2006). Curcumin is the main ingredient (70–80%) in commercially available

W.W. Quitschke (✉)
Department of Psychiatry and Behavioral Science,
State University of New York at Stony Brook,
Stony Brook, NY 11794-8101, USA
e-mail: wolfgang.quitschke@sbumed.org

M. Diederich and K. Noworyta (eds.), *Natural Compounds as Inducers of Cell Death: Volume 1*, DOI 10.1007/978-94-007-4575-9_5,

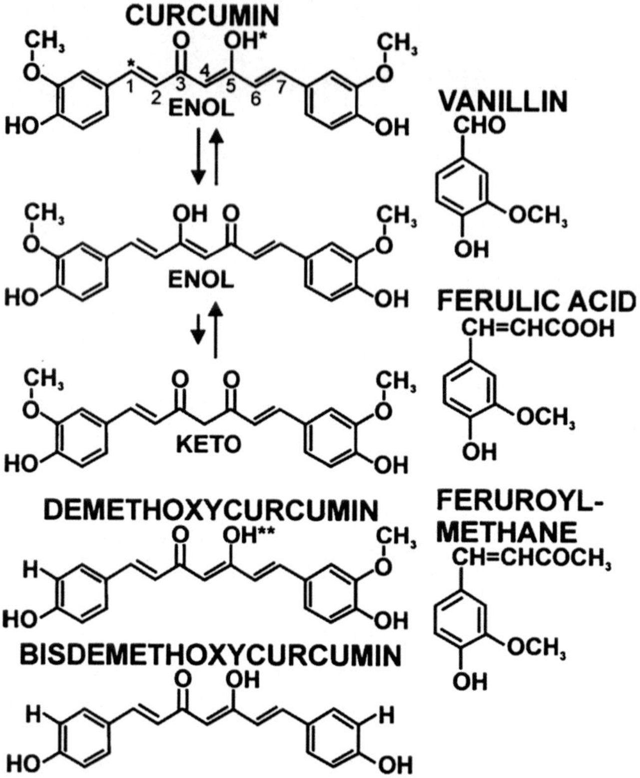

Fig. 5.1 Structure of curcuminoids (curcumin, demethoxy-, and bisdemethoxycurcumin) and the chemical degradation products of curcumin (vanillin, ferulic acid, and feruloylmethane). The keto-enol equilibria of curcumin are indicated. *: A glutathione conjugation site at position C1 and an alternative *in vitro* enol glucuronidation site at position C5 [or C3]. **: Alternative modification site for demethoxycurcumin at position C5 (Zeng et al. 2007)

curcumin preparations (Huang et al. 1995; Marczylo et al. 2007). Structurally, curcumin (diferuloylmethane; 1,7-bis(4-hydroxy-3-methoxy phenyl)-1,6-heptadiene-3,5,-dione; curcumin I) is composed of two feruloyl chromophores joined by a methylene group. Curcumin contains a diketone structure that exists in a tautomeric equilibrium with two possible enol structures through intramolecular hydrogen transfer. Indeed, in most organic solvents the enol form predominates (Payton et al. 2007). Since the resulting two enol tautomers are in equilibrium, the single hydrogen atom shared by the two possible keto-enol structures becomes delocalized (Balasubramanian 2006; Mague et al. 2004). In addition to curcumin, turmeric contains two additional structurally related congeners that lack either one (demethoxycurcumin [DMC], curcumin II, 15–25%) or both (bisdemethoxycurcumin [BDMC], curcumin III, 3–10%) methoxy groups in the phenyl rings (Fig. 5.1). Collectively, these compounds are referred to as curcuminoids. However, the term 'curcumin' is often used interchangeably.

Curcuminoids have been implicated in numerous medicinal applications. These include inhibition of tumor propagation, protection against Alzheimer disease and antiinflammatory properties [reviews: (Aggarwal and Sung 2009; Anand et al. 2007, 2008a; Epstein et al. 2010; Hatcher et al. 2008; Villegas et al. 2008)]. *In vitro*, curcumin slows the rate of cell division or induces apoptosis in a concentration dependent manner. These effects are observed at curcumin concentrations ranging from 10 to 100 μM depending on cell culture system. Inhibition of Alzheimer-associated plaque formation and resolution of preexisting plaques has been reported at lower concentrations in the 1 μM range both *in vivo* and *in vitro* (Frautschy et al. 2001; Garcia-Alloza et al. 2007; Lim et al. 2001; Ono et al. 2004; Yang et al. 2005). One conundrum associated with the biological effects of curcumin is its exceedingly poor bioavailability (Yang et al. 2008). Following oral uptake of curcumin, the measured plasma concentration is extremely low, not exceeding transient levels of about 1 μM. It is therefore unclear how the effects observed in *in vivo* studies can be explained in terms of the biological effects observed *in vitro*. Bioavailability is dependent on numerous factors. These include solubility, chemical stability, uptake, metabolism, and excretion. The inter-relationship between these factors on the bioavailability of curcuminoids is here examined.

5.2 Curcumin Solubility and Chemical Stability

It might be assumed that curcumin bioavailability through oral uptake is dependent on the compound being in solution before being absorbed into the bloodstream by the intestinal tract. The solubility properties of curcumin and its chemical stability therefore warrant some further consideration.

Curcumin is virtually insoluble in aqueous buffers at pH 5 [$<10^{-8}$ M] (Tønnesen 2002). In this laboratory, the solubility of curcumin in deionized water, phosphate-buffered saline, pH 7, with or without 1% dimethyl sulfoxide (DMSO), was found not to exceed 1 μM (personal observations), Astoundingly higher solubility values in water have been reported (Leung and Kee 2009; Maiti et al. 2007; Wang et al. 1997), although it is not clear how these values were obtained. The water solubility of curcumin is greatly enhanced in alkaline solutions (~3 mM). This is accomplished by ionization through successive dissociation of protons from the three ionizable hydroxyl groups (two phenolic and one enolic, [Fig. 5.1]). The acidic constants have been variably determined as ranging from pKA_1 (enolic) = 7.7–8.55, pKA_2 (phenolic) = 8.1–10.41 and pKA_3 (phenolic) = 9–10.69 (Bernabé-Pineda et al. 2004; Jovanovic et al. 1999; Priyadarsini et al. 2003; Shen and Ji 2007; Tang et al. 2002; Tønnesen and Karlsen 1985a). However, curcumin is chemically unstable in alkaline solutions and undergoes spontaneous decomposition. The main decomposition products are vanillin, ferulic acid, and feruroyl methane. Vanillin is derived from further decomposition of feruloyl methane, which may in turn undergo condensation into yellow products with spectral absorption characteristics similar to curcumin (Tønnesen and Karlsen 1985a, b; Wang et al. 1997). On the other hand, curcumin is exceedingly stable at acidic pH. In aqueous solutions containing 10% methanol, degradation half-lives ranged from 6.6×10^3 h at pH 1.23, 4.6 h at pH 7.3, to 2.5×10^{-2} h at pH 10.84 when incubated at 31.5°C (Tønnesen and Karlsen 1985a). The pH-dependent stability of curcumin was confirmed by Wang et al. (1997) although in this report 90% of the curcumin decomposed within 30 min when incubated with 0.1 M phosphate buffer (pH 7.2) at 37°C.

In contrast, the solubility and stability of curcumin in aqueous solutions is greatly enhanced by the presence of bovine serum albumin [BSA] (Barik et al. 2003; Blasius et al. 2004; Pfeiffer et al. 2003; Quitschke 2008; Wang et al. 1997). Spectroscopic studies on BSA and human serum albumin [HSA] have indicated that this occurs through complex formation of curcumin (Zsila et al. 2003) via the interactions with both polar domains (Mandeville et al. 2009) and the hydrophobic domain surrounding Trp 214 [HSA] or Trp 213 [BSA] (Barik et al. 2003; Mandeville et al. 2009; Sahoo et al. 2008; Wang et al. 2005). The overall binding constant was estimated to be $4–5 \times 10^5$ M^{-1}. A different study identified two different curcumin-HSA interaction sites: A high- and a low-affinity site with equilibrium constants of 2×10^5 M^{-1} and 2.1×10^4 M^{-1}, respectively (Pulla Reddy et al. 1999). As a result of the interaction with serum albumin, the stability of curcumin is greatly increased. Indeed, the rate of curcumin decomposition in HSA solutions was 16-fold lower than in comparable phosphate buffered solutions at pH 7.4 (Leung and Kee 2009). It is likely that this is the reason why curcumin is similarly stabilized in solutions containing serum supplements (Blasius et al. 2004; Pfeiffer et al. 2003; Quitschke 2008; Wang et al. 1997). The solubility of curcuminoids in serum albumin solutions is also greatly enhanced with a maximum solubility of about 2.5 mM in 5% BSA (Quitschke 2008). Although the interaction of curcumin with serum albumin and other plasma proteins (Leung and Kee 2009) may have limited relevance to its bioavailability by oral uptake, it offers other alternatives for curcumin delivery, such as by intravenous injection (Quitschke 2008).

The complex formation of curcumin with serum components is also crucial in the context of cell culture experiments, where this interaction may be the only source of curcumin solubility and stability in an otherwise aqueous nutrient solution. It is a little appreciated fact that curcumin pre-dissolved in an organic solvent will precipitate upon addition to an aqueous medium. In the serum-free culture medium, the soluble fraction of curcumin would then approach the solubility limit in aqueous solutions at physiological pH, i.e. ~1 μM. The remainder remains in a suspension that is readily pelleted under standard microcentrifuge conditions. The presence of serum in the culture medium increases curcumin solubility proportionally to the serum concentration in the culture medium (usually 5–10%). However, the solubilization process takes time and requires continuous mixing for optimal results (Quitschke 2008). The kinetics of solubilization has not been established under conditions where the dissolved curcumin is simply added to the medium prior to incubation. Since the interaction of suspended curcumin with cells has not been adequately characterized, results from cell culture experiments addressing issues relating to the dose-dependent effects of curcumin should be interpreted with caution.

In contrast to its poor solubility in water, curcumin is readily dissolved in several organic solvents. Such solvents include alcohols, ketones, esters, and organic acids. The solubility of curcumin in these solvents has not been systematically determined, but it generally ranges from 1 to 30 mM. The common property of these solvents is that they have amphiphilic properties. According to the same principle, curcumin is also to varying degrees soluble in e.g. chloroform, acetonitrile, detergents, and polyethylene glycol (PEG). However, the solvent in which the highest levels of curcumin solubility can be achieved may conceivably be dimethyl sulfoxide (DMSO). In this solvent, curcumin concentrations as high as 1 M can be achieved. The most common solvents used for media dilution in cell culture experiments are ethanol and DMSO. The solubility of curcumin in organic solvents also forms the basis for its extraction from the powdered root of *Curcuma longa* (Braga et al. 2003; Verghese 1993). The stability of curcumin in organic solvents usually poses no practical problem, in particular when stored at −20°C. However, photochemical degradation of curcumin in such solvents has been reported and the degradation products are different from those observed in aqueous solutions (Tønnesen et al. 1986). The half-life (2–95 h) was solvent-dependent and increased with the concentration of curcumin in solution.

In the literature, curcumin is often referred to as being lipophilic. Assuming that lipophilic is defined as a tendency to dissolve in non-polar solvents, this description is not entirely correct. Indeed, curcumin does not to any significant extent dissolve in strictly non-polar solvents such as diethylether or mineral oil. An example that best illustrates this situation is provided by a comparison of curcumin solubility in heptane and heptanoic acid. The solubility of curcumin is exceedingly low in heptane compared to its approximately 3,000-fold higher solubility in heptanoic acid. Furthermore, the solubility of curcumin decreases with increasing aliphatic chain length (unpublished results). These observations justify a careful qualification of the lipophilic nature of the interaction of curcumin with cells and serum proteins. Clearly, curcumin does not have an affinity for hydrophobic moieties alone, but requires the balanced presence of hydrophilic residues as was suggested with its interaction with serum albumin (Mandeville et al. 2009). It is therefore more accurate to describe the solubility behavior of curcumin as amphipathic (Sun et al. 2008).

5.3 Curcumin Uptake, Tissue Distribution, and Excretion

After oral ingestion, curcumin travels through the gastrointestinal tract. It is first exposed to the acidic content of the stomach, followed by the somewhat alkaline environment of the small intestines. It is there mixed with digestive fluids from the pancreas and bile from the gall bladder. Before being eliminated through the bowel, it also encounters the intestinal flora. The entire process takes place at 37°C . This provides ample opportunity for curcumin to be solubilized via complex formation with digestive proteins (pancreas) or interaction with organic molecules (bile). On the other hand, it also exposes curcumin to potential chemical degradation, although the effect of light can be excluded here. The results on systemic availability addressed in this section are limited to the administration of standard curcumin preparations either in solid form (powder, capsules), as suspensions (oil, water) or in solutions (e.g. alkaline, organic solvents) for i.v. and i.p. injection. Special formulations and curcumin co-administered with other compounds are discussed in subsequent sections.

In an early systematic investigation of curcumin metabolism (Holder et al. 1978), tritiated curcumin was injected into rats either intravenously (i.v.) or intraperitoneally (i.p.). The excretion products of curcumin were then determined in urine and feces. Within 72 h after i.p. injection, about 73% of the radioactivity was excreted in the feces and 11% in the urine with no significant amount remaining in the tissues. Most of the excreted radioactivity was in the form of metabolized curcumin. The presence of the i.p. injected compound in feces suggested elimination via the bile. This was supported by the observation that 6 h after i.v. injection of [H^3]-curcumin, about 85% of the radioactivity was recovered in the bile (Holder et al. 1978).

In another study on curcumin bioavailability (Wahlström and Blennow 1978), 1 g/kg of curcumin suspended in arachis oil was administered to rats by gavage in a single dose. The majority of the curcumin (65–85%) was excreted in the feces within 3 days while negligible amounts (<0.01%) were measured in the urine. Curcumin was detected in the plasma after 3 h in only one of four animals. A small proportion of curcumin (0.00056%) was found to be excreted in the bile and 0.015% was distributed in liver, kidneys and body fat. Most of the administered curcumin was located to the small intestines. After i.v injection of curcumin (in 0.1 N NaOH), the results were different, although the amount administered was not specified. In this case, 2.1% of the curcumin was excreted as free curcumin in the bile within 3 h and 20% as conjugated curcumin, with a concomitant increase in bile flow. At the same time, the relative amount in liver was 3.1% and in the kidneys 0.5%. The concentration of both free and conjugated curcumin in plasma reached a level of about 10 μg/ml within 5 min and declined to undetectable levels within 60 min (Wahlström and Blennow 1978).

Ravindranath and Chandrasekhara (1980) administered a single dose of 400 mg curcumin by gavage and 40% of the curcumin was excreted unchanged in the feces over a 5 day period. No free curcumin was detected in the urine while conjugated products were increased for 7 days. Although it was implied, it was not established whether the conjugates were necessarily derived from curcumin. No curcumin was detected in blood from the heart or portal veins. The amount of curcumin in the gastrointestinal tract decreased from 96% to 38% during the 24-h period after administration. The difference was interpreted as representing curcumin absorption (Ravindranath and Chandrasekhara 1980). The uptake and excretion of curcumin after oral uptake was further investigated by the same group using tritiated curcumin. Three doses (400, 80, and 10 mg) of [H^3]-curcumin suspended in water with 0.01% Tween 20 was administered to rats by gavage and the excretion of radioactivity was monitored for 12 days. The main route of excretion was via the feces, which accounted for 59–99% of the total amount of radioactivity administered, of which about 34% was in the form of unmodified curcumin. Most of the radioactivity was excreted during the first 3 days after oral intake. Very little radioactivity (1–4%) was eliminated via the urin (Ravindranath and Chandrasekhara 1982).

More recent studies on the systemic uptake of curcumin reported a maximum serum concentration of 500 ng/ml (1.36 μM), which was attained less than 1 h following the oral administration of 100–300 mg/ml of curcumin suspended in water-Tween-20 (Liu et al. 2006; Maiti et al. 2007). Thereafter, the serum concentration of curcumin declined linearly to undetectable levels over 6 h. Very similar results were obtained by Shoba et al. (1998) except that after administering a nearly tenfold higher dose of curcumin (2 g/kg), the maximum serum concentration more than doubled to 1.35 μg/ml (3.67 μM). In the same study, a single 2 g (~30 mg/kg) dose of curcumin administered to humans resulted in negligible serum concentrations in the low nM range (Shoba et al. 1998).

Marczylo et al. (2009) determined the urine, plasma and tissue distribution of curcumin 20 min after oral intake (340 mg/kg) in the rat. The highest levels of curcumin was found in the rat intestinal mucosa (1,400 μg/g) followed by liver (3.7 μg/g), heart (0.8 μg/g) and kidney (0.2 μg/g). Plasma and urine levels reached 16.1 and 2 ng/ml, respectively. Most of the curcumin was present as glucuronides of either the parental compound or its reduction products (Marczylo et al. 2009).

A systematic investigation of the uptake of curcumin was carried out on mice to evaluate their potential application in Alzheimer disease (Begum et al. 2008). For acute oral administration by gavage, mice were given two doses of curcumin (148 μg, ~6 mg/kg) on two consecutive days. For chronic oral administration, curcumin was mixed with food at two different concentrations (~1.25 mg/day and ~10 mg/day) for 4 months. The mice were subsequently analyzed for the presence of curcumin in plasma and brain tissue. Following acute administration, no curcumin was detected in the plasma, while the level in the brain was 0.519 μg/g. In contrast, after chronic administration, plasma concentrations of 35 ng/ml (low dose) and 171 ng/ml (high dose) were recorded. The comparable respective values for brain curcumin levels were 0.469 and 0.525 μg/g. After chronic oral administration of curcumin, the reduction product tetrahydrocurcumin was detected in both plasma and brain tissue at 10–25% of the curcumin level, indicating some degree of metabolic conversion. These results indicate that the plasma concentration after oral uptake of curcumin is dose-dependent while the concentration in brain is largely constant (0.469 and 0.525 μg/ml), even after acute administration of curcumin (0.519 μg/g). Delivery of curcumin by single intramuscular (i.m.; 3 mg/kg) or i.p. (6 mg/kg) injections yielded higher plasma levels (127 ng/ml, i.p.; 238 ng/ml, i.m.) than those obtained by acute oral administration. The brain concentrations (0.739 μg/g, i.p.; 1.162 μg/g, i.m.) were consistently higher than those obtained by either acute or chronic oral administration.

The distribution of curcumin into other tissues of mice and rats has been further investigated following oral uptake (Marczylo et al. 2009; Padhye et al. 2009a; Suresh and Srinivasan 2010) and i.p. or i.v. injection (Perkins et al. 2002; Yang et al. 2007). As expected, the by far highest levels are found in the intestines both after oral ingestion and i.p. injection. High curcumin concentrations are also recorded in the liver. The distribution in other organs and tissues vary between studies (Table 5.1). In general, tissue levels of curcumin are much higher than comparable plasma levels.

A very recent article on the systemic distribution and excretion in rats after oral uptake of curcumin suspended in peanut oil (500 mg/kg) reported vastly higher values of curcumin serum levels than comparable previous studies. Six days after uptake, a maximum curcumin serum concentration of 83.8 μg/ml (228 μM!) was reported. Interestingly, the comparable curcumin content of total blood was 490.3 μg. Assuming that whole blood contains about 50% serum, almost all of the blood curcumin would be accounted for in the serum fraction. This suggests that curcumin does not adhere to other cellular components to any significant degree. The values for the tissue distribution (liver, kidney, intestine) of curcumin is in the same range as those reported by others, although the data are difficult to compare since they are reported in μg/whole tissue (Table 5.1). 36.5% of administered curcumin was eliminated in the feces and 0.173% in the urine (Suresh and Srinivasan 2010).

These and additional studies on the distribution of curcumin in plasma and tissues in mice and rats after either oral intake or i.v. and i.p. injections are summarized in Table 5.1. The plasma concentrations for both species range from 16.1 to 500 ng/ml (43 nM–1.36 μM) after a single oral dose by gavage. Vastly higher initial plasma concentrations up to 10,000 ng/ml (27 μM) can be achieved by i.p or i.v. injection. However, the plasma levels of curcumin and their metabolites are exceedingly transient and generally decline to undetectable levels within 4–12 h. Curcumin levels in tissues vary greatly, but they are generally much higher (10–100-fold, p.o.) than corresponding plasma levels. Particularly after oral intake, but also after i.p injections, the highest curcumin levels are consistently observed in the intestines followed by the liver.

Much of the information on the systemic availability of curcumin in humans was obtained from clinical trials for a range of conditions (Baum et al. 2007, 2008; Cheng et al. 2001; Dhillon et al. 2008; Garcea et al. 2004; Garcea et al. 2005; Lao et al. 2006; Sharma et al. 2001, 2004) and complementary to animal studies (Shoba et al. 1998). These results are summarized in Table 5.2. Plasma curcumin concentrations ranged from undetectable to the highest levels of about 1.75 μM, which are comparable to those observed in animal studies.

In summary, data from both animal and human studies suggest that the plasma curcumin levels following oral uptake are relatively low ranging from undetectable levels to concentrations of up to 1.75 μM, (Tables 5.1 and 5.2). The primary route of elimination is via the feces. Here the curcumin may pass either unmodified without prior uptake or via the bloodstream into the bile after modification in the liver. Urinary excretion is by comparison of secondary importance. As most of these studies indicate, free curcumin is a minor species in circulation and elimination. Instead, curcumin is vigorously modified to generate reduction and conjugation products. However, in animal studies the reported tissue concentrations after oral uptake are quite significant reaching levels as high as in the mM range in the intestines and about 10 μM in the liver after oral uptake (Marczylo et al. 2009). Even in the brain, which is the organ with the lowest reported concentration of curcumin, levels of 1–3 μM are consistently detected. Higher levels of systemic curcumin are obtained

Table 5.1 Curcumin levels in plasma and tissues (animal studies)

Dose (Species), route	Cmax[a] (ng/ml) plasma	Tmax (h) plasma	Tissue (μg/g)	Reference
340 mg/kg (rat), p.o	~87	0.5–1	na	Marczylo et al. (2007)
340 mg/kg (rat), p.o	16.1	0.25	Intestine: 1,400 Liver: 3.67 Kidney: 0.21 Heart: 0.807	Marczylo et al. (2009)
2 g/kg (rat), oral	1350	0.83	na	Shoba et al. (1998)
100 mg/kg (rat), p.o	266.7	1.62	na	Liu et al. (2006)
~2.3 g/kg (rat), p.o	Trace	0.25–24	na	Ravindranath and Chandrasekhara (1980)
1 g/kg (rat), oral	Trace-nd	0–1	na	Wahlström and Blennow (1978)
Not specified (rat), i.v.	~100	<0.08		
1 g/kg, p.o	500	0.75 h	na	Maiti et al. (2007)
~6 mg/kg (mouse), p.o	n.d	4[b]	Brain: 0.519	Begum et al. (2008)
~6 mg/kg (mouse) i.p.	127 1		Brain: 0.739	
~3 mg/kg (mouse), i.m.	238		Brain: 1.162	
50 mg/kg (mouse), i.v.	nd	na	na	Wang et al. (2008)
100 mg/kg (rat), p.o	64.6	2	na	Takahashi et al. (2009)
50 mg/kg (mouse), p.o	~40	1.5	na	Narayanan et al. (2009)
10 mg/kg (rat), i.v.	~10,000	<0.08	na	Ma et al. (2007)
250 mg/kg (rat), p.o	90.3	0.5	na	Shaikh et al. (2009)
400 mg/kg (rat), oral	nd (<20)	na	na	Xu et al. (2006)
100 mg/kg (rat), p.o	~200	~0.5	na	Asai and Miyazawa (2000)
1 g/kg (mouse), oral	220	1	na	Pan et al. (1999)
100 mg/kg (mouse), i.p.	2,250 (600)	0.25 (1)	Intestine: 117.04 Liver: 26.9 Kidney: 7.51 Spleen: 26.06 Brain: 0.41	
250 mg/kg (mouse), p.o	220	1		Padhye et al. (2009a)
0.5% in diet (mouse), p.o.	~1.8	ss	Intestine (s): 88.3	Perkins et al. (2002)
100 mg/kg (mouse), i.p.	9,200	ns (<4)	Intestine (l): 263.1 Intestine: 73.6 Liver: 26.9 Lungs: 5.9 Heart: 3.4 Muscle: 3.1 Kidney:28.7 Brain: 0.41	

(continued)

Table 5.1 (continued)

Dose (Species), route	Cmax[a] (ng/ml) plasma	Tmax (h) plasma	Tissue (μg/g)	Reference
500 mg/kg (rat), p.o.	60	0.7	na	Yang et al. (2007)
10 mg/kg (rat), i.v.	360	ns (<0.08)		
500 mg/kg (rat), p.o.	83,800	6	Intestine: 11,830 Liver: 135.2 Kidney: 9.03 Note: whole tissue	Suresh and Srinivasan (2010)

Abbreviations: *p.o.* per os, *i.v.* intravenous, *i.p.* intraperitoneal, *nd* not detected, *na* not available, *ns* not specified, *ss* steady state, *s* small, *l* large
[a]Total curcuminoids, including metabolites
[b]Time of measurement

Table 5.2 Plasma curcumin levels in humans

Oral dose curcumin	Peak plasma level (ng/ml)[a]	Reference
36–180 mg/day	nd	Sharma et al. (2001)
3.6 g/day	4.2	Sharma et al. (2004)
0.45,1.8,3.6 g/day	nd-trace	Garcea et al. (2004)
1 g/day	198[b]	Baum et al. (2008)
4 g/day	328[b]	
4 g/day	188	Cheng et al. (2001)
6 g/day	236	
8 g/day	651	
10,12 g/day	nd-trace	Vareed et al. (2008)
1 g/day	155	Baum et al. (2007)
4 g/day	294	
1,2,4,6,8,10,12 g/day	nd-trace	Lao et al. (2006)
3.6 g/day	Trace	Garcea et al. (2005)
8 g/day	nd	Dhillon et al. (2008)
2 g	Trace	Shoba et al. (1998)
2 g	150	Antony et al. (2008)

Abbreviations: *nd* not detected
[a]Total curcuminoids, including metabolic products
[b]Calculated median value

by alternate routes of administrations such as i.v., i.m., and i.p. injections. Overall, the systemic availability of curcumin as judged by plasma levels does not seem high enough to achieve many of the effects observed in cell culture. However, the relatively high levels in tissues reach concentrations that justify the suspicion that biological effects are indeed feasible. In particular, a potential for the treatment and prevention of Alzheimer disease exists due to the much lower levels of curcumin required to affect biochemical changes related to this disorder. It therefore seems appropriate to consider tissue distribution, rather than plasma levels, when evaluating the therapeutic potential of curcumin.

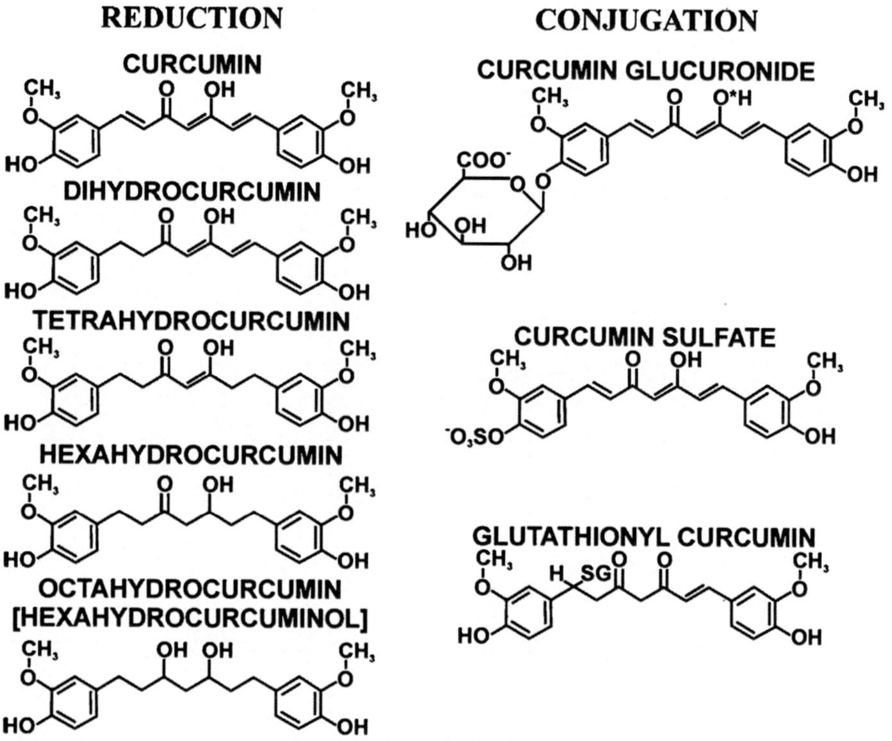

Fig. 5.2 Structures of curcumin phase I (reduction) and phase II (conjugation) metabolites as described in the text. *: Alternative *in vitro* glucuronidation site

5.4 Curcumin Metabolism

As suggested in the preceding section, curcumin undergoes metabolic transformation *in vivo*. This transformation takes place via both phase I and phase II metabolic pathways. The phase I metabolism of curcumin generates exclusively reduction products such as dihydrocurcumin, tetrahydrocurcumin, hexahydrocurcumin and octahydrocurcumin [hexahydrocurcuminol] (Fig. 5.2). The phase II metabolites are primarily curcumin mono-glucuronide, curcumin mono-sulfate, or mixed curcumin glucuronide-sulfate conjugated at either of the phenolic residues (Fig. 5.2). The phase I metabolites may also be similarly conjugated. The results from the following section are summarized in Table 5.3.

In an early study on curcumin metabolism, [H^3]-curcumin was administered to rats by i.p. injection. As discussed above, within 6 h after i.v. injection of [H^3]-curcumin about 85% of the radioactivity was recovered in the bile and 95% of this was accounted for by glucuronidated conjugates of curcumin. The conjugated fraction was deglucuronidated and further fractionated into tetrahydrocurcumin (50%), hexahydrocurcumin (42%), and a smaller amount of dihydroferulic acid (4%). Consequently, the main

Table 5.3 Curcumin metabolism (*in vivo* and *in vitro*)

Species (Route of administration)	Source	Conjugate	Conjugated compound	Reference
In vivo				
Rat (i.v.)	Feces	Glucuronides	Tetrahydrocurcumin Hexahydrocurcumin Dihydroferulic acid	Holder et al. (1978)
Mouse (i.p.)	Plasma	Glucuronides	Dihydrocurcumin Tetrahydrocurcumin Hexahydrocurcumin	Pan et al. (1999)
Rat (p.o.)	Plasma	Glucuronide + glucuronide-sulfate		Asai and Miyazawa (2000)
Rat (p.o. or i.v.)	Plasma	Glucuronide + glucuronide-sulfate + sulfate	Curcumin	Ireson et al. (2001)
Rat (p.o.)	Plasma Urine	Glucuronide + sulfate	Curcuminoids	Marczylo et al. (2009)
Mouse (p.o.)	Plasma	Glucuronides	Curcumin Dihydrocurcumin Tetrahydrocurcumin	Pan et al. (1999)
Human (p.o.)	Plasma	Glucuronides	Curcuminoids Tetrahydrocurcumin Ferulic acid Vanillic acid	Baum et al. (2007)

In vitro				
Rat (liver)	Slice	Glucuronide + sulfate	Hexahydrocurcumin Tetrahydrocurcumin Octahydrocurcumin	Hoehle et al. (2006)
Rat (Liver)	Cells	–	Hexahydrocurcumin Octahydrocurcumin	Ireson et al. (2001)
Rat (liver)	Cytosol	–	Reduction products	Hoehle et al. (2006)
Rat (liver)	Microsomes	Glucuronide	Curcumin	
Rat (liver, intestine)	Microsomes	Glucuronide	Liver < Intestine (fourfold)	Pfeiffer et al. (2007)
Human (liver, intestine)	Microsomes	Glucuronide	Liver = Intestine	
Rat (liver, intestine)	Microsomes	Glucuronide	Liver > Intestine (60-fold)	Ireson et al. (2002)
Human (liver, intestine)	Microsomes		Liver < Intestine (2.7-fold)	
Rat (liver, intestine)	Microsomes	Glucuronide	Liver > Intestine (threefold)	Wang et al. (2008)
Rat (liver, kidney, intestine)	Cytosol	Sulfate	Liver > Kidney >>> Intestine	Asai and Miyazawa (2000)
Rat (liver, intestine)	Cytosol	Sulfate	Liver > Intestine (sevenfold)	Narayanan et al. (2009)
Human (liver, intestine)	Cytosol		Liver < Intestine (2.6-fold)	

Abbreviations: *p.o.* per os, *i.v.* intravenous, *i.p.* intraperitoneal excretion products in the bile had been formed by reduction and subsequent glucuronidation of curcumin (Holder et al. 1978). Wahlström and Blennow (1978) found that after i.v. injection, 2.1% of the administered curcumin excreted in the bile was in the free and 20.1% (i.e. ~90% of the total) in the conjugated form. By comparison, using perfused livers, 49% of the curcumin was excreted in the bile in the conjugated form. In suspensions of isolated hepatocytes, added curcumin disappeared from the medium as a result of rapid metabolism (Wahlström and Blennow 1978). Although these metabolic products were not identified, it may be concluded from other similar studies (see below) that they represented phase I metabolites of curcumin.

An *in vitro* study used everted intestinal sacs from rats that were incubated with curcumin on the mucosal (luminal) side to determine the potential for intestinal absorption. Much of the curcumin disappeared from the mucosal side, but was not detectable in the serosal fluid (Ravindranath and Chandrasekhara 1981). In addition, little curcumin was recovered in the intestinal tissue. Instead, a structurally related, less polar, colorless compound was detected in both the intestinal tissue and in the serosal fluid (Ravindranath and Chandrasekhara 1981). It may again be surmised that this compound represents either reduction or more likely, chemical degradation products of curcumin, since these no longer absorb light in the 420 nm range. It was concluded that curcumin undergoes vigorous metabolic transformation during uptake in the intestinal tract, which may limit its systemic availability.

After i.p. injection of curcumin in mice, Pan et al. (1999) identified a range of curcumin metabolic products by reversed phase chromatography. It was proposed that curcumin undergoes sequential phase I reduction to dihydrocurcumin, tetrahydrocurcumin and hexahydrocurcumin. Glucuronidated phase II metabolites included curcumin-glucuronide and glucuronidated reduction products. Indeed, about 99% of the curcumin and >85% of the tetrahydrocurcumin in plasma was conjugated (Pan et al. 1999). Except for the additional identification of the reduction product dihydrocurcumin, these metabolic products were essentially the same as those identified by Holder et al. (1978). Interestingly, the presence of the other major conjugation product, curcumin sulfate, was not reported in either study.

Curcumin sulfate was first detected as a major metabolite in rat plasma after curcumin administration by gavage (Asai and Miyazawa 2000). In this instance, about 99% of the plasma curcumin was present in either the glucuronidated form (~42%) or as a mixed glucuronide/sulfate conjugate (~58%). It was also found that the curcumin congeners DMC and BDMC were similarly processed. In contrast to the data reported by Holder et al. (1978) and Pan et al. (1999), this study did not detect tetrahydrocurcumin or its conjugates as metabolic products. This discrepancy was interpreted as resulting from the difference in the methods of curcumin administration (i.e., oral vs. i.p and i.v.). Accordingly, curcumin would be differently processed depending on whether it bypassed or was absorbed by the alimentary tract.

Another study investigated the metabolism of curcumin following oral or i.v. injected curcumin in rats. In both cases, the presence of curcumin-glucuronide, -sulfate and mixed -glucuronide/sulfate was demonstrated. Judging from an HPLC chromatogram from plasma extract following i.v. injection, curcumin-glucuronide and mixed curcumin-glucuronide/sulfate were represented in approximately equal proportions, whereas the level of curcumin-sulfate was lower (~10% of total conjugates). In contrast, incubating curcumin with rat or human hepatocyte suspensions yielded primarily the reduction product hexahydrocurcumin. A proportion of hexahydrocurcumin was further reduced to the newly identified hexahydrocurcuminol (octahydrocurcumin). Consequently, primarily the reduction products of curcumin were generated in liver cell suspensions, whereas the conjugated products predominated *in vivo* (Ireson et al. 2001).

Curcumin reduction products and glucuronidation have also been demonstrated in cell free systems and liver tissue slices from the rat (Hoehle et al. 2006). The major metabolite in rat liver slices was hexahydrocurcumin. Sex differences were noted in the conversion to octa- and tetrahydrocurcumin. Liver slices from male rats produced octahydrocurcumin more efficiently, whereas slices from female rats generated more tetrahydrocurcumin. Most of the hydrocurcumins were in the glucuronidated form with a significant proportion sulfate. DMC and BDMC were similarly metabolized (Hoehle et al. 2006). In contrast, an *in vivo* study on the metabolism of DMC in rats uncovered seven additional reduction products in urine and feces after oral intake. These included primarily 5-O-methyl- and 5-dehydroxy-hexahydrodemethoxycurcumins (Fig. 5.1). The distribution of these additional reduction products differed in urine and feces. Since DMC is the only asymmetric curcuminoid, the two enol isomers could be distinguished by NMR. The isomer with the enol group in the C5 position was found to predominate (Zeng et al. 2007). This is consistent with the observation that methylation and dehydroxylation occurs primarily at this site.

Cytosol extracts from rat liver or alcohol dehydrogenase supplemented with NADH produced the full spectrum of unconjugated curcumin reduction products while microsomal fractions supplemented with uridine diphosphate glucuronic acid produced the glucuronidated products (Hoehle et al. 2006). Similar results were obtained by Ireson et al. (2002). The glucuronidation of curcumin was further quantitated in cell-free microsomal preparations from liver and intestine (Pfeiffer et al. 2007). While human microsomal preparations from intestines and liver yielded similar glucuronidation activities, the activity in microsomes from rat intestine was about fourfold higher than from liver (Pfeiffer et al. 2007). In contrast, Ireson et al. (2002) detected a 60-fold higher glucuronidation activity in rat liver than intestine. In human microsomal preparations, the activity was about 2.7-fold higher in the intestine than in the liver. Similarly, Asai and Miyazawa (2000) found an approximately threefold higher glucuronidation activity in enzyme preparations from rat liver compared to both small and large intestine.

The glucuronidation of curcumin is catalyzed by UDP-glucuronosyltransferase and this enzyme exists in multiple isoforms (Tukey and Strassburg 2000). Microsomes expressing nine UGT isoforms that are also expressed in human liver and intestines were expressed in baculovirus-infected cells and analyzed for their ability to differentially activate curcuminoid glucuronidation. Although most of the isoforms were to some extent able to affect curcuminoid glucuronidation, the highest activities for the native curcuminoids were found with isoforms UGT1A1, 1A8, and 1A10

(Hoehle et al. 2007; Pfeiffer et al. 2007). Using hexahydrocurcumin as a substrate the highest activities were found with isoforms UGT1A8, 1A9, and 2B7. Both the native and the hydrogenated form of BDMC appeared to be poorer substrates for UGT than the two other curcuminoids (Hoehle et al. 2007).

Sulfation is accomplished with the cytosolic enzyme sulfotransferase [SULT] (Nagata and Yamazoe 2000). SULT activity was primarily detected in enzyme preparations from rat liver and kidney with little or no activity in either large or small intestines (Asai and Miyazawa 2000). Similar results were obtained by Ireson et al. (2002) with cytosol preparations from rat livers showing a sevenfold higher sulfation activity than rat intestines. In contrast, SULT activities in human intestinal preparations were about 2.6-fold higher than those in the liver. Furthermore, the presence of the two SULT isoforms SULT1A1 and SULT1A3 were identified by Western blot analysis in human intestinal and liver tissue (Ireson et al. 2002).

Both glucuronidated and sulfated curcumin were also identified in the plasma from peripheral and portal circulation in humans after oral ingestion of curcumin (Garcea et al. 2004). In one study, the ratio of glucuronidated/sulfated product was found to be 1.92 (Vareed et al. 2008). Baum et al. (2007) detected no curcuminoids or metabolic products unless the plasma had been pretreated with glucuronidase. In addition, the reduction product tetrahydrocurcumin was identified together with significant amounts of ferulic acid and vanillic acid (Baum et al. 2007).

Glutathione conjugation of curcumin mediated by glutathione S-transferase has also been reported in cell-free preparations from human intestine and liver and in cultured Caco-2 cells. In contrast to the phenolic glucuronide and sulfate conjugation, this conjugation takes place on the (C1) unsaturated carbonyl site of curcumin (Usta et al. 2007) [Figs. 5.1 and 5.2]. A glucuronidation product at the enol site of curcumin was also identified in cell free preparations by Pfeiffer et al. (2007) [Fig. 5.1]. However, since these conjugation products have not been unequivocally identified *in vivo*, their biological significance remains uncertain.

Based on these data, it seems likely that after oral uptake, a portion of the free curcumin is first glucuronidated and/or sulfated in the intestinal mucosa concomitant with systemic uptake. Further phase I reduction may then take place in the liver, where the curcumin reduction products may also be conjugated prior to excretion via the bile (feces) and to a much lesser extent the kidneys. The remaining free curcumin that escapes conjugation in the intestines is then likely complexed with albumin and other serum proteins as it is transferred to the bloodstream. Upon entering the capillary circulation, the free curcumin can then be released to individual cells, where they can exert their biological effects. Supporting this notion is a careful examination of the data reported by Marczylo et al. (2009). The published chromatograms seem to suggest that the composition of curcuminoids in plasma and urine differs from that in tissues. All curcuminoids in urine and the majority in plasma are conjugated. In contrast, the parent compounds seem to predominate in the organs. It is therefore conceivable that curcumin in plasma reflects residual curcumin that has escaped cellular binding and has been metabolized in the liver. Circulating curcumin may also reflect metabolic products from other cells and tissues. For example, Baum et al. (2007) identified significant amounts of the additional curcumin-derived products vanillic acid and ferulic acid in plasma and Holder (1978) reported the presence of dihydroferulic acid in bile. Although these compounds are identical or structurally related to those formed by chemical decomposition, it is conceivable that alternative metabolic processes exist other than the reduction processes that typically occur in the liver. The conspicuously low and rapidly declining plasma levels may reflect rapid tissue binding followed by gradual slow release of unconventional metabolic products.

5.5 Strategies for Increasing Curcumin Bioavailability

The limited uptake of curcumin in the intestinal tract may conceivably be due to its low solubility. Strategies to overcome this obstacle include the development of formulations that improve the solubilization of curcumin. A further problem is its rapid conversion to biologically less active conjugates followed by excretion via the bile or urine. Inhibiting this metabolic conversion and thereby increasing the half-life of available curcumin in circulation offers the additional potential possibility for enhancing its bioavailability. In addition, the design of structural analogues that retain or enhance the biological activity of curcumin and show a better solubilization profile in water is vigorously pursued.

5.5.1 Inhibition of Metabolic Enzymes

Piperine is an alkaloid derived from black pepper that has been shown to enhance the oral bioavailability by oral uptake of a wide range of drugs and supplements, including phenytoin (Pattanaik et al. 2006), theophylline, propranolol, (Bano et al. 1991), coenzyme Q10 (Badmaev et al. 2000), β-lactam antibiotics (Hiwale et al. 2002), and curcumin (Shoba et al. 1998) [For review, see (Srinivasan 2007)]. The mechanism for this effect remains obscure, but it may involve synergistic interactions between piperine and the co-administered substances, inhibition of gastrointestinal passage (Bajad et al. 2001), or the inhibition of metabolic enzymes.

Most relevant for the effect on curcumin metabolism are earlier reports that piperine inhibits the activity of UGT both *in vivo* and *in vitro* (Atal et al. 1985; Reen and Singh 1991; Singh et al. 1986). The inhibition of UGT was more pronounced in cell-free preparations from rat intestine than liver (Reen and Singh 1991). However, a more recent systematic *in vitro* study on the inhibition of metabolic enzymes from human liver preparations and the intestinal cell line LS180 showed no inhibition of acetaminophen glucuronidation or sulfation by piperine (Volak et al. 2008). However, piperine inhibited UGT activity *in vivo* and *in vitro* and this effect was enhanced *in vivo* by the co-administration of curcumin and capsaicin (Suresh and Srinivasan 2006). Interestingly, curcuminoids by themselves inhibited both glucuronidation and sulfation (Volak et al. 2008). Similarly, Basu et al. reported the inhibition of UGTs with mouse duodenal microsomes after oral uptake of curcumin and in LS180 cells by preventing PKC-mediated phosphorylation of UGT (Basu et al. 2004, 2007). These effects were limited primarily to the intestinal mucosa. Administration of curcuminoids and piperine (50 μM) together did not appreciably change the IC_{50} values for glucuronidation (11 μM) or sulfation (4.1 μM) vs. curcuminoids alone (10 and 4.3 μM, respectively). Both curcuminoids and piperine also specifically inhibited multiple cytochrome P_{450} enzymes (Oetari et al. 1996; Suresh and Srinivasan 2006; Volak et al. 2008). Another *in vitro* study found that a 100 μM concentration of piperine inhibited the glucuronidation of (−)-epigallocatechin-3-gallate from green tea by 40% with microsomes from the mouse intestinal tract but not with liver (Lambert et al. 2004).

Although these studies are not conclusive, they seem to suggest a role for piperine in the inhibition of glucuronidation in the intestinal mucosa. The observation that there is a stronger inhibition of UGTs from intestinal tissue than liver seems to support this notion. However, the fact that curcuminoids by themselves also inhibit both sulfation and glucuronidation suggests that this effect alone may not be responsible for the increase in bioavailability from the co-administration of curcumin and piperine as observed in several studies.

Oral administration of curcumin (2 g/kg) and piperine (20 mg/kg) in rats, transiently increased the level of serum curcumin by about 154%. In humans, the effect was more profound. Ingestion of 2 g of curcumin and 20 mg of piperine increased the serum curcumin level 20-fold versus the intake of curcumin alone (Shoba et al. 1998). A cross-over study with six human subjects ingesting 2 g of curcumin with 5 mg of piperine showed an initial rapid increase to a maximum after 60 min to serum curcumin levels that were about threefold higher than without piperine. That level remained stable and declined after 140 min following ingestion. In contrast, curcumin levels without piperine gradually increased for 140 min after uptake followed by a rapid decline (Anand et al. 2007). A study coincidental to developing probes for Alzheimer β-amyloid plaque imaging found increased levels (45–75%) of radiolabeled [18^F]-fluoropropyl substituted curcumin in blood, brain, and spleen after co-injection with piperine in mice. However, these effects were transient and had already been neutralized within 30–60 min (Ryu et al. 2006).

These *in vivo* studies show that the simultaneous administration of curcumin and piperine may have some beneficial effects on the bioavailability of curcumin. Although seemingly impressive, these effects are exceedingly short-lived and terminate within 30–120 min. Clearly, more studies are required to assess the therapeutic potential of co-administered curcumin and piperine. These include studies of chronic intake and perhaps using higher doses of piperine, which has a favorable toxic profile when ingested orally [review: (Srinivasan 2007)].

5.5.2 *Formulations for Enhanced Solubilization*

Numerous attempts have been made to improve curcumin bioavailability and stability by enhancing its solubility properties. In addition to curcumin solubilization with albumin solutions and serum as described earlier, these include the encapsulation in liposomes, micelles, or nanoparticles, complex formation with phospholipids, cyclodextrin, or metals.

Liposomal micelles characteristically contain amphiphilic polymers with hydrophobic and hydrophilic blocks of varying composition. Under appropriate conditions these polymers self-assemble into micelles in aqueous solutions (Letchford et al. 2008). Such micelles dramatically improve the solubility and chemical stability of curcumin in aqueous media compared to free curcumin (Tønnesen 2002). As determined by *in vitro* dialysis, curcumin release from micelles (98.7%) was slower than that of free curcumin (68%) in distilled water after 6 h. However, in the presence of serum albumin, the situation was reversed [36% and 70.8%, respectively] (Ma et al. 2007). Kunwar et al., found comparable binding of liposomal and albumin solubilized curcumin to cultured cells (Kunwar et al. 2006). Liposomal preparations increased the chemical stability of curcumin in phosphate buffered saline, whereas the stability was similar to free curcumin in plasma and cell culture medium containing fetal bovine serum (Chen et al. 2009). It is most likely that this is due to the stabilization of free curcumin by binding to albumin and other serum components. Curcumin encapsulated in liposomes were found to have similar properties to conventional preparations in cell culture studies (Li et al. 2005). After i.v. injection of liposomal curcumin in mice (40 mg/kg curcumin), the liposomal preparation inhibited pancreatic carcinoma, colorectal cancer and tumor angiogenesis (Li et al. 2005, 2007). However, these studies did not specifically address the *in vivo* bioavailability of liposomal curcumin preparations.

A study administering liposomal-encapsulated curcumin (1 mg/100 ml) by i.v. injection into mice reported a peak plasma concentration of 8.79 pM after 4 h. The level declined to undetectable levels after 48 h. By comparison, DMSO solubilized curcumin was never detected in the plasma. Low concentrations of curcumin (0.009–0.070 μM) were also detected in the liver after both liposomal and DMSO-solubilized curcumin injection (Wang et al. 2008). In a different study, micellar curcumin was compared to curcumin solubilized in a formulation (DPD) of N,N-dimethylacetamide [15%], PEG400 [45%], and 5% dextrose [40%] by i.v. injection into rats. A rapid decrease in curcumin plasma concentration with both formulations was observed within 2 h of injection. However, liposomal curcumin concentrations remained relatively stable for 24 h [$t_{1/2}$ = 60.5 h], whereas curcumin solubilized in DPD rapidly declined to unquantifiable levels [$t_{1/2}$ = 0.57 h]. In addition, other pharmacokinetic parameters such as clearance, volume distribution, and mean residence time were more favorable for micellar curcumin by orders of magnitude (Ma et al. 2007). Two hours after oral ingestion by rats, curcumin solubilized as a phospholipid complex had a higher serum concentration (~700 ng/ml) than conventional curcumin (~260 ng/ml). Similar ratios persisted after 16 h (~300 vs. 100 ng/ml). However, it needs to be pointed out that the administered dose for the phospholipid-curcumin complex (300 mg/kg) was three times higher than the dose for conventional curcumin [100 mg/kg] (Liu et al. 2006), although similar results were obtained by Maiti et al. (2007) using the same amount of conventional curcumin and phospholipid-curcumin complex [1 g/kg]. In this case, the maximal concentration was reached within 0.75–2 h after uptake with serum concentrations of 0.5 μg/ml for conventional curcumin and

1.2 μg/ml for phospholipid-curcumin with concomitant increases in elimination half-life (Maiti et al. 2007).

In cell culture studies, PLGA [poly(lactic-co-glycolic acid)]-encapsulated curcumin was shown to improve cellular uptake by as much as sixfold compared to free curcumin (Mukerjee and Vishwanatha 2009; Yallapu et al. 2010). Similar results were noted with different formulations of nanoparticles (Bisht et al. 2007; Thangapazham et al. 2008). After oral application in rats of PLGA-encapsulated curcumin (100 mg/kg), a maximal serum curcumin concentration of 260.5 ng/ml was achieved at 2 h after ingestion, compared to only 90.3 ng/ml at 0.5 h after ingestion of a higher dose (250 mg/kg) of suspended curcumin, together with a longer plasma half-life. The effect on suspended curcumin was further enhanced by the co-administration of piperine (Shaikh et al. 2009). Using nanoparticles composed of polymers of N-isopropylacrylamide, vinylpyrrolidone, and acrylic acid in a mouse model, Bisht et al. (2010) found reduced tumor growth and metastasis after i.p. administration of encapsulated curcumin [25 mg/kg](Bisht et al. 2010) in combination with gemcitabine. Maximum plasma concentrations (~13,000 ng/ml) were reached by less than 5 h after injection and declined to undetectable levels by 24 h. By comparison, plasma levels after injection of curcumin suspended in corn oil were essentially undetectable (Bisht et al. 2010).

The inclusion of curcumin into casein micelles was found to have a similar cytotoxic profile as free curcumin on HeLa cells (Sahu et al. 2008). Curcumin has also been used as an adjuvant in the nanoemulsion delivery of paclitaxel (Ganta et al. 2010) and as a model cream base (Teichmann et al. 2007; Tiyaboonchai et al. 2007).

The interaction of curcumin and phosphatidylcholine from egg and soy was characterized by fluorescence spectroscopy. The determined equilibrium constants were 32.5 and 26.4 μM, respectively (Began et al. 1999). Rats receiving curcumin [340 mg/kg] formulated with phosphatidylcholine orally showed fivefold higher serum concentrations than those receiving standard curcumin. Similarly, liver concentrations were also higher while the curcumin concentration was somewhat lower in the intestinal tract in rats receiving phosphatidylcholine than standard curcumin formulations (Marczylo et al. 2007).

Cyclodextrins are cyclic compounds containing 6–8 glucose monomers (α, β, and γ) with both central less polar and outer more hydrophilic moieties. The glucose residues can be further methylated or hydroxypropylated (Tomren et al. 2007; Tønnesen et al. 2002). It is often assumed that curcumin forms an inclusion complex within the hydrophobic central cavity. However, it is also possible that curcumin, due to its amphophilic character, forms different complexes by interaction with both the hydrophilic and hydrophobic residues of cyclodextrins (Loftsson et al. 2004). In one study, curcumin solubility was increased by complexation with various cyclodextrins by a factor of at least 10^4. At the same time, hydrolytic stability of curcumin was increased while photodecomposition was increased compared to curcumin in organic solvents. The highest level of solubility was achieved with a 10% solution of hydroxypropyl γ-cyclodextrin [5.35 mM] (Tomren et al. 2007) or with a supersaturated solution of hydroxypropyl β-cyclodextrin complex [~16 mM] (Yadav et al. 2009). The stoichiometric ratios of curcumin/cyclodextrins was generally found to be 1:2

(Baglole et al. 2005; Tang et al. 2002; Yadav et al. 2009). This lead Baglole et al. (2005) to propose a structure in which each phenolic ring of the curcumin molecule is immersed into the hydrophobic cavity of the cyclodextrin structure. An *in vivo* study on dextran sulfate induced colitis in rats found improvement in rats treated with both conventional curcumin and curcumin-cyclodextrin complexes with the curcumin-cyclodextrin complexes being more effective (Yadav et al. 2009). Cell culture studies with hydroxypropyl-γ-cyclodextrin of curcumin showed that the curcumin-cyclodextrin complex had superior antiproliferative and anti-inflammatory effects to free curcumin (Yadav et al. 2010). Although none of these studies addressed the systemic availability of curcumin-cyclodextrin complexes, this form of curcumin solubilization nevertheless seems to have profound therapeutic potential as judged by its therapeutic effectiveness by oral uptake and their potential for high levels of curcumin solubilization. I.v. injections may further extend the therapeutic usefulness of cyclodextrin complexes due to their relatively favorable toxic profile (Stella and He 2008).

Alternative methods for curcumin solubilization include complex formation with metals (Eybl et al. 2006; John et al. 2002; Kurien and Scofield 2009; Mohammadi et al. 2005; Sui et al. 1993; Thompson et al. 2004; Valentini et al. 2009; Zebib et al. 2010) or heat solubilization, which has been reported to increase curcumin solubility 12-fold (Kurien and Scofield 2009). Although these formulations show biological activity in cell culture studies and *in vivo*, their effectiveness in enhancing bioavailability (Eybl et al. 2006) remains to be established. Another approach to increase curcumin solubility and approve oral absorption is by solid dispersion with polyvinylpyrrolidone K30 [PVP K30]. This was found to increase curcumin solubility at least 880-fold (Kaewnopparat et al. 2009; Paradkar et al. 2004; Xu et al. 2006). With an oral dose of 400 mg/kg PVP K30 dispersed curcumin in rats, peak plasma levels of 200 ng/ml were reached by 45 min after uptake (Xu et al. 2008). Another curcumin formulation of proprietary composition (BCM-95 CG) was used in a pilot cross-over study to determine its bioavailability (Antony et al. 2008). After ingesting a single dose of BCM-95 CG formulated curcumin (2 g), the maximum serum concentration of curcumin (457 ng/ml) and plasma half life (4.96 h) increased about threefold compared to the ingestion of standard curcumin ($C_{max} = 150$ ng/ml, $t_{1/2} = 2.63$ h). These effects were further enhanced by the co-administration of piperine. These results are summarized in Table 5.4.

5.5.3 *Design of Structural Analogues*

Synthetic modifications in curcumin structure have been introduced to generate a multitude of compounds variably referred to as derivatives, analogues or curcumin-related. Recent examples of modifications are substitutions at the C4 carbon between the keto groups (Padhye et al. 2009b; Yanagisawa et al. 2010), substitutions at the benzene rings (Shibata et al. 2009), conjugations at the aromatic hydroxyl groups

Table 5.4 Curcumin carriers and adjuvants: effect on plasma levels

Dose (Species), uptake	Vehicle	Concentration ratios at T_{max} (Peak): vehicle/ standard	Reference
2 g/kg (rat), p.o.	Piperine (20 mg)	1.54	Shoba et al. (1998)
2 g (human), p.o.		20	
2 g (human), p.o.	Piperine (5 mg)	3	Anand et al. (2007)
1 mg (mouse), i.v.	Liposome	8.79 pM/undetectable	Wang et al. (2008)
100 mg (rat), p.o.	Phospholipid	2.33	Liu et al. (2006)
1 g/kg (rat), p.o.	Phospholipid	2.4	Maiti et al. (2007)
250/100 mg/kg (rat), p.o.	Nanoparticle	2.9	Shaikh et al. (2009)
250 mg/kg (rat), p.o.	Piperine	1.34	
25 mg/kg (mouse), i.p.	Nanoparticle	13 μg/ml/undetectable	Bisht et al. (2010)
340 mg/kg (rat), p.o.	Phosphatidylcholine	5	Marczylo et al. (2007)
2 g (human), p.o.	BCM-95 CG	3	Antony et al. (2008)

Abbreviations: *p.o.* per os, *i.v.* intravenous, *i.p.* intraperitoneal

(Harish et al. 2010; Li et al. 2009; Majhi et al. 2010), modifications of the keto groups and substitutions at the phenyl and methoxy sites (Basile et al. 2009; Cen et al. 2009), and elimination of the aromatic hydroxyl and methoxy groups (Nardo et al. 2009). These structural changes are introduced to identify curcumin-related compounds with enhanced biological activity or bioavailability profiles. Indeed, curcumin derivatives have been described with implications for the treatments of cancer (Basile et al. 2009; Cen et al. 2009; Li et al. 2009; Majhi et al. 2010; Padhye et al. 2009b; Shibata et al. 2009), Alzheimer disease (Yanagisawa et al. 2010), and Parkinson disease (Harish et al. 2010). Most of these studies have been carried out *in vitro* with specific cell lines. However, Shibata et al. (2009) found improved survival in a mouse model for colorectal cancer with curcumin (191 days) and a curcumin derivative (213 days) compared to control mice (166.5 days). After oral uptake of a single dose (250 mg/kg), Padhye et al. (2009a) found a tenfold higher retention and distribution of fluorocurcumins into the pancreas of mice compared to curcumin. These are only a few examples of recently published curcumin derivatives with therapeutic potential. For extensive reviews on the multitude of structural modifications of curcumin and their biological effects, see Anand et al. (2008b) and Padhye et al. (2010).

5.6 Conclusion

The available data from both animal and human studies indicate that after oral uptake, a portion of the ingested curcumin is absorbed in the intestines. Here it is partially conjugated into curcumin glucuronide or sulfate by the microsomal UGT and cytosolic SULT phase II metabolic enzymes. Upon entering the circulation, the unmodified curcumin is most likely complexed with albumin and other serum constituents due to its low water solubility. Some of the unmodified curcumin is then transported to cells and tissues, where it can be detected at surprisingly high concentrations (1–10 μM) or it will be further reduced by phase I cytosolic metabolic enzymes in the liver to generate the curcumin reduction products. Conversion of curcumin by cells and tissues other than the liver is also likely, perhaps yielding unconventional metabolic products. These metabolic products are further conjugated in the liver and excreted in the feces via the bile and to a much lesser extent, the kidneys. These processes result in very low levels of mostly modified circulating curcumin, suggesting poor bioavailability. However, perhaps a better indicator of bioavailability is the concentration of curcumin in tissues, where it exists at levels high enough to exert biological effects similar to those described in *in vitro* studies. If tissue distribution is used as a criterion, curcumin may indeed have therapeutic potential. A major problem with oral curcumin intake is that much of the ingested material passes through the intestinal tract without being absorbed. Enhancing the solubility of curcumin may improve this situation, provided that the solubilization procedure retains its effectiveness throughout the intestinal tract. Another advantage of solubilized curcumin is the prospect of rendering it into a safe injectable form. In particular, i.v. injection can potentially deliver high controlled levels of curcumin directly into the circulation without exposing it to the metabolic enzymes of the intestines. Co-administration of piperine may further increase the half-life of circulating unmodified curcumin. Overall, the available data seem to suggest that curcumin has a better therapeutic potential than is suggested by its low plasma levels. The synthesis of potent analogues may further improve its effectiveness.

References

Aggarwal BB, Sung B (2009) Pharmacological basis for the role of curcumin in chronic diseases: an age-old spice with modern targets. Trends Pharmacol Sci 30:85–94

Anand P, Kunnumakkara AB, Newman RA, Aggarwal BB (2007) Bioavailability of curcumin: problems and promises. Mol Pharm 4:807–818

Anand P, Sundaram C, Jhurani S, Kunnumakkara AB, Aggarwal BB (2008a) Curcumin and cancer: an "old-age" disease with an "age-old" solution. Cancer Lett 267:133–164

Anand P, Thomas SG, Kunnumakkara AB, Sundaram C, Harikumar KB, Sung B, Tharakan ST, Misra K, Priyadarsini IK, Rajasekharan KN, Aggarwal BB (2008b) Biological activities of curcumin and its analogues (Congeners) made by man and Mother Nature. Biochem Pharmacol 76:1590–1611

Antony B, Merina B, Iyer VS, Judy N, Lennertz K, Joyal S (2008) A pilot cross-over study to evaluate human oral bioavailability of BCM-95CG (biocurcumax). A novel bioenhanced preparation of curcumin. Indian J Pharm Sci 70:445–449

Asai A, Miyazawa T (2000) Occurrence of orally administered curcuminoid as glucuronide and glucuronide/sulfate conjugates in rat plasma. Life Sci 67:2785–2793

Atal CK, Dubey RK, Singh J (1985) Biochemical basis of enhanced drug bioavailability by piperine: evidence that piperine is a potent inhibitor of drug metabolism. J Pharmacol Exp Ther 232:258–262

Badmaev V, Majeed M, Prakash L (2000) Piperine derived from black pepper increases the plasma levels of coenzyme Q10 following oral supplementation. J Nutr Biochem 11:109–113

Baglole KN, Boland GB, Wagner BD (2005) Fluorescence enhancement of curcumin upon inclusion into parent and modified cyclodextrins. J Photochem Photobiol A 173:230–237
Bajad S, Bedi KL, Singla AK, Johri RK (2001) Piperine inhibits gastric emptying and gastrointestinal transit in rats and mice. Planta Med 67:176–179
Balasubramanian K (2006) Molecular orbital basis for yellow curry spice curcumin's prevention of Alzheimer's disease. J Agric Food Chem 54:3512–3520
Bano G, Raina RK, Zutshi U, Bedi KL, Johri RK, Sharma SC (1991) Effect of piperine on bioavailability and pharmacokinetics of propranolol and theophylline in healthy volunteers. Eur J Clin Pharmacol 41:615–617
Barik A, Priyadarsini KI, Mohan H (2003) Photophysical studies on binding of curcumin to bovine serum albumins. Photochem Photobiol 77:597–603
Basile V, Ferrari E, Lazzari S, Belluti S, Pignedoli F, Imbriano C (2009) Curcumin derivatives: molecular basis of their anti-cancer activity. Biochem Pharmacol 78:1305–1315
Basu NK, Kole L, Kubota S, Owens IS (2004) Human UDP-glucuronosyltransferases show atypical metabolism of mycophenolic acid and inhibition by curcumin. Drug Metab Dispos 32:768-773
Basu NK, Kole L, Basu M, McDonagh AF, Owens IS (2007) Targeted inhibition of glucuronidation markedly improves drug efficacy in mice - a model. Biochem Biophys Res Commun 360:7–13
Baum L, Cheung SK, Mok VC, Lam LC, Leung VP, Hui E, Ng CC, Chow M, Ho PC, Lam S, Woo J, Chiu HF, Goggins W, Zee B, Wong A, Mok H, Cheng WK, Fong C, Lee JS, Chan MH, Szeto SS, Lui VW, Tsoh J, Kwok TC, Chan IH, Lam CW (2007) Curcumin effects on blood lipid profile in a 6-month human study. Pharmacol Res 56:509–514
Baum L, Lam CW, Cheung SK, Kwok T, Lui V, Tsoh J, Lam L, Leung V, Hui E, Ng C, Woo J, Chiu HF, Goggins WB, Zee BC, Cheng KF, Fong CY, Wong A, Mok H, Chow MS, Ho PC, Ip SP, Ho CS, Yu XW, Lai CY, Chan MH, Szeto S, Chan IH, Mok V (2008) Six-month randomized, placebo-controlled, double-blind, pilot clinical trial of curcumin in patients with Alzheimer disease. J Clin Psychopharmacol 28:110–113
Began G, Sudharshan E, Udaya Sankar K, Appu Rao AG (1999) Interaction of curcumin with phosphatidylcholine: a spectrofluorometric study. J Agric Food Chem 47:4992–4997
Begum AN, Jones MR, Lim GP, Morihara T, Kim P, Heath DD, Rock CL, Pruitt MA, Yang F, Hudspeth B, Hu S, Faull KF, Teter B, Cole GM, Frautschy SA (2008) Curcumin structure-function, bioavailability, and efficacy in models of neuroinflammation and Alzheimer's disease. J Pharmacol Exp Ther 326:196–208
Bernabé-Pineda M, Ramírez-Silva MT, Romero-Romo M, González-Vergara E, Rojas-Hernández A (2004) Determination of acidity constants of curcumin in aqueous solution and apparent rate constant of its decomposition. Spectrochim Acta A Mol Biomol Spectrosc 60:1091–1097
Bisht S, Feldmann G, Soni S, Ravi R, Karikar C, Maitra A (2007) Polymeric nanoparticle-encapsulated curcumin ("nanocurcumin"): a novel strategy for human cancer therapy. J Nanobiotechnol 5:3
Bisht S, Mizuma M, Feldmann G, Ottenhof NA, Hong SM, Pramanik D, Chenna V, Karikari C, Sharma R, Goggins MG, Rudek MA, Ravi R, Maitra A (2010) Systemic administration of polymeric nanoparticle-encapsulated curcumin (NanoCurc) blocks tumor growth and metastases in preclinical models of pancreatic cancer. Mol Cancer Ther 9(8):2255–2264
Blasius R, Duvoix A, Morceau F, Schnekenburger M, Delhalle S, Henry E, Dicato M, Diederich M (2004) Curcumin stability and its effect on glutathione S-transferase P1-1 mRNA expression in K562 cells. Ann N Y Acad Sci 1030:442–448
Braga ME, Leal PF, Carvalho JE, Meireles MA (2003) Comparison of yield, composition, and antioxidant activity of turmeric (Curcuma longa L.) extracts obtained using various techniques. J Agric Food Chem 51:6604–6611
Cen L, Hutzen B, Ball S, DeAngelis S, Chen CL, Fuchs JR, Li C, Li PK, Lin J (2009) New structural analogues of curcumin exhibit potent growth suppressive activity in human colorectal carcinoma cells. BMC Cancer 9:99
Chen C, Johnston TD, Jeon H, Gedaly R, McHugh PP, Burke TG, Ranjan D (2009) An in vitro study of liposomal curcumin: stability, toxicity and biological activity in human lymphocytes and Epstein-Barr virus-transformed human B-cells. Int J Pharm 366:133–139

Cheng AL, Hsu CH, Lin JK, Hsu MM, Ho YF, Shen TS, Ko JY, Lin JT, Lin BR, Ming-Shiang W, Yu HS, Jee SH, Chen GS, Chen TM, Chen CA, Lai MK, Pu YS, Pan MH, Wang YJ, Tsai CC, Hsieh CY (2001) Phase I clinical trial of curcumin, a chemopreventive agent, in patients with high-risk or pre-malignant lesions. Anticancer Res 21:2895–2900

Dhillon N, Aggarwal BB, Newman RA, Wolff RA, Kunnumakkara AB, Abbruzzese JL, Ng CS, Badmaev V, Kurzrock R (2008) Phase II trial of curcumin in patients with advanced pancreatic cancer. Clin Cancer Res 14:4491–4499

Epstein J, Sanderson IR, Macdonald TT (2010) Curcumin as a therapeutic agent: the evidence from in vitro, animal and human studies. Br J Nutr 103:1545–1557

Eybl V, Kotyzova D, Leseticky L, Bludovska M, Koutensky J (2006) The influence of curcumin and manganese complex of curcumin on cadmium-induced oxidative damage and trace elements status in tissues of mice. J Appl Toxicol 26:207–212

Frautschy SA, Hu W, Kim P, Miller SA, Chu T, Harris-White ME, Cole GM (2001) Phenolic anti-inflammatory antioxidant reversal of Abeta-induced cognitive deficits and neuropathology. Neurobiol Aging 22:993–1005

Ganta S, Devalapally H, Amiji M (2010) Curcumin enhances oral bioavailability and anti-tumor therapeutic efficacy of paclitaxel upon administration in nanoemulsion formulation. J Pharm Sci 99:4630–4641

Garcea G, Jones DJ, Singh R, Dennison AR, Farmer PB, Sharma RA, Steward WP, Gescher AJ, Berry DP (2004) Detection of curcumin and its metabolites in hepatic tissue and portal blood of patients following oral administration. Br J Cancer 90:1011–1015

Garcea G, Berry DP, Jones DJ, Singh R, Dennison AR, Farmer PB, Sharma RA, Steward WP, Gescher AJ (2005) Consumption of the putative chemopreventive agent curcumin by cancer patients: assessment of curcumin levels in the colorectum and their pharmacodynamic consequences. Cancer Epidemiol Biomark Prev 14:120–125

Garcia-Alloza M, Borrelli LA, Rozkalne A, Hyman BT, Bacskai BJ (2007) Curcumin labels amyloid pathology in vivo, disrupts existing plaques, and partially restores distorted neurites in an Alzheimer mouse model. J Neurochem 102:1095–1104

Harish G, Venkateshappa C, Mythri RB, Dubey SK, Mishra K, Singh N, Vali S, Bharath MM (2010) Bioconjugates of curcumin display improved protection against glutathione depletion mediated oxidative stress in a dopaminergic neuronal cell line: implications for Parkinson's disease. Bioorg Med Chem 18:2631–2638

Hatcher H, Planalp R, Cho J, Torti FM, Torti SV (2008) Curcumin: from ancient medicine to current clinical trials. Cell Mol Life Sci 65:1631–1652

Hiserodt R, Hartman TG, Ho C-T, Rosen RT (1996) Characterization of powdered turmeric by liquid chromatography-mass spectrometry and gas chromatography-mass spectrometry. J Chromatogr A 740:51–63

Hiwale AR, Dhuley JN, Naik SR (2002) Effect of co-administration of piperine on pharmacokinetics of beta-lactam antibiotics in rats. Indian J Exp Biol 40:277–281

Hoehle SI, Pfeiffer E, Solyom AM, Metzler M (2006) Metabolism of curcuminoids in tissue slices and subcellular fractions from rat liver. J Agric Food Chem 54:756–764

Hoehle SI, Pfeiffer E, Metzler M (2007) Glucuronidation of curcuminoids by human microsomal and recombinant UDP-glucuronosyltransferases. Mol Nutr Food Res 51:932–938

Holder GM, Plummer JL, Ryan AJ (1978) The metabolism and excretion of curcumin (1,7-bis-(4-hydroxy-3-methoxyphenyl)-1,6-heptadiene-3,5-dione) in the rat. Xenobiotica 8:761–768

Huang MT, Ma W, Lu YP, Chang RL, Fisher C, Manchand PS, Newmark HL, Conney AH (1995) Effects of curcumin, demethoxycurcumin, bisdemethoxycurcumin and tetrahydrocurcumin on 12-O-tetradecanoylphorbol-13-acetate-induced tumor promotion. Carcinogenesis 16:2493–2497

Ireson C, Orr S, Jones DJ, Verschoyle R, Lim CK, Luo JL, Howells L, Plummer S, Jukes R, Williams M, Steward WP, Gescher A (2001) Characterization of metabolites of the chemopreventive agent curcumin in human and rat hepatocytes and in the rat in vivo, and evaluation of their ability to inhibit phorbol ester-induced prostaglandin E2 production. Cancer Res 61:1058–1064

Ireson CR, Jones DJ, Orr S, Coughtrie MW, Boocock DJ, Williams ML, Farmer PB, Steward WP, Gescher AJ (2002) Metabolism of the cancer chemopreventive agent curcumin in human and rat intestine. Cancer Epidemiol Biomark Prev 11:105–111

Jayaprakasha GK, Jagan Mohan Rao L, Sakariah KK (2002) Improved HPLC method for the determination of curcumin, demethoxycurcumin, and bisdemethoxycurcumin. J Agric Food Chem 50:3668–3672
John VD, Kuttan G, Krishnankutty K (2002) Anti-tumour studies of metal chelates of synthetic curcuminoids. J Exp Clin Cancer Res 21:219–224
Jovanovic SV, Steenken S, Boone CW, Simic MG (1999) H-atom transfer is a preferred mechanism of curcumin. J Am Chem Soc 121:9677–9681
Kaewnopparat N, Kaewnopparat S, Jangwang A, Maneenaun D, Chuchome T, Panichayupakaranant P (2009) Increased solubility, dissolution and physicochemical studies of curcumin-polyvinylpyrrolidone K-30 solid dispersions. World Acad Sci Eng Technol 55:229–234
Kunwar A, Barik A, Pandey R, Priyadarsini KI (2006) Transport of liposomal and albumin loaded curcumin to living cells: an absorption and fluorescence spectroscopic study. Biochim Biophys Acta 1760:1513–1520
Kurien BT, Scofield RH (2009) Increasing the solubility of the nutraceutical curcumin by heat and inhibition of oxidative modification. Mol Nutr Food Res 53:308
Lambert JD, Hong J, Kim DH, Mishin VM, Yang CS (2004) Piperine enhances the bioavailability of the tea polyphenol (−)-epigallocatechin-3-gallate in mice. J Nutr 134:1948–1952
Lao CD, Ruffin MTt, Normolle D, Heath DD, Murray SI, Bailey JM, Boggs ME, Crowell J, Rock CL, Brenner DE (2006) Dose escalation of a curcuminoid formulation. BMC Complement Altern Med 6:10
Letchford K, Liggins R, Burt H (2008) Solubilization of hydrophobic drugs by methoxy poly(ethylene glycol)-block-polycaprolactone diblock copolymer micelles: theoretical and experimental data and correlations. J Pharm Sci 97:1179–1190
Leung MH, Kee TW (2009) Effective stabilization of curcumin by association to plasma proteins: human serum albumin and fibrinogen. Langmuir 25:5773–5777
Li L, Braiteh FS, Kurzrock R (2005) Liposome-encapsulated curcumin: in vitro and in vivo effects on proliferation, apoptosis, signaling, and angiogenesis. Cancer 104:1322–1331
Li L, Ahmed B, Mehta K, Kurzrock R (2007) Liposomal curcumin with and without oxaliplatin: effects on cell growth, apoptosis, and angiogenesis in colorectal cancer. Mol Cancer Ther 6:1276–1282
Li J, Wang Y, Yang C, Wang P, Oelschlager DK, Zheng Y, Tian DA, Grizzle WE, Buchsbaum DJ, Wan M (2009) Polyethylene glycosylated curcumin conjugate inhibits pancreatic cancer cell growth through inactivation of Jab1. Mol Pharmacol 76:81–90
Lim GP, Chu T, Yang F, Beech W, Frautschy SA, Cole GM (2001) The curry spice curcumin reduces oxidative damage and amyloid pathology in an Alzheimer transgenic mouse. J Neurosci 21:8370–8377
Liu A, Lou H, Zhao L, Fan P (2006) Validated LC/MS/MS assay for curcumin and tetrahydrocurcumin in rat plasma and application to pharmacokinetic study of phospholipid complex of curcumin. J Pharm Biomed Anal 40:720–727
Loftsson T, Masson M, Brewster ME (2004) Self-association of cyclodextrins and cyclodextrin complexes. J Pharm Sci 93:1091–1099
Ma Z, Shayeganpour A, Brocks DR, Lavasanifar A, Samuel J (2007) High-performance liquid chromatography analysis of curcumin in rat plasma: application to pharmacokinetics of polymeric micellar formulation of curcumin. Biomed Chromatogr 21:546–552
Mague JT, Alworth WL, Payton FL (2004) Curcumin and derivatives. Acta Crystallogr C 60:o608–o610
Maiti K, Mukherjee K, Gantait A, Saha BP, Mukherjee PK (2007) Curcumin-phospholipid complex: preparation, therapeutic evaluation and pharmacokinetic study in rats. Int J Pharm 330:155–163
Majhi A, Rahman GM, Panchal S, Das J (2010) Binding of curcumin and its long chain derivatives to the activator binding domain of novel protein kinase C. Bioorg Med Chem 18:1591–1598
Mandeville JS, Froehlich E, Tajmir-Riahi HA (2009) Study of curcumin and genistein interactions with human serum albumin. J Pharm Biomed Anal 49:468–474

Marczylo TH, Verschoyle RD, Cooke DN, Morazzoni P, Steward WP, Gescher AJ (2007) Comparison of systemic availability of curcumin with that of curcumin formulated with phosphatidylcholine. Cancer Chemother Pharmacol 60:171–177

Marczylo TH, Steward WP, Gescher AJ (2009) Rapid analysis of curcumin and curcumin metabolites in rat biomatrices using a novel ultraperformance liquid chromatography (UPLC) method. J Agric Food Chem 57:797–803

Mohammadi K, Thompson KH, Patrick BO, Storr T, Martins C, Polishchuk E, Yuen VG, McNeill JH, Orvig C (2005) Synthesis and characterization of dual function vanadyl, gallium and indium curcumin complexes for medicinal applications. J Inorg Biochem 99:2217–2225

Mukerjee A, Vishwanatha JK (2009) Formulation, characterization and evaluation of curcumin-loaded PLGA nanospheres for cancer therapy. Anticancer Res 29:3867–3875

Nagata K, Yamazoe Y (2000) Pharmacogenetics of sulfotransferase. Annu Rev Pharmacol Toxicol 40:159–176

Narayanan NK, Nargi D, Randolph C, Narayanan BA (2009) Liposome encapsulation of curcumin and resveratrol in combination reduces prostate cancer incidence in PTEN knockout mice. Int J Cancer 125:1–8

Nardo L, Andreoni A, Bondani M, Masson M, Hjorth Tonnesen H (2009) Studies on curcumin and curcuminoids. XXXIV. Photophysical properties of a symmetrical, non-substituted curcumin analogue. J Photochem Photobiol B 97:77–86

Oetari S, Sudibyo M, Commandeur JN, Samhoedi R, Vermeulen NP (1996) Effects of curcumin on cytochrome P450 and glutathione S-transferase activities in rat liver. Biochem Pharmacol 51:39–45

Ono K, Hasegawa K, Naiki H, Yamada M (2004) Curcumin has potent anti-amyloidogenic effects for Alzheimer's beta-amyloid fibrils in vitro. J Neurosci Res 75:742–750

Padhye S, Banerjee S, Chavan D, Pandye S, Swamy KV, Ali S, Li J, Dou QP, Sarkar FH (2009a) Fluorocurcumins as cyclooxygenase-2 inhibitor: molecular docking, pharmacokinetics and tissue distribution in mice. Pharm Res 26:2438–2445

Padhye S, Yang H, Jamadar A, Cui QC, Chavan D, Dominiak K, McKinney J, Banerjee S, Dou QP, Sarkar FH (2009b) New difluoro Knoevenagel condensates of curcumin, their Schiff bases and copper complexes as proteasome inhibitors and apoptosis inducers in cancer cells. Pharm Res 26:1874–1880

Padhye S, Chavan D, Pandey S, Deshpande J, Swamy KV, Sarkar FH (2010) Perspectives on chemopreventive and therapeutic potential of curcumin analogs in medicinal chemistry. Mini Rev Med Chem 10:372–387

Pan MH, Huang TM, Lin JK (1999) Biotransformation of curcumin through reduction and glucuronidation in mice. Drug Metab Dispos 27:486–494

Paradkar A, Ambike AA, Jadhav BK, Mahadik KR (2004) Characterization of curcumin-PVP solid dispersion obtained by spray drying. Int J Pharm 271:281–286

Pattanaik S, Hota D, Prabhakar S, Kharbanda P, Pandhi P (2006) Effect of piperine on the steady-state pharmacokinetics of phenytoin in patients with epilepsy. Phytother Res 20:683–686

Payton F, Sandusky P, Alworth WL (2007) NMR study of the solution structure of curcumin. J Nat Prod 70:143–146

Perkins S, Verschoyle RD, Hill K, Parveen I, Threadgill MD, Sharma RA, Williams ML, Steward WP, Gescher AJ (2002) Chemopreventive efficacy and pharmacokinetics of curcumin in the min/+ mouse, a model of familial adenomatous polyposis. Cancer Epidemiol Biomark Prev 11:535–540

Pfeiffer E, Hoehle S, Solyom AM, Metzler M (2003) Studies on the stability of turmeric constituents. J Food Eng 56:257–259

Pfeiffer E, Hoehle SI, Walch SG, Riess A, Solyom AM, Metzler M (2007) Curcuminoids form reactive glucuronides in vitro. J Agric Food Chem 55:538–544

Priyadarsini KI, Maity DK, Naik GH, Kumar MS, Unnikrishnan MK, Satav JG, Mohan H (2003) Role of phenolic O-H and methylene hydrogen on the free radical reactions and antioxidant activity of curcumin. Free Radic Biol Med 35:475–484

Pulla Reddy AC, Sudharshan E, Appu Rao AG, Lokesh BR (1999) Interaction of curcumin with human serum albumin–a spectroscopic study. Lipids 34:1025–1029
Quitschke WW (2008) Differential solubility of curcuminoids in serum and albumin solutions: implications for analytical and therapeutic applications. BMC Biotechnol 8:84
Ravindranath V, Chandrasekhara N (1980) Absorption and tissue distribution of curcumin in rats. Toxicology 16:259–265
Ravindranath V, Chandrasekhara N (1981) In vitro studies on the intestinal absorption of curcumin in rats. Toxicology 20:251–257
Ravindranath V, Chandrasekhara N (1982) Metabolism of curcumin–studies with [3H]curcumin. Toxicology 22:337–344
Reen RK, Singh J (1991) In vitro and in vivo inhibition of pulmonary cytochrome P450 activities by piperine, a major ingredient of piper species. Indian J Exp Biol 29:568–573
Ryu EK, Choe YS, Lee KH, Choi Y, Kim BT (2006) Curcumin and dehydrozingerone derivatives: synthesis, radiolabeling, and evaluation for beta-amyloid plaque imaging. J Med Chem 49:6111–6119
Sahoo BK, Ghosh KS, Dasgupta S (2008) Investigating the binding of curcumin derivatives to bovine serum albumin. Biophys Chem 132:81–88
Sahu A, Kasoju N, Bora U (2008) Fluorescence study of the curcumin-casein micelle complexation and its application as a drug nanocarrier to cancer cells. Biomacromolecules 9:2905–2912
Shaikh J, Ankola DD, Beniwal V, Singh D, Kumar MN (2009) Nanoparticle encapsulation improves oral bioavailability of curcumin by at least 9-fold when compared to curcumin administered with piperine as absorption enhancer. Eur J Pharm Sci 37:223–230
Sharma RA, McLelland HR, Hill KA, Ireson CR, Euden SA, Manson MM, Pirmohamed M, Marnett LJ, Gescher AJ, Steward WP (2001) Pharmacodynamic and pharmacokinetic study of oral Curcuma extract in patients with colorectal cancer. Clin Cancer Res 7:1894–1900
Sharma RA, Euden SA, Platton SL, Cooke DN, Shafayat A, Hewitt HR, Marczylo TH, Morgan B, Hemingway D, Plummer SM, Pirmohamed M, Gescher AJ, Steward WP (2004) Phase I clinical trial of oral curcumin: biomarkers of systemic activity and compliance. Clin Cancer Res 10:6847–6854
Shen L, Ji HF (2007) Theoretical study on physicochemical properties of curcumin. Spectrochim Acta A Mol Biomol Spectrosc 67:619–623
Shibata H, Yamakoshi H, Sato A, Ohori H, Kakudo Y, Kudo C, Takahashi Y, Watanabe M, Takano H, Ishioka C, Noda T, Iwabuchi Y (2009) Newly synthesized curcumin analog has improved potential to prevent colorectal carcinogenesis in vivo. Cancer Sci 100:956–960
Shoba G, Joy D, Joseph T, Majeed M, Rajendran R, Srinivas PS (1998) Influence of piperine on the pharmacokinetics of curcumin in animals and human volunteers. Planta Med 64:353–356
Singh J, Dubey RK, Atal CK (1986) Piperine-mediated inhibition of glucuronidation activity in isolated epithelial cells of the guinea-pig small intestine: evidence that piperine lowers the endogeneous UDP-glucuronic acid content. J Pharmacol Exp Ther 236:488–493
Srinivasan K (2007) Black pepper and its pungent principle-piperine: a review of diverse physiological effects. Crit Rev Food Sci Nutr 47:735–748
Stella VJ, He Q (2008) Cyclodextrins. Toxicol Pathol 36:30–42
Sui Z, Salto R, Li J, Craik C, Ortiz de Montellano PR (1993) Inhibition of the HIV-1 and HIV-2 proteases by curcumin and curcumin boron complexes. Bioorg Med Chem 1:415–422
Sun Y, Lee CC, Hung WC, Chen FY, Lee MT, Huang HW (2008) The bound states of amphipathic drugs in lipid bilayers: study of curcumin. Biophys J 95:2318–2324
Suresh D, Srinivasan K (2006) Influence of curcumin, capsaicin, and piperine on the rat liver drug-metabolizing enzyme system in vivo and in vitro. Can J Physiol Pharmacol 84:1259–1265
Suresh D, Srinivasan K (2010) Tissue distribution & elimination of capsaicin, piperine & curcumin following oral intake in rats. Indian J Med Res 131:682–691
Takahashi M, Uechi S, Takara K, Asikin Y, Wada K (2009) Evaluation of an oral carrier system in rats: bioavailability and antioxidant properties of liposome-encapsulated curcumin. J Agric Food Chem 57: 9141–9146

Tang B, Ma L, Wang HY, Zhang GY (2002) Study on the supramolecular interaction of curcumin and beta-cyclodextrin by spectrophotometry and its analytical application. J Agric Food Chem 50:1355–1361

Tayyem RF, Heath DD, Al-Delaimy WK, Rock CL (2006) Curcumin content of turmeric and curry powders. Nutr Cancer 55:126–131

Teichmann A, Heuschkel S, Jacobi U, Presse G, Neubert RH, Sterry W, Lademann J (2007) Comparison of stratum corneum penetration and localization of a lipophilic model drug applied in an o/w microemulsion and an amphiphilic cream. Eur J Pharm Biopharm 67:699–706

Thangapazham RL, Puri A, Tele S, Blumenthal R, Maheshwari RK (2008) Evaluation of a nanotechnology-based carrier for delivery of curcumin in prostate cancer cells. Int J Oncol 32:1119–1123

Thompson KH, Bohmerle K, Polishchuk E, Martins C, Toleikis P, Tse J, Yuen V, McNeill JH, Orvig C (2004) Complementary inhibition of synoviocyte, smooth muscle cell or mouse lymphoma cell proliferation by a vanadyl curcumin complex compared to curcumin alone. J Inorg Biochem 98:2063–2070

Tiyaboonchai W, Tungpradit W, Plianbangchang P (2007) Formulation and characterization of curcuminoids loaded solid lipid nanoparticles. Int J Pharm 337:299–306

Tomren MA, Masson M, Loftsson T, Tonnesen HH (2007) Studies on curcumin and curcuminoids XXXI. Symmetric and asymmetric curcuminoids: stability, activity and complexation with cyclodextrin. Int J Pharm 338:27–34

Tønnesen HH (2002) Solubility, chemical and photochemical stability of curcumin in surfactant solutions. Studies of curcumin and curcuminoids XXVIII. Pharmazie 57:820–824

Tønnesen HH, Karlsen J (1985a) Studies on curcumin and curcuminoids VI. Kinetics of curcumin degradation in aqueous solution. Z Lebensm Unters Forsch 180:402–404

Tønnesen HH, Karlsen J (1985b) Studies on curcumin and curcuminoidsV. Alkaline degradation of curcumin. Z Lebensm Unters Forsch 180:132–134

Tønnesen HH, Karlsen J, van Henegouwen GB (1986) Studies on curcumin and curcuminoids VIII. Photochemical stability of curcumin. Z Lebensm Unters Forsch 183:116–122

Tønnesen HH, Másson M, Loftsson T (2002) Studies of curcumin and curcuminoids. XXVII. Cyclodextrin complexation: solubility, chemical and photochemical stability. Int J Pharm 244:127–135

Tukey RH, Strassburg CP (2000) Human UDP-glucuronosyltransferases: metabolism, expression, and disease. Annu Rev Pharmacol Toxicol 40:581–616

Usta M, Wortelboer HM, Vervoort J, Boersma MG, Rietjens IM, van Bladeren PJ, Cnubben NH (2007) Human glutathione S-transferase-mediated glutathione conjugation of curcumin and efflux of these conjugates in Caco-2 cells. Chem Res Toxicol 20:1895–1902

Valentini A, Conforti F, Crispini A, De Martino A, Condello R, Stellitano C, Rotilio G, Ghedini M, Federici G, Bernardini S, Pucci D (2009) Synthesis, oxidant properties, and antitumoral effects of a heteroleptic palladium(II) complex of curcumin on human prostate cancer cells. J Med Chem 52:484–491

Vareed SK, Kakarala M, Ruffin MT, Crowell JA, Normolle DP, Djuric Z, Brenner DE (2008) Pharmacokinetics of curcumin conjugate metabolites in healthy human subjects. Cancer Epidemiol Biomark Prev 17:1411–1417

Verghese J (1993) Isolation of curcumin from curcuma longa L. Rhizome. Flavour Fragr J 8:315–319

Villegas I, Sanchez-Fidalgo S, Alarcon de la Lastra C (2008) New mechanisms and therapeutic potential of curcumin for colorectal cancer. Mol Nutr Food Res 52:1040–1061

Volak LP, Ghirmai S, Cashman JR, Court MH (2008) Curcuminoids inhibit multiple human cytochromes P450, UDP-glucuronosyltransferase, and sulfotransferase enzymes, whereas piperine is a relatively selective CYP3A4 inhibitor. Drug Metab Dispos 36:1594–1605

Wahlström B, Blennow G (1978) A study on the fate of curcumin in the rat. Acta Pharmacol Toxicol (Copenh) 43:86–92

Wang YJ, Pan MH, Cheng AL, Lin LI, Ho YS, Hsieh CY, Lin JK (1997) Stability of curcumin in buffer solutions and characterization of its degradation products. J Pharm Biomed Anal 15:1867–1876

Wang F, Yang J, Wu X, Liu S (2005) Study of the interaction of proteins with curcumin and SDS and its analytical application. Spectrochim Acta A Mol Biomol Spectrosc 61:2650–2656
Wang D, Veena MS, Stevenson K, Tang C, Ho B, Suh JD, Duarte VM, Faull KF, Mehta K, Srivatsan ES, Wang MB (2008) Liposome-encapsulated curcumin suppresses growth of head and neck squamous cell carcinoma in vitro and in xenografts through the inhibition of nuclear factor kappaB by an AKT-independent pathway. Clin Cancer Res 14:6228–6236
Xu D-H, Wang S, Jin J, Mei X-T, Xu SB (2006) Dissolution and absorption researches of curcumin in solid dispersion with the polymer PVP. Asian J Pharmacodyn Pharmacokinet 6:343–349
Xu DH, Wang S, Mei XT, Luo XJ, Xu SB (2008) Studies on solubility enhancement of curcumin by Polyvinylpyrrolidione K30. Zhong Yao Cai 31:438–442
Yadav VR, Suresh S, Devi K, Yadav S (2009) Effect of cyclodextrin complexation of curcumin on its solubility and antiangiogenic and anti-inflammatory activity in rat colitis model. AAPS PharmSciTech 10:752–762
Yadav VR, Prasad S, Kannappan R, Ravindran J, Chaturvedi MM, Vaahtera L, Parkkinen J, Aggarwal BB (2010) Cyclodextrin-complexed curcumin exhibits anti-inflammatory and antiproliferative activities superior to those of curcumin through higher cellular uptake. Biochem Pharmacol 80:1021–1032
Yallapu MM, Gupta BK, Jaggi M, Chauhan SC (2010) Fabrication of curcumin encapsulated PLGA nanoparticles for improved therapeutic effects in metastatic cancer cells. J Colloid Interface Sci 351:19–29
Yanagisawa D, Shirai N, Amatsubo T, Taguchi H, Hirao K, Urushitani M, Morikawa S, Inubushi T, Kato M, Kato F, Morino K, Kimura H, Nakano I, Yoshida C, Okada T, Sano M, Wada Y, Wada KN, Yamamoto A, Tooyama I (2010) Relationship between the tautomeric structures of curcumin derivatives and their Abeta-binding activities in the context of therapies for Alzheimer's disease. Biomaterials 31:4179–4185
Yang F, Lim GP, Begum AN, Ubeda OJ, Simmons MR, Ambegaokar SS, Chen PP, Kayed R, Glabe CG, Frautschy SA, Cole GM (2005) Curcumin inhibits formation of amyloid beta oligomers and fibrils, binds plaques, and reduces amyloid in vivo. J Biol Chem 280:5892–5901
Yang KY, Lin LC, Tseng TY, Wang SC, Tsai TH (2007) Oral bioavailability of curcumin in rat and the herbal analysis from Curcuma longa by LC-MS/MS. J Chromatogr B Analyt Technol Biomed Life Sci 853:183–189
Yang CS, Sang S, Lambert JD, Lee MJ (2008) Bioavailability issues in studying the health effects of plant polyphenolic compounds. Mol Nutr Food Res 52(Suppl 1):S139–S151
Zebib B, Mouloungui Z, Noirot V (2010) Stabilization of curcumin by complexation with divalent cations in glycerol/water system. Bioinorg Chem Appl 2010:292760
Zeng Y, Qiu F, Liu Y, Qu G, Yao X (2007) Isolation and identification of phase 1 metabolites of demethoxycurcumin in rats. Drug Metab Dispos 35:1564–1573
Zsila F, Bikadi Z, Simonyi M (2003) Unique, pH-dependent biphasic band shape of the visible circular dichroism of curcumin-serum albumin complex. Biochem Biophys Res Commun 301:776–782

Part II
Natural Compounds from Animal Origins

Chapter 6
Melatonin in Cell Fate Decisions: Mechanistic Perspectives and Therapeutical Potential

M. Sánchez-Hidalgo, J.M. Guerrero, I. Villegas, and Catalina Alarcón De La Lastra

Abstract Melatonin, an indolamine derived from the amino-acid tryptophan via synthesis of serotonin, is secreted by the pineal gland in cyclical periods. In mammals, melatonin is involved in physiological processes, such as sleep/wake regulation in the circadian cycle. It has antioxidant oncostatic and anti-inflammatory properties, functions as an immunomodulator, and stimulates bone metabolism. In particular, the antitumor effects of melatonin, have been studied in multiple cancer cell types including melanoma, breast and prostate cancer, lymphoma, ovarian and colorectal cancer. This chapter summarizes the numerous observations about melatonin anticancer effects in both *in vivo* and *in vitro* studies published in recent years as well as the action mechanisms of melatonin involved in its anticarcinogenic activity focusing on the signalling pathways that regulate programmed cell death. In the majority of studies, melatonin has shown to inhibit development and/or growth of various experimental animal tumors and human cancer cell lines *in vitro* promoting apoptosis in contrast to the obvious inhibition of apoptotic processes in normal cells (focused in immune cells and neurons). Furthermore, if melatonin uniformly induced apoptosis in cancer cells, the findings could have important clinical utility given that many tumors show resistance to drug treatment due to their resistance to undergo apoptosis.

M. Sánchez-Hidalgo (✉) • I. Villegas • C.A. De La Lastra
Department of Pharmacology, Faculty of Pharmacy, University of Seville,
Profesor García González Street 2, 41012 Seville, Spain
e-mail: hidalgosanz@us.es

J.M. Guerrero
Instituto de Biomedicina de Sevilla (IBis), Hospital
Universitario Virgen del Rocio/CSIC/Universidad de Sevilla,
Department of Medical Biochemistry and Molecular Biology,
University of Seville School of Medicine, Seville, Spain

M. Diederich and K. Noworyta (eds.), *Natural Compounds as Inducers of Cell Death: Volume 1*, DOI 10.1007/978-94-007-4575-9_6,

6.1 Melatonin Biosynthesis, Catabolism and Regulation

Melatonin (N-actetyl-5-methoxy-tryptamine), also known as "*the chemical expression of darkness*", is an indolamine derived from the amino-acid tryptophan via synthesis of serotonin (Fig. 6.1). Melatonin first isolated by Lerner et al. in 1958 (Lerner et al. 1960) and is produced by the pineal gland and secreted into the blood in a circadian manner; pineal production of melatonin is low level during daytime and higher at night.

The enzymatic machinery for melatonin biosynthesis in pinealocytes was first identified by Axelrod in 1974 (Axelrod 1974). Its biosynthesis is mediated by the sequential action of arylalkylamine- N-acetyltransferase (AA-NAT) and hydroxyindole-O-methyltransferase (HIOMT). In mammals, the regulation of pineal melatonin biosynthesis is mediated by the retinohypothalamic tract, which projects from the retina to the suprachiasmatic nucleus (SCN), the endogenous circadian oscillator. The primary neurotransmitter, noradrenalin, is released during the night from the postganglionic sympathetic fibers of the superior cervical ganglion that terminate in the pinealocytes where it couples to β-adrenergic receptors. This leads to an activation of adenylate cyclase with a consequent rise in cAMP levels, promoting the *novo* protein synthesis and stimulating the rate-limiting enzyme in melatonin production, arylalkylamine-N-acetyltransferase (AA-NAT) (Klein et al. 1981). As a result, AA-NAT N-acetylates serotonin to N-acetylserotonin (NAS) and as long as NAS is generated, is quickly *O*-methylated by hydroxyindole-*O*-methyltransferase (HIOMT) to finally produce melatonin (Axelrod and Weissbach 1960). Stimulation of α-adrenergic receptors potentates the β stimulation; calcium ions, phosphatidylinositol, diacylglycerol and protein kinase C (PKC) participate in this mechanism (Sugden 1989). The dramatic rise in AA-NAT (10–100-fold) drives melatonin synthesis which is released during periods of darkness in a circadian manner (Reiter 1991). In contrast, the nocturnal increase in pineal HIOMT activity is weak but significant. HIOMT gene expression is high during daytime but displays an additional twofold increase at night.

The amplitude of nocturnal melatonin secretion is believed to be genetically determined and shows considerable interindividual differences. Thus, some subjects produce more melatonin during their life than others. In addition, the secretory dynamic of melatonin attenuates gradually with age, resulting in a loss of nocturnal peak of melatonin with nearly undetectable plasma levels at 20–22 months of age in rodents (Reiter 1980) and at 60–70 years old in humans (Touitou et al. 1985).

Once synthesized and released into blood at night, melatonin is transferred through biological membranes and it is found throughout the organism in all tissues of the body within a very short period. This presence does not necessarily indicate an endogenous synthesis because the high lipophilic nature permits its transfer. To date, extrapineal melatonin synthesis has been demonstrated only in retina, harderian gland, brain, gut, ovary, testes, inner ear and immune system including

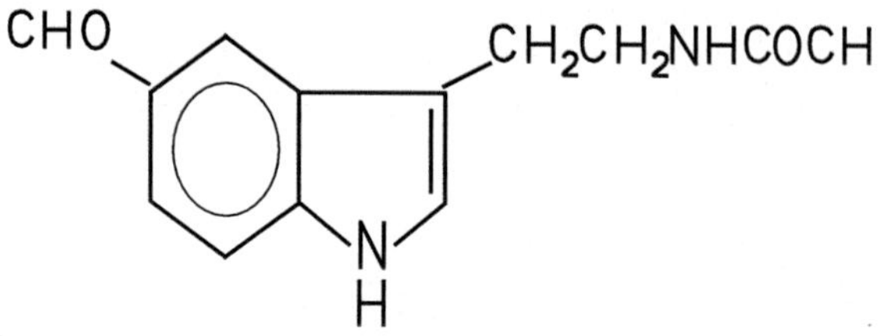

Fig. 6.1 Chemical structure of melatonin

bone marrow, lymphocytes, macrophages and, more recently, in thymus (Hardeland 2008). In general, while pineal melatonin seems to act as a typical hormone reaching target cells through the bloodstream, extrapineal melatonin may play a key role as an intra-, auto- and paracrine signal molecule in those tissues where it is synthesized.

Circulating melatonin is metabolized mainly in the liver where it is first hydroxylated by cytochrome P_{450} mono-oxygenases and thereafter conjugated with sulphate to be excreted as 6-sulfatoxymelatonin (Claustrat et al. 2005). Glucuronide conjugation is extremely limited. Melatonin can also be metabolized nonenzymatically by free radicals and a few other oxidants. It is converted into cyclic 3-hydroxymelatonin when it directly scavenges two hydroxyl radicals (Tan et al. 1998). In the brain, a fraction of melatonin is metabolized to kynuramine derivatives such us N-acetyl-N-formyl-5-metoxykynuramine (AFMK) and N-acetyl-5-methoxykynuramine (AMK). This is of interest as the antioxidant and anti-inflammatory properties of melatonin are shared by these metabolites.

Actually, melatonin is considered one of the hormones most ubiquitous among living beings. This great functional versatility is reflected in its wide distribution within phylogenetically distant organisms from bacteria to humans. It has also been reported in plants and because substances normally found in foods do not fall under jurisdiction of the US Food and Drug Administration melatonin was classed a dietary supplement.

6.2 Melatonin Action Mechanisms

Melatonin exerts its cellular effects via: i) binding to specific membrane G-protein-coupled receptors, ii) direct interaction with cytosol proteins (i.e. calmodulin, protein kinase C (PKC)), iii) neutralization of free radicals including scavenging properties and iv) nuclear receptors belonging to the RZR/ROR orphan receptor superfamily and more recently, v) serving as a potential co-factor for quinone reductase-2 (QR-2) (Hardeland 2008) (Fig. 6.2).

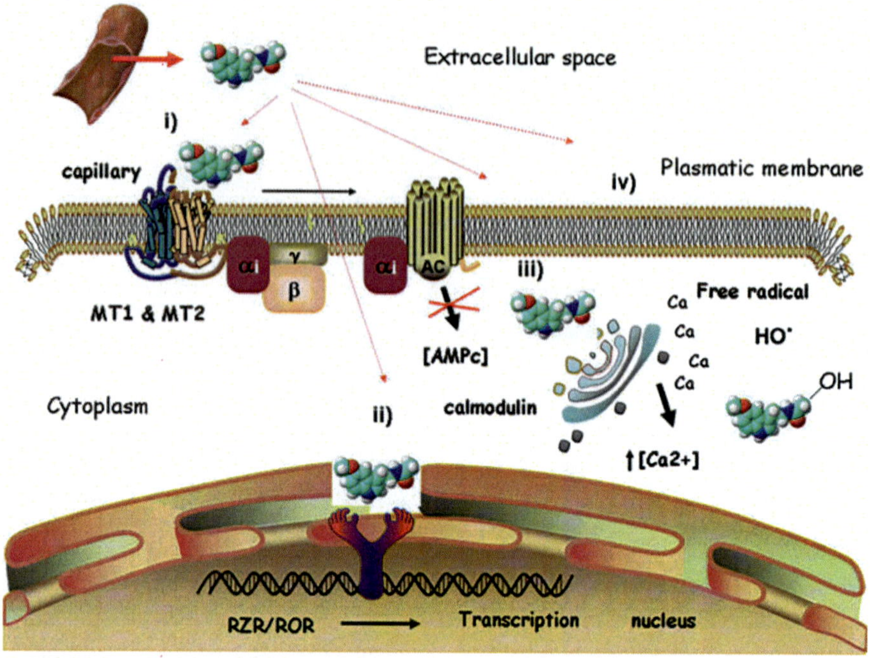

Fig. 6.2 Melatonin action mechanisms: i) binding to specific membrane G-protein-coupled receptors (MT1 and MT2), ii) direct interaction with cytosol proteins (i.e calmodulin), iii) neutralization of free radicals and iv) nuclear receptors belonging to the RZR/ROR orphan receptor superfamily

6.3 Potencial Beneficial Actions of Melatonin

Melatonin is involved in diverse physiological processes, such as sleep/wake regulation in the circadian cycle and seasonal behaviour, sexual development and retinal physiology. In addition, melatonin has antioxidant, oncostatic, anti-aging and anti-inflammatory properties, functions as an immunomodulator, participates in cardiovascular, neurological and gastrointestinal homeostasis systems and stimulates bone metabolism (Pandi-Perumal et al. 2006).

6.3.1 Melatonin in Reproduction and Sexual Maturation

Melatonin participates in the regulation of reproductive function in seasonal mammals by its inhibitory action at various levels of the hypothalamic-pituitary-gonadal axis. Melatonin has been shown to down-regulate gonadotropin-releasing hormone (GnRH) gene expression in a cyclical pattern over a 24 h period (Roy et al. 2001). In seasonal breeders, reproductive performance is timed by variations in the photoperiod, effects that are mediated by corresponding changes in melatonin. Both surgical and functional pinealectomy decrease significantly plasmatic melatonin levels and accelerate the development in the puberty. On the contrary, short day exposition or exogenous melatonin administration delayed the sexual maturation in experimental animals (Brainard et al. 1986) due to inhibitory role of melatonin on the hypothalamus and on pubertal maturation. In humans, pineal tumours are associated with an abnormal pubertal maturation.

6.3.2 Melatonin as a Chronobiotic Agent

Melatonin acts as an endogenous synchronizer of the different circadian rhythms generated in the organism. The first evidence of its chronobiotic role was established in birds and reptiles and afterwards in rats, hamsters and humans (Webb and Puig-Domingo 1995). In mammals, melatonin synchronizes circadian rhythms in fetal and neonatal stages and can also entrain free-running rhythms both in normal individuals and in blind people. The mechanisms, by which melatonin exerts its chronobiotic function, are not totally well established; nevertheless, expression of melatonin receptors in SCN suggests a direct action of melatonin in the endogenous circadian clock to consequently influence in the circadian rhythms.

Its chronobiotic properties have been shown to have value in treating various circadian rhythm sleep disorders such as *jet lag* or shift-work sleep disorder. Melatonin promotes sleep which has been demonstrated to be useful for treating insomnia symptoms in elderly and depressive patients and also exhibits a remarkable role as photoperiodic molecule in seasonal reproduction. Melatonin may mediate some of the tranquillizing effects of meditation and melatonin treatment has been shown to be useful for treating delayed sleep phase syndrome, mood disorders.

6.3.3 Melatonin as an Immunomodulator

During the last three decades, a great number of reports have documented the existence of a relationship between melatonin/pineal and the immune system in different birds and mammals, including humans. *In vivo* and *in vitro* data confirming this relationship have been provided as follows: (i) correlation between melatonin production and circadian and seasonal variations in the immune system, (ii) effects of surgical or functional pinealectomy on the immune system, (iii) effects of melatonin administration *in vivo* on the immune system, (iv) *in vitro* regulation of immune cell activity by melatonin and (v) presence of melatonin receptors in the immune system (Carrillo-Vico et al. 2006).

The seasonal changes in immune function observed in animals and humans are likely to be mediated by the changes in the duration of melatonin secretion (Guerrero and Reiter 2002). On the other hand, both surgical and functional pinealectomy are directly correlated with weight loss and abnormal development in the primary immune organs of mammals and birds.

According to the immunomodulatory role of exogenous melatonin, the majority of the studies published have confirmed melatonin administration promotes a clear immuno-enhancement in terms of immune tissue morphology due to its ability to increasing weight of thymus and spleen both under basal and immunosuppressive conditions. Melatonin administration enhances both innate and cellular immunity.

In human neutrophils, melatonin modulates the respiratory burst (Pieri et al. 1998). Both melatonin and its metabolite, AFMK, inhibit lipopolysaccharide (LPS)-mediated production of tumor necrosis factor alpha (TNFα) and IL-8 in neutrophils (Silva et al. 2004). Melatonin stimulates the production of progenitor cells for granulocytes-macrophages and melatonin also stimulates the production of natural killer (NK) cells and CD4+ cells and inhibits CD8+ cells. The production and release of various cytokines from NK and T-helper lymphocytes also are enhanced by melatonin. Thus, melatonin regulates IL-2 and IFNγ production in lymphocytes T CD4+ (Th1), activates IL-1, IL-6, IL-12, TNFα, NO and other oxygen reactive species (ROS) production in monocytes while diminishes IL-10 production in human macrophages and monocytes, abolishes lipoxygenase expression in B lymphocytes likewise stimulates α1 timusine and timuline peptides in thymus (Guerrero et al. 1997; Guerrero and Reiter 2002). Melatonin also participates in the regulation of apoptosis of T (Sainz et al. 1995) and B cells (Yu et al. 1981).

Melatonin also acts on the hematopoietic system via induction of T-helper cell (Th)-derived opioid cytokines (MIOS system), which exert significant colony-stimulating activity (Maestroni et al. 1994). In peripheral blood mononuclear cells (PBMCs)/ T-cells melatonin increases IL-2, IFNγ and IL-12 production while decreases IL-10 production (Garcia-Maurino et al. 1997). *In vivo* studies have also revealed the adjuvant-like properties of melatonin due to its ability to enhance antibody production (Regodon et al. 2005).

The cells and organs of the immune system are remarkable sources of melatonin, and high concentrations of melatonin and/or its biosynthetic enzymatic machinery has been described in human, mouse and rat bone marrow (Tan et al. 1999; Conti et al. 2000), as well as, in human immunocompetent cells (Pozo et al. 1997; Carrillo-Vico et al. 2004) and human thymus (Naranjo et al. 2007). Carrillo-Vico et al, found that cultured human lymphocytes synthesize and release large amounts of melatonin, which acts as intra-, auto-, and/or paracrine substance, via the modulation of the IL-2/IL-2R system by its membrane and/or nuclear receptors (Carrillo-Vico et al. 2005a).

Recent reports have revealed the presence of melatonin binding sites in the immune system both in membrane and nuclear fractions (Carrillo-Vico et al. 2005b). In human lymphocytes, the signal transduction for melatonin involves a pertussis toxin-sensitive G protein (Garcia-Perganeda et al. 1997). As mentioned above, melatonin has also been reported to interact with the RZR/ROR subfamily of nuclear receptors, which are present in different rodent and human immunocompetent cells (Pozo et al. 1997; Carrillo-Vico et al. 2003). Finally, the development of several specific melatonin membrane and nuclear receptor agonists and antagonists has allowed the characterization of several physiology roles for both melatonin membrane and nuclear receptors in the immune system (Carrillo-Vico et al. 2006).

On the other hand, melatonin treatment has demonstrated delaying the onset of disease in several viral infections (Bonilla et al. 2004) and improves the survival rate of rodents after administration of a lethal dose of LPS (Cuzzocrea and Reiter 2001), through the inhibition of pro-inflammatory factors such as cytokines and nitric oxide (NO), as well as to decrease lipid peroxidation levels and apoptosis (Escames et al. 2006). Its beneficial effect has been also confirmed in a study conducted in newborn infants in which melatonin improved clinical outcome and prevented death due to septic shock (Gitto et al. 2001). According to the autoimmune diseases such as rheumatoid arthritis, multiple sclerosis, systemic lupus and Crohn's disease, the effects of melatonin are controversial and may not always be beneficial.

6.3.4 *Melatonin as an Antioxidant*

Since the discovery of melatonin as an antioxidant in 1993 (Tan et al. 1993), numerous *in vitro* and *in vivo* studies have documented the ability of both physiological and pharmacological concentrations of melatonin to protect against free radical destruction. Melatonin is a potent free radical scavenger which was originally shown to detoxify the highly toxic hydroxyl radical (·OH). Since this discovery, its scavenging repertoire has been expanded to include H_2O_2, HOCl, $^1O_2$, O_2^-, NO·, $ONOO^-$ and others (Reiter et al. 2007). The large subcellular distribution of melatonin allows its interaction with almost any kind of molecule, reducing oxidative damage in both lipid and aqueous environments. This is supported experimentally by numerous studies in which melatonin has been demonstrated to protect lipids in the cellular membranes, proteins in the cytosol and DNA in the nucleus from free radical damage (Reiter et al. 2004).

Melatonin can also develop its antioxidant action due to its ability to induce the expression and/or the activity of the main antioxidant enzymes. Thus, it up-regulates antioxidative enzymes such as glutathione peroxidase, glutathione reductase and glucose 6-phosphate dehydrogenase, superoxide dismutase and catalase.

The efficacy of melatonin in functioning in this antioxidant capacity relates also to its efficacy in reducing electron leakage from the mitochondrial electron transport chain (Leon et al. 2005) and its synergistic interactions with other antioxidant (Lopez-Burillo et al. 2003). In recent years, it has become apparent that when melatonin scavenges radicals and related reactants, the products generated are also free radical scavengers thereby greatly exaggerating the antioxidant potential of melatonin.

Examples of situations in which melatonin has been found to lower induced oxidative damage include ischaemia reperfusion injury (in brain, heart, liver, gut, lung and urinary bladder), toxic drug exposure, bacterial toxin exposure, schistosomias, heavy metal toxicity, amyloid β (Aβ) protein exposure (as a model of Alzheimer's disease), I-methyl-4-phenyl-1,2,3,6-tetrahydropyridine (MPTP) exposure (as a model of Parkinsonism) among others (Reiter et al. 2004). Melatonin has also been successfully used as an adjuvant treatment in neonates with sepsis (a high free radical condition) (Gitto et al. 2001). In humans, melatonin has also been shown to be beneficial in skin erythema due to exposure to ultraviolet radiation (Bangha et al. 1996), iron and erythropoietin administration (Shamir et al. 2001) and tardive dyskinesia (Herrera et al. 2001).

6.3.5 Melatonin and Aging

The consequences of aging are also seen in melatonin production. The mean nighttime serum melatonin concentration is low during the first 6 months of life, increasing to a peak value at 1–3 years of age and diminished on individuals age 15–20 years with a gradually declination gradually with age, resulting in a loss of nocturnal peak of melatonin with nearly undetectable plasma levels at 60–70 year-old humans. Thus, if serum melatonin levels contribute to the antioxidant capacity, such ability would be reduced in advanced age. Nevertheless, there are variations in the amplitude of the nocturnal concentrations of melatonin among individuals which indicate that some subjects produce significantly less melatonin during lifetime than others which may have significance in terms of aging. High and young secretors have plasma levels of melatonin ranging from 54 to75 pg/mL whereas low and elderly secretors range from 18 to 40 pg/mL.

Since Pierpaoli and Maestroni showed, for first time, that exogenous nocturnal administration of melatonin or engraftment of young homologous pineals to old syngeneic mice adjacent to the thymus resulted in a significant enhancement of survival and juvenile characters in mice, due to its immunostimulatory property (Pierpaoli and Maestroni 1987), several studies have been performed to elucidate the effects of melatonin on life-span progression in different species (Anisimov et al. 2006). Pinealectomy seems to accelerate the aging process reducing animal survival while pineal graft in rodents exhibits surprising results in increasing life-span and recovering juvenile characters (Anisimov 2003).

Although the role of melatonin during aging is not fully understood and the relation is difficult to document, several properties of the indolamine indicate that it may be beneficial in aging. In fact, there are reports that confirm that exogenous administration of this indoleamine is able to reduce the inflammatory and oxidative processes associated to the age as well as exert an immunomodulatory effect. There are reports that document this reduced melatonin concentrations in the pineal gland and serum during advancing age (Reiter 1986; Bondarenko 1992).

Aging is also characterized by sleep disturbances and a decline in immune system function, so-called inmmunosenescence, in which melatonin seems to play a remarkable role. It has been demonstrated that melatonin administration improves sleep disorders (Cajochen et al. 2003) and has an immune reconstituting effect in aging (Arlt and Hewison 2004).

Recent studies have suggested that age-related decline in melatonin concentration involves a loss of its antioxidant ability against damage produced by free radicals

(Reiter et al. 2002). Oxidative damage plays a remarkable role in the pathogenesis of neurodegenerative and hepatic diseases, commonly manifested in the elderly population. Given the high incidence of hepatic pathologies during aging, recent studies have described the protective effect of exogenous melatonin treatment against age-related oxidative damage in hepatocytes and liver from rats (Castillo et al. 2005; Kireev et al. 2007). Melatonin also prevents age-related oxidative DNA damage in the brain of female senescence-accelerated SAM-P/6 mice (Morioka et al. 1999), restores mitochondrial respiratory control index, ADP/O ratio, state 3 and DNP-dependent uncoupled respiration (Okatani et al. 2002). Furthermore, melatonin induces the senescence-associated reductions of complex I and IV activities in liver mitochondria from SAMP8 (Okatani et al. 2002). Melatonin also counteracts LPS-induced inhibition of complexes I and IV. In general, the actions of melatonin were greater in old than in young animals (Escames et al. 2003).

Numerous studies have suggested that melatonin may provide protection against aging through the enhancement of immune function and its antioxidant property. Therefore, the loss of this potent antioxidant during aging may be consequential of the onset of age-related diseases as well as sleep disorders, cancer and immunological disturbances commonly manifested in elderly. In fact, some studies in rodents have suggested that such diminished melatonin secretion may accelerate aging.

6.3.6 Melatonin and Cancer

In relation to its oncostatic properties, there is evidence that tumor initiation, promotion or progression may be restrained by the night-time physiological surge of melatonin in the blood or extracellular fluid (Blask et al. 2005). Nevertheless, in the majority of studies melatonin has been shown to inhibit development and/or growth of various experimental animal tumors and some human cell lines *in vitro*, its role in human malignancy is not clear. When administered in physiological (nM) and pharmacological concentrations (μM-mM), melatonin exhibits a growth inhibitory effect in estrogen-positive, MCF7 human breast cancer cell lines (Blask et al. 2005). The antitumor effect of melatonin has been also described in hepatoma which seems to result from MT1/MT2-dependent inhibition of linoleic acid uptake, thereby preventing the formation of its mitogenic metabolite, 13-hydroxyoctadecadienoic acid (Blask et al. 2005). Several reports have suggested the antiproliferative effects of melatonin by binding to nuclear receptors altering the transcription of several genes that play a role in cellular proliferation (Carlberg 2000). Melatonin has been shown to increase calmodulin degradation due to direct binding as well as causing redistribution of calmodulin, thereby inhibiting cell cycle progression (Blask et al. 2002). A final well-documented function of melatonin is its direct and indirect antioxidant properties leading to a decrease in DNA damage (Blask et al. 2002). Inhibition of NF-κB by melatonin may be another potential mechanism associated to apoptosis and cytokine activity modulation.

Melatonin has been demonstrated to exhibit oncostatic properties against a variety of tumor cells including prostate cancer, uterus cancer, endometrial carcinoma, ovarian carcinoma cell lines, human melanoma, intestine tumors and lung cancer (Jung and Ahmad 2006). In addition, depressed nocturnal melatonin concentrations or nocturnal excretion of the main melatonin metabolite 6-sulfatoxymelatonin were found in various tumor types including breast cancer, prostate cancer, colorectal cancer (CRC), endometrial cancer, cervical cancer, lung cancer and stomach cancer. However, in other types such as Hodgkin's sarcoma, osteosarcoma, ovarian cancer and others, melatonin levels were not changed or showed great variations among individuals (Bartsch et al. 2002).

Several clinical studies suggest that administration of melatonin (in high doses either alone or in combination with IL-2) is able to favourably influence the course of advanced malignant disease in humans and lead to an improvement in their quality of life (Lissoni et al. 2001). Likewise, recent epidemiologic studies have suggested that women who work exclusively at night for long periods have a significantly elevated risk of breast cancer (Blask et al. 2005).

6.4 Melatonin as Inducer of Cell Death in Cancer

Apoptosis and necrosis represent two major mutually different mechanisms of cell death. Necrosis is defined as uncontrolled process of cellular break-up executed as a consequence of massive and irreversible damage. However, apoptosis is controlled to a certain degree reversible process of programmed cell disintegration that usually doesn't induce inflammatory reaction. Although the understanding of detail signalling pathways that execute apoptosis is incomplete, this process is controlled by numerous proteins and protein complexes that, when activated by various triggers, induce sequential activation of the effector mechanisms. Apoptosis is triggered by two major apoptosis-initiating pathways, designated as the intrinsic (also known as inner or mitochondria-mediated) and extrinsic (also known as outer or receptor-mediated) pathways. Both pathways converge to a final apoptosis execution step resulting in the cleavage of cell regulatory and structural molecules (Green and Kroemer 2004; Thorburn 2004).

Apoptosis is an essential physiological process throughout the life of multi-cellular organisms important in the development and in the maintenance of tissue homeostasis. Apoptosis is involved in controlling of cell number and proliferation during embryogenesis, detection of activated lymphocytes at the end of the immune response, elimination of self-reactive lymphocytes, in controlled destruction of damaged, aged, infected, transformed, and other harmful cells (Nagata 1997).

The defect in apoptosis and in apoptotic regulatory mechanisms can result in various pathological states, including malignant transformation, tumor progression or autoimmune and neurodegenerative disorders. Apoptosis represents a major causative factor in the development and progression of cancer. Some types of cancer are characterized by defects in apoptosis leading to immortal clones of cells.

This ability of tumor cells to evade engagement of apoptosis can play a significant role in their resistance to conventional therapeutic regimens. Further understanding of the different signalling pathways that control apoptosis in the different tumor types will help with the discovery of novel targeted agents and the design of clinical trials that are based on the molecular defects specific to the targeted tumor. Consequently, in the search of new anticancer targets, melatonin seems to play a remarkable role on inhibition of several human cancer cells lines growth. In fact, melatonin proapoptotic action has been described in a variety of both *in vitro* and *in vivo* studies (Tables 6.1 and 6.2, respectively). In contrast, there is evidence that melatonin may actually inhibit apoptotic processes in normal cells (focused in immune cells and neurons).

6.4.1 *In Vitro Studies*

Given the importance of the apoptotic program in the treatment of cancer, the role of melatonin in influencing apoptosis in tumor cells attracted attention because it seems that it can actually increase apoptosis in some tumor cells. Melatonin proapoptotic action has been described in a great variety of human cancer cell types including human breast cancer cell line MCF-7, human colon cancer, hepatocarcinoma H22, Jurkat, human B cells lymphoma, human neuroblastoma cells and, more recently, in human myeloid HL-60 cells and human pancreatic carcinoma PANC-1 cells. The action mechanisms involved in melatonin pro-apoptotic effects in experimental *in vitro* studies has been reviewed and compiled in great detail in Table 6.1.

To date, the results obtained appear promising; furthermore, if melatonin uniformly induced apoptosis in human cancer cells, the findings could have relevant clinical utility.

6.4.2 *In Vivo Studies*

There is evidence on suppressive effect of melatonin on the development of spontaneous and chemically induced carcinogenesis at various sites in mice and rats as well as on the tumor growth *in vitro*. In addition, for a variety of tumors their growth is accelerated in pinealectomized animals. The inhibitory effect of melatonin is well established in relation to mammary tumors and colon cancer. Nevertheless, there are some interesting data on the effect of melatonin on tumors of other localizations (for review see Anisimov et al. 2006). The mechanism of the oncostatic action is complex and probably includes: (1) modulation of the endocrine system; (2) modulation of the immune system; (3) the direct oncostatic action of melatonin on tumor cells. The latter includes the antioxidative action which probably plays an important role in the countering the DNA damage during the radiation challenge or the exposure to chemical carcinogens. It also includes the antiproliferative and pro-apoptotic

Table 6.1 Mechanisms and efficacious concentrations of melatonin in preclinical *in vitro* models related to different types of cancer

Reference	Experimental system	Mechanism/s of action	Efficacious concentrations
CRC			
Ko et al. (2007)	HT29, COLO205, COLO320HSR, COLO320DM, HL-60, Jurkat, RAW264.7, J774A.1, NIH3T3, A431, HaCaT, glioma C6 and MCF-7 cell lines	Significantly inhibition of GOS-induced ROS production through blocking the occurrence of apoptosis	50–100 μM
González-Puga et al. (2005)	HT-29	Strong antiproliferative effect at millimolar concentrations Induction of apoptotic cell death Melatonin generally enhanced the antiproliferative effects of devazepide, lorglumide and proglumide (cholecystokinin (CCK) antagonists) and increased the proglumide-induced apoptosis The synergism between melatonin and CCK-A antagonists to reduce cell proliferation was mainly due to a cell growth decrease	10^{-9}–10^{-3} M
Wenzel et al. (2005)	HT-29	Melatonin did not affect any of the apoptosis markers when given alone at a concentration of 1 mM Combination of flavone and melatonin increased caspase-3-like activity 30-fold and 80% of cells exhibited fragmentation of DNA when compared to untreated controls Melatonin potentiated flavone-induced apoptosis by enhancing the level of oxidizable substrates that can be transported into mitochondria in the presence of flavones	50 μM–1 mM
Winczyk et al. (2002)	Murine transplantable Colon 38 cancer	Melatonin and UCM 386 decreased the cell proliferation, but administration of melatonin and UCM 386 together did not change the inhibitory effect of melatonin alone. That oncostatic effect of melatonin depends on acting via both MT(2) and RZR/ROR nuclear receptors	–

Prostate cancer			
Leja-Szpak et al. (2010)	PANC-1	Stimulation of Bcl-2/Bax and caspase-9 proteins levels (pro-apoptotic effects probably by interaction with the Mel-1 A/B receptors)	10^{-12}–10^{-8} M (physiological concentration)
Pirozhok et al. (2010)	LNCaP 22RV1 PC3 DU145 human fibroblasts and BPH-1, as reference cell lines	No inhibitory effects on cellular viability in the concentration range 10^{-8} to 10^{-3} M A marked concentration-dependent decrease in cellular viability at supraphysiologic concentrations (10^{-3} to 10^{-2} M)	10^{-8}–10^{-2} M
Joo and Yoo (2009)	LNCaP	Melatonin-induced apoptosis was JNK- and p38-dependent, but ERK-independent. Significantly inhibition of the growth of cells in a dose- and time-dependent manner. Induction of both an early stage of apoptosis and a late apoptosis/secondary necrosis, which indicated induction of serial stages of apoptosis in cells Melatonin markedly activated c-JUN N-terminal kinase (JNK) and p38 kinase, whereas extracellular signal-regulated kinase (ERK) was not responsive to melatonin	0–3 mM
Sainz et al. (2008)	LNCaP	Elevation of the p21 protein levels and increasing of the antioxidant capacity of prostate cancer cells Significantly augmentation of hrTNFα induced cell death by decreasing NFkB activation Bcl-2 and survivin down-regulation appeared to be associated to apoptosis stimulation under NFkappaB inhibition No promotion of the irradiation-induced cell death due to an increment in intracellular glutathione content	0–1 mM
Renal cancer			
Um and Kwon (2010)	Caki, HT29, MDA231	Attenuates oxaliplatin-induced apoptosis in cancer cells by inhibition of GSH depletion and Mcl-1 downregulation	0.1, 0.5 and 1 mM

(continued)

Table 6.1 (continued)

Reference	Experimental system	Mechanism/s of action	Efficacious concentrations
Liver cancer			
Fan et al. (2010)	HepG2	The synergism of melatonin and doxorubicin inhibited the cell growth and induced cell apoptosis	10^{-8}–10^{-5} mol/L
	Bel-7402	That cooperative apoptosis induction was associated with decreased expression of Bcl-2 as well as increased expression of Bax and Caspase3	
Ozdemir et al. (2009)	HepG2	Without effect on apoptosis	$5{\cdot}10^{-5}$ M, $5{\cdot}10^{-4}$ M, 10^{-3} M
Martín-Renedo et al. (2008)	HepG2	Reduction in cell number in a dose- and time-dependent manner	10^{3}–10^{4} μM
		Induction of apoptosis with increasing of caspase-3 activity and poly(ADP-ribose) polymerase proteolysis. Proapoptotic effects were related to cytosolic cytochrome c release, upregulation of Bax and induction of caspase-9 activity	
		Elevation of caspase-8 activity but no significant change in Fas-L expression	
		Upregulation of JNK 1,-2 and -3 and p38, members of the MAPK family	
		Growth inhibition altered the percentage or cells in G0-G1 and G2/M phases indicating cell cycle arrest in the G2/M phase. The reduced cell proliferation and alterations of cell cycle were coincident with a significant increase in the expression of p53 and p21 proteins	
She et al. (2004)	H22	Melatonin inhibits the proliferation of cells by arrest and apoptosis, and the mechanism perhaps interferes with increasing p53 that results in down-regulation of cyclin E indirectly and stimulates the expression of Fas gene	10^{-6} M

Qin et al. (2004)	H22	Inhibition of the growth cells by inducing apoptosis and extending the length of cell cycle of the tumor cells	–
Gong et al. (2003)	H22	Induction of apoptosis in a concentration- and time-dependent manner, showing the participation of bcl-2 and bax	–
Pandey et al. (2003)	5123tc NT2	Melatonin was capable of inhibiting the increased ROS production and apoptosis in serum-deprived cells	100 μM
Hermann et al. (2002)	HEPA 1–6	A dose-dependent inhibition of the proliferative activity (from 640 μM to 3 mM), possibly caused by a prolonged activation of mitogen-activated protein kinase (concentrations of 320 μM and less had no effect on cell proliferation). Apoptosis was found to be enhanced by melatonin (75% more than with the solvent alone, $P<0.001$). The inhibitory effect of tamoxifen (25 μM) was markedly enhanced by the coincubation with melatonin (1.3 mM) up to 75% ($P<0.001$)	100–3,200 μM
Nervous system cancer			
Astrocytoma and myeloma	132 1 N1	Antiapoptotic effects (melatonin dose ≥10 μmol/L):	1 mmol/l
Radogna et al. (2009)	U937	In astrocytoma cells melatonin's antiapoptotic effect occurs in a receptor- and a LOX-independent ways but with possible involvement of the PLC pathway In U937 monocytes, antiapoptotic effect requires the cooperation of additional mechanisms involving LOX	
Astroglioma Feng and Zhang (2004)	C6	Melatonin protects C6 cells from Aβ-induced apoptosis by decreasing the percentage of apoptotic cells as well as reducing DNA fragmentation. In addition to the beneficial effects of providing direct antioxidant protection to neurons, melatonin may enhance neuroprotection against Aβ-based neurotoxicity by promoting the survival of glial cells via an augmentation of their antioxidant capacity	10^{-7}–10^{-5} M

(continued)

Table 6.1 (continued)

Reference	Experimental system	Mechanism/s of action	Efficacious concentrations
Malignant glioma cells Martín et al. (2009)	A172 U87 MG	Melatonin effectively increased cell sensitivity to TRAIL-induced cell apoptosis in both type of cells. The effect seems to be related to a modulation of PKC activity which in turns decreases Akt activation leading to an increase in death receptor 5 (DR5) levels and a decrease in the antiapoptotic proteins survivin and bcl-2 levels	1 mM
Neuroblastoma Pizarro et al. (2008)	B65	Melatonin inhibited dopaminergic B65 proliferation, induced cell apoptosis, and modulated cell cycle progression by inhibiting the transcriptional activity of cyclins and cdks related to the progression of the G1-phase	0.1–1 mM
Neuroblastoma Suresh et al. (2006)	SHSY5Y	Pretreatment with melatonin blocked the effects of lead (Pb) on GSH content and caspase-3 activity (antiapoptotic effect), and showed significant improvement in reducing the level of PGE2	10 μM
Neuroblastoma García-Santos et al. (2006)	SK-N-MC	Induction of apoptosis in a dose and time-dependent manner, following the classical caspase 3-dependent pattern. Effective concentrations ranged from 100 to 1 mM. Apoptosis was accompanied by an arrest of cells in G2/M and, in a lesser extent, in S phase of the cell cycle	0.1 μM–1 mM
Neuroblastoma Deng et al. (2005)	N2a	Exposure of the cells to wortmannin resulted in an obvious lipid peroxidation, reduction of cell viability, cell process retraction, and plasma vacuolation, but with no obvious cell apoptosis. Preincubation of the cells with melatonin attenuated differentially wortmannin-induced oxidative stress as well as GSK-3 overactivation and tau hyperphosphorylation	25, 50, and 100 μmol/L

Neuroblastoma and glioma	SKNSH	Melatonin can partly inhibit the cytotoxicity of H_2O_2 and Aβ through its role as a free radical scavenger	10 μM
An et al. (2000)	U251		
Neuroblastoma	N1E-115	The melatonin effects on altered cytoskeletal organization induced by OA were dose-dependent and were not abolished by luzindole (a melatonin antagonist)	10^{-11}, 10^{-9}, 10^{-7}, or 10^{-5} M
Benitez-King et al. (2003)		Melatonin prevented the increased lipid peroxidation and augmented apoptosis induced by OA	
Neuroblastoma	SHSY5Y	Melatonin (50 μM) exhibited a profile of proapoptotic gene expression, increasing the level of bax, caspase-6, fas ligand, and the cell-cycle inhibitor gadd45 genes, while decreasing antiapoptotic bcl-2 and bcl-xL	1–50 μM
Weinreb et al. (2003)		Conversely, the low neuroprotective concentration (1 μM) induced an antiapoptotic response	
Neuroblastoma	SH-SY5Y	Melatonin in physiological concentrations did not exhibit protective properties against neurotoxicity of 24-hydroxycholesterol	10–500 μM
Kölsch et al. (2001)			
Neuroblastoma	SH-SY5Y	HIV-1 protease-induced cyto- and neurotoxicity were prevented by melatonin	60 μM
Hawkins et al. (1999)			
Neuroblastoma	N2a	Melatonin was remarkably effective in preventing death of cultured neuroblastoma cells as well as oxidative	50 μM
Pappolla et al. (1997)	PC12		
Pheochromocytoma	PC12	Any apparent cell death	100 μM
Raza et al. (2008)		No increase in cellular oxidative stress in PC12 cells	
		The mitochondrial functions and redox pools remained stable and there was no increase in ROS production	

(continued)

Table 6.1 (continued)

Reference	Experimental system	Mechanism/s of action	Efficacious concentrations
Pheochromocytoma	PC12	Protection from the apoptotic action of the fungicide maneb by inhibition of both caspase-3/7 activation and disruption of the mitochondrial transmembrane potential. The anti-apoptotic action of melatonin might be Bcl-2-independent	1 nM
Ishido (2007)		Inhibition of maneb-induced aggregation of alpha-synuclein	
Other types of cancer			
Bone cancer	SK-N-MC	Potentiation of cell death, mainly the extrinsic apoptotic pathway: there was a significant increase in the activation of caspase-3, -8, -9 and Bid when melatonin was combined with vincristine or ifosfamide, compared to the individual treatments	Melatonin (50 μM–1 mM) combined with vincristine (5–10 nM) or with ifosfamide (100 μM–1 mM)
Casado-Zapico et al. (2010)		MAPK or PKB/Akt were not involved in apoptosis induced by these agents separately or when combined	
Lymphoma	BL41	Melatonin was able to reduce stress-induced apoptosis in normal lymphocytes and in the lymphoma BL41 cells	1 mmol/l
Paternoster et al. (2009)	E2r	Interestingly, melatonin did not reduce apoptosis in E2r, suggesting that the latent infection with EBV might likely interfere with melatonin's action on apoptosis	
	PBML	The main mechanism of resistance to apoptosis of E2r was the hyperactivation of 5-lipoxygenase and specifically its product 5-HETE	
Leukemia	Jurkat E6-1	Melatonin enhances radiation-induced apoptosis in cells, possibly through the regulation of p53 expression, which supported the prooxidant actions of melatonin in specific cancer types	1 mM
Jang et al. (2009)			

Leukemia Büyükavci et al. (2006)	Jurkat , MOLT-4, CMK, HL-60, Daudi, K562	Melatonin had inhibitory and sometimes apoptotic actions in cancer cells, while in normal cells it typically reduced apoptosis and free radical formation	10^{-5} and 10^{-3} M
Leukemia Trubiani et al. (2005)	RAMOS-1	The apoptotic effect of melatonin was associated with cell-cycle arrest, downregulation of Bcl-2, mitochondrial membrane depolarization, cytochrome c release and activation of caspase-3	2 mM
Leukemia and cervix adenocarcinoma Majsterek et al. (2005)	Normal human lymphocytes K562 HeLa	Melatonin protected both normal and cancer cells against genotoxic treatment and apoptosis induced by idarubicin. The results from the caspase-3 activity and DNA fragmentation in the presence of melatonin confirmed its high a protective effect against idarubicin-induced damage and apoptosis. However, melatonin did not displayed a selectivity toward normal and cancer cells in vitro	50 μM
Ovarian carcinoma Petranka et al. (1999)	BG-1	Melatonin at concentrations of 10^{-9}–10^{-7} M caused a 20–25% reduction in cell number. Melatonin also resulted in a similar reduction in [3H]-thymidine incorporation with no significant increase in cell death Melatonin at 10^{-7} and 10^{-5} M failed to enhance cell death, suggesting a reduction in the cell number by reducing cell proliferation High concentrations of melatonin did not cause apoptosis Growth inhibition by melatonin did not alter the percentage of cells in G1 versus S/G2/M	10^{-9}–10^{-5} M
Tumor skin Cho et al. (2007)	Ultraviolet-B (UVB)-irradiated HaCaT	Modulation of the expression of apoptosis related genes in UVB-irradiated HaCaT cells, resulting in increasing cell survival	10 nM

(continued)

Table 6.1 (continued)

Reference	Experimental system	Mechanism/s of action	Efficacious concentrations
Inducible Ha-ras oncogene	Ha-ras-transformed NIH/3 T3	Melatonin significantly suppressed ras-triggered cell growth by inhibiting the increase of ROS and GSH	1 mM
Chuang et al. (2003)		Melatonin effectively blocked cell apoptosis, but cell growth was also slowed without affecting Ras expression	
		Cotreatment of ras-related cancer cells with melatonin and BSO stops cell growth as well as apoptosis	
Lung and laryngeal carcinomas	Human keratinocytes	Melatonin intensified cytotoxicity of doxorubicin in all cell lines, significantly decreasing cell numbers and promoting apoptosis. The effect was melatonin concentration-dependent. Melatonin decreased the proportion of cells with necrotic lesions	0.1 and 1.0 mM
Fic et al. (2007)	(primary culture) A-549 HEp-2		
Breast cancer	MCF-7	Two distinct apoptotic processes was triggered: an early, TGFβ1 and caspase-independent response, and a late apoptotic TGFβ1-dependent process in which activated caspase-7 was likely to be the terminal effector	1 nM (physiological concentration)
Cucina et al. (2009)			
Breast cancer	MDA-MD-231	Reduction in cell number and augmentation of apoptosis, in combination with troglitazone	1 mM
Korkmaz et al. (2009)			
Breast cancer	MCF-7A	Ineffective alone or in combination with valproic acid, in the first (MCF-7A) subline examined	1 or 10 nM
Jawed et al. (2007)	MCF-7B	Significant synergistic inhibition of cell proliferation in MCF-7B in combination with valproic acid, suggesting induction of apoptosis (similar apoptotic changes were not seen in cells treated with just melatonin)	
Breast cancer	MCF-7	Melatonin enhanced the inhibitory effect that retinoids induced on cell proliferation as well as on the apoptotic pathway in a dose-dependent manner	10^{-5} M
Czeczuga-Semeniuk et al. (2002)			

Breast cancer Cos et al. (2002)	MCF-7	Melatonin reduced cell proliferation by modulating cell cycle length through the control of the p53-p21 pathway, but without clearly inducing apoptosis	1 nM
Breast cancer Eck-Enriquez et al. (2000)	MCF-7	Treatment with melatonin for 24 h before the addition of atRA decreased the protein levels of the death suppressor, Bcl-2, and increased, although with different time courses, the levels of the death promoters, Bax and Bak. However, there was no change in the levels of the tumor suppressor gene, p53 Sequentially treatment with melatonin and atRA also demonstrated an enhanced sensitivity to the apoptotic effects of atRA, suggesting an induction of apoptosis by modulation of members of the Bcl-2 family of proteins	10^{-9} M
Breast cancer Eck et al. (1998)	MCF-7 MDA-MB-231 BT-20	Sequential treatment with melatonin and atRA resulted in the complete cessation of MCF-7 and T47D cell growth as well as a reduction in the number of cells to below the initial plating density. This cytocidal effect on MCF-7 cells was due to the activation pathways leading to apoptosis as evidenced by decreased ER and Bcl-2 and increased Bax and TGF-β1 expression, and was in contrast to the growth-suppressive effects seen with either hormone alone	10^{-9} M
	T47D	The apoptotic effect of this sequential treatment appeared to be both cell and regimen specific as (a) ER-negative MDA-MB-231 and BT-20 breast tumour cells were unaffected, and (b) the simultaneous administration of melatonin and atRA was not associated with apoptosis in any of the breast cancer cell lines studied	

(continued)

Table 6.1 (continued)

Reference	Experimental system	Mechanism/s of action	Efficacious concentrations
Prolactinoma			
Yang et al. (2007)	Primary cultured prolactinoma cells from E(2)-induced rat pituitary prolactin-secreting tumor	Physiological (10^{-11}–10^{-9} M) or low pharmacological (10^{-8}–10^{-6} M) concentrations of melatonin did not demonstrate a significant effect. With high pharmacological (10^{-5}, 10^{-4} and 10^{-3} M) concentrations, melatonin increased caspase-3 activity, Bax mRNA expression, and cytochrome c protein expression. Conversely, Bcl-2 mRNA expression and mitochondrial membrane potential were inhibited by melatonin treatment. These results suggested that melatonin inhibited tumor growth by inducing apoptosis directly via the damage of mitochondria	10^{-11}–10^{-3} M
Ascites carcinoma			
El-Missiry and Abd El-Aziz (2000)	EAC	There was gradual decrease in the cells viability with increasing the melatonin concentration in a dose dependent type Melatonin not only delayed the progression of cells from G(0)/G(1) phase to S-phase of the cell cycle but also reduced DNA synthesis during cell cycle, suggesting an induction of apoptosis	10^{-9}, 10^{-6}, 10^{-3} M

132 1N1 human astrocytoma cell line, *5123tc* rat hepatoma cell line, *A172* and *U87 MG* human glioma cell lines, *A431* squamous cell carcinoma cell line, *A-549* non-small cell lung cancer cell line, *atRA* alltrans-retinoic acid, *B65* rat dopaminergic neuroblastoma cell line, *BG-1* ovarian adenocarcinoma cell line, *Bid* pro-apoptotic bcl-2 family protein that is cleaved and activated by activated caspase-8, *BL41* EBV-negative B-cell line obtained from a Burkitt's lymphoma carrying a mutant form of the p53 gene, *BPH-1* benign prostatic hyperplasia epithelial cell line, *C6* rat astroglioma cells, *Caki* human renal cancer cells, *CMK*, HL-60 and Jurkat human myeloid leukemia cell line, *Daudi* human B lymphoblastic cell line, *E2r* clone obtained after infection of the parental BL41 cell line with a nondefective B95–8 EBV strain, *EAC* Ehrlich ascites carcinoma cells, *GOS* gossypol, is a polyphenolic compound isolated from cotton seeds, *GSK-3* glycogen synthase kinase-3, *H22* mouse hepatocarcinoma cells, *HaCaT* human keratinocyte cell line, *HeLa* cervix adenocarcinoma cells, *HEp-2* laryngeal cancer cell line, *HEPA 1–6* mouse hepatoma cell line, *HepG2* and *Bel-7402* human hepatoma cell lines, *HT29, COLO205, COLO320HSR* and *COLO320DM cells* human colorectal carcinoma cells, *Jurkat E6-1* human T lymphoblastic leukemia cell line, *K562* human leukemic cell line, *LNCaP* (hormone-dependent), *22RV1* (hormone-responding), *PC3* and *DU145* (hormone-independent) prostate cancer cell lines, *MOLT-4* human T lymphoblastic leukemia cell line, *MAPK* and *PKB/Akt* mitogen-activated protein kinase or protein kinase B/Akt (both involved in the extrinsic apoptosis pathway), *MCF-7* and *T47D* (ER)-positive human breast cancer cells, *MCF-7A* and *MCF-7B* a sublines of human MCF-7 breast cancer cells, *MDA-MB-231* and *BT-20* ER-negative human breast cancer cell lines, *N1E-115* mouse neuroblastoma cell line, *N2a* neuroblastoma cell line, *NIH/3T3* mouse fibroblast-derived 7–4 cells, *NIH3T3* fibroblast cell line, *NT2* human teratocarcinoma cell line, *OA* okadaic acid (a potent specific inhibitor of serine/threonine protein phosphatases 1 and 2A), *PANC-1* human pancreatic carcinoma cells, *PBML* human peripheral blood mononuclear leukocytes, *PC12* rat sympathetic pheochromocytoma cell line, *RAMOS-1* human leukaemic cells, *RAW264.7* and *J774A.1* murine macrophage cell lines, *RZR/ROR* nuclear orphan receptors (a subfamily within the superfamily of nuclear hormone receptors), *SHSY5Y* human neuroblastoma cell line, *SK-N-MC* human Ewing sarcoma cancer cells, *SK-N-MC* and *SKNSH* human neuroblastoma cell lines, *TGF-β1* transforming growth factor beta 1, *U251* human glioma cell line, *U937* human monocytic myeloma cell line, *UCM 386* antagonist of membrane MT(1) receptor and partial agonist of membrane MT(2) receptor

Table 6.2 Dose of melatonin and mechanisms of apoptosis in preclinical animal models related to different types of cancer

Referernce	Model	Daily dose	Route	Mechanism/s of action
CRC				
Anisimov et al. (2000)	Female LIO rats	Five days a week during the night time (from 18.00 h to 08.00 h) melatonin, 20 mg/l		Pro-apoptotic effect (TUNEL-method)
Kossoy et al. (2000)	Rats		Fed	Pro-apoptotic effect Activation of Fas signaling
Winczyk et al. (2001, 2002)	Male mice	10 or 100 μg in the evening for 6 days	Subcutaneous	Pro-apoptotic effect (TUNEL-method) mediated by RZR/ROR receptors
Tanaka et al. (2008)	Male F344 rats	0.4, 2 or 10 ppm MEL in drinking water for 17 weeks		Modulation of apoptosis by reduction expression of nuclear factor kappa B, tumor necrosis factor alpha, interleukin-1beta and STAT3
Hepatoma				
Cini et al. (1998)	Rat	Of 0.34 mg/kg at 19:00 h every evening, starting the day before tumor transplantation and continuing throughout the animal's life	i.m.	No changes in the apoptotic index (TUNEL-method)
Dziegiel et al. (2003)	Rat	10 mg/kg	Subcutaneous	Decrease in the apoptotic index (TUNEL method)
Prostate cancer				
Xi et al. (2001)	Male BALB/c athymic nude mice	Daily melatonin (4 microg/g body weight) ,1 h before room lighting was switched	i.p.	No changes in the apoptotic index (TUNEL-method)

Bladder cancer				
Zupancic et al. (2008)	Male ICR mice	(10 mg/kg)	i.p.	Inhibition of apoptosis no active caspase-3 immunohistochemistry
Tripathi and Jena (2010)	Male Sprague–Dawley rat	(10 mg/kg)	i.p.	Inhibition of apoptosis
Breast cancer				
Melancon et al. (2005)	Rat	500–1,000 μg/day in the afternoon	Subcutaneous injection	Pro-apoptotic effect
el-Aziz et al. (2005)	Rat	2,500 μg/Kg body weight/day	Subcutaneous injection	Pro-apoptotic effect increased tumour necrosis factor reduction of (TNF)-alpha, tissue caspase-3 activity and percentage of DNA fragmentation
Prolactinoma				
Yang et al. (2006)	Rat	0.125, 0.25, 0.50 or 1.0 mg melatonin/day/rat at 17:30–18:00 h	Subcutaneous injection	Pro-apoptotic effect (TUNEL-method) Bax and cytochrome c protein overexpression Down expression of Bcl-2, and mitochondrial membrane potential
Lung cancer				
Maestroni et al. (1994)	Female C57BL/6 mice	1 mg/kg body weight/day	Subcutaneous injection	Prevention of etoposide-induced apoptosis in bone marrow cells

effects exerted via melatonin membrane and nuclear receptors expressed by tumor cells (Pawlikowski et al. 2002; Hill et al. 2009). However, in a series of studies contradictory results have also been observed as it has been shown that melatonin may inhibit apoptosis. In this section we will review available data on anticarcinogenic effects of melatonin and its effects on the modulation of apoptosis in experimental *in vivo* studies (Table 6.2).

6.4.2.1 Colon Cancer

The inhibitory effects of exogenous melatonin on colon oncogenesis have been investigated by several authors. For instance, Anisimov et al. (2000) demonstrated the suppression of 1,2-dimethylhydrazine (DMH)-induced colon carcinogenesis by melatonin in female LIO rats which received from the day of the 1st injection of the carcinogen 5 days a week during the night time (from 18.00 to 08.00 h) melatonin, 20 mg/l. The reduction of multiplicity of colon tumors under the influence of melatonin was correlated with the significant inhibitory effect of the pineal hormone on mitotic index and with stimulating effect of melatonin on the relative number of apoptotic cells (TUNEL-method) in colon tumors. Kossoy et al. (2000) evaluated histologically and immunohistochemically the splenic immune response to 1,2-dimethylhydrazine (DMH)-induced colon carcinogenesis in melatonin fed rats. The anti-carcinogenic properties of melatonin were evidenced by the expansion of the splenic zones by 106–125%, compared to those from DMH-treated rats, and the numbers of CD8+ lymphocytes and Fas-positive cells increased sharply, concluding that anti-carcinogenic and pro-apoptotic effects of melatonin were related to activation of several elements of the host's lymphatic system and pro-apoptotic Fas signaling respectively.

Winczyk et al. (2001) studied the effects of melatonin and the thiazolidinedione derivative CGP 52608 on apoptosis of Colon 38 cancer in male mice implanted subcutaneously with a suspension of Colon 38 cells. Ten days after induction of tumors, the animals were treated with melatonin in subcutaneous injections in daily doses of 10 or 100 μg in the evening for 6 days. Melatonin increased significantly the number of apoptotic cells in tumors. This finding confirms our earlier observation that melatonin exerts a pro-apoptotic effect on murine colonic cancer cells. In addition authors suggested that RZR/ROR receptors are involved the in the pro-apoptotic effect of melatonin. In a later study, by Winczyk et al. (2002) investigated whether CGP 55644 (an antagonist of the nuclear RZR/RORalpha receptor) changed the oncostatic and proapoptotics effects of Melatonin on murine Colon 38 cancer. The experiment was performed on adult male B6D2F1 mice. Melatonin or CGP were given either alone or combined during 10 days and, the proliferation/apoptosis (P/A) ratio were determined. It was found that melatonin increased the apoptotic index, but CGP decreased it. In addition, CGP given together with the hormone blocked its proapoptotic effect. Based on our data, they concluded that nuclear RZR/RORalpha receptors participated in the oncostatic action of melatonin.

In another study by Tanaka et al. (2008) using an azoxymethane (AOM)/dextran sodium sulfate (DSS) in Male F344 rats. Animals were given 0.4, 2 or 10 ppm MEL in drinking water for 17 weeks. Colonic adenocarcinoma was developed at week 20 which was significantly inhibited by the administration with MEL dose-dependently. MEL exposure modulated the mitotic and apoptotic indices in the colonic adenocarcinomas that developed and lowered the immunohistochemical expression of nuclear factor kappa B, tumor necrosis factor alpha, interleukin-1beta and STAT3 in the epithelial malignancies. These results indicated the beneficial effects of MEL on colitis-related colon carcinogenesis and a potential application for inhibiting colorectal cancer development in the inflamed colon (Tanaka et al. 2008).

6.4.2.2 Bladder Cancer

Repeated cyclophosphamide (CP) chemotherapy increases the risk of developing bladder cancer, which could be due to the extremely rapid proliferation of urothelial cells observed in hyperplastic urothelium induced by CP treatment. Zupancic et al. (2008) investigated the effect of melatonin on the development of urothelial hyperplasia induced by repeated CP treatment. Male ICR mice were injected with CP (150 mg/kg) or melatonin (10 mg/kg) with CP once a week for 3, 4 and 5 weeks. Repeated doses of CP caused the development of hyperplastic urothelium and increased proliferation and apoptotic indices regarding Ki-67 and active caspase-3 immunohistochemistry, respectively. Melatonin co-treatment prevented the development of hyperplastic urothelium, statistically significantly decreased proliferation and apoptotic indices after four and five doses of CP and caused higher differentiation state of superficial urothelial cells. Similar results were found by Tripathi and Jena (2010) who in male Sprague–Dawley rats. Melatonintreatment (10 mg/kg) reduced the bladder damage and significantly decrease in the percentage of TUNEL positive cells as compared with CP-treated group.

6.4.2.3 Hepatoma

Cini et al. (1998) tested the effects of daily melatonin treatment on the growth of the ascites hepatoma in rats, determining survival time, cell number and cell cycle phases at various stages of tumor development. MLT was injected intramuscularly at a dose of 0.34 mg/kg, equivalent to a daily dose of 0.048 mg/rat at 1,900 h every evening, starting the day before tumor transplantation and continuing throughout the animal's life. Melatonin inhibited cellular proliferation, doubled mean life-time and increased survival. Thymidine incorporation in hepatoma cells from treated rats decreased significantly without changes in the apoptotic index (TUNEL-method). Flow cytometric analysis showed that melatonin slowed cell cycle progression by increasing the number of cells in phase G0G1. Thus, similar to in vitro models, melatonin's oncostatic action in vivo appears to be directed to specific cell cycle mechanisms, which remain to be elucidated.

Different results were found by Dziegiel et al. (2003) in a study about the cytostatic efficiency of doxorubicin (DOX) applied together with melatonin to rats with transplantable Morris hepatoma. Melatonin was administered subcutaneously before and after every injection of a cytostatic drug at a dose of 10 mg/kg b.w. Administration of melatonin together with DOX decreased the extent of tumour necrosis and the apoptotic tumour cells but, on the other hand, decreased the number of apoptotic cardiomyocytes.

6.4.2.4 Prostate Cancer

Prostate cancer is one of the most common malignancies among elderly males in the developed countries of South and East Asia, Europe and the United States. Although some studies have shown a relationship between high dietary fat intake and increased testosterone levels, the cause of prostate cancer remains unknown. Nevertheless, mechanistically, apoptosis is closely involved in the initiation, progression and metastasis of prostate cancer. Therefore, potential anti-prostate cancer strategies may include effective apoptosis induction or enhancement via novel apoptosis inducers (Joo and Yoo 2009). Xi et al. (2001) demonstrated the antiproliferative effects of melatonin on prostate cancer cell proliferation and apoptosis in athymic nude mice xenograft models of LNCaP and PC-3 cells. Daily i.p. melatonin (4 μg/g body weight), 1 h before room lighting was switched off, was given to nude mice before or after tumor cell inoculation. Melatonin inhibited the growth of LNCaP tumors, without affecting the growth of PC-3 xenografts, in nude mice. It induced significant decreases in the expression of PCNA, cyclin A, and PSA in LNCaP tumors. Detection and quantitation of apoptosis were performed by the TUNEL reaction. When melatonin or saline treatment was initiated 10 days before LNCaP cell inoculation, no significant differences in the number of apoptotic cells/HPF in prostate tumors were found between the saline treated group and melatonin-treated group. Similarly, the number of apoptotic cells/HPF in LNCaP tumors from saline-treated animals was not significantly different from those derived from melatonin-treated animals when the animals were injected 10 days after tumor cell transplantation.

6.4.2.5 Breast Cancer and Prolactinoma

Substantial evidence has accumulated demonstrating that the pineal hormone melatonin exerts an inhibitory influence on the growth of breast cancer cells *in vitro* and the development and growth of carcinogen-induced rat mammary tumors *in vivo* (Nowfar et al. 2002). This oncostatic activity has been explained on the basis of its antiestrogenic property. An interesting study by Melancon et al. (2005) demonstrated **a** significant increase in tumor regression induced in N-nitroso-N-methylurea-induced mammary tumors in rats treated with the combination of melatonin and 9-cis-retinoic acid (9cRA). Melatonin was administered by subcutaneous injection in the late afternoon. Treatment groups included: control melatonin 500 μg/day, melatonin 1,000 μg/day, melatonin 500 μg/day+9cRA and melatonin 1,000 μg/day+9cRA. Rats treated with the lower dose of melatonin 500 μg+9cRA showed the greatest degree of tumor regression (78%), with 54% undergoing complete regression and a significant increase in apoptotic cells observed by TUNEL Assay. Furthermore, tumor multiplicity and burden were significantly decreased by the combination of melatonin and 9cRA. These data demonstrated that the combined use of Melatonin and 9cRA produced additive or synergistic effects, which were more efficacious than 9cRA alone. This combination of melatonin and 9cRA could be a potentially useful clinical treatment regimen for breast cancer since it allows the use of lower doses of retinoic acid, thus, avoiding the toxic side effects associated with the use of high dose retinoids.

In 7, 12-di-methylbenz(a)anthracene (DMBA) model of mammary carcinoma, melatonin was daily injected subcutaneously in a dose of 250 μg/100 g body weight for 3 months from 14 days before the intake of DMBA and then continued until the end of the experiments. Melatonin reduced the carcinogenic effects of DMBA. The protective effect in melatonin treated group was associated with decreased levels of markers of tumorigenicity, endocrine derangement and oxidative stress. Also, it was associated with increased levels of markers of apoptotic activity: tumour necrosis factor (TNF)-alpha, tissue caspase-3 activity and percentage of DNA fragmentation and ultrastructural features of apoptosis (el-Aziz et al. 2005). In a later study by Yang et al. (2006) the *in vivo* effects of melatonin on proliferation and apoptosis of 17-beta-estradiol (E2)-induced pituitary prolactin secreting tumor (prolactinoma) were investigated in rats kept in 12 L/12 D (lights on: 06:00–18:00 h). As melatonin was shown to induce apoptosis of breast and liver tumor cells, we examined whether melatonin would induce apoptosis of rat pituitary prolactinoma cells. 0.125, 0.25, 0.50 or 1.0 mg melatonin/day/rat was administrated subcutaneously at 17:30–18:00 h. The weight of prolactinomas was measured. Apoptosis was evaluated using the TdT-mediated dUTP nick-end labeling method. It was found that treatment with 0.25 and 0.50 mg melatonin for 97 days inhibited prolactinoma cell proliferation and increased prolactinoma cell apoptosis. Furthermore, melatonin induced mRNA expression of Bax and cytochrome c protein expression. Conversely, mRNA expression of Bcl-2, and mitochondrial membrane potential were inhibited by melatonin treatment. These results suggest that melatonin inhibits the proliferation and induces apoptosis of rat pituitary prolactin-secreting tumor via perturbation of mitochondria physiology.

6.4.2.6 Lung Cancer

Although melatonin has been shown to inhibit urethane-induced carcinogenesis tumors in murine lung in mice (Vesnushkin et al. 2006), previous report by Perissin et al. (1989) observed opposite results in mice bearing Lewis lung carcinoma. Additionally, we have not found any preclinic study about the effects of melatonin administration on apoptosis *in vivo* experimental models of lung cancer. Although Maestroni et al. (1994) investigated whether melatonin could affect tumor growth and/or hematopoiesis in mice transplanted with Lewis lung carcinoma and treated with cyclophosphamide or etoposide. These agents were injected i.p. for 5 days at two different cumulative doses (cyclophosphamide, 40 and 160 mg/kg body weight; etoposide, 20 and 40 mg/kg body weight) from day 8 through day 12 after tumor transplantation. Melatonin was injected s.c. at a dose of 1 mg/kg body weight/day, from day 8 throughout the experiments and from days 8 through 12 or from day 13 onwards. Melatonin did not influence tumor growth but selectively counteracted bone marrow toxicity when administered together with the cancer chemotherapy compounds without interfering with their anticancer action. *In vitro*, melatonin proved to counteract apoptosis in bone marrow cells incubated with etoposide.

References

An Y, Liu E, Liu X et al (2000) Protective effect of melatonin on neural cells against the cytotoxicity of oxyradicals. Chin Med Sci J 15(1):40–44

Anisimov VN (2003) Effects of exogenous melatonin – a review. Toxicol Pathol 31:589–603

Anisimov VN, Popovich IG, Shtylik AV et al (2000) Melatonin and colon carcinogenesis. III. Effect of melatonin on proliferative activity and apoptosis in colon mucosa and colon tumors induced by 1,2-dimethylhydrazine in rats. Exp Toxicol Pathol 52(1):71–76

Anisimov VN, Popovich IG, Zabezhinski MA et al (2006) Melatonin as antioxidant, geroprotector and anticarcinogen. Biochim Biophys Acta 1757(5–6):573–589

Arlt W, Hewison M (2004) Hormones and immune function: implications of aging. Aging Cell 3:209–216

Axelrod J (1974) The pineal gland: a neurochemical transducer. Science 184:1341–1348

Axelrod J, Weissbach H (1960) Enzymatic O-methylation of N-acetylserotonin to melatonin. Science 131:1312

Bangha E, Elsner P, Kistler GS (1996) Suppression of UV-induced erythema by topical treatment with melatonin (N-acetyl-5-methoxytryptamine). A dose response study. Arch Dermatol Res 288:522–526

Bartsch C, Bartsch H, Karasek M (2002) Melatonin in clinical oncology. Neuro Endocrinol Lett 23(1):30–38

Benitez-King G, Túnez I, Bellon A et al (2003) Melatonin prevents cytoskeletal alterations and oxidative stress induced by okadaic acid in N1E-115 cells. Exp Neurol 182(1):151–159

Blask DE, Sauer LA, Dauchy RT (2002) Melatonin as a chronobiotic/anticancer agent: cellular, biochemical, and molecular mechanisms of action and their implications for circadian-based cancer therapy. Curr Top Med Chem 2:113–132

Blask DE, Brainard GC, Dauchy RT et al (2005) Melatonin-depleted blood from premenopausal women exposed to light at night stimulates growth of human breast cancer xenografts in nude rats. Cancer Res 65:11174–11184

Bondarenko LO (1992) The comparative evaluation of the effect of the season on the formation of a nighttime melatonin peak in young sexually mature and old rats. Fiziol Zh 38:111–114

Bonilla E, Valero N, Chacin-Bonilla L et al (2004) Melatonin and viral infections. J Pineal Res 36:73–79

Brainard GC, Podolin PL, Leivy SW et al (1986) Near-ultraviolet radiation suppresses pineal melatonin content. Endocrinology 119(5):2201–2205

Büyükavci M, Ozdemir O, Buck S et al (2006) Melatonin cytotoxicity in human leukemia cells: relation with its pro-oxidant effect. Fundam Clin Pharmacol 20(1):73–79

Cajochen C, Krauchi K, Wirz-Justice A (2003) Role of melatonin in the regulation of human circadian rhythms and sleep. J Neuroendocrinol 15:432–437

Carlberg C (2000) Gene regulation by melatonin. Ann N Y Acad Sci 917:387–396

Carrillo-Vico A, Garcia-Perganeda A, Naji L et al (2003) Expression of membrane and nuclear melatonin receptor mRNA and protein in the mouse immune system. Cell Mol Life Sci 60:2272–2278

Carrillo-Vico A, Calvo JR, Abreu P et al (2004) Evidence of melatonin synthesis by human lymphocytes and its physiological significance: possible role as intracrine, autocrine, and/or paracrine substance. FASEB J 18:537–539

Carrillo-Vico A, Guerrero JM, Lardone PJ et al (2005a) A review of the multiple actions of melatonin on the immune system. Endocrine 27:189–200

Carrillo-Vico A, Lardone PJ, Fernandez-Santos JM et al (2005b) Human lymphocyte-synthesized melatonin is involved in the regulation of the interleukin-2/interleukin-2 receptor system. J Clin Endocrinol Metab 90:992–1000

Carrillo-Vico A, Reiter RJ, Lardone PJ et al (2006) The modulatory role of melatonin on immune responsiveness. Curr Opin Investig Drugs 7:423–431

Casado-Zapico S, Rodriguez-Blanco J, García-Santos G et al (2010) Synergistic antitumor effect of melatonin with several chemotherapeutic drugs on human Ewing sarcoma cancer cells: potentiation of the extrinsic apoptotic pathway. J Pineal Res 48(1):72–80

Castillo C, Salazar V, Ariznavarreta C et al (2005) Effect of melatonin administration on parameters related to oxidative damage in hepatocytes isolated from old Wistar rats. J Pineal Res 38:240–246

Cho JW, Kim CW, Lee KS (2007) Modification of gene expression by melatonin in UVB-irradiated HaCaT keratinocyte cell lines using a cDNA microarray. Oncol Rep 17(3):573–577

Chuang JI, Chang TY, Liu HS (2003) Glutathione depletion-induced apoptosis of Ha-ras-transformed NIH3T3 cells can be prevented by melatonin. Oncogene 22(9):1349–1357

Cini G, Coronnello M, Mini E et al (1998) Melatonin's growth-inhibitory effect on hepatoma AH 130 in the rat. Cancer Lett 125(1–2):51–59

Claustrat B, Brun J, Chazot G (2005) The basic physiology and pathophysiology of melatonin. Sleep Med Rev 9(1):11–24

Conti A, Conconi S, Hertens E et al (2000) Evidence for melatonin synthesis in mouse and human bone marrow cells. J Pineal Res 28:193–202

Cos S, Mediavilla MD, Fernández R et al (2002) Does melatonin induce apoptosis in MCF-7 human breast cancer cells in vitro? J Pineal Res 32(2):90–96

Cucina A, Proietti S, D'Anselmi F et al (2009) Evidence for a biphasic apoptotic pathway induced by melatonin in MCF-7 breast cancer cells. J Pineal Res 46(2):172–180

Cuzzocrea S, Reiter RJ (2001) Pharmacological action of melatonin in shock, inflammation and ischemia/reperfusion injury. Eur J Pharmacol 426:1–10

Czeczuga-Semeniuk E, Wołczyński S, Anchim T et al (2002) Effect of melatonin and all-trans retinoic acid on the proliferation and induction of the apoptotic pathway in the culture of human breast cancer cell line MCF-7. Pol J Pathol 53(2):59–65

Deng YQ, Xu GG, Duan P et al (2005) Effects of melatonin on wortmannin-induced tau hyperphosphorylation. Acta Pharmacol Sin 26(5):519–526

Dziegiel P, Podhorska-Okolow M, Surowiak P, Ciesielska U, Rabczynski J, Zabel M (2003) Influence of exogenous melatonin on doxorubicin-evoked effects in myocardium and in transplantable Morris hepatoma in rats. In Vivo 17(4):325–328

Eck KM, Yuan L, Duffy L et al (1998) A sequential treatment regimen with melatonin and all-transretinoic acid induces apoptosis in MCF-7 tumour cells. Br J Cancer 77(12):2129–2137

Eck-Enriquez K, Kiefer TL, Spriggs LL, Hill SM (2000) Pathways through which a regimen of melatonin and retinoic acid induces apoptosis in MCF-7 human breast cancer cells. Breast Cancer Res Treat 61(3):229–239

El-Aziz MA, Hassan HA, Mohamed MH et al (2005) The biochemical and morphological alterations following administration of melatonin, retinoic acid and Nigella sativa in mammary carcinoma: an animal model. Int J Exp Pathol 86(6):383–396

El-Missiry MA, Abd El-Aziz AF (2000) Influence of melatonin on proliferation and antioxidant system in Ehrlich ascites carcinoma cells. Cancer Lett 15(2):119–125

Escames G, Leon J, Macias M et al (2003) Melatonin counteracts lipopolysaccharide-induced expression and activity of mitochondrial nitric oxide synthase in rats. FASEB J 17:932–934

Escames G, Acuna-Castroviejo D, Lopez LC et al (2006) Pharmacological utility of melatonin in the treatment of septic shock: experimental and clinical evidence. J Pharm Pharmacol 58:1153–1165

Fan LL, Sun GP, Wei W et al (2010) Melatonin and doxorubicin synergistically induce cell apoptosis in human hepatoma cell lines. World J Gastroenterol 16(12):1473–1481

Feng Z, Zhang JT (2004) Protective effect of melatonin on beta-amyloid-induced apoptosis in rat astroglioma C6 cells and its mechanism. Free Radic Biol Med 37(11):1790–1801

Fic M, Podhorska-Okolow M, Dziegiel P et al (2007) Effect of melatonin on cytotoxicity of doxorubicin toward selected cell lines (human keratinocytes, lung cancer cell line A-549, laryngeal cancer cell line Hep-2). In Vivo 21(3):513–518

Garcia-Perganeda A, Pozo D, Guerrero J.M, Calvo J.R (1997) Signal transduction for melatonin in human lymphocytes, involvement of a pertussis toxin-sensitive G protein. J Immunol 159(8): 774–781

García-Santos G, Antolín I, Herrera F et al (2006) Melatonin induces apoptosis in human neuroblastoma cancer cells. J Pineal Res 41(2):130–135

Gitto E, Karbownik M, Reiter RJ et al (2001) Effects of melatonin treatment in septic newborns. Pediatr Res 50:756–760

Gong LH, Ren DH, Xiong M et al (2003) Melatonin in in vitro apoptosis of H22 hepatocarcinoma cells. Zhonghua Zhong Liu Za Zhi 25(6):550–554

González-Puga C, García-Navarro A, Escames G et al (2005) Selective CCK-A but not CCK-B receptor antagonists inhibit HT-29 cell proliferation: synergism with pharmacological levels of melatonin. J Pineal Res 39(3):243–250

Green DR, Kroemer G (2004) The pathophysiology of mitochondrial cell death. Science 305:626–629

Guerrero JM (1997) Melatonin enhances IL-2, IL-6, and IFN-gamma production by human circulating CD4+ cells: a possible nuclear receptor-mediated mechanism involving T helper type 1 lymphocytes and monocytes. J Immunol 159:574–581

Guerrero JM, Reiter RJ (2002) Melatonin-immune system relationships. Curr Top Med Chem 2:167–179

Hardeland, R (2008) Melatonin, hormone of darkness and more, occurrence, control mechanisms, actions and bioactive metabolites. Cell Mol Life Sci 65(13):2001–2018

Hawkins V, Shen Q, Chiueh CC (1999) Kynostatin and 17beta-estradiol prevent the apoptotic death of human neuroblastoma cells exposed to HIV-1 protease. J Biomed Sci 6(6):433–438

Hermann R, Podhajsky S, Jungnickel S et al (2002) Potentiation of antiproliferative effects of tamoxifen and ethanol on mouse hepatoma cells by melatonin: possible involvement of mitogen-activated protein kinase and induction of apoptosis. J Pineal Res 33(1):8–13

Herrera J, Nava M, Romero F et al (2001) Melatonin prevents oxidative stress resulting from iron and erythropoietin administration. Am J Kidney Dis 37:750–757

Hill SM, Frasch T, Xiang S et al (2009) Molecular mechanisms of melatonin anticancer effects. Integr Cancer Ther 8(4):337–346

Ishido M (2007) Melatonin inhibits maneb-induced aggregation of alphasynuclein in rat pheochromocytoma cells. J Pineal Res 42(2):125–130

Jang SS, Kim WD, Park WY (2009) Melatonin exerts differential actions on X-ray radiation-induced apoptosis in normal mice splenocytes and Jurkat leukemia cells. J Pineal Res 47(2):147–155

Jawed S, Kim B, Ottenhof T et al (2007) Human melatonin MT1 receptor induction by valproic acid and its effects in combination with melatonin on MCF-7 breast cancer cell proliferation. Eur J Pharmacol 560(1):17–22

Joo SS, Yoo YM (2009) Melatonin induces apoptotic death in LNCaP cells via p38 and JNK pathways: therapeutic implications for prostate cancer. J Pineal Res 47(1):8–14

Jung B, Ahmad N (2006) Melatonin in cancer management: progress and promise. Cancer Res 66:9789–9793

Kireev RA, Tresguerres AC, Castillo C et al (2007) Effect of exogenous administration of melatonin and growth hormone on pro-antioxidant functions of the liver in aging male rats. J Pineal Res 42(1):64–70

Klein DC, Namboodiri MA, Auerbach DA (1981) The melatonin rhythm generating system: developmental aspects. Life Sci 28:1975–1986
Ko CH, Shen SC, Yang LY et al (2007) Gossypol reduction of tumor growth through ROS-dependent mitochondria pathway in human colorectal carcinoma cells. Int J Cancer 8:1670–1679
Kölsch H, Ludwig M, Lütjohann D et al (2001) Neurotoxicity of 24-hydroxycholesterol, an important cholesterol elimination product of the brain, may be prevented by vitamin E and estradiol-17beta. J Neural Transm 108(4):475–488
Korkmaz A, Tamura H, Manchester LC et al (2009) Combination of melatonin and a peroxisome proliferatoractivated receptor-gamma agonist induces apoptosis in a breast cancer cell line. J Pineal Res 46(1):115–116
Kossoy G, Ben-Hur H, Popovich I et al (2000) Melatonin and colon carcinogenesis. IV. Effect of melatonin on proliferative activity and expression of apoptosis-related proteins in the spleen of rats exposed to 1,2-dimethylhydrazine. Oncol Rep 7(6):1401–1405
Leja-Szpak A, Jaworek J, Pierzchalski P et al (2010) Melatonin induces pro-apoptotic signaling pathway in human pancreatic carcinoma cells (PANC-1). J Pineal Res 49(3):248–255
Leon J, Acuna-Castroviejo D, Escames G et al (2005) Melatonin mitigates mitochondrial malfunction. J Pineal Res 38:1–9
Lerner AB, Case JD, Takahashi Y (1960) Isolation of melatonin and 5-methoxyindole-3-acetic acid from bovine pineal glands. J Biol Chem 235:1992–1997
Lissoni P, Rovelli F, Malugani F et al (2001) Anti-angiogenic activity of melatonin in advanced cancer patients. Neuro Endocrinol Lett 22:45–47
Lopez-Burillo S, Tan DX, Mayo JC et al (2003) Melatonin, xanthurenic acid, resveratrol, EGCG, vitamin C and alpha-lipoic acid differentially reduce oxidative DNA damage induced by Fenton reagents: a study of their individual and synergistic actions. J Pineal Res 34:269–277
Maestroni GJ, Covacci V, Conti A (1994) Hematopoietic rescue via T-cell-dependent, endogenous granulocyte-macrophage colony-stimulating factor induced by the pineal neurohormone melatonin in tumor-bearing mice. Cancer Res 54(9):2429–2432
Majsterek I, Gloc E, Blasiak J et al (2005) A comparison of the action of amifostine and melatonin on DNA-damaging effects and apoptosis induced by idarubicin in normal and cancer cells. J Pineal Res 38(4):254–263
Martín V, García-Santos G, Rodriguez-Blanco J et al (2009) Melatonin sensitizes human malignant glioma cells against TRAIL-induced cell death. Cancer Lett 287(2):216–223
Martín-Renedo J, Mauriz JL, Jorquera F et al (2008) Melatonin induces cell cycle arrest and apoptosis in hepatocarcinoma HepG2 cell line. J Pineal Res 45(4):532–540
Melancon K, Cheng Q, Kiefer TL et al (2005) Regression of NMU-induced mammary tumors with the combination of melatonin and 9-cis-retinoic acid. Cancer Lett 227(1):39–48
Morioka N, Okatani Y, Wakatsuki A (1999) Melatonin protects against age-related DNA damage in the brains of female senescence-accelerated mice. J Pineal Res 27:202–209
Nagata S (1997) Apoptosis by death factor. Cell 88:355–365
Naranjo MC, Guerrero JM, Rubio A et al (2007) Melatonin biosynthesis in the thymus of humans and rats. Cell Mol Life Sci 64:781–790
Nowfar S, Teplitzky SR, Melancon K et al (2002) Tumor prevention by 9-cis-retinoic acid in the N-nitroso-Nmethylurea model of mammary carcinogenesis is potentiated by the pineal hormone melatonin. Breast Cancer Res Treat 72(1):33–43
Okatani Y, Wakatsuki A, Reiter RJ (2002) Melatonin protects hepatic mitochondrial respiratory chain activity in senescence-accelerated mice. J Pineal Res 32:143–148
Ozdemir F, Deniz O, Kaynar K et al (2009) The effects of melatonin on human hepatoma (Hep G2) cell line. Bratisl Lek Listy 110(5):276–279
Pandey S, Lopez C, Jammu A (2003) Oxidative stress and activation of proteasome protease during serum deprivation-induced apoptosis in rat hepatoma cells; inhibition of cell death by melatonin. Apoptosis 8(5):497–508
Pandi-Perumal SR, Srinivasan V, Maestroni GJ et al (2006) Melatonin: nature's most versatile biological signal? FEBS J 273:2813–2838

Pappolla MA, Sos M, Omar RA et al (1997) Melatonin prevents death of neuroblastoma cells exposed to the Alzheimer amyloid peptide. J Neurosci 17(5):1683–1690
Paternoster L, Radogna F, Accorsi A et al (2009) Melatonin as a modulator of apoptosis in B-lymphoma cells. Ann N Y Acad Sci 1171:345–349
Pawlikowski M, Winczyk K, Karasek M (2002) Oncostatic action of melatonin: facts and question marks. Neuro Endocrinol Lett 23(1):24–29
Perissin L, Zorzet S, Rapozzi V et al (1989) Effect of different light cycles and stress on urinary excretion of melatonin and tumor spread in mice bearing Lewis lung carcinoma. Pharmacol Res 21:131–135
Petranka J, Baldwin W, Biermann J et al (1999) The oncostatic action of melatonin in an ovarian carcinoma cell line. J Pineal Res 26(3):129–136
Pieri C, Recchioni R, Moroni F et al (1998) Melatonin regulates the respiratory burst of human neutrophils and their depolarization. J Pineal Res 24:43–49
Pierpaoli W, Maestroni GJ (1987) Melatonin: a principal neuroimmunoregulatory and anti-stress hormone: its anti-aging effects. Immunol Lett 16:355–361
Pirozhok I, Meye A, Hakenberg OW et al (2010) Serotonin and melatonin do not play a prominent role in the growth of prostate cancer cell lines. Urol Int 84(4):452–460
Pizarro JG, Yeste-Velasco M, Esparza JL et al (2008) The antiproliferative activity of melatonin in B65 rat dopaminergic neuroblastoma cells is related to the downregulation of cell cycle-related genes. J Pineal Res 45(1):8–16
Pozo D, Delgado M, Fernandez-Santos JM et al (1997) Expression of the Mel1a-melatonin receptor mRNA in T and B subsets of lymphocytes from rat thymus and spleen. FASEB J 11:466–473
Qin L, Wang X, Duan Q et al (2004) Inhibitory effect of melatonin on the growth of H22 hepatocarcinoma cells by inducing apoptosis. J Huazhong Univ Sci Technolog Med Sci 24(1):19–21, 31
Radogna F, Nuccitelli S, Mengoni F et al (2009) Neuroprotection by melatonin on astrocytoma cell death. Ann N Y Acad Sci 1171:509–513
Raza H, John A, Brown EM et al (2008) Alterations in mitochondrial respiratory functions, redox metabolism and apoptosis by oxidant 4-hydroxynonenal and antioxidants curcumin and melatonin in PC12 cells. Toxicol Appl Pharmacol 226(2):161–168
Regodon S, Martin-Palomino P, Fernandez-Montesinos R et al (2005) The use of melatonin as a vaccine agent. Vaccine 23:5321–5327
Reiter RJ (1980) Photoperiod: its importance as an impeller of pineal and seasonal reproductive rhythms. Int J Biometeorol 24:57–63
Reiter RJ (1986) Normal patterns of melatonin levels in the pineal gland and body fluids of humans and experimental animals. J Neural Transm 21:35–54
Reiter RJ (1991) Melatonin: the chemical expression of darkness. Mol Cell Endocrinol 79:C153–C158
Reiter RJ, Tan DX, Manchester LC et al (2002) Melatonin reduces oxidant damage and promotes mitochondrial respiration: implications for aging. Ann N Y Acad Sci 959:238–250
Reiter RJ, Tan DX, Gitto E et al (2004) Pharmacological utility of melatonin in reducing oxidative cellular and molecular damage. Pol J Pharmacol 56:159–170
Reiter RJ, Tan DX, Terron MP et al (2007) Melatonin and its metabolites: new findings regarding their production and their radical scavenging actions. Acta Biochim Pol 54:1–9
Roy D, Angelini NL, Fujieda H et al (2001) Cyclical regulation of GnRH gene expression in GT1-7 GnRH-secreting neurons by melatonin. Endocrinology 142:4711–4720
Sainz RM, Mayo JC, Uria H et al (1995) The pineal neurohormone melatonin prevents in vivo and in vitro apoptosis in thymocytes. J Pineal Res 19:178–188
Sainz RM, Reiter RJ, Tan DX et al (2008) Critical role of glutathione in melatonin enhancement of tumor necrosis factor and ionizing radiation-induced apoptosis in prostate cancer cells in vitro. J Pineal Res 45(3):258–270
Shamir E, Barak Y, Shalman I et al (2001) Melatonin treatment for tardive dyskinesia: a double-blind, placebo-controlled, crossover study. Arch Gen Psychiatry 58:1049–1052
She MH, Chen BB, Wang XM et al (2004) p53-dependent antiproliferation and apoptosis of H22 cell induced by melatonin. Ai Zheng 23(7):803–807

Silva SO, Rodrigues MR, Carvalho SR et al (2004) Oxidation of melatonin and its catabolites, N1-acetyl-N2 -formyl-5-methoxykynuramine and N1-acetyl-5-methoxykynuramine, by activated leukocytes. J Pineal Res 37:171–175
Sugden D (1989) Melatonin biosynthesis in the mammalian pineal gland. Experientia 45:922–932
Suresh C, Dennis AO, Heinz J et al (2006) Melatonin protection against lead-induced changes in human neuroblastoma cell cultures. Int J Toxicol 25(6):459–464
Tan DX, Poeggeler B, Reiter RJ et al (1993) The pineal hormone melatonin inhibits DNA-adduct formation induced by the chemical carcinogen safrole in vivo. Cancer Lett 70:65–71
Tan DX, Manchester LC, Reiter RJ et al (1998) A novel melatonin metabolite, cyclic 3-hydroxymelatonin: a biomarker of in vivo hydroxyl radical generation. Biochem Biophys Res Commun 253:614–620
Tan DX, Manchester LC, Reiter RJ et al (1999) Identification of highly elevated levels of melatonin in bone marrow: its origin and significance. Biochim Biophys Acta 1472:206–214
Tanaka T, Yasui Y, Tanaka M et al (2008) Melatonin suppresses AOM/DSS-induced large bowel oncogenesis in rats. Chem Biol Interact 177(2):128–136
Thorburn A (2004) Death receptor-induced cell killing. Cell Signal 16:139–144
Touitou Y, Fevre-Montange M, Proust J et al (1985) Age- and sex-associated modification of plasma melatonin concentrations in man. Relationship to pathology, malignant or not, and autopsy findings. Acta Endocrinol (Copenh) 108:135–144
Tripathi DN, Jena GB (2010) Effect of melatonin on the expression of Nrf2 and NF-kappaB during cyclophosphamide-induced urinary bladder injury in rat. J Pineal Res 48(4):324–331
Trubiani O, Recchioni R, Moroni F et al (2005) Melatonin provokes cell death in human B-lymphoma cells by mitochondrial-dependent apoptotic pathway activation. J Pineal Res 39(4):425–431
Um HJ, Kwon TK (2010) Protective effect of melatonin on oxaliplatin-induced apoptosis through sustained Mcl-1 expression and anti-oxidant action in renal carcinoma Caki cells. J Pineal Res 49(3):283–290
Vesnushkin GM, Plotnikova NA, Semenchenko AV et al (2006) Melatonin inhibits urethane-induced carcinogenesis tumors in murine lung. Vopr Onkol 52(2):164–168
Webb SM, Puig-Domingo M (1995) Role of melatonin in health and disease. Clin Endocrinol (Oxf) 42:221–234
Weinreb O, Mandel S, Youdim MB (2003) cDNA gene expression profile homology of antioxidants and their antiapoptotic and proapoptotic activities in human neuroblastoma cells. FASEB J 17(8):935–937
Wenzel U, Nickel A, Daniel H (2005) Melatonin potentiates flavone-induced apoptosis in human colon cancer cells by increasing the level of glycolytic end products. Int J Cancer 116(2):236–242
Winczyk K, Pawlikowski M, Karasek MJ (2001) Melatonin and RZR/ROR receptor ligand CGP 52608 induce apoptosis in the murine colonic cancer. J Pineal Res 31(2):179–182
Winczyk K, Pawlikowski M, Lawnicka H et al (2002) Effects of melatonin and melatonin receptors ligand N-[(4-methoxy-1 H-indol-yl)methyl]propanamide on murine Colon 38 cancer growth in vitro and in vivo. Neuro Endocrinol Lett 23(1):50–54
Xi SC, Siu SW, Fong SW et al (2001) Inhibition of androgen-sensitive LNCaP prostate cancer growth in vivo by melatonin: association of antiproliferative action of the pineal hormone with mt1 receptor protein expression. Prostate 46(1):52–61
Yang QH, Xu JN, Xu RK et al (2006) Inhibitory effects of melatonin on the growth of pituitary prolactin-secreting tumor in rats. J Pineal Res 40(3):230–235
Yang QH, Xu JN, Xu RK et al (2007) Antiproliferative effects of melatonin on the growth of rat pituitary prolactin-secreting tumor cells in vitro. J Pineal Res 42(2):172–179
Yu HS, Pang SF, Tang PL (1981) Increase in the level of retinal melatonin and persistence of its diurnal rhythm in rats after pinealectomy. J Endocrinol 91:477–481
Zupancic D, Jezernik K, Vidmar G (2008) Effect of melatonin on apoptosis, proliferation and differentiation of urothelial cells after cyclophosphamide treatment. J Pineal Res 44:299–306

Chapter 7
Pharmacologically Active Compounds from Ticks and Other Arthropods and Their Potential Use in Anticancer Therapy

Mária Kazimírová

Abstract Arthropods represent a rich source of various biologically and pharmacologically active molecules and were also shown to possess cytotoxic and cytolytic effects on tumor cell lines as well as anti-angiogenic activities. Cytotoxic and apoptosis-inducing factors were found, e.g., in some butterflies, beetles and saprophagous flies, however, venomous and blood feeding animals contain the widest array of pharmacologically active compounds. Antitumor and anti-angiogenic compounds have been detected in saliva of ticks and blood feeding insects quite recently. For example, an antigen 5-like protein (tabRTS) containing the RTS-disintegrin motif with anti-angiogenic properties was isolated from horsefly salivary glands. However, and in contrast to blood feeding dipterans (e.g., horseflies or mosquitoes), hard ticks (Ixodida) as a distinct group of blood feeding arthropods remain attached to their hosts for several days to weeks. Tick salivary compounds are secreted into the host during feeding and are involved in the modulation of host haemostasis and immune responses and thus are essential for completion of the feeding process and tick survival. During the extended feeding period, expression of new proteins is switched on in salivary glands of hard ticks. By exploring the proteins expressed in tick salivary glands (sialome), novel sequences with similarities to disintegrin metalloproteases and thrombospondin were discovered, suggesting that tick salivary peptides can be involved in disruption of platelet aggregation, cell-matrix interactions and/or inhibition of angiogenesis. These findings suggest that tick saliva modulates negatively angiogenesis-dependent wound healing and tissue repair, allowing ticks to feed for prolonged periods. Antihemostatic factors in tick saliva represent another source of promising anticancer therapeutics. Ixolaris, a tissue factor inhibitor from ticks blocks tumor growth and angiogenesis in a glioblastoma model. The inhibitory effect of ixolaris is most probably due to downregulation of the vascular endothelial

M. Kazimírová (✉)
Institute of Zoology, Slovak Academy of Sciences,
Dúbravská cesta 9, 845 06 Bratislava, Slovakia
e-mail: maria.kazimirova@savba.sk

M. Diederich and K. Noworyta (eds.), *Natural Compounds as Inducers of Cell Death: Volume 1*, DOI 10.1007/978-94-007-4575-9_7,

growth factor and reduced tumor vascularization. Amblyomin-X, a tick Kunitz-type serine protease inhibitor induces tumor mass regression and decreased number of metastatic processes in a murine melanoma model, indicating that the compound selectively acts on tumor cells by inducing apoptosis. Generally, the diversity of arthropod bioactive molecules is very wide and needs further extensive exploration with the perspective to discover novel compounds with potential use as pharmaceuticals in anticancer therapy.

Keywords Arthropods • Insects • Ticks • Angiogenesis • Tumor growth

7.1 Introduction

Cancer still causes one of five deaths worldwide. Surgery, chemotherapy and radiotherapy provide inadequate protection and instead, affect normal cells along with the cancer cells. The search for cancer treatment by application of natural products has been practiced over a long period and several new cytotoxic molecules on natural basis have been discovered and further developed to pharmaceuticals. During the last decades a number of promising molecules with anticancer activities have been discovered in animal venoms and some of them are in clinical trials and may emerge be future drugs in cancer therapy (e.g., Kuczer et al. 2008; Gomes et al. 2010).

Animal venoms represent a rich source of various biologically and pharmacologically active molecules (e.g., Andrade et al. 2005; Pimenta and de Lima 2005; Steen et al. 2006; Kuczer et al. 2008; Hovius et al. 2008; Gomes et al. 2010). During the process of evolution, animal venoms have developed in various groups of animals, having various functions in defence systems against predators as well as in the evolution of (ecto)parasite – host relationships (Fry et al. 2009). Among parasites, blood feeding and tissue dwelling arthropods (ticks, insects) represent distinct groups. To facilitate blood feeding and ensure further development and reproduction, blood feeding organisms have developed special mechanisms to counteract the defence systems of their hosts, such as hemostasis, itch/pain and innate and acquired immune responses, by a wide variety of active compounds, involving inhibitors of factors of the coagulation pathways, inhibitors of platelet aggregation, vasodilators and immunomodulatory and immunosuppressive molecules. These compounds are secreted via their saliva into to host skin while taking a blood meal. The diversity of pharmacologically active molecules expressed in the salivary glands of hematophagous arthropods is very large and the functions of a lot of molecules have still not been elucidated (Charlab et al. 1999; Ribeiro and Francischetti 2003; Valenzuela 2004; Andrade et al. 2005; Tu et al. 2005; Koh and Kini 2009; Francischetti et al. 2010).

Insects comprise approximately 85% of animal species (Chernysh et al. 2002) and represent the richest source of candidate molecules for development of new therapeutics. Among the bioactive peptides derived from insects, antimicrobial peptides and anticoagulants have been best characterized (Bulet et al. 1999; Koh and Kini 2009). The limited number of compounds with antitumor properties identified in insects and other arthropods (see Table 7.1) were shown to possess mainly cytotoxic and cytolytic effects on tumor cell lines, apoptosis inducing properties (e.g., Cohen and Quistad 1998; Kuhn-Nentwig 2003) and/or anti-angiogenic activities (e.g., Ma et al. 2010; Francischetti et al. 2010; Carneiro-Lobo et al. 2009).

According to Pimenta and Lima (2005), toxins present in animal venoms can be classified based on their chemical nature, their pharmacological or biological properties, their molecular level effects and their sub-molecular binding sites. According to this classification, toxins comprise, e.g., various peptides and proteins, glycoproteins, alkaloids and biogenic amines and can act as neurotoxins, myotoxins, antimicrobial compounds, vasoactive peptides (vasodilators or vasoconstrictors), and exert hemolytic, cytolytic, necrotic, hemorrhagic, anti-inflammatory, antitumoral or analgesic activities. Moreover, venom compounds can act as ion channel ligands, agonists or antagonists of receptors, enzymes or inhibitors of enzymes.

Ixodid ticks as a distinct group of blood feeding arthropods remain attached to their hosts for several days to weeks. Tick salivary compounds are involved in the modulation of host haemostasis and immune responses and are essential for completion of the feeding process and tick survival (e.g., Ribeiro 1995). During the extended blood meal, expression of new proteins with a wide range of biological activities is switched on in tick salivary glands. Considering the peculiar feeding habits and complex biology of ticks, they are characterized in more details below.

Generally, isolation and identification of arthropod salivary molecules is often slow and difficult. High-throughput approaches involving molecular biology techniques, proteomics, transcriptomics and functional genomics to study salivary components of blood feeding arthropods have been introduced and will enable to test predicted and novel functions of arthropod molecules (e.g., Valenzuela 2002, 2004).

7.2 Ticks (Acari)

The salivary glands of ticks are multifunctional complex organs. They enable the feeding ticks to concentrate blood nutrients by returning excess water and ions via saliva to the host. In addition, salivary glands of ticks produce a cocktail of molecules that regulate secretion of salivary proteins and modulate host defence mechanisms (Ribeiro and Francischetti 2003; Valenzuela 2004). After a tick attaches to a host, expression of a series of new genes and synthesis of proteins is initiated in their salivary glands that reflect the stages of the feeding process. Argasid (soft) ticks feed rapidly and penetrate deeply in the host skin and do not secrete factors enabling strong attachment to the host. In contrast, almost all ixodid (hard) ticks produce cement proteins that ensure firm attachment of the tick to the host and seal the area around the mouth parts to the wound site. As feeding progresses, the amount of secreted saliva increases and salivary glands undergo a remarkable and rapid structural reorganization. At the peak of the feeding process, the glands can increase 25-fold in size and protein content. Once the tick is engorged and detaches, the glands degenerate through a process of cell apoptosis.

Table 7.1 Examples of pharmacologically active compounds with antitumor potential in arthropods

Species	Molecule	Target and/or function	Reference
30 arthropods	Crude extracts	Cytotoxic effects	Cohen and Quistad (1998)
Ticks			
Haemaphysalis longicornis	Troponin I-like molecule	Inhibition of angiogenesis	Fukumoto et al. (2006)
Haemaphysalis longicornis	Haemagin	Disruption of angiogenesis and wound healing; inhibition of vascular endothelial cell proliferation and induction of apoptosis	Islam et al. (2009)
Amblyomma americanum	Calreticulin	Inhibition of angiogenesis	Jaworski et al. (1995)
Amblyomma cajannense	Amblyomin-X	Induction of tumor cell death	Chudzinski-Tavassi et al. (2010)
Ixodes scapularis	Salivary gland extracts	Inhibition of endothelial cell proliferation and angiogenesis	Francischetti et al. (2005a)
Ixodes scapularis	Ixolaris	Blocking of TF activity; inhibition of tumor growth, downregulation of VEGF and reduced tumor vascularization	Carneiro-Lobo et al. (2009)
Ixodes ricinus	Metalloproteases Metis family	Involvement in tissue remodeling or disruption through digestion of structural components	Decrem et al. (2008)
Ixodes ricinus	Salivary gland extracts	Antiproliferative activities	Kazimírová et al. (2006)
Rhipicephalus appendiculatus *Dermacentor reticulatus* *Amblyomma variegatum*		Growth factor binding	Hajnická et al. (2011)
Insects			
Scorpions, various species	Venom	Various mechanisms, induction of apoptosis, cytotoxicity	Gomes et al. (2010)
Heterometrus bengalensis	Bengalin	Cytotoxicity, apoptosis	Das Gupta et al. (2010)
Various insects	Crude extracts	Cytotoxic effects	Ahn et al. (2000)
Musca domestica	Crude extract	Antitumor activity	Hou et al. (2007)
	Cecropin, antimicrobial peptide	Apoptosis-inducing activity	Jin et al. (2010)

(continued)

Table 7.1 (continued)

Species	Molecule	Target and/or function	Reference
Sarcophaga bullata	Lectin	Cytotoxic effects	Itoh et al. (1985)
Calliphora vicina	Alloferon	Antiviral and antitumor peptides	Chernysch et al. (2002)
Drosophila virilis	SK-84, antimicrobial peptide	Antiproliferative activities	Lu and Chen (2010)
Tabanus bovinus	Crude whole body extracts	Cytotoxic effects, anti-angiogenic activities	Ahn et al. (2000), Kwak et al. (2002)
Tabanus yao	TabRTS	Inhibitor for angiogenesis	Ma et al. (2010)
Lepidoptera (Pieridae)	Pierisins	Apoptosis-inducing protein; cytotoxic activity based on DNA ADP-ribosylating activity	Matsumoto et al. (2008), Watanabe et al. (1999)
Antheraea yamamai	Any–GS (VII)	Antiproliferative	Yang et al. (2004)
Hyalophora cecropia	Cecropins and their derivatives, antimicrobial peptides	Cytotoxic and antiproliferative activities	Moore et al. (1994), Suttmann et al. (2008)
Coleoptera	Derivatives of 43-mer defensins	Cytotoxic and antiproliferative activities	Iwasaki et al. (2009)
Mylabris phalerata	Buthanol extracts	Apoptosis-inducing activity	Huh et al. (2003)
Mylabris soo.	Cantharidin	Cytotoxic and apoptosis inducing ctivities	Liu and Chen (2009)
Honey bee	Melittin	Cell cycle arrest and apoptosis	Ip et al. (2008a, b), Oršolić (2012)

The insertion of the tick mouthparts (hypostome) to the host skin causes damage of the epidermis and rupture of blood vessels. Injury of the host skin would normally lead to formation of a hemostatic plug by activation of the coagulation cascade and vasoconstriction as well as to inflammatory responses and finally to wound healing and tissue remodelling. Wound healing is a cascade of processes and involves three phases — inflammatory, proliferative, and maturation and remodeling (e.g., Midwood et al. 2004). Briefly, in the inflammatory phase, mechanisms of the innate response of the organism to injury are involved. Platelet aggregation and activation of the coagulation cascade lead to formation of a blood clot that serves in prevention of local hemorrhage and functions as a provisional matrix for the wound healing. Following hemostasis, bacteria and tissue debris are phagocytosed and removed, and chemical signals that modulate migration, proliferation and differentiation of cells involved in the proliferative phase and signals that trigger synthesis and degradation of extracellular matrix (ECM) proteins are released. During the proliferative phase, granulation tissue is formed and the process involves proliferation of endothelial cells (EC), fibroblast accumulation, collagen synthesis and formation of a new network of blood vessels (angiogenesis). Epithelial cells finally cover the wound (epithelialisation). Macrophages produce cytokines that stimulate fibroplasia and angiogenesis. During angiogenesis, the vascular basement membrane and the fibrin or interstitial matrix are degraded by ECs, and these cells start to migrate into the matrix and proliferate by forming new capillary-like tubes. Fibroblasts produce new ECM that supports additional cell ingrowth. Blood vessels provide oxygen and nutrients and ensure sustained cell metabolism. The integrity of the granulation tissue depends on the presence of lipid mediators, the activity of target cells and growth factors which originate from plasma or are released into the wound by activated platelets, infiltrated peripheral blood monocytes and macrophages or by injured and activated parenchymal cells. The temporary fibrin matrix also promotes formation of granulation tissue. Fibroblasts and ECs express integrin receptors and invade the fibrin/fibronectin-rich clot in the wound and start synthesizing a permanent ECM. Maturation and remodeling is the final phase of wound healing and occurs when the wound has closed. During contraction, the wound size is decreasing due to the activity of myofibroblasts. Collagen is remodeled and realigned along tension lines. Cellular activity is reduced and cells that are not needed are removed by apoptosis. The number of blood vessels in the wound decrease.

Angiogenesis is an important process in wound healing (Folkman 2003; Carmeliet 2003; Laurens et al. 2006). It is a complex process, in which proliferation of ECs is stimulated by growth factors (VEGF or FGF-2) and migration of ECs into the ECM occurs while new capillaries are formed. EC migration is controlled by proteolytic enzymes of the plasminogen activator/plasmin system and by matrix metalloproteinases. The cells proliferate and elongate. Vessel stabilization occurs thanks to interaction with pericytes and reconstitution of the basement membrane. Integrins (e.g., $alpha_{pi\,b}$ $beta_3$, $alpha_5 beta_1$, alpha $Vbeta_3$, and alpha $Vbeta_5$) are important in wound healing and angiogenesis as they facilitate binding of EC to ECM fibrin(ogen), vitronectin, and fibronectin. Except wound healing, angiogenesis plays also an important role in the development and progression of tumor metastasis, thus tick compounds impairing wound healing have probably also an antitumor potential.

The wound healing response of the host would normally disrupt tick feeding and cause rejection of the tick, with detrimental consequences to tick viability and reproduction. However, ticks complete their blood meal thanks to the presence of a wide range of physiologically active molecules in their salivary glands Fig. 7.1. These molecules evolved during the host-parasite co-evolution and are crucial in overcoming haemostatic and immune responses of the hosts and, in addition, they support transmission of tick-borne pathogens (e.g., Ribeiro and Francischetti 2003; Brossard and Wikel 2004; Nuttall and Labuda 2004; Ramamoorthi et al. 2005; Andrade et al. 2005; Steen et al. 2006).

Saliva of ixodid ticks were shown to contain factors that bind cytokines (IL-2, IL-4) and chemokines [CXCL8 (IL-8), CCL2 (MCP-1), CCL3 (MIP-1a), CCL5 (RANTES),

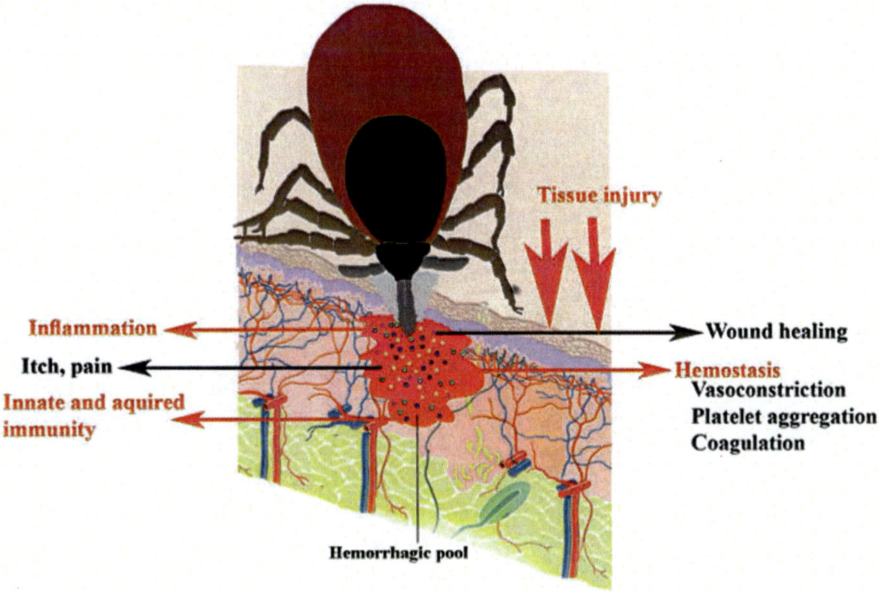

Fig. 7.1 Hard ticks (Ixodidae) insert their mouthparts into the skin of their hosts and remain attached for several days to weeks. In the wound at the tick attachment site, a hemorrhagic pool is created. Ticks secrete biologically active salivary compounds to the wound and counteract host defence mechanisms involved in wound healing, hemostasis, innate and acquired immunity, itch and pain. Among blood feeding animals, ticks, due to their unique feeding habits and prolonged blood-meal, produce the richest cocktail of pharmacologically active substances with potential use in treatment of various disorders

CCL11 (eotaxin)] which are involved in host immune and wound healing responses and neutralize their biological activities (Hajnická et al. 2005; Frauenschuh et al. 2007; Déruaz et al. 2008). Targeting of factors involved in wound healing (angiogenesis, growth factors) appears to be another strategy adopted by ixodid ticks to suppress inflammation and succeed in blood feeding (Francischetii et al. 2010; Hajnická et al. 2011).

The network of signal molecules involved in regulation of the wound healing processes includes cytokines and chemokines (Werner and Grose 2003) and, in addition, a number of growth factors like epidermal growth factor (EGF), fibroblast growth factor (FGF-2), platelet-derived growth factor (PDGF), transforming growth factor beta (TGF-β1), granulocyte macrophage colony stimulating factor (GM-CSF), hepatocyte growth factor (HGF) and vascular endothelial growth factor (VEGF) (e.g., Barrientos et al. 2008). Compounds of salivary gland extracts of various hard ticks seem to bind growth factors in a species-specific manner, e.g., salivary gland extracts derived from *Amblyomma variegatum* bind TGF- β1, PDGF, FGF-2 and HGF, from *Dermacentor reticulatus* and *Rhipicephalus appendiculatus* react with TGF-β1, FGF-2 and HGF, and from *Ixodes ricinus* and *I. scapularis* with PDGF. Salivary gland extracts of the tick species that react with PDGF (*A. variegatum* and *I. ricinus*) also display antiproliferative activities and affect changes in cell morphology in a number of cell lines. These activities correlate with disruption of the actin cytoskeleton, but have not been detected in those tick species that did not target PDGF (Hajnická et al. 2011).

Generally, the composition of tick saliva is complex and redundant at the same time, which reflects complex and redundant host defence responses. As already stated, tick saliva contains inhibitors of blood coagulation and platelet aggregation as well as vasodilatory and immuno-modulatory substances (Wikel and Alarcon-Chaidez 2001; Brossard and Wikel 2004; Andrade et al. 2005; Steen et al. 2006). The blood feeding strategy of ticks on one hand, and the pool and mode of action of the pharmacologically active compounds contained in their saliva and salivary glands on the other hand, are mostly species-specific. The activity, mechanisms of action and characteristics of these compounds have been studied more intensively during the last two decades. The aim of such studies was to identify the active compounds and prepare them in recombinant form, with their perspective usage as pharmaceuticals (Titus et al. 2006; Maritz-Olivier et al. 2007; Hovius et al. 2008). Recent progress in transcriptome research in hard ticks has disclosed hundreds of different proteins expressed in their salivary glands, whereby for the majority not known function has been ascribed and they include many novel and unique protein families (Francischetti et al. 2010).

By exploring the proteins expressed in salivary glands of ticks (sialomes), novel sequences with similarities to disintegrin metalloproteases and thrombospondin were discovered, indicating that tick salivary peptides can be involved in disruption of platelet aggregation, cell-matrix interactions and/or inhibition of angiogenesis (Valenzuela et al. 2002; Francischetti et al. 2005a, b; Fukumoto et al. 2006). These findings suggest that tick saliva is a negative modulator of angiogenesis-dependent wound healing and tissue repair, allowing ticks to feed for prolonged periods (Francischetti et al. 2005a, b). In addition, calreticulin with potent anti-angiogenesis properties was also detected in salivary glands of the hard tick *Amblyomma americanum* (Jaworski et al. 1995). The presence of the N-terminus of calreticulin was also found in saliva of *Ixodes scapularis* and a potent inhibitory activity on both endothelial cell proliferation and chick aorta sprouting formation was demonstrated in saliva of this tick (Valenzuela et al. 2002; Francischetti et al. 2005a).

In a study involving four hard tick species (*Ixodes ricinus, Dermacentor reticulatus, Rhipicephalus appendiculatus* and *Amblyomma variegatum*), dose-dependent inhibitory effects of salivary gland extracts on the proliferation of HeLa cells were demonstrated (Kazimírová et al. 2006). The results suggested that salivary gland extracts of various hard tick species might contain different compounds to suppress cell proliferation and induce apoptosis, whereas the presence and amounts of the active compounds might change during tick feeding. Inhibition of cell proliferation by salivary gland extracts of these ticks was most probably related to suppression of proliferation rather than to cytotoxic or cytolytic effects. The active compounds are most probably proteins as the anti-proliferative effects of salivary gland extracts were abolished by their incubation at 100°C.

Thrombospondin-like molecules were also detected in tick sialome (Valenzuela et al. 2002). The role of the thrombospondin-1 (TSP1) in tumor cell adhesion, motility and proliferation was discussed by Roberts (1996) who stated contradictory effects of TSP1 on tumor growth indicating that the activities are most probably cell-specific.

Platelet aggregation inhibitors and disintegrin metalloproteases present in tick salivary glands and participating in the inhibition of wound healing after a tick bite could potentially also be involved in the suppression of tumor cell proliferation (Mans et al. 2002; Valenzuela et al. 2002; Decrem et al. 2008).

Disintegrins contained in tick saliva inhibit platelet aggregation and are also important for successful tick feeding (Decrem et al. 2008; Francischetti et al. 2005a; Harnnoi et al. 2007). In the sialome of *Ixodes scapularis* two cysteine-rich peptides (ISL 929 and ISL 1373) with homology to the cysteine-rich domain of disintegrin metalloproteinases, a family of structurally and evolutionarily related negative regulators of integrins have been identified (Valenzuela et al. 2002; Ribeiro et al. 2006; Guo et al. 2009). ISL 929 and ISL 1373 belong to the ixostatin family (short-coding cysteine-rich-peptides). These peptides code for cysteine-rich peptides which are similar to the cysteine-rich domains of the ADAMTS (a disintegrin and metalloprotease with thrombospondin motifs) proteins, i.e., enzymes that, among other functions, cleave cartilage and inhibit angiogenesis. However, the function of peptides belonging to the ixostatin family is largely unknown, although they might be involved in inhibition of angiogenesis/tissue repair (Ribeiro et al. 2006; Francischetti et al. 2005a, b). For example, polymorphonuclear leukocytes treated with the saliva of *I. scapularis* and recombinant ISL 929 and ISL 1373 displayed reduced expression of β_2 integrins and impaired adherence (Guo et al. 2009).

The effects of coagulation inhibitors on tumor cells and an association between cancer and thrombosis have been recognized and described, however, the manner by which tumor growth is regulated by coagulation in vivo remains largely unclear (Nierodzik and Karpatkin 2006). Thrombin is known to activate tumor cell adhesion to platelets, endothelial cells, and subendothelial matrix proteins, enhance tumor cell growth, increase tumor cell seeding and spontaneous metastasis, and stimulate angiogenesis in tumors. Thus, tumor malignancy may be regulated by a procoagulant/anticoagulant pathway. Thrombin (thrombosis) contributes to increased malignancy by activating platelet-tumor aggregation, tumor adhesion to subendothelial matrix, tumor growth and metastasis, and tumor-associated angiogenesis, and in addition, thrombin serves to preserve and/or activate dormant tumor cells. Tick saliva is known to contain a wide array of molecules with antithrombin activities, like savignin (Nienaber et al. 1999), madanin (Iwanaga et al. 2003), variegin (Koh et al. 2007) or boophilin (Macedo-Ribeiro et al. 2008) (for review see e.g., Koh and Kini 2009; Francischetti et al. 2010) which also could be considered as candidates in the development of drugs for administration in anticancer adjuvant therapy.

Francischetti et al. (2005a) demonstrated for the first time that saliva of the hard tick *Ixodes scapularis* dose-dependently inhibited microvascular endothelial cell proliferation. The process was accompanied by a change in cell shape (shrinkage of the cytoplasm with loss of cell-cell interactions) and apoptosis. The effect of saliva appeared to be mediated by endothelial cell $\alpha_5\beta_1$ integrin, suggesting that a metalloprotease is responsible for the antiproliferation activity. These findings suggest that tick saliva is a negative modulator of angiogenesis-dependent wound healing and tissue repair, allowing ticks to feed for a prolonged period. Prior to this discovery, inhibition of angiogenesis was an unidentified biologic property of tick saliva or of any blood-sucking arthropods studied so far. Thus tick saliva may be regarded as an additional source of angiogenesis inhibitors with potential applications in anticancer therapy.

During vessel wall injury, membrane-bound tissue factor (TF) is exposed and blood coagulation is initiated (Gomez and McVey 2006). Abnormal elevated TF expression has been documented in several tumor types including high grade tumors (glioblastomas) and indicates a potential role for TF in progression of this disease, and suggests that anticoagulants could be used as adjuvants for its treatment. Ixolaris, a TF pathway inhibitor, belonging to a novel group of tick anticoagulants, was isolated from *I. scapularis* ticks (Francischetti et al. 2002). Ixolaris is a Kunitz-like serine proteinase inhibitor that interacts with zymogen FX through a precursor state of the heparin-binding exosite, displaying potent and long-lasting antithrombotic activity. It was hypothesized that Ixolaris might interfere with progression of glioblastoma due to its potent activity against *in vitro* procoagulant properties and *in vivo* tumor growth of U87-MG glioblastoma cells. Along with inhibition of tumor growth, Ixolaris caused downregulation of VEGF and vessel density in the tumor mass. The results suggest that Ixolaris is among the promising candidates for development of antitumor therapeutics (Carneiro-Lobo et al. 2009).

Amblyomin-X, a Kunitz-type serine protease inhibitor present in salivary glands of *Amblyomma cajannense* (Batista et al. 2010), inhibits the activity of coagulation Factor Xa (FXa) and, in addition, displays cytotoxic activity by decreasing tumor mass and reducing metastasis in a murine melanoma model. Moreover, Amblyomin-X displays a pro-apoptotic activity in SK-Mel-28 (melanoma) or Mia-PaCa-2 (pancreas adenocarcinoma) cell lines. Treatment of the tumor cell lines with Amblyomin-X resulted in alterations of expression of a number of genes related to cell cycle. Amblyomin-X most probably acts on tumor cells selectively by targeting the ubiquitin-proteasome system and induces apoptotic cell death (Chudzinski-Tavassi et al. 2010).

Haemangin, a novel Kunitz-type inhibitor from salivary glands of *Haemaphysalis longicornis* was shown to disrupt angiogenesis and wound healing via inhibition of vascular endothelial cell proliferation and induction of apoptosis (Islam et al. 2009). In addition, haemangin was shown to inactivate trypsin, chymotrypsin, and plasmin, indicating its antiproteolytic potential on angiogenic cascades. Analysis of haemangin-specific gene expression kinetics at different blood feeding stages of adult *H. longicornis* ticks revealed a dramatic up-regulation prior to feeding completion, which seems to be linked to the ingestion of the blood-meal. The study also provided the first insights into transcriptional responses of human microvascular endothelial cells to Haemangin. DNA microarray data revealed that Haemangin altered the expression of 3,267 genes, including those involved in angiogenesis, which further support the anti-angiogenic function of the compound. Moreover, the study provided novel information on the blood feeding strategies of hard ticks that enable them to feed for a prolonged period and ensure full blood-meals through modulation of angiogenesis and wound healing processes.

Troponin I (TnI) (Feldman and Rouleau 2002) is a novel cartilage-derived angiogenesis inhibitor that inhibits endothelial cell proliferation and angiogenesis, and was shown to inhibit metastasis of a wide variety of tumors *in vivo*. Despite evidence of its efficacy, little has been known about the mode of action of TnI as an anti-proliferative and anti-angiogenic agent. It has been demonstrated that TnI inhibits both bFGF-stimulated and basal levels of endothelial cell proliferation, and it was hypothesized that this inhibition occurs, at least in part, through an interaction of TnI with the cell surface bFGF receptor on capillary endothelial cells, suggesting that the compound competes with bFGF for interaction with the bFGF receptor. In a cDNA expression library prepared from *H. longicornis* a cDNA encoding 27/30 kDa proteins was cloned and assigned as P27/30 gene. The predicted amino acid sequence of the P27/30 gene showed high homology with the *Drosophila melanogaster* troponin I clone E2, suggesting that *H. longicornis* P27/30 is a troponin I-like protein (You et al. 2001). To investigate the inhibitory effects of tick troponin-like molecules on angiogenesis, recombinant HLTnI was prepared. In an assay for testing the activity of VEGF, significant inhibition of formation of capillaries in a culture of human vascular endothelial cells (HUVEC) by HLTnI was demonstrated. The results indicate that HLTnI is a potent inhibitor of angiogenesis (Fukumoto et al. 2006).

The effects of *Dermacentor variabilis* saliva on basal- and platelet-derived growth factor (PDGF)-stimulated cell migration and extracellular signal-regulated kinase (ERK) signalling in fibroblasts was also examined (Kramer et al. 2008). The study revealed a delay in repair of injured cell monolayers after pre-treatment with tick saliva, which was not associated with reductions in cell number. In a migration assays, tick saliva suppressed both basal and PDGF-stimulated fibroblast migration. Tick saliva also reduced ERK activity stimulated with PDGF. It was suggested that the delayed repair of injured cell monolayers was a result of inhibition of fibroblast migration normally elicited by chemotactic signals. Moreover, tick saliva suppressed ERK activation in injured renal epithelial OK cells. Thus it appears that ticks ensure prolonged feeding and maintenance of the feeding lesion in the host skin also by suppression of ERK activation and fibroblast migration, both being important events in the wound healing process. The fact that the effects of tick saliva on ERK activity stimulated by injury- and growth factors are not cell-type specific suggests that some compounds in tick saliva might also control the invasiveness of cancer cells.

7.3 Scorpions

Scorpions (Arachnida, Scorpionidea) are the most venomous representatives of the class Arachnida and contain compounds that affect cell proliferation and induce apoptosis (for review see Gomes et al. 2010). Venom of the scorpion *Buthus martensii* was shown to suppress proliferation and induce cell death of malignant glioma U251-MG cells, but did not affect human hepatocellular carcinoma cells. The glioma cell death was determined as apoptosis and is most probably related to modulation of ion channels in glioma cells (Wang and Ji 2005). Moreover, scorpion venoms contain chlorotoxins that specifically bind to glioma cells and thus have a potential to be used in treatment of glioma (Lyons et al. 2002). Hyaluronidase and serine proteinase-like proteins (e.g. BMK-CBP) have also been isolated from scorpion venom and have anticancer effects. Dose-dependent cell binding activity of BMK-CBP, e.g., with the breast cancer cell line MCF-7 was demonstrated and the substance is most probably related to the anticancer potential of the scorpion venom (Gao et al. 2008).

Isolated protein fractions of the scorpion *junceus* venom showed different cytotoxic effects on tumor cell lines of epithelial origin (HeLa, Hep-2, NCI-H292) and induced apoptosis, but the mode of their action has not been elucidated (Díaz García et al. 2010). On the other hand, cytotoxic activity of the venom of the species *Heterometrus bengalensis* on human leukemic cells was explained by induction of DNA fragmentation. Recently, a 72 kDa novel scorpion venom protein named bengalin has been purified from *H. bengalensis* venom (Das Gupta et al. 2010). The protein shows antiproliferative and apoptogenic effects on human leukemic cell lines U937 and K562. In addition, the protein elicits loss of mitochondrial membrane potential, and subsequent release of cytochrome c into the cytosol, decrease in expression of heat shock proteins HSP70 and HSP90, activation of caspase-9 and caspase-3 and induction of cleavage of poly(ADP-ribose) polymerase. It was also demonstrated that the antiproliferative and apoptogenic effects of bengalin were related to inhibition of HSPs expression. Based on these results it was hypothesised that the molecular mechanism of the anticancer potential of bengalin might be mediated by the mitochondrial death cascade.

7.4 Spiders and Centipedes

Cohen and Quistad (1998) assessed venoms from 30 arthropods (including 26 spider species) for cytotoxicity by using cultured cells of three mammalian sources (murine neuroblastoma and macrophages and human osteosarcoma). The most cytotoxic venoms were derived from predatory jumping spiders (Salticidae, *Phidippus* sp.) and a centipede (*Scolopendra* sp.). The cytotoxicity of the *Phidippus ardens* venom was instantaneous and evidenced by dramatic disruption of cell membranes resulting in cell collapse. Surprisingly, the venoms of spiders from the families Loxoscelidae and Theridiidae that have been known for their use in medical practice, exerted only moderate cytotoxicity to cultured mammalian neuroblastoma cells. In contrast, the venom of the centipede *Scolopendra* sp. was highly toxic to the three mammalian cell cultures. It is suggested that the cytotoxic compounds in spider venom that cause disruption of cell membranes are not neuroactive peptides or acylpolyamines, but most probably enzymes and their mode of action needs further investigation.

7.5 Honey Bee

The therapeutic properties of bee venom (bee venom therapy) have been well known for a long period. Bee venom therapy has been applied in traditional medicine, for instance, in treatment of arthritis, rheumatism, pain and skin diseases. Bee venom contains a wide variety of biologically active substances, like peptides (e.g. melittin, apamin, adolapin, mast-cell-degranulating peptide, phospholipase A2), amines (e.g., histamine, epinephrine), and nonpeptide substances. Among various effects, anticancer potential of bee venom has also been demonstrated and melittin appears to be the main compound responsible for cytotoxic and apoptogenic activities (for review see, e.g., Son et al. 2007; Oršolić 2012).

The cytotoxic effect of bee venom is most probably due to activation of phospholipase A2 by melittin, but suppression of expression of matrix metalloproteinase-9 which is important in invasion of cancer cells and metastasis seems to be another important anticancer property of melittin (Park et al. 2010). A wide range of cancer cells (e.g., renal, lung, liver, prostate, bladder, mammary cancer cells and leukemia cells) were shown to be affected by melittin. Besides the cytotoxic effects, induction of apoptosis by bee venom has been reported for a number of cancer cell lines, however, the underlying molecular mechanisms have not been completely elucidated. Several death mechanisms of cancer cells induced by bee venom or its component melittin have been reported, including activation of caspase and matrix metalloproteinases (MMP) (see Son et al. 2007). For example, in human breast cancer MCF7 cells, bee venom probably induces apoptosis through the mitochondrial-dependent pathway (Ip et al. 2008a), while in human cervical cancer Ca Ski cells, apoptosis is induced via a Fas receptor pathway, also involving mitochondrial-dependent pathways (Ip et al. 2008b). In leukemic U937 cells, melittin appears to induce apoptosis through downregulating Akt signal pathways (Moon et al. 2008).

7.6 Beetles (Coleoptera)

The beetle *Mylabris phalerata* (Chrysomelidae) is known as an insect crude extracts of which have been used in anticancer therapy in oriental medicine. A butanol fraction prepared from the beetle extract displayed low cytotoxic activity on human monocytic leukemic U937 cells, but induced morphological changes leading to apoptosis and activated the caspase cascade and release of cytochrome c from mitochondria into the cytosol. The anticancer activity of *M. phalerata* fraction is most probably due to apoptosis rather than cytotoxicity (Huh et al. 2003).

Cantharidin, a highly toxic compound, has been isolated from *M. phalerata* and a number of other beetle species and has been used in anticancer therapy due to its cytotoxic activities (Liu and Chen 2009). However, because of its toxicity clinical application of cantharidin has been limited. On the other hand, synthetic analogues of cantharidin due to their reduced toxicity on non-malignant cells are promising new drugs. They were shown to induce apoptosis, e.g., in leukemia cell lines through activation of the caspase-dependent pathway (Kok et al. 2006).

Modified 43-mer defensins (D-9-mer peptides) with antibacterial properties which were derived from the coconut rhinoceros beetle *Oryctes rhinoceros,* are also among promising candidates for drugs in anticancer therapy. The synthesized peptides displayed antiproliferative effects on mouse myeloma cell lines and cytotoxic activities based on disrupting the membrane of the cancer cells (Iwasaki et al. 2009).

7.7 Diptera

Peptides, referred to as alloferons, were isolated from bacteria-challenged larvae of the blow fly *Calliphora vicina* (Chernysh et al. 2002). *In vitro*, alloferon demonstrated stimulatory activity on natural killer lymphocytes and *in vivo* this peptide displayed antiviral and antitumor activities.

Anticancer potential was also demonstrated in extracts of the housefly *Musca domestica,* showing high in vitro antitumor activity against the human colon cancer cell line CT26 (Hou et al. 2007), but the antitumor mechanisms are still unclear. Studies on apoptogenic activities of the antimicrobial peptide cecropin isolated from *M. domestica* in BEL-7402 (human hepatocellular carcinoma cell line) revealed that cell death is most probably induced through the extrinsic apoptotic pathway by upregulation of Fas, Fas-L, and caspase-8 and -3 (Jin et al. 2010).

Lectin of the fleshfly, *Sarcophaga peregrina* was reported to show cytotoxicity against murine ascetic and solid tumors *in vivo* (Itoh et al. 1985), suggesting that also these insects could be a good source of new biologically active substances, including anticancer agents.

Recently, a novel glycine-rich antimicrobial peptide has been purified from *Drosophila virilis* larvae and further characterised (Lu and Chen 2010). The peptide was named SK84 and, except antibacterial activity, exerts specific inhibitory effects on proliferation of cancer cell lines (human leukemia THP-1, liver cancer HepG2, breast cancer MCF-7).

Potent antitumor and anti-angiogenic activities were also demonstrated in whole body extracts of the blood feeding horse fly *Tabanus bovinus* (Ahn et al. 2000; Kwak et al. 2002). Strong correlation between cytotoxicity and L-amino acid oxidase (LAO) activity in the crude extracts suggests that LAO may be one of the cytotoxic components associated with apoptosis. Except cytotoxic effects, anti-angiogenic activities of *T. bovinus* extracts were also demonstrated (Kwak et al. 2002), suggesting that the antitumor and anti-metastatic properties of horsefly extracts might be mediated by the anti-angiogenic mechanism.

Recently, an antigen 5-like protein (named tabRTS) was purified and characterized from the salivary glands of the horsefly *Tabanus yao* (Ma et al. 2010). TabRTS contains the SCP domain (Sc7 family of extracellular protein domain) and an Arg-Thr-Ser (RTS) disintegrin motif at the C-terminus of tabRTS. The RTS motif is positioned in a loop bracketed by cysteine residues similarly as detected in RTS-disintegrins contained in the venom of snakes belonging to Crotalidae and Viperidae, which act as angiogenesis inhibitors. TabRTS significantly inhibited angiogenesis *in vitro* and *in vivo* in the endothelial Cell Tube formation assay and chicken chorioallantoic membrane (CAM) angiogenesis assay, respectively. This study revealed the first angiogenesis inhibitor protein containing the RTS motif from invertebrates, a possible novel type of RTS-disintegrin.

7.8 Lepidoptera

Anticancer factors were detected also in some butterflies (Costa-Neto 2005). A pentapeptide Any–GS (VII) isolated from larvae of the silkmoth *Antheraea yamamai* suppress proliferation of hepatoma cells, most probably due to cell cycle arrest rather than to an apoptotic/necrotic activity (Yang et al. 2004).

Cabbage butterflies, *Pieris rapae* and *Pieris brassicae,* contain cytotoxic proteins, designated as pierisin-1 and -2, inducing apoptosis in several cancer cell lines (Koyama et al. 1996; Kono et al. 1997, 1999; Watanabe et al. 1998, 1999; Matsushima-Hibiya et al. 2000). The proteins exhibit DNA ADP-ribosylating activity. Similar activities have also been detected in other species of the Pieridae family, but not all (Matsumoto et al. 2008). Recently, further pierisins (Pierisin-3, Pierisin-4) beloning to the pierisin protein family have been found in other representatives of the Pieridae family (Yamamoto et al. 2009) and their anticancer potential was confirmed.

Antimicrobial peptides Cecropin A and B, belonging to the Cecropin-family, were originally isolated from the hemolymph of the silk moth *Hyalophora cecropia* and, besides their antimicrobial activities, they display specific antitumor activities against a number of cancer cell lines, like mammalian leukemia, lymphoma, colon carcinoma (Moore et al. 1994; Chen et al. 1997). In addition, cecropins as well as the structurally and functionally related antimicrobial peptide Magainin II exert cytotoxic and antiproliferative effects on human bladder cancer cell lines (Lehmann et al. 2006; Suttmann et al. 2008). The mode of action of cecropins is most probably related to disruption of cancer cell membranes and subsequent cytolysis and destruction.

7.9 Concluding Remarks

Salivary glands of blood feeding ticks and insects as well as venoms and extracts of other arthropods represent a rich source of various pharmacologically active compounds that, in blood feeding organisms, primarily facilitate blood feeding and interfere with host defence systems. In addition to antihemostatics and immunomodulators, arthropods produce a number of other molecules with a wide range of biological activities, such as cardiotoxic factors and neutotoxins, various enzymes and enzyme inhibitors, protein homologues, and in addition, they also contain factors that regulate would healing and angiogenssis and display cytotoxic and cytolytic activities. Novel arthropod-derived molecules may be useful for development of pharmaceuticals for treatment of cancer. However, the isolation and identification of such molecules is often slow and difficult. High-throughput genomic and proteomic approaches for cloning salivary and venom cDNA have resulted in the discovery of genes and proteins not previously reported in blood feeding and venomous arthropods. These allow not only the isolation of factors with known activities, but also the characterization of novel molecules, for which the biological function is unknown.

Acknowledgments This work was supported by the Slovak Research and Development Agency (contract no. APVV-51-004505).

References

Ahn MY, Ryu KS, Lee YW, Kim YS (2000) Cytotoxicity and L-amino acid oxidase activity of crude insect drugs. Arch Pharm Res 23:477–481

Andrade BB, Teixeira CR, Barral A, Barral-Netto M (2005) Haematophagous arthropod saliva and host defense system: a tale of tear and blood. Anais da Academia Brasileira de Ciências (Ann Braz Acad Sci) 77:665–693

Barrientos S, Stojadinovic O, Golinko MS, Brem H, Tomic-Canic M (2008) Growth factors and cytokines in wound healing. Wound Rep Reg 16:585–601

Batista IFC, Ramos OHP, Ventura JS, Junqueira-de-Azevedo ILM, Ho PL, Chudzinski-Tavassi AM (2010) A new Factor Xa inhibitor from *Amblyomma cajennense* with a unique domain composition. Arch Biochem Biophys 493:151–156

Brossard M, Wikel SK (2004) Tick immunobiology. Parasitology 129:S161–S176

Bulet P, Hetru M, Dimarcq J-L, Hoffmann D (1999) Antimicrobial peptides in insects; structure and function. Dev Comp Immunol 23:329–344

Carmeliet P (2003) Angiogenesis in health and disease. Nat Med 9:653–660

Carneiro-Lobo TC, Konig S, Machado DE, Nasciutti LE, Forni MF, Francischetti IM, Sogayar MC, Monteiro RQ (2009) Ixolaris, a tissue factor inhibitor, blocks primary tumor growth and angiogenesis in a glioblastoma model. J Thromb Haemost 7:1855–1864

Charlab R, Valenzuela JG, Rowton ED, Ribeiro JMC (1999) Toward an understanding of the biochemical and pharmacological complexity of the saliva of a hematophagous sand fly *Lutzomyia longipalpis*. Proc Natl Acad Sci USA 96:15155–15160

Chen HM, Wang W, Smith D, Chan SC (1997) Effects of the anti-bacterial peptide cecropin B and its analogs, cecropins B-1 and B-2, on liposomes, bacteria, and cancer cells. Biochim Biophys Acta 1336:171–179

Chernysh S, Kim SI, Bekker G, Pleskach VA, Filatova NA, Anikin VB, Platonov VG, Bulet P (2002) Antiviral and antitumor peptides from insects. Proc Natl Acad Sci USA 99:12628–12632

Chudzinski-Tavassi AM, De-Sá-Júnior PL, Simons SM, Maria DA, de Souza VJ, de Fátima Correia Batista I, Faria F, Durães E, Moraes Reis E, Demasi M (2010) A new tick Kunitz type inhibitor, Amblyomin-X, induces tumor cell death by modulating genes related to the cell cycle and targeting the ubiquitin-proteasome system. Toxicon 56:1145–1154. doi:10.1016/j.toxicon.2010.04.019

Cohen E, Quistad GB (1998) Cytotoxic effects of arthropod venoms on various cultured cells. Toxicon 36:353–358

Costa-Neto EMA (2005) Animal-based medicines: biological prospection and the sustainable use of zootherapeutic resources. An Acad Bras Cienc 77:33–43

Das Gupta S, Gomes A, Debnath A, Saha A, Gomes A (2010) Apoptosis induction in human leukemic cells by a novel protein Bengalin, isolated from Indian black scorpion venom: through mitochondrial pathway and inhibition of heat shock proteins. Chem Biol Interact 183:293–303

Decrem Y, Beaufays J, Blasioli V, Lahaye K, Brossard M, Vanhamme L, Godfroid E (2008) A family of putative metalloproteases in the salivary glands of the tick *Ixodes ricinus*. FEBS J 275:1485–1499

Déruaz M, Frauenschuh A, Alessandri AL, Dias JM, Coelho FM, Russo RC, Ferreira BR, Graham GJ, Shaw JP, Wells TN, Teixeira MM, Power CA, Proudfoot AE (2008) Ticks produce highly selective chemokine binding proteins with antiinflammatory activity. J Exp Med 205:2019–2031

Díaz García A, Morier Díaz L, Rodríguez Sánchez H, Caballero Lorenzo Y (2010) Cytotoxicity of *Rhopalurus junceus* Cuban scorpion venom and its fractions on human tumor cell lines. Labiofam. Revista Institucional del Grupo Empresarial de Producciones Biofarmaceúticas y Químicas 1(2010):12–18

Feldman L, Rouleau C (2002) Troponin I inhibits capillary endothelial cell proliferation by interaction with the cell's bFGF receptor. Microvasc Res 63:41–49

Folkman J (2003) Fundamental concepts of the angiogenic process. Curr Mol Med 3:643–651

Francischetti IMB, Valenzuela JG, Andersen JF, Mather TN, Ribeiro JMC (2002) Ixolaris, a novel recombinant tissue factor pathway inhibitor (TFPI) from the salivary gland of the tick, *Ixodes scapularis*: identification of factor X and factor Xa as scaffolds for the inhibition of factor VIIa/Tissue factor complex. Blood 99:3602–3612

Francischetti IMB, Mather TN, Ribeiro JMC (2005a) Tick saliva is a potent inhibitor of endothelial cell proliferation and angiogenesis. Thromb Haemost 94:167–174

Francischetti IM, My Pham V, Mans BJ, Andersen JF, Mather TN, Lane RS, Ribeiro JM (2005b) The transcriptome of the salivary glands of the female western black-legged tick *Ixodes pacificus* (Acari: Ixodidae). Insect Biochem Mol Biol 35:1142–1161

Francischetti IMB, Sá-Nunes A, Mans BJ, Santos IM, Ribeiro JMC (2010) The role of saliva in tick feeding. Front Biosci 14:2051–2088

Frauenschuh A, Power CA, Déruaz M, Ferreira BR, Silva JS, Teixeira MM, Dias JM, Martin T, Wells TN, Proudfoot AE (2007) Molecular cloning and characterization of a highly selective chemokine-binding protein from the tick *Rhipicephalus sanguineus*. J Biol Chem 282:27250–27258

Fry BG, Roelants K, Champagne DE, Scheib H, Tyndall JDA, King GK, Nevalainen TJ, Norman JA, Lewis RJ, Norton RS, Renjifo C, Rodrıguez de la Vega RC (2009) The toxicogenomic multiverse: convergent recruitment of proteins into animal venoms. Annu Rev Genomics Hum Genet 10:483–511

Fukumoto S, Sakaguchi T, You M, Xuan X, Fujisaki K (2006) Tick troponin I-like molecule is a potent inhibitor for angiogenesis. Microvasc Res 71:218–221

Gao R, Zhang Y, Gopalakrishnakone P (2008) Purification and N-terminal sequence of a serine proteinase-like protein (BMK-CBP) from the venom of the Chinese scorpion (*Buthus martensii* Karsch). Toxicon 52:348–353

Gomes A, Bhattacharjee P, Mishra R, Biswas AK, Dasgupta SC, Giri B (2010) Anticancer potential of animal toxins and venoms. Ind J Exp Biol 48:93–103

Gomez K, McVey JH (2006) Tissue factor initiated blood coagulation. Front Biosci 11:1349–1359

Guo X, Booth CJ, Paley MA, Wang X, DePonte K, Fikrig E, Narasimhan S, Montgomery RR (2009) Inhibition of neutrophil function by two tick salivary proteins. Infect Immun 77:2320–2329

Hajnická V, Vančová I, Kocáková P, Slovák M, Gašperík J, Sláviková M, Hails RS, Labuda M, Nuttall PA (2005) Manipulation of host cytokine network by ticks: a potential gateway for pathogen transmission. Parasitology 130:333–342

Hajnická V, Vančová-Štibrániová I, Slovák M, Kocáková P, Nuttall PA (2011) Ixodid tick salivary gland products target host wound healing growth factors. Int J Parasitol 41:213–223. doi:10.1016/j.ijpara.2010.09.005

Harnnoi T, Sakaguchi T, Nishikawa Y, Xuan X, Fujisaki K (2007) Molecular characterization and comparative study of 6 salivary gland metalloproteases from the hard tick, *Haemaphysalis longicornis*. Comp Biochem Physiol B 147:93–101

Hou L, Shi Y, Zhai P, Le G (2007) Antibacterial activity and in vitro anti-tumor activity of the extract of the larvae of the housefly (*Musca domestica*). J Ethnopharmacol 111:227–231
Hovius JWR, Levi M, Fikrig E (2008) Salivating for knowledge: potential pharmacological agents in tick saliva. PLoS Med 5:0202–0208
Huh J-E, Kang K-S, Ahn K-S, Kim DH, Saikie I, Kim S-H (2003) *Mylabris phalerlata* induces apoptosis by caspase activation following cytochrome c release and Bid cleavage. Life Sci 73:2249–2262
Ip SW, Liao SS, Lin SY, Lin JP, Yang JS, Lin ML, Chen GW, Lu HF, Lin MW, Han SM, Chung JG (2008a) The role of mitochondria in bee venom-induced apoptosis in human breast cancer MCF7 cells. In Vivo 22:237–245
Ip SW, Wei HC, Lin JP, Kuo HM, Liu KC, Hsu SC, Yang JS, Mei-Dueyang CTH, Han SM, Chung JG (2008b) Bee venom induced cell cycle arrest and apoptosis in human cervical epidermoid carcinoma Ca Ski cells. Anticancer Res 28:833–842
Islam MK, Tsuji N, Miyoshi T, Alim MA, Huang X, Hatta T, Fujisaki K (2009) The Kunitz-like modulatory protein haemangin is vital for hard tick blood-feeding success. PLoS Pathog 5:e1000497. doi:10.1371/journal.ppat.1000497
Itoh A, Iizuka K, Natori S (1985) Antitumor effect of *Sarcophaga* lectin on murine transplanted tumors. Jpn J Cancer Res (Gann) 76:1027–1033
Iwanaga S, Okada M, Isawa H, Morita A, Yuda M, Chinzei Y (2003) Identification and characterization of novel salivary thrombin inhibitors from the ixodidae tick, *Haemaphysalis longicornis*. Eur J Biochem 270:1926–1934
Iwasaki T, Ishibashi J, Tanaka H, Sato M, Asaoka A, Taylor D, Yamakawa M (2009) Selective cancer cell cytotoxicity of enantiomeric 9-mer peptides derived from beetle defensins depends on negatively charged phosphatidylserine on the cell surface. Peptides 30:660–668
Jaworski DC, Simmen FA, Lamoreaux W, Coons LB, Muller MT, Needham GR (1995) A secreted calreticulin protein in ixodid tick (*Amblyomma americanum*) saliva. J Insect Physiol 41:369–375
Jin X, Mei H, Li X, Ma Y, Zeng A-H, Wang Y, Lu X, Chu F, Wu Q, Zhu J (2010) Apoptosis-inducing activity of the antimicrobial peptide cecropin of *Musca domestica* in human hepatocellular carcinoma cell line BEL-7402 and the possible mechanism. Acta Biochim Biophys Sin 2010:259–265
Kazimírová M, Dovinová I, Rolníková T, Tóthová L, Hunáková Ľ (2006) Anti-proliferative activity and apoptotic effect of tick salivary gland extracts on human HeLa cells. Neuroendocrinol Lett 27(suppl 2):48–52
Koh CY, Kini RM (2009) Molecular diversity of anticoagulants from haematophagous animals. Thromb Haemost 102:437–453
Koh CY, Kazimirova M, Trimnell A, Takac P, Labuda M, Nuttall PA, Kini RM (2007) Variegin, a novel fast and tight binding thrombin inhibitor from the tropical bont tick. J Biol Chem 282:29101–29113
Kok SH, Chui CH, Lam WS, Chen J, Lau FY, Wong RS, Cheng GY, Tang WK, Cheng CH, Tang JC, Chan AS (2006) Mechanistic insight into a novel synthetic cantharidin analogue in a leukaemia model. Int J Mol Med 18:375–379
Kono T, Watanabe M, Koyama K, Sugimura T, Wakabayashi K (1997) Anti-cancer substance in *Pieris brassicae*. Proc Jpn Acad 73B:192–194
Kono T, Watanabe M, Koyama K, Kishimoto T, Fukushima S, Sugimura T, Wakabayashi K (1999) Cytotoxic activity of pierisin, from the cabbage butterfly, *Pieris rapae*, in various human cancer cell lines. Cancer Lett 137:75–81
Koyama K, Wakabayashi K, Masutani M, Koiwai K, Watanabe M, Yamazaki S, Kono T, Miki K, Sugimura T (1996) Presence in *Pieris rapae* of cytotoxic activity against human carcinoma cells. Jpn J Cancer Res 87:1259–1262
Kramer C, Nahmias Z, Norman DD, Mulvihill TA, Coons LB, Cole JA (2008) *Dermacentor variabilis:* regulation of fibroblast migration by tick salivary gland extract and saliva. Exp Parasitol 119:391–397
Kuczer M, Dziubasik K, Łuczak M, Majewska A, Kamysz W, Saniewska A, Konopińska D (2008) The search for new biological activities for selected insect peptides. Pestycydy 1–2:5–11

Kuhn-Nentwig L (2003) Antimicrobial and cytolytic peptides of venomous arthropods. Cell Mol Life Sci 60:2651–2668

Kwak DH, Kim JK, Kim JY, Jeong HY, Keum KS, Han SH, Rho YI, Woo WH, Jung KY, Choi BK, Choo YK (2002) Anti-angiogenic activities of *Cnidium officinale* Makino and *Tabanus bovinus*. J Ethnopharmacol 81:373–379

Laurens N, Koolwijk P, de Maat MP (2006) Fibrin structure and wound healing. J Thromb Haemost 4:932–939

Lehmann J, Retz M, Sidhu SS, Suttmann H, Sell M, Paulsen F, Harder J, Unteregger G, Stöckle M (2006) Antitumor activity of the antimicrobial peptide Magainin II against bladder cancer cell lines. Eur Urol 50:141–147

Liu D, Chen Z (2009) The effects of cantharidin and cantharidin derivates on tumour cells. Anticancer Agents Med Chem 9:392–396

Lu J, Chen Z-w (2010) Isolation, characterization and anti-cancer activity of SK84, a novel glycine-rich antimicrobial peptide from *Drosophila virilis*. Peptides 31:44–50

Lyons SA, O'Neal J, Sontheimer H (2002) Chlorotoxin, a scorpion-derived peptide, specifically binds to gliomas and tumors of neuroectodermal origin. Glia 39:162–173

Ma D, Gao L, An S, Song Y, Wu J, Xu X, Lai R (2010) A horsefly saliva antigen 5-like protein containing RTS motif is an angiogenesis inhibitor. Toxicon 55:45–51

Macedo-Ribeiro S, Macedo-Ribeiro S, Almeida C, Calisto BM, Friedrich T, Mentele R, Stürzebecher J, Fuentes-Prior P, Pereira PJ (2008) Isolation, cloning and structural characterisation of boophilin, a multifunctional Kunitz-type proteinase inhibitor from the cattle tick. PLoS One 3:e1624

Mans BJ, Louw AI, Neitz AWH (2002) The RGD integrin recognition motif of savignygrin, a platelet aggregation inhibitor from the soft tick, *Ornithodoros savignyi* is presented on the Kunitz-BPTI fold. J Biol Chem 277:21371–21378

Maritz-Olivier C, Stutzer C, Jongejan F, Neitz AW, Gaspar AR (2007) Tick anti-hemostatics: targets for future vaccines and therapeutics. Trends Parasitol 23:397–407

Matsumoto Y, Nakano T, Yamamoto M, Matsushima-Hibiya Y, Odagiri K-I, Yata O, Koyama K, Sugimura T, Wakabayashi K (2008) Distribution of cytotoxic and DNA ADP-ribosylating activity in crude extracts from butterflies among the family Pieridae. Proc Natl Acad Sci 105:2516–2520

Matsushima-Hibiya Y, Watanabe M, Kono T, Kanazawa T, Koyama K, Sugimura T, Wakabayashi K (2000) Purification and cloning of pierisin-2, an apoptosis-inducing protein from the cabbage butterfly, *Pieris brassicae*. Eur J Biochem 267:5742–5750

Midwood KS, Williams LV, Schwarzbauer JE (2004) Tissue repair and the dynamics of the extracellular matrix. Int J Biochem Cell Biol 36:1031–1037

Moon DO, Park SY, Choi YH, Kim ND, Lee C, Kim GY (2008) Melittin induces Bcl-2 and caspase-3-dependent apoptosis through downregulation of Akt phosphorylation in human leukemic U937 cells. Toxicon 51:112–120

Moore AJ, Devine DA, Bibby MC (1994) Preliminary experimental anticancer activity of cecropins. Pept Res 7:265–269

Nienaber J, Gaspar AR, Neitz AW (1999) Savignin, a potent thrombin inhibitor isolated from the salivary glands of the tick *Ornithodoros savignyi* (Acari: Argasidae). Exp Parasitol 3:82–91

Nierodzik ML, Karpatkin S (2006) Thrombin induces tumor growth, metastasis, and angiogenesis: evidence for a thrombin-regulated dormant tumor phenotype. Cancer Cell 10:355–362

Nuttall PA, Labuda M (2004) Tick-host interactions: saliva-activated transmission. Parasitology 129:S177–S189

Oršolić N (2012) Bee venom in cancer therapy. Cancer and Metastasis Rev 31:173–194

Park JH, Jeong YJ, Park KK, Cho HJ, Chung IK, Min KS, Kim M, Lee KG, Yeo JH, Park KK, Chang YC (2010) Melittin suppresses PMA-induced tumor cell invasion by inhibiting NF-κB and AP-1-dependent MMP-9 expression. Mol Cells 29:209–215

Pimenta AM, De Lima ME (2005) Small peptides, big world: biotechnological potential in neglected bioactive peptides from arthropod venoms. J Pept Sci 11:670–676

Ramamoorthi N, Narasimhan S, Pal U, Bao F, Yang XF, Fish D, Anguita J, Norgard MV, Kantor FS, Anderson JF, Koski RA, Fikrig E (2005) The Lyme disease agent exploits a tick protein to infect the mammalian host. Nature 436:573–577

Ribeiro JMC (1995) How ticks make a living. Parasitol Today 11:91–93
Ribeiro JMC, Francischetti IMB (2003) Role of arthropod saliva in blood feeding: sialome and post-sialome perspectives. Annu Rev Entomol 48:73–88
Ribeiro JM, Alarcon-Chaidez F, Francischetti IM, Mans BJ, Mather TN, Valenzuela JG, Wikel SK (2006) An annotated catalog of salivary gland transcripts from *Ixodes scapularis* ticks. Insect Biochem Mol Biol 36:111–129
Roberts DR (1996) Regulation of tumor growth and metastasis by thrombospondin-1. FASEB J 10:1183–1191
Son DJ, Lee JW, Lee YH, Song HS, Lee CK, Hong JT (2007) Therapeutic application of anti-arthritis, pain-releasing, and anti-cancer effects of bee venom and its constituent compounds. Pharmacol Ther 115:246–270
Steen NA, Barker SC, Alewood PF (2006) Proteins in the saliva of the Ixodida (ticks): pharmacological features and biological significance. Toxicon 47:1–20
Suttmann H, Retz M, Paulsen F, Harder J, Zwergel U, Kamradt J, Wullich B, Unteregger G, Stöckle M, Lehmann J (2008) Antimicrobial peptides of the Cecropin-family show potent antitumor activity against bladder cancer cells. BMC Urol 8:5. doi:10.1186/1471-2490-8-5
Titus RG, Bishop JV, Mejia JS (2006) The immunomodulatory factors of arthropod saliva and the potential for these factors to serve as vaccine targets to prevent pathogen transmission. Parasite Immunol 28:131–141
Tu AT, Motoyashi T, Azimov DA (2005) Bioactive compounds in tick and mite venoms (saliva). Toxin Rev 24:143–174
Valenzuela JG (2002) High-throughput approaches to study salivary proteins and genes from vectors of disease. Insect Biochem Mol Biol 32:1199–1209
Valenzuela JG (2004) Exploring tick saliva: from biochemistry to "sialomes" and functional genomics. Parasitology 129:S83–S94
Valenzuela JG, Francischetti IMB, Pham VM, Garfield MK, Mather TN, Ribeiro JMC (2002) Exploring the sialome of the tick *Ixodes scapularis*. J Exp Biol 205:2843–2864
Wang WX, Ji YH (2005) Scorpion venom induces glioma cell apoptosis in vivo and inhibits glioma tumor growth in vitro. J Neurooncol 73(1):1–7
Watanabe M, Kono T, Koyama K, Sugimura T, Wakabayashi K (1998) Purification of pierisin, an inducer of apoptosis in human gastric carcinoma cells, from cabbage butterfly, *Pieris rapae*. Jpn J Cancer Res 89:556–561
Watanabe M, Kono T, Matsushima Hibiya Y, Kanazawa T, Nishisaka N, Kishimoto T, Koya K, Sugimura T, Wakabayashi K (1999) Molecular cloning of an apoptosis-inducing protein, pierisin, from cabbage butterfly: possible involvement of ADP ribosylation in its activity. Proc Natl Acad Sci 96:10608–10613
Werner S, Grose R (2003) Regulation of wound healing by growth factors and cytokines. Physiol Rev 83:835–870
Wikel SK, Alarcon-Chaidez FJ (2001) Progress toward molecular characterization of ectoparasite modulation of host immunity. Vet Parasitol 101:275–287
Yamamoto M, Nakano T, Matsushima-Hibiya Y, Totsuka Y, Takahashi-Nakaguchi A, Matsumoto Y, Sugimura T, Wakabayashi K (2009) Molecular cloning of apoptosis-inducing Pierisin-like proteins, from two species of white butterfly, *Pieris melete* and *Aporia crataegi*. Comp Biochem Physiol B 154:326–333
Yang P, Abe S, Zhao Y-P, An Y, Suzuki K (2004) Growth suppression of rat hepatoma cells by a pentapeptide from *Antheraea yamamai*. J Insect Biotechnol Sericol 73:7–13
You M, Xuan X, Tsuji N, Kamio T, Igarashi I, Nagasawa H, Mikami T, Fujisaki K (2001) Molecular characterization of a troponin I-like protein from the hard tick *Haemaphysalis longicornis*. Insect Biochem Mol Biol 32:67–73

Part III
Polyphenols as Inducers of Cell Death

Chapter 8
Induction of Apoptosis by Polyphenolic Compounds in Cancer Cells

Didem Turgut Cosan and Ahu Soyocak

Abstract Apoptosis, one of the main types of programmed cell death, is a kind of defense mechanism that eliminates the cells that are abnormal or not needed and plays a critical role for the development and maintenance of tissue homeostasis. Apoptosis can be triggered by various physiological and pathological stimuli. Apoptotic pathways require activation of caspases, a group destructive cystein proteases responsible for the cleavage of the key cellular proteins. Recent studies indicate that are two main apoptotic pathways, including extrinsic or death receptor pathway and intrinsic or mitochondrial pathway. Many natural compounds induce apoptosis in various cancer cells by acting through these pathways. These compounds are either antioxidants or inducers of antioxidant defense mechanism. Polyphenols (alone or in combination) are major constituents of plant-derived antioxidants that induce apoptosis by variety of mechanisms in cancer cells and reduce the risk of cancer. This chapter is focused on the effects of polyphenols such as resveratrol, quercetin and tannic acid on apoptosis in various cancers such as breast, colon and prostate cancers.

8.1 Introduction

Apoptosis or programmed cell death plays a major role in the control of normal development in multicellular organisms and tissue homeostasis. Defects in the mechanism of apoptosis might lead to various abnormalities ranging from autoimmune diseases to cancer (Lorenzo and Susin 2004). On the other hand, induction of apoptosis might act as a protective mechanism against cancer. This mechanism is responsible for the apoptosis-related degradation and death of cells and occurs via various activation signals (D'Archivio et al. 2008). Apoptosis is mainly the result of

D. Turgut Cosan (✉) • A. Soyocak
Department of Medical Biology, Eskisehir Osmangazi University,
26480 Eskisehir, Turkey
e-mail: dcosan@gmail.com; asoyocak@gmail.com

M. Diederich and K. Noworyta (eds.), *Natural Compounds as Inducers of Cell Death: Volume 1*, DOI 10.1007/978-94-007-4575-9_8,

two pathways activated by intracellular and extracellular signals and is characterized with several morphological changes including cell shrinkage, nuclear DNA fragmentation and membrane blebbing (Debatin 2004). The cytoplasmic (extrinsic) pathway of apoptosis activated by extracellular signals occurs via the death receptors that belong to a subgroup of TNF receptor super family. Activation of these receptors located on the cell membrane of target cell by related ligands induces the apoptotic pathway (Sprick and Walczak 2004; Bradshaw and Edward Dennis 2003). Mitochondrial (intrinsic) pathway of apoptosis activated by intracellular signals is triggered by release of cytochrome-c to cytoplasm from intermembrane area of mitochondria and activation of the apoptosome complex consisting of cytosolic factor Apaf-1, ATP and active caspase 9. Caspases and members of the Bcl-2 protein family are involved in both of these apoptotic pathways. Caspases are members of a cystein protease family and are synthesized in the form of inactive zymogens activated by proteolytic cleavage. Overall caspases act as initiator (caspase 2,8,9,10) and effectors (caspase 3,6,7) in the apoptotic process. Members of the Bcl-2 family consist of proteins that either trigger (proapoptotic) or prevent (antiapoptotic) apoptosis. Among this family, while proteins including Bcl-2, Bcl-X_L and Mcl-1 prevent apoptosis, other proteins including Bax, Bad, Bid, Bak, Bcl-xs trigger apoptosis (Bradshaw and Edward Dennis 2003; Burlacu 2003; Twomey and McCarthy 2005). In addition, there are several other proteins that are involved in the apoptotic cell death whose names and functions have been summarized in Table 8.1.

Many natural compounds including polyphenols induce apoptosis in various cancer cells by acting through these pathways. Polyphenols are major constituents of plant-derived antioxidants that induce apoptosis by a variety of mechanisms in cancer cells and reduce the risk of cancer.

Polyphenols in diet are extremely important for their favorable effects on health particularly due to their anti-cancer features (Ramos 2008). These polyphenols are found in fruits, vegetables, seeds and beverages and are classified as stillbens (e.g. resveratrol), flavonoids (e.g. quercetin), tannins (e.g. tannic acid), phenolic acids and analogues, lignans and others according to their chemical structures (Ramos 2008; Huang et al. 2010).

Most dietary polyphenolic compounds including resveratrol, quercetin and tannic acid have an inhibitory role on carcinogenesis with the induction of apoptosis by several different mechanisms. The present chapter will focus the molecular basis of chemopreventive activity of some polyphenols (resveratrol, quercetin and tannic acid), addressing their effects on the induction of apoptosis in cancer cells (Fig. 8.1). Abbreviations are listed in Table 8.2.

8.1.1 Induction of Apoptosis by Resveratrol

Apoptotic effects of resveratrol (3,5,4′ trihydroxystilbene), a member of the stilben family, has been investigated in cancer cell lines in several studies. Other effects of resveratrol are summarized in Table 8.3.

Table 8.1 Proteins involved in apoptosis

Apoptotic proteins	Function	References
Death ligands (*e.g. FasL,TNFα,TRAIL*) Death receptor (*Fas(CD95),TNFR1,TRAILR*)	These are effective in the cytoplasmic (extrinsic) pathway of apoptosis. The extrinsic pathway is initiated by the interaction between the specific ligands and the surface receptors which are able to deliver a death signal from the extracellular microenvironment to the cytoplasm. Induction of apoptosis through extrinsic pathway is therefore very rapid	Bradshaw and Edward Dennis (2003) and Reuter et al. (2008)
Caspase family (e.g. Capase 3,6,7,2,8,9,10)	Caspases are members of a cystein protease family and are synthesized in the form of inactive zymogens activated by proteolytic cleavage. The intracellular transmission of the apoptotic signal is regulated by caspase family	Bradshaw and Edward Dennis (2003) and Holdenrieder and Stieber (2004)
Bcl-2 family (e.g. Bcl-2,Bcl-xl, Mcl-1,Bax, Bad, Bid, Bak, Bcl-xs, Noxa, PUMA)	Bcl-2 family proteins can target the mitochondria and regulated membrane permeabilization	Debatin (2004) and Bradshaw and Edward Dennis (2003)
Smac/Diablo	Smac/DIABLO, a mitochondrial protein, can block IAP mediated caspase inhibition by binding XIAP	Bradshaw and Edward Dennis (2003)
HtrA2/Omi	Omi/HtrA2 is a mitochondrial serine protease that is released into the cytosol during apoptosis to antagonize inhibitors of apoptosis (IAPs) and contribute to cell death	Yang et al. (2003)
AIF	AIF is released from mitochondria in apoptotic conditions, it triggers cell death either directly, through interaction with DNA, or indirectly, through reactive oxygen species production	Lorenzo and Susin (2004)
IAP (e.g. Survivin, IXAP)	IAPs are blocks activity of caspases and may target active caspases for degradation	Debatin (2004) and Bradshaw and Edward Dennis (2003)
c-FLIP	FLIP molecules constitute one of the negative regulators of death receptor induced apoptosis	Los and Walczak (2002)
Cytochrome c	The mitochondrial pathway is initiated by the release of apoptogenic factors such as cytochrome c, from the mitochondrial intermembrane space. The release of cytochrome c into the cytosol triggers caspase-3 activation through formation of the cytochrome-c/Apaf-1/caspase-9–containing apoptosome complex	Debatin (2004)

(continued)

Table 8.1 (continued)

Apoptotic proteins	Function	References
Apaf-1	Apaf1 plays a central role in the common events of mitochondria-dependent apoptosis in most death pathways. Apaf-1 mediated clustering of caspase-9 into in apoptosome requires the presence of cytochrome c	Los and Walczak (2002) and Yoshida et al. (1998)
P21 (WAF-1/CIP-1)	p21 is a potent cyclin-dependent kinase inhibitor (CKI). p21 plays an essential role in growth arrest after DNA damage	Reuter et al. (2008), Gartel and Tyner (2002), and Coqueret (2003)
P27 (Kip-1)	p27 is a potent cyclin-dependent kinase inhibitor (CKI). Following anti-mitogenic signals or DNA damage, p27 bind to cyclin-CDK complexes to inhibit their catalytic activity and induce cell-cycle arrest	Coqueret (2003) and Aggarwal and Shishodia (2006)
P38	The induction of apoptosis is accompanied by immediate and sustained activation of p38 mitogen-activated protein kinase (MAPK) Activation of the p38 signaling pathway occurs upstream of caspase activation	Kralova et al. (2008)
P53	P53 is a tumor-suppressor and transcription factor. It is a critical regulator in many cellular processes including cell signal transduction, cellular response to DNA-damage, genomic stability, cell cycle control, and apoptosis	Aggarwal and Shishodia (2006)
PI3K	The phosphatidylinositol-3-kinase (PI3K) signaling pathway is crucial for many aspects of cell growth and survival and is frequently disrupted in human cancers	Reuter et al. (2008)
Akt	Act inactivates pro-apoptotic factors like Bad, which controls the release of cytochrome c, procaspase-9 and Forkhead transcription factors. Akt also activates anti-apoptotic genes, including cyclic-AMP response element-binding protein (CREB) and IκB kinase (IKK) leading to NF- B nuclear localization and the subsequent transcription of survival genes, such as Bcl-xL, caspase inhibitors and c-Myb	Reuter et al. (2008)
pRb	The retinoblastoma protein (Rb) has been recognized as an important cell cycle regulator actively involved in preventing cells from undergoing apoptosis. The activity of Rb is regulated through its phosphorylation state by cell cycle-dependent protein kinases (CDKs) and CDK inhibitors (CDKIs)	Fan and Steer (1999)

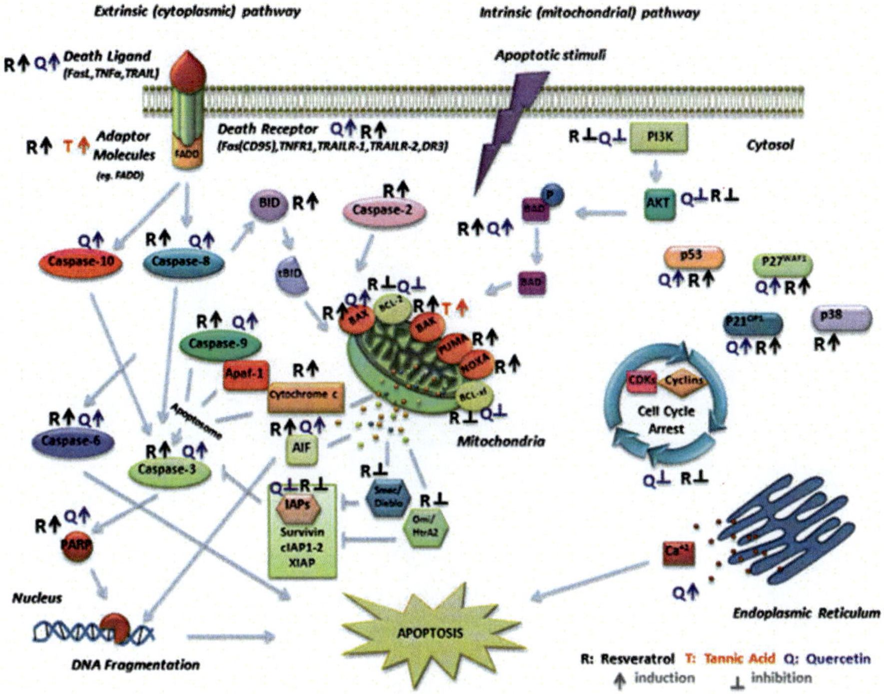

Fig. 8.1 The effects of dietary polyphenolic compounds, including resveratrol, quercetin and tannic acid, in regulation of various molecules in intrinsic and extrinsic pathways of apoptosis. Apoptosis can be triggered in a cell through either the intrinsic or extrinsic pathways. Dietary polyphenols exert their effects by altering levels or activity of single or multiple apoptotic pathways depending on a cancer type or the structure of the compounds

8.1.1.1 Breast Cancer Cells and Resveratrol

Resveratrol induces apoptotic process in several breast cancer cell lines by up- or down-regulating certain pro- and anti-apoptotic proteins, respectively, that have a role in the intrinsic pathway (e.g., Bcl-2, Bcl-XL, Bak and Bax). For instance resveratrol inhibits expression of Bcl-XL anti-apoptotic protein and increases levels of bak and bax proapoptotic proteins(Nakagawa et al. 2001; Kim et al. 2004; Pozo-Guisado et al. 2005; Sakamoto et al. 2010). Moreover, resveratrol induces apoptosis by increasing the activities of caspase 3 and 9 (Nakagawa et al. 2001; Kim et al. 2004; Alkhalaf et al. 2008; Sareen et al. 2007). Analysis of the resveratrol-induced mechanisms in T47D breast cancer cells indicate that it induces apoptosis by activating death receptor pathway via FADD (CD95) in the extrinsic pathway (Clement et al. 1998).

Alkhalaf et al. (2008) have shown that resveratrol induces PARP degradation with caspase 3 activation in MDA-MD-231 breast cancer cell line (Alkhalaf et al. 2008). Furthermore, it has been reported that resveratrol induces apoptosis in T47D

Table 8.2 Abbreviations

AIF	Apoptosis inducing factor
AMPK	5′ adenosine monophosphate (AMP)-activated protein kinase
Apaf-1	Apoptosis protease activation factor-1
Bad	BCL2-antagonist of cell death
Bak	BCL2-antagonist/killer
Bax	BCL2-associated X protein
Bcl-2	B-cell leukemia/lymphoma 2
Bcl-X_L/BCL2L1	BCL2-like 1
Bid	BH3 interacting domain death agonist
Caspase	Cysteine-aspartic-acid-protease
Cdc	Cell division cycle
Cdk	Cyclin-dependent kinase
CIP1	Cdk-interacting protein 1
DD	Death domain
DR	Death receptor
EGCG	Epigallocatechin gallate
EGFR	Epidermal growth factor
ERK	Extracellular signal regulated kinase
ER	Estrogen receptor
FADD	Fas-associated DD Kinase
FasR (CD95/APO-1)	Fas receptor
FLICE	FADD like interleukin-1 β converting enzyme
FLIP	FLICE like inhibitory protein
HSP-70	Heat shock protein 70
Omi/HtrA2	High temperature requirement protein A2(Omi)
IAP	Inhibitor of apoptosis protein
I B	Inhibitor of *K*B
JNK	c-jun N-terminal kinase
MAP	Mitogen-activated protein
Mcl-1	Myeloid cell leukemia sequence 1
NF- B	Nuclear factor- *Kappa* B
NO	Nitric oxide
NOS	Nitric oxide synthase
Noxa	NADPH oxidase activator 1
P21 (Waf-1/Cip-1)	Cyclin-dependent kinase inhibitor (CDKI)
P27 (Kip-1)	Cyclin-dependent kinase inhibitor 1B
P38	Mitogen-activated protein kinase
P53	Tumor suppressor protein
PARP	Poly (ADP-ribose) polymerase
PI3K	Phosphoinositide 3-kinase
Stat 3	Signal transducer and activator of transcription 3
Akt	Related to protein kinase A and C (RAC), Protein kinase B (PKB)
pRb	Retinoblastoma protein
PUMA	p53 up-regulated modulator of apoptosis
ROS	Reactive oxygen species
Smac/Diablo	Second mitochondria-derived activator of caspase/Direct IAP binding protein

(continued)

Table 8.2 (continued)

AIF	Apoptosis inducing factor
TNF	Tumor necrosis factor
TNFR	TNF receptor
TRAIL	Tumor necrosis factor related apoptosis inducing ligand
TRAIL-R	TRAIL receptor
WAF1	Wild type p53 activated protein-1
XIAP	X-linked Inhibitor of apoptosis protein

breast cancer cells that is associated with activation of p53 (Alkhalaf 2007). Pozo-Guisado et al. (2002) showed that resveratrol induces CDK inhibitors, such as p27 and p21 in MCF-7 breast cancer cells, suggesting that resveratrol also inhibits cell cycle progression (Pozo-Guisado et al. 2002).

Furthermore, resveratrol has been shown to induce activity of JNKs and p38 of the MAP kinase family as well as inhibiting NF-kB, PI3K and Akt (Pozo-Guisado et al. 2005; Sakamoto et al. 2010; Filomeni et al. 2007; Li et al. 2006). At higher doses, resveratrol is also capable of inhibiting the proliferation of breast cancer cells and reducing their growth and viability (Nakagawa et al. 2001; Pozo-Guisado et al. 2002; Schmitt et al. 2002; Mgbonyebi et al. 1998; Scarlatti et al. 2003). Studies have reported that resveratrol-induced growth inhibition is associated with changes in cell cycle at several levels including sub-G1, sub G0/G1, G1/S and G2/M (Nakagawa et al. 2001; Kim et al. 2004; Sakamoto et al. 2010; Pozo-Guisado et al. 2002; Scarlatti et al. 2003; Wang et al. 2009a).

Resveratrol can induce antiproliferative and apoptotic effects in highly metastatic and invasive breast cancer cell line, MDA-MB-231, by induction of ceramide, which is the mediator of various intracellular processes including proliferation, apoptosis, differentiation, and aging (Scarlatti et al. 2003).

8.1.1.2 Colon Cancer Cells and Resveratrol

Several studies demonstrated that both the intrinsic and extrinsic apoptotic pathways contribute to cell death induced by resveratrol treatment (Kim et al. 2009a; Cosan et al. 2009). Studies in CaCo-2, HCT-116, SW620, and HT-29 colon cancer cells have demonstrated that resveratrol inhibits cell proliferation and commits cells to apoptosis (Szendel et al. 2000; Wolter et al. 2001; Juan et al. 2008; Zhang et al. 2009). Delmas et al. (2003) have reported that resveratrol activates certain caspases in SW480 human colon cancer cells and might trigger apoptosis by inducing the redistribution of Fas receptor on cell membrane (Delmas et al. 2003). Trincheri et al. (2007) have shown that resveratrol activates the intrinsic pathway in DLD1 and HT29 cell lines, whereas the study by Pohland et al. (2006) suggested that apoptosis occurred via the death receptor dependent pathway in HCT 116 cells with Bax and Bak deficiency (Trincheri et al. 2007; Pohland et al. 2006). However, Mahyar et al. (2002) have shown that resveratrol triggers apoptosis through both Bax-dependent and independent mechanisms in HCT 116 cells (Mahyar-Roemer et al. 2002). In study on HCT 116 cells,

Table 8.3 Polyphenolic compounds and their known biological activities

Polyphenolic compounds (representative pheolics)	Sources	Biological activities of polyphenolic compounds
Resveratrol 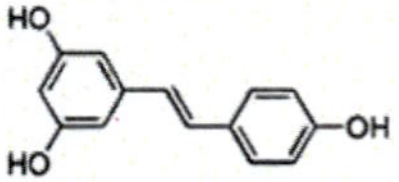	*Berries* (Corre et al. 2005; Azız et al. 2003; Gusman et al. 2001)	*Alteration of eicosanoid synthesis* (Corre et al. 2005; Azız et al. 2003; Gusman et al. 2001)
	Grapes (Corre et al. 2005; Azız et al. 2003; Gusman et al. 2001)	*Antibacterial activities* (Gusman et al. 2001)
	Groundnuts (Pervaız 2003)	*Anticarcinogenic activities* (Corre et al. 2005; Ignatowicz and Baer-Dubowska 2001)
		Anticoagulant properties (Corre et al. 2005; Ignatowicz and Baer-Dubowska 2001)
	Peanuts (Corre et al. 2005); Azız et al. 2003; Gusman et al. 2001)	*Antiinflammatory activities* (Corre et al. 2005; Azız et al. 2003; Gusman et al. 2001; Ignatowicz and Baer-Dubowska 2001)
	Polygonum cuspidatum (Corre et al. 2005; Azız et al. 2003; Pervaız 2003)	*Antimutajen properties* (Azız et al. 2003)
	Red wine (Azız et al. 2003)	*Antioxidant properties* (Corre et al. 2005; Azız et al. 2003; Gusman et al. 2001; Ignatowicz and Baer-Dubowska 2001; Pervaız 2003)
		Cardioprotective (Corre et al. 2005; Pervaız 2003)
		Chelation of copper (Azız et al. 2003; Gusman et al. 2001)
		Inhibition of lipid peroxidation (Corre et al. 2005; Azız et al. 2003; Gusman et al. 2001)
		Inhibition of platelet aggregation (Corre et al. 2005; Azız et al. 2003; Pervaız 2003)
		Neuroprotective (Pervaız 2003)
		Oestrogenic/anti-oestrogenic activity (Gusman et al. 2001)
		Vasorelaxing activities (Corre et al. 2005; Azız et al. 2003)

Quercetin 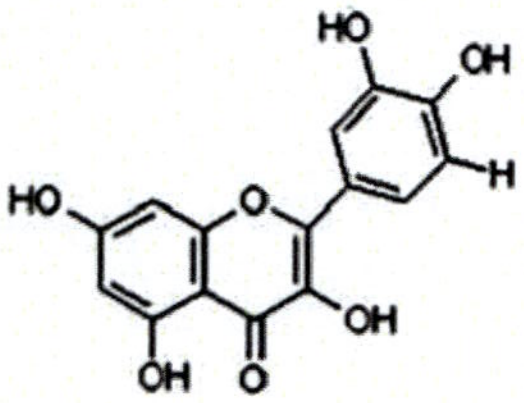	*Apples* (Bischoff 2008; Aherne and O'Brien 2002; Middleton et al. 2000) *Berries* (Bischoff 2008; Aherne and O'Brien 2002) *Broccoli* (Bischoff 2008; Aherne and O'Brien 2002) *Cherries* (Bischoff 2008; Aherne and O'Brien 2002) *Citrus fruits* (Bischoff 2008) *Grapes* (Bischoff 2008; Aherne and O'Brien 2002) *Onions* (Bischoff 2008; Aherne and O'Brien 2002; Middleton et al. 2000) *Red wine* (Aherne and O'Brien 2002) *Tea* (Bischoff 2008; Aherne and O'Brien 2002) *Tomato* (Aherne and O'Brien 2002)	*Antiallergic activity* (Bischoff 2008) *Anticataract effects* (Bischoff 2008) *Antihypertensive activity* (Perez-Vizcaino et al. 2009) *Antiinflammatory activity* (Bischoff 2008) *Antimicrobial effects* (Bischoff 2008) *Antineurodegenerative effects* (Bischoff 2008) *Antioxidant activity* (Bischoff 2008; Middleton et al. 2000) *Antiplatelet activity* (Bischoff 2008) *Antitumor effects* (Bischoff 2008) *Antiviral activity* (Middleton et al. 2000) *Inhibition of lipid peroxidation* (Middleton et al. 2000)
Tannic acid 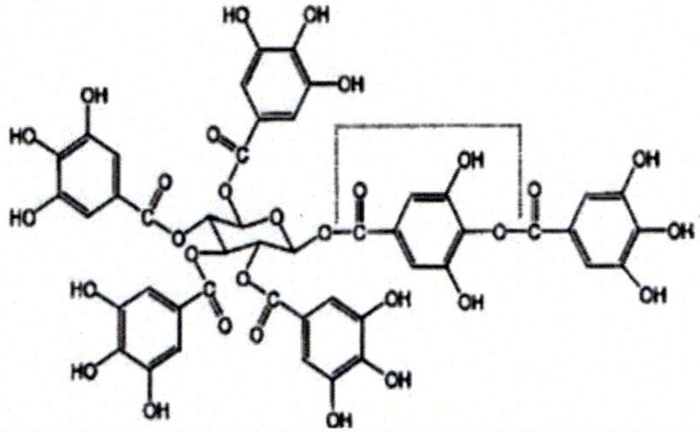	*Beans* (Naus et al. 2007) *Coffee* (Taffetani et al. 2005) *Grapes* (Naus et al. 2007) *Nuts* (Naus et al. 2007; Taffetani et al. 2005) *Red wine* (Taffetani et al. 2005) *Tea* (Taffetani et al. 2005)	*Antiangiogenic activity* (Chen et al. 2003) *Antibacterial activity* (Chung et al. 1998) *Anticarcinogenic* (Chung et al. 1998; Khan and Hadi 1998) *Antimicrobial activity* (Chung et al. 1998) *Antimutagenic activity* (Khan and Hadi 1998) *Antioxidant properties* (Chung et al. 1998; Khan and Hadi 1998; Khan et al. 2000) *Antiproliferative effects* (Taffetani et al. 2005) *Chemopreventive effects* (Chen et al. 2003) *Prooxidant properties* (Khan et al. 2000)

Mahyar et al. (2001), have reported that apoptosis induced through the mitochondrial pathway and that resveratrol up- regulated Bax independently of p53 (Mahyar-Roemer et al. 2001). Studies on various colon cancer cell lines demonstrated that resveratrol induces the release of cytochrome c from mitochondria (Kim et al. 2009a; Trincheri et al. 2007).

The effects of resveratrol on caspases have been studied in colon cancer cells. Several studies have shown that resveratrol effects caspases 2, 3, 6, 8 and 9 (Kim et al. 2009a; Wolter et al. 2001; Juan et al. 2008; Mahyar-Roemer et al. 2002; Lee et al. 2006; Mohan et al. 2006). A study performed on DLD-1 and HT-29 colon cancer cells have shown the effects of resveratrol on cathepsin D, a lysosomal protease that emerges in the later stages of apoptosis. Thus, it might be suggested that lysosomes constitute one of the targets of resveratrol (Trincheri et al. 2007). Resveratrol reduced mitotic activity by affecting cell cycle proteins in colon cancer cells. It has been reported that resveratrol inhibits the cell cycle. These effects of resveratrol on cell cycle have been shown to be associated with alterations in the expression of cyclins and CDKs (Wolter et al. 2001). However, a study performed with CaCo-2 cell line has demonstrated that although resveratrol causes inhibition of cell growth and accumulation of cells in S/G2 phase, it has no effects on cytotoxicity or apoptosis (Schneider et al. 2000). Caspase 6 activation has been reported to be an important factor in apoptosis triggered by resveratrol in HCT116 colon cancer cells with or without p53 (Lee et al. 2009a). Resveratrol also inhibits Wnt signaling markedly at low doses; an effect considered to be a consequence of regulation of intracellular beta-catenin localization (Hope et al. 2008). Overall, studies suggest that resveratrol exerts its effects through multiple pathways leading to induction of apoptosis and inhibition of cell growth.

8.1.1.3 Prostate Cancer Cells and Resveratrol

Studies have shown that resveratrol induces apoptosis by up-regulating TRAILR1/DR4 and TRAILR2/DR5 in the death receptor pathway in LNCaP prostate cancer cell line (Shankar et al. 2007a, b). Aziz et al. (2006) have shown that resveratrol can induce apoptotic molecules including Bax, Bak, Bid and Bad in the intrinsic pathway, and commit cells to apoptosis in LNCaP cell line (Aziz et al. 2006). In study on LNCap, PC3 and DU145 prostate cancer cell line, resveratrol alters release of Smac/Diablo, cytochrome c, AIF, Omi/HtrA2, PuMA and Noxa by causing loss of mitochondrial membrane potential (Shankar et al. 2007a; b). Studies have shown that resveratrol activates caspases in prostate cancer cells. In androgen responsive LNCaP and androgen insensitive PC3 prostate cancer cells, resveratrol induces apoptosis by activating both caspase 9 and caspase 3 (Shankar et al. 2007b; Benitez et al. 2007a). Resveratrol increases expression of proapoptotic proteins in LNCaP cells, while down-regulating antiapoptotic molecules cIAP1-2, XIAP, Bcl-xl, survivin and Bcl-2 (Shankar et al. 2007b). It also has antiproliferative effects on prostate cancer cells and decreases cell viability (Aziz et al. 2006; Benitez et al. 2007a, b; Hsieh and Wu 1999). In a study performed with Du-145 prostate cancer cells, suppressive effects of resveratrol on proliferation have been suggested to be mediated by HSPs70- (Cardile et al. 2003).

Resveratrol might inhibit certain molecules in cell survival pathways including PI3K, Akt and NF-κB (Shankar et al. 2007b; Aziz et al. 2006; Benitez et al. 2007b; 2009). Scarlatti et al. (2007) have shown that resveratrol induced cell cycle arrest and promoted apoptosis in prostate cancer cells (Benitez et al. 2009). Kotha et al. (2006) have reported that resveratrol inhibits the activity of Src tyrosine kinase in malign cells and thus blocks the activation of Stat 3 proteins. As a result of the treatment of malign cells expressing active-Stat3 with resveratrol, human breast (MDA-MB-231) and prostate carcinoma (DU145) cell lines were inhibited at G0-G1 phase of cell cycle. However, resveratrol inhibited S phase of the cell cycle in human breast cancer (MDA-MB-468) and induced cell death via apoptosis (Kotha et al. 2006).

Narayanan et al. (2003) showed that resveratrol alters the cell cycle regulation including cyclins, cdks, p53 and cdk inhibitors and expression of genes associated with apoptosis (Narayanan et al. 2003). Joe et al. (2002) reported that resveratrol induces marked growth inhibition in MCF7 and SW480 cell lines (Joe et al. 2002). Hsieh (2009) has been demonstrated that resveratrol achieves its anti-cancer activity in prostate cancer cells by suppressing cell proliferation, inhibiting proceeding of cell cycle and thus inducing apoptosis in androgen responsive LNCaP and androgen resistant (or insensitive) DU145 and PC-3 CaP cells (Hsieh 2009).

Antiproliferative and proapoptotic effects of resveratrol in breast cancer cells might be due to accumulation of ceramide. However, Sala et al. (2003) have demonstrated that resveratrol might exhibit antiproliferative/proapoptotic effects secondary to endogen ceramide accumulation in androgen receptor (AR) negative prostate cancer cell line PC3 (Sala et al. 2003).

8.1.2 Induction of Apoptosis by Quercetin

Quercetin (3,5,7,3′,4′-pentahidroksiflavon) is a flavonoid commonly found in vegetables and fruits (Table 8.3). Its effects in the molecular mechanisms of apoptosis have been investigated in several cancer cell lines.

8.1.2.1 Breast Cancer Cells and Quercetin

Several studies indicate that quercetin induces apoptosis in breast cancer cells (Chou et al. 2010; Choi et al. 2001; Hatipoglu et al. 2010). Quercetin, induces apoptosis through modulation of various pathways in a manner similar to other phenolic compounds and causes reduction in Bcl-2, and elevation Bax and AIF levels in MCF-7, MDA-MB-231 and MDA-MB-453 breast cancer cells (Chou et al. 2010; Chien et al. 2009; Choi et al. 2008). Chou et al. (2010) reported that quercetin decreased levels of Bcl-2 protein and increased the activation of caspase-6, -8 and –9 in MCF-7 cells (Chou et al. 2010). Chien et al. (2009) showed that quercetin treatment promoted activation of caspase-3, -8 and −9 in MDA-MB-231 cells (Chien et al. 2009). Other studies showed that quercetin induces growth inhibition and decrease proliferation and cell viability in breast cancer cells (Chou et al. 2010; Choi et al. 2001; Hatipoglu et al. 2010; Chien et al. 2009; Choi et al. 2008; Jeong et al. 2009; Rodgers and Grant 1998; Lee et al. 2009b; Hakimuddin et al. 2004). Quercetin affects the cell cycle by increasing the levels of Cdk inhibitors including p53, $p21^{CIP1/waf1}$ and $p27^{Kip1}$ (Chou et al. 2010; Choi et al. 2001; Jeong et al. 2009). In MDA-MB-231 cells, quercetin was shown to increase levels of cytosolic calcium, which is known to trigger apoptosis. (Chien et al. 2009). In addition, Costillo-pichardo et al. (2009) have demonstrated that combination of various grape polyphenols induce apoptosis and are more effective than single use of resveratrol, quercetin, or catechin in inhibition of cell proliferation, cell cycle progression, and cell migration in the highly metastatic ER (−) MDA-MB-435 cell line (Castillo-Pichardo et al. 2009).

8.1.2.2 Colon Cancer Cells and Quercetin

Studies have shown that quercetin induces TRAIL-mediated apoptosis in colon adenocarcinoma cells (Psahoulia et al. 2007). Kim WK et al. (2005) have reported that Bcl-2 was reduced while Bax remained unchanged in HT9 and SW480 colon cancer cells after administration of quercetin (Kim et al. 2005). Quercetin has been shown to decrease cell viability, increase differentiation, inhibit cell proliferation and induce apoptosis in colon cancer cells (Kim et al. 2005; Xavier et al. 2009; Wenzel et al. 2004; Kim et al. 2010; Van Erk et al. 2004; Shan et al. 2009). Van Erk et al. (2005) showed that in CaCo-2 cell lines, quercetin down-regulates cell cycle genes (CDC6, CDK4, cyclin D1), reduces the number of cells in G1 phase, and increases the sub-G1 population (Van Erk et al. 2004). Proapoptotic effector caspase 3 and PARP cleavage increases with the effect of quercetin (Kim et al. 2005; Wenzel et al. 2004). Kim et al. (2010) shown that quercetin causes upregulation of proteins including AMPK, p53 and p21 in HT-29 colon cancer cell line (Kim et al. 2010). Shan et al. (2009) have been reported that quercetin down-regulates survivin genes in SW480 colon cancer cells (Shan et al. 2009). Kim et al. (2005) have demonstrated that in CO115 cells quercetin decreased Akt phosphorylation, but did not alter that of phospho-ERK (Xavier et al. 2009). Overall available data suggest that quercetin exerts its effects by multiple mechanism in cells and not only induces apoptosis but also inhibits survival pathways and cell cycle progression.

8.1.2.3 Prostate Cancer Cells and Quercetin

Studies in prostate cancer cell lines demonstrated that quercetin induces TRAIL-mediated cytotoxicity in these cells (Kim et al. 2008; Jung et al. 2010). However, one study has suggested that quercetin does not alter levels of TRAIL receptors including DR4, DR5, DcR2 in prostate adenocarcinoma cells (Kim and Lee 2007). Another study has suggested that TRAIL-induced apoptosis was associated with the up-regulation of DR5 receptor (Jung et al. 2010). This discrepancy might be due to the utilization of different cell lines by different studies. It is also possible that the dose of the compounds, or the time of the treatment may cause different findings by different investigators. Kim et al. (2008), quercetin leads to TRAIL induced apoptosis with the inhibition of survivin, an antiapoptotic protein, expression. Although, survivin is down-regulated with quercetin, the expressions of apoptosis inhibitor proteins, FLIP and IAP, are not altered in prostate cancer cell line (Kim et al. 2008). On the other hand, quercetin has been shown to inhibit activity (phosphorylation) of PI3K/Akt signaling pathway in DU-145, LNCaP, PC3 prostate cancer cell lines (Kim and Lee 2007; Senthilkumar et al. 2010; Lee et al. 2008). Quercetin decreases levels of Bcl-2, Bcl-xl, while increases levels of Bax, Bad and caspases including 3, 8, 9, 10 and PARP cleavage in several prostate cell lines (Kim et al. 2008; Jung et al. 2010; Kim and Lee 2007; Senthilkumar et al. 2010; Lee et al. 2008; Vijayababu et al. 2005; Vijayababu et al. 2006a, b). In addition, quercetin inhibits proliferation and cell viability and induces cell cycle arrest (Vijayababu et al. 2005; Aalinkeel et al. 2008). It has been demonstrated that cdc2/cdk1, cyclin B1 and D1 expressions were decreased and G2/M transition was blocked with quercetin (Senthilkumar et al. 2010; Vijayababu et al. 2005). Some studies suggested that quercetin exerts its effects independent of p53. Quercetin induces p21/Cip1 CDK-inhibitor expression, suggesting that it blocks cell cycle progression (Vijayababu et al. 2005, 2006a; b). Quercetin induced apoptosis and inhibition of migration and invasion are synergistically enhanced when combined with EGCG (Tang et al. 2010). Overeall, studies indicate that quercetin is highly effective in inducing apoptosis and inhibition of cell growth in different prostate cancer cells regardless of androgen receptor status. The other important feature of quercetin is that this compound also have multiple effects in prostate cancer cells, ranging from inhibition of cell proliferation, cell cycle to induction of apoptosis.

8.1.3 Induction of Apoptosis by Tannic Acid

Tannins are polyphenolic compounds with molecular weights between 500 and 3000 Da. They are classified into two categories including hydrolyzed and condensed tannins. Hydrolyzed tannins are commonly termed as tannic acids and contain either gallotannin or ellagic tannin (Nam et al. 2001) (Table 8.3).

8.1.3.1 Breast Cancer Cells and Tannic Acid

Recent studies have shown that pomegranate extracts containing tannic acid inhibited the growth of breast, prostate, colon and lung cancer cells (Adhami et al. 2009). In our study performed with MCF-7 breast cancer cell line, we demonstrated that treatment of cells with various doses of tannic acid induced apoptosis and increased the level of FADD and Bak proteins in extrinsic and intrinsic pathways, respectively (data not published). In the study by Uchiumi et al, they examined the effects of biological activities of tannic acid on breast tumor, and found that tannic acid inhibits promoter of mouse mammary tumor virus (Uchiumi et al. 1998). In another study of our group, we observed that tannic acid reduces the overall activity of NOS that is responsible for the synthesis of NO in colon adenocarcinoma cells (CaCo-2) and breast adenocarcinoma cells (MCF-7) (Cosan et al. 2010). Sirivastava et al, have reported that tannic acid might be a potential inhibitor of NOS activity due to its antioxidant features (Srivastava et al. 2000).

8.1.3.2 Colon Cancer Cells and Tannic Acid

Our laboratory has investigated the effects of tannic acid on apoptosis in CaCo-2 colon cancer cell line, Bak in intrinsic pathway and FADD protein in extrinsic pathway by administration of tannic acid in various doses. We found that tannic acid led to an increased apoptotic index and dose and time independent increase in Bak and FADD proteins (Cosan et al. 2009). In the study of Seeram et al. (2005), antiproliferative effects of punicalagin, total pomegranate tannin and ellagic acid were demonstrated in human colon (HT-29, HCT116, SW480, SW620), oral (KB, CAL27) and prostate (RWPE-1, 22Rv1) cancer cells. In addition punicalagin, total pomegranate tannin and ellagic acid were reported to induce apoptosis in HT-29, HCT116 colon cancer cell lines (Seeram et al. 2005). However, the mechanisms by which tannic acid induce apoptosis remains to be elucidated by further studies.

8.1.3.3 Prostate Cancer Cells and Tannic Acid

Various studies have been conducted in order to understand the effects and mechanisms of polyphenols in prostate cancer. In one of these studies, Romero et al. (2002), have found that tannic acid inhibits growth of LNCaPs prostate cancer cells and induces apoptosis (Romero et al. 2002). Bawadi et al. (2005) have demonstrated the anti-angiogenic activity of water-soluble condense tannins isolated from black bean in HEL 299 normal human fibroblast lung cells, Caco-2 colon, MCF-7 and Hs578T breast and DU 145 human prostate cancer cell lines. Furthermore, they found that the condense tannin at lower doses does not have an effect on growth of normal cells however induces death of cancer cells by means of apoptosis in a dose-dependent manner (Bawadi et al. 2005).

Chemopreventive effects of tannic acid might be due to suppression the growth of cancer cells. Currently, there are only very few studies with tannic acid with regard to its role in cancer chemoprevention. However in vitro studies showed that tannic acid inhibits cell proliferation and induces apoptosis in several cancer cell lines. In one of the these studies, Devi et al. (1993) have demonstrated that tannic acid has the highest effect on proliferation in several natural plant polyphenols tested in normal and abnormal human lymphocytes (Devi and Das 1993). Ramanathan et al. (1992), has demonstrated that together with various flavonoids, tannic acid inhibits growth of HeLa and Raji lymphoma cells (Ramanathan et al. 1992). Pan et al. (1999) have shown that penta-O-galloyl-beta-D-glucose is structurally related to (−)-epigallocatechin gallate and is isolated from hydrolyzed tannin, induces apoptosis in HL-60 human acute leukemia (AML) cells by activation of caspase 3 (Pan et al. 1999). Wang et al. (2000), have found that the anti tumor effect of Cuphiin D1 (CD1) which is a macrocyclic hydrolysable tannin induces apoptosis by inhibiting Bcl-2 expression in HL60 leukemia cells, and G1-arrest (accumulation of cells in G1 phase of cell cycle) and decreasing number of cells in G2/M phase (Wang et al. 2000). Chen et al. (2009) have demonstrated tannic acid induced apoptotic death has been observed in HL-60 AML cells in a dose- and time-dependent manner and that this effects were associated with an increase in sub-G1 fraction, chromosome condensation, and DNA fragmentation. Furthermore, it has been stated that tannic acid leads to apoptosis by activation of caspase cascade and cleavage of PARP followed by the disruption of mitochondrial membrane potential, and release of cytochrome c (Chen et al. 2009). Sakagami et al. (2000), have indicated that hydrolyzable tannins lead to induction of apoptotic cell death in human oral squamous cell carcinoma and salivary gland tumor as indicated by the activation of caspases, cytokeratin 18 cleavage and DNA fragmentation (Sakagami et al. 2000). Marienfeld et al. (2003), have found out that tannic acid inhibits in vitro proliferation and cell cycle progression and increases expression of cyclin-dependent kinase inhibitor $p27^{KIP1}$ in malignant human cholangiocytes (Marienfeld et al. 2003).

More interestingly, administration of tannic acid with a diet in C3H mice was shown to be highly effective in prevention of self developing liver tumors depending on dosage. These data clearly suggested that tannic acid can be used as a chemical prevention method against certain tumors (Nam et al. 2001). However, more studies need to be performed to demonstrate the role of tannic acid as a chemopreventive agent in different carcinogenesis models.

Ubiquitin proteasome system plays a critical role in specific degradation of cellular proteins. The most significant functions of proteasomes are to promote tumor cell proliferation and protect tumor cells against apoptosis. Tannic acids effective in the ubiquitin-proteasome system, which plays an important role in destruction of cell proteins. The ubiquitin-proteasome system can modulate levels of proteins such as p53, pRb, p21, $p27^{Kip1}$, IKB-α and Bax that are involved in regulation of cell proliferation and cell death. Inhibition of proteasomes by tannic acid in Jurkat T cancer cells, stimulates apoptosis by accumulation of kinase inhibitor $p27^{Kip1}$, proapoptotic protein Bax and suppression of cell cycle in G1 phase (Nam et al. 2001).

8.1.4 Induction of Apoptosis by Other Polyphenols

Dietary polyphenols are the compounds found in fruits, vegetables and seeds. There are approximately 8.000 different polyphenols that are classified according to their chemical and structural features. The idea that these polyphenols might have a role in the prevention of cancer and can be used as chemical inhibitors of cancer justified

Table 8.4 Effects of other dietary polyphenols on apoptotic pathways in breast, prostate and colon cancer cells

Other dietary polyphenols	Sources	Cancer cells type	Apoptosis effects
Apigenin	Plant seeds fruits and vegetables (Aggarwal and Shishodia 2006)	Breast cancer cells (MDA-MB-453,SK-BR-3) (Choi and Kim 2009a, b)	Induced apoptosis (Choi and Kim 2009a, b; Chung et al. 2007; Kaur et al. 2008) Triggered caspase activation (Choi and Kim 2009a; Shukla and Gupta 2008)
		Colon cancer cells (HT29-APC, HT29-GAL) (Chung et al. 2007)	Released cytochrome c (Choi and Kim 2009a) Expression of Bax (Choi and Kim 2009b; Shukla and Gupta 2008)
		Prostate cancer cells (22Rv1, PC-3) (Shukla and Gupta 2008; Kaur et al. 2008)	Decreased levels of Bcl-XL,Bcl-2 (Shukla and Gupta 2008) Inhibited cell proliferation (Choi and Kim 2009b) Induced cell cycle arrest (Choi and Kim 2009b; Chung et al. 2007) Regulation of CDK1 and p21(Cip1) (Choi and Kim 2009b) Increased accumulation of p53 (Choi and Kim 2009b) Inactivation of Akt (Kaur et al. 2008)
Capsaicin	Red peppers (Chou et al. 2009)	Breast cancer cells (MCF-7, T47D, BT-474, SKBR-3, MDA-MB231) (Chou et al. 2009; Thoennissen et al. 2010)	Induced apoptosis (Thoennissen et al. 2010; Kim et al. 2009b; Yang et al. 2009; Kim et al. 2007) Induced cellular apoptosis through a caspase independent pathway (Chou et al. 2009) Induced apoptosis through mitochondrial and death receptor pathways
		Colon cancer cells (HCT116, Colo320DM, LoVo, HT-29) (Kim et al. 2007, 2009b; Yang et al. 2009)	Induced apoptosis via ROS generation (Sánchez et al. 2007) Activation of caspase 3 (Yang et al. 2009)
		Prostate cancer cells(PC-3) (Sánchez et al. 2007)	Inhibited cell growth (Chou et al. 2009; Thoennissen et al. 2010; Kim et al. 2009b) Decreased cell viability (Yang et al. 2009) Induced cell cycle arrest (Thoennissen et al. 2010) AMPK activation (Kim et al. 2007) JNK activation (Sánchez et al. 2007) ERK activation (Sánchez et al. 2007)

Curcumin	Curcuma longa (Teiten et al. 2010)	Breast cancer cells (MDA-MB-231, BT-483,MCF-7) (Liu et al. 2009; Chiu and Su 2009; Duvoix et al. 2005)	Induced apoptosis (Chiu and Su 2009; Duvoix et al. 2005; Teiten et al. 2010; Lee et al. 2009c; Watson et al. 2008; Hilchie et al. 2010; Srivastava et al. 2007)
			Inhibited expressions of Bcl-2, Bcl-XL, survivin and XIAP (Shankar et al. 2007c)
			Induced expressions of Bax, Bak, PUMA, Bim, and Noxa and death Receptors (TRAIL R1/DR4 and TRAIL-R2/DR5) (Shankar et al. 2007c)
			Down-regulation of NFkappaB inducinggenes (Liu et al. 2009)
			Activation of caspase-3, -8,-9 (Shankar et al. 2007)
		Colon cancer cells (HT-29, HCT-116) (Lee et al. 2009c; Watson et al. 2008)	Decreased protein expression of p53 and Bcl-2 (Chiu and Su 2009)
			Activation of p38 mitogen-activated protein kinase (MAPK) (Hilchie et al. 2010)
			Activation of c-jun N-terminal kinase (JNK) (Hilchie et al. 2010)
		Prostate cancer cells (PC3, LNCaP) (Teiten et al. 2010; Hilchie et al. 2010; Srivastava et al. 2007; Shankar et al. 2007c)	Inhibited cell proliferation (Liu et al. 2009; Chiu and Su 2009)
			Induced cell cycle arrest (Liu et al. 2009; Chiu and Su 2009; Srivastava et al. 2007)
			Induced expression of cyclin-dependent kinase (CDK) inhibitors p16(/INK4a), p21(/WAF1/CIP1) and p27(/KIP1) (Srivastava et al. 2007)
			Inhibited expression of cyclin E and cyclin D1 (Srivastava et al. 2007)
			Decreased pAkt and COX-2 (Lee et al. 2009c)
			Increased p-AMPK (Lee et al. 2009c)
			Activation of p38 mitogen-activated protein kinase (MAPK) (Hilchie et al. 2010)

(continued)

Table 8.4 (continued)

Other dietary polyphenols	Sources	Cancer cells type	Apoptosis effects
Daidzein	Soybean (Hsu et al. 2010)	Breast cancer cells (MCF-7, MDA-MB-453) (Jin et al. 2010; Choi and Kim 2008)	Induced apoptosis (Jin et al. 2010; Hsu et al. 2010)
			Activation of caspase-3,-9,-7 (Jin et al. 2010; Choi and Kim 2008; Guo et al. 2004)
			Down-regulation of bcl-2 (Jin et al. 2010)
			Up-regulation of bax (Jin et al. 2010; Hsu et al. 2010)
		Colon cancer cells (LoVo) (Guo et al. 2004)	Released cytochrome c (Jin et al. 2010)
			Inhibited cell proliferation (Jin et al. 2010; Choi and Kim 2008)
		Prostate cancer cells (LnCap, PC3) (Hsu et al. 2010; Wang et al. 2009b)	Arrested cell cycle (Choi and Kim 2008; Guo et al. 2004)
			Increased expression of the CDK inhibitors p21(Cip1), p57(Kip2) (Choi and Kim 2008)
			DNA fragmentation (Guo et al. 2004)
			Increased p53 protein expression (Wang et al. 2009b)
Delphinidin	Pigmented fruits and vegetables (berries, pomengranates etc.) (Afaq et al. 2008; Yun et al. 2009)	Breast cancer cells (AU-565, MCF-10A) (Afaq et al. 2008)	Induced apoptosis (Afaq et al. 2008; Yun et al. 2009; Bin Hafeez et al. 2008)
			Activation of caspase-3,-8,-9 (Afaq et al. 2008; Yun et al. 2009
			Increased Bax (Afaq et al. 2008; Yun et al. 2009)
			Decreased Bcl-2 protein (Afaq et al. 2008; Yun et al. 2009; Bin Hafeez et al. 2008)
		Colon cancer cells (HCT116) (Yun et al. 2009)	Cleavage of PARP protein (Afaq et al. 2008; Yun et al. 2009)
			Suppressed NF- B pathway (Yun et al. 2009)
			Decreased cell viability (Yun et al. 2009)
			Arrested cell cycle in the G2/M phase (Yun et al. 2009)
		Prostate cancer cells (PC3, LNCaP, C4-2, 22Rnu1) (Bin Hafeez et al. 2008; Hafeez et al. 2008)	Activation of PI3K (Afaq et al. 2008)
			Inhibited EGF-induced autophosphorylation of EGFR, AKT and MAPK (Afaq et al. 2008)
			Inhibition of NFkappaB signaling (Yun et al. 2009; Bin Hafeez et al. 2008)
			Decreased expression of NFkappaB/p65 and PCNA (Hafeez et al. 2008)

Diallylpolysulfides	Garlic (Busch et al. 2010)	HCT116 human colon cancer cells (Busch et al. 2010)	Induced apoptosis (Busch et al. 2010) Arrested cell cycle (Busch et al. 2010) Decreased cell viability (Busch et al. 2010)
Ellagic acid	Avacado Red berries	Breast cancer cells (MCF-7, Hs578T, WA-4) (Losso et al. 2004; Dai et al. 2010)	Induced apoptosis (Losso et al. 2004) Decreased ATP production (Losso et al. 2004)
	Grapes Strawberries	Colon cancer cells (CaCo-2) (Losso et al. 2004)	Arrested cell cycle progression in the G0/G1 phase (Dai et al. 2010) Decreased levels of pro-MMP-2,-9 (Losso et al. 2004)
	Raspberries Nuts (Aggarwal and Shishodia 2006; Losso et al. 2004)	Prostate cancer cells (Du-145) (Losso et al. 2004)	Decreased levels of VEGF (Losso et al. 2004)
Epigallocatechin Gallate (EGCG)	Green tea (Thangapazham et al. 2007; Hastak et al. 2005)	Breast cancer cells (MDA-MB-231, MCF-7) (Thangapazham et al. 2007; Tang et al. 2007)	Induced apoptosis (Thangapazham et al. 2007; Hastak et al. 2005) Increased caspase-9 activity (Tang et al. 2007) Increased Bax (Thangapazham et al. 2007) Reduced Bcl-2 (Thangapazham et al. 2007)
		Colon Cancer Cells (HCT116, HT-29) (Thakur et al. 2010; Hwang et al. 2007)	Increased levels of Bax (Hastak et al. 2005) PARP cleavage (Thangapazham et al. 2007) Arrested cell growth (Hastak et al. 2005)
		Prostate cancer cells (LnCaP) (Hastak et al. 2005)	Inhibited cell proliferation (Thangapazham et al. 2007; Tang et al. 2007) Arrested cell cycle in the G1 phase (Hastak et al. 2005) Induced p53, p21 and PUMA (Thakur et al. 2010; Hastak et al. 2005) Decreased AKT phosphorylation (Thangapazham et al. 2007; Tang et al. 2007) Suppression of survivin (Tang et al. 2007) Decreased COX-2 expression (Hwang et al. 2007) Activation of AMPK (Hwang et al. 2007)

(continued)

Table 8.4 (continued)

Other dietary polyphenols	Sources	Cancer cells type	Apoptosis effects
Genistein	Soy beans	Breast cancer cells (MDA-MB-231, MCF-7) (Ferenc et al. 2010; Li et al. 2008; Tophkhane et al. 2007)	Induced apoptosis (Hsu et al. 2010; Li et al. 2008; Fan et al. 2010; Lu and Yu 2005)
			Induced caspase-3 activity (Li et al. 2008)
			Down-regulation of Bcl-2 (Ferenc et al. 2010; Li et al. 2008)
			Up-regulation of Bax (Ferenc et al. 2010; Li et al. 2008; Fan et al. 2010; Lu and Yu 2005)
	Chickpea	Colon cancer cells (SW480,HT-29) (Fan et al. 2010; Lu and Yu 2005)	Increased cytochrome c release (Tophkhane et al. 2007)
			Inhibited cell growth (Li et al. 2008; Fan et al. 2010)
			Inhibited proliferation (Lu and Yu 2005)
		Prostate cancer cells (LnCap, PC3) (Hsu et al. 2010; Wang et al. 2009b)	Arrested cell cycle (Hsu et al. 2010; Wang et al. 2009b; Tophkhane et al. 2007; Fan et al. 2010; Lu and Yu 2005)
	Kudzu root (Aggarwal and Shishodia 2006; Li et al. 2008)		Inhibited NF-kappaB activity via the MEK5/ERK5 pathway (Li et al. 2008)
			Down-regulation of expression of VEGFand PCNA (Fan et al. 2010; Lu and Yu 2005)
			Up-regulation of expression of p21 (Fan et al. 2010)
Luteolin	Tea	Colon cancer cells (HT-29, COLO205, HCT116) (do Lim et al. 2007; Shi et al. 2004)	Induced apoptosis (do Lim et al. 2007; Chiu and Lin 2008)
	Fruits		Repressed cell proliferation (Chiu and Lin 2008)
	Vegetables		Inhibited cell growth (Chiu and Lin 2008)
	Celery	Prostate cancer cells (LNCaP, DU145, PC-3) (Chiu and Lin 2008)	Arrested cell cycle (do Lim et al. 2007)
	Green pepper perilla leaf (Aggarwal and Shishodia 2006; do Lim et al. 2007)		Suppressed expression of NF-kappaB (Shi et al. 2004)

Lycopene	Tomato (Aggarwal and Shishodia 2006)	Breast cancer cells (MCF-7 and MDA-MB-231) (Wang and Zhang 2007a; Chalabi et al. 2006)	Induced apoptosis (Wang and Zhang 2007a; Chalabi et al. 2006; Palozza et al. 2010; Wang and Zhang 2007b)
			Down-regulation of bcl-2 (Wang and Zhang 2007b)
			Up-regulation of bax (Wang and Zhang 2007b)
		Colon cancer cells (HuCC) (Salman et al. 2007)	Inhibited cell growth (Wang and Zhang 2007a)
			Antiproliferative effect (Salman et al. 2007; Wang and Zhang 2007b)
		Prostate cancer cells (LNCaP, PC3) (Palozza et al. 2010; Wang and Zhang 2007b)	Arrested cell cycle progression (Wang and Zhang 2007a; Chalabi et al. 2006; Palozza et al. 2010; Wang and Zhang 2007b)
			Decreased cyclin D1 and phospho-AKT levels (Palozza et al. 2010)
			Increased p21, p27 and p53 levels (Palozza et al. 2010)
Silibinin (Silymarine)	Silybum marianum L. (Aggarwal and Shishodia 2006)	Breast cancer cells (MCF-7) (Wang et al. 2008)	Induced apoptosis (Wang et al. 2008; Agarwal et al. 2007)
			Up-regulation of FADD (Wang et al. 2008)
		Colon cancer cells (HT-29) (Agarwal et al. 2003)	Activated mitochondrial death pathway (Wang et al. 2008)
			Activation of caspase (Agarwal et al. 2007)
		Prostate cancer cells (DU145) (Agarwal et al. 2007)	Arrested cycle cell (Agarwal et al. 2003)
			Inhibited cell growth (Agarwal et al. 2003)

the need to investigate their mechanisms (Saunders and Wallace 2010; Han et al. 2007; Ramos 2007). Other polyphenols, their effects and the mechanisms by which they induce apoptosis in breast, colon and prostate cancer cell line are summarized in Table 8.4.

8.2 Conclusions and Future Directions

In this chapter, we summarized the findings of recent studies and the effects of resveratrol, quercetin and tannic acid on apoptosis in cancer cells. Experimental data obtained from recent studies have indicated that polyphenols have antiproliferative effects through different mechanisms, including inhibition of cell signaling and survival pathways in addition to their effects on different apoptotic pathways. However, the exact mechanisms by which these compounds exert their effects have not been well understood. Considering their beneficial effects in prevention of cancer or as novel potential therapeutic agents more research are needed to determine their mechanism of action in normal and cancer cells. Furthermore, more in vivo studies are also required to evaluate the efficacy of these polyphenols alone and in combination with standard therapies in various human tumor models. It is also critical to elucidate mechanisms of induction of apoptosis and antiproliferative effects as well as determining the in vivo effective doses and administration schedules of these compound for using them as potential chemopreventive and novel potential anticancer agents.

References

Aalinkeel R, Bindukumar B, Reynolds JL, Sykes DE, Mahajan SD et al (2008) The dietary bioflavonoid, quercetin, selectively induces apoptosis of prostate cancer cells by down-regulating the expression of heat shock protein 90. Prostate 68(16):1773–1789

Adhami VM, Khan N, Mukhtar H (2009) Cancer chemoprevention by pomegranate: laboratory and clinical evidence. Nutr Cancer 61(6):811–815

Afaq F, Zaman N, Khan N, Syed DN, Sarfaraz S et al (2008) Inhibition of epidermal growth factor receptor signaling pathway by delphinidin, an anthocyanidin in pigmented fruits and vegetables. Int J Cancer 123(7):1508–1515

Agarwal C, Singh RP, Dhanalakshmi S, Tyagi AK, Tecklenburg M et al (2003) Silibinin upregulates the expression of cyclin-dependent kinase inhibitors and causes cell cycle arrest and apoptosis in human colon carcinoma HT-29 cells. Oncogene 22(51):8271–8282

Agarwal C, Tyagi A, Kaur M, Agarwal R (2007) Silibinin inhibits constitutive activation of Stat3, and causes caspase activation and apoptotic death of human prostate carcinoma DU145 cells. Carcinogenesis 28(7):1463–1470

Aggarwal BB, Shishodia S (2006) Molecular targets of dietary agents for prevention and therapy of cancer. Biochem Pharmacol 14;71(10):1397–1421

Aherne SA, O'Brien NM (2002) Dietary flavonols: chemistry, food content, and metabolism. Nutrition 18:75–81

Alkhalaf M (2007) Resveratrol-induced apoptosis is associated with activation of p53 and inhibition of protein translation in T47D human breast cancer cells. Pharmacology 80(2–3):134–143

Alkhalaf M, El-Mowafy A, Renno W, Rachid O, Ali A et al (2008) Resveratrol-induced apoptosis in human breast cancer cells is mediated primarily through the caspase-3-dependent pathway. Arch Med Res 39(2):162–168

Azız MH, Kumar R, Ahmad N (2003) Cancer chemoprevention by resveratrol: in vitro and in vivo studies and the underlying mechanisms. Int J Oncol 23:17–28

Aziz MH, Nihal M, Fu VX, Jarrard DF, Ahmad N (2006) Resveratrol caused apoptosis of human prostate carcinoma LNCaP cells is mediated via modulation of phosphatidylinositol 3′-kinase/Akt pathway and Bcl-2 family proteins. Mol Cancer Ther 5:1335–1341

Bawadi HA, Bansode RR, Trappey A 2nd, Truax RE, Losso JN (2005) Inhibition of Caco-2 colon, MCF-7 and Hs578T breast, and DU 145 prostatic cancer cell proliferation by water-soluble black bean condensed tannins. Cancer Lett 218(2):153–162

Benitez DA, Pozo-Guisado E, Alvarez-Barrientos A, Fernandez-Salguero PM, Castellon EA (2007a) Mechanisms involved in resveratrol-induced apoptosis and cell cycle arrest in prostate cancer–derived cell lines. J Androl 28(2):282–293

Benitez DA, Pozo-Guisado E, Clementi M, Castello'n E, Fernandez-Salguero PM (2007b) Non-genomic action of resveratrol on androgen and oestrogen receptors in prostate cancer: modulation of the phosphoinositide 3-kinase pathway. Br J Cancer 96:1595–1604

Benitez DA, Hermoso MA, Pozo-Guisado E, Fernández-Salguero PM, Castellón EA (2009) Regulation of cell survival by resveratrol involves inhibition of NFκB-regulated gene expression in prostate cancer cells. Prostate 69:1045–1054

Bin Hafeez B, Asim M, Siddiqui IA, Adhami VM, Murtaza I et al (2008) Delphinidin, a dietary anthocyanidin in pigmented fruits and vegetables: a new weapon to blunt prostate cancer growth. Cell Cycle 7(21):3320–3326

Bischoff SC (2008) Quercetin: potentials in the prevention and therapy of disease. Curr Opin Clin Nutr Metab Care 11:733–740

Bradshaw R, Edward Dennis E (2003) Apoptosis signaling: a means to an End. Handb Cell Signal 3(331):431–439

Burlacu A (2003) Regulation of apoptosis by Bcl-2 family proteins. J Cell Mol Med 7(3):249–257

Busch C, Jacob C, Anwar A, Burkholz T, Aicha L Ba, Cerella C, Diederich M, Brandt W, Wessjohann L, Montenarh M (2010) Diallylpolysulfides induce growth arrest and apoptosis. Int J Oncol 36(3):743–749

Cardile V, Scifo C, Russo A, Falsaperla M, Morgia G et al (2003) Involvement of HSP70 in resveratrol-induced apoptosis of human prostate cancer. Anticancer Res 23(6C):4921–4926

Castillo-Pichardo L, Martínez-Montemayor MM, Martínez JE, Wall KM, Cubano LA et al (2009) Inhibition of mammary tumor growth and metastases to bone and liver by dietary grape polyphenols. Clin Exp Metastasis 26(6):505–516

Chalabi N, Delort L, Le Corre L, Satih S, Bignon YJ et al (2006) Gene signature of breast cancer cell lines treated with lycopene. Pharmacogenomics 7(5):663–672

Chen X, Beutler JA, McCloud TG, Loehfelm A, Yang L et al (2003) Tannic acid is an inhibitor of CXCL12 (SDF-1α)/CXCR4 with antiangiogenic activity. Clin Cancer Res 9:3115–3123

Chen KS, Hsiao YC, Kuo DY, Chou MC, Chu SC et al (2009) Tannic acid-induced apoptosis and-enhanced sensitivity to arsenic trioxide in human leukemia HL-60 cells. Leuk Res 33(2):297–307

Chien SY, Wu YC, Chung JG, Yang JS, Lu HF et al (2009) Quercetin-induced apoptosis acts through mitochondrial- and caspase-3-dependent pathways in human breast cancer MDA-MB-231 cells. Hum Exp Toxicol 28(8):493–503

Chiu FL, Lin JK (2008) Downregulation of androgen receptor expression by luteolin causes inhibition of cell proliferation and induction of apoptosis in human prostate cancer cells and xenografts. Prostate 68(1):61–71

Chiu TL, Su CC (2009) Curcumin inhibits proliferation and migration by increasing the Bax to Bcl-2 ratio and decreasing NF-kappaBp65 expression in breast cancer MDA-MB-231 cells. Int J Mol Med 23(4):469–475

Choi EJ, Kim GH (2008) Daidzein causes cell cycle arrest at the G1 and G2/M phases in human breast cancer MCF-7 and MDA-MB-453 cells. Phytomedicine 15(9):683–690

Choi EJ, Kim GH (2009a) Apigenin Induces Apoptosis through a Mitochondria/Caspase-Pathway in Human Breast Cancer MDA-MB-453 Cells. J Clin Biochem Nutr 44(3):260–265

Choi EJ, Kim GH (2009b) Apigenin causes G(2)/M arrest associated with the modulation of p21(Cip1) and Cdc2 and activates p53-dependent apoptosis pathway in human breast cancer SK-BR-3 cells. J Nutr Biochem 20(4):285–290

Choi JA, Kim JY, Lee JY, Kang CM, Kwon HJ et al (2001) Induction of cell cycle arrest and apoptosis in human breast cancer cells by quercetin. Int J Oncol 19(4):837–844

Choi EJ, Bae SM, Ahn WS (2008) Antiproliferative effects of quercetin through cell cycle arrest and apoptosis in human breast cancer MDA-MB-453 cells. Arch Pharm Res 31(10):1281–1285

Chou CC, Wu YC, Wang YF, Chou MJ, Kuo SJ et al (2009) Capsaicin-induced apoptosis in human breast cancer MCF-7 cells through caspase-independent pathway. Oncol Rep 21(3):665–671

Chou CC, Yang JS, Lu HF, Ip SW, Lo C et al (2010) Quercetin-mediated cell cycle arrest and apoptosis involving activation of a caspase cascade through the mitochondrial pathway in human breast cancer MCF-7 cells. Arch Pharm Res 33(8):1181–1191

Chung KT, Wong TY, Wei CI, Huang YW, Lin Y (1998) Tannins and human health: a review. Crit Rev Food Sci Nutr 38(6):421–464

Chung CS, Jiang Y, Cheng D, Birt DF (2007) Impact of adenomatous polyposis coli (APC) tumor suppressor gene in human colon cancer cell lines on cell cycle arrest by apigenin. Mol Carcinog 46(9):773–782

Clement MV, Hirpara JL, Chawdhury SH, Pervaiz S (1998) Chemopreventive agent resveratrol, a natural product derived from grapes, triggers CD95 signaling-dependent apoptosis in human tumor cells. Blood 92:996–1002

Coqueret O (2003) New roles for p21 and p27 cell-cycle inhibitors: a function for each cell compartment? Trends Cell Biol 13:65–70

Corre LL, Chalabi N, Delort L, Bingon YJ, Bernard-Gallon DJ (2005) Resveratrol and breast cancer chemoprevention: molecular mechanisms. Mol Nutr Food Res 49:462–471

Cosan D, Soyocak A, Basaran A, Degirmenci I, Gunes HV (2009) The effects of resveratrol and tannic acid on apoptosis in colon adenocarcinoma cell line. Saudi Med J 30(2):191–195

Cosan DT, Bayram B, Soyocak A, Basaran A, Gunes HV et al (2010) Role of phenolic compounds in nitric oxide synthase activity in colon and breast adenocarcinoma. Cancer Biother Radiopharm 25(5):577–580

D'Archivio M, Santangelo C, Scazzocchio B, Varì R, Filesi C, Masella R, Giovannini C (2008) Modulatory effects of polyphenols on apoptosis induction: relevance for cancer prevention. Int J Mol Sci 2(9):213–228

Dai Z, Nair V, Khan M, Ciolino HP (2010) Pomegranate extract inhibits the proliferation and viability of MMTV-Wnt-1 mouse mammary cancer stem cells in vitro. Oncol Rep 24(4):1087–1091

Debatin K-M (2004) Apoptosis pathways in cancer and cancer therapy. Cancer Immunol Immunother 53:153–159

Delmas D, Rébé C, Lacour S, Filomenko R, Athias A et al (2003) Resveratrol-induced apoptosis is associated with Fas redistribution in the rafts and the formation of a death-inducing signaling complex in colon cancer cells. J Biol Chem 278(42):41482–41490

Devi MA, Das NP (1993) In vitro effects of natural plant polyphenols on the proliferation of normal and abnormal human lymphocytes and their secretions of interleukin-2. Cancer Lett 69:191–196

do Lim Y, Jeong Y, Tyner AL, Park JH (2007) Induction of cell cycle arrest and apoptosis in HT-29 human colon cancer cells by the dietary compound luteolin. Am J Physiol Gastrointest Liver Physiol 292(1):G66–G75

Duvoix A, Blasius R, Delhalle S, Schnekenburger M, Morceau F et al (2005) Chemopreventive and therapeutic effects of curcumin. Cancer Lett 223(2):181–190

Fan G, Steer CJ (1999) The role of retinoblastoma protein in apoptosis. Apoptosis 4:21–29

Fan YZ, Li GH, Wang YH, Ren QY, Shi HJ (2010) Effects of genistein on colon cancer cells in vitro and in vivo and its mechanism of action. Zhonghua Zhong Liu Za Zhi 32(1):4–9

Ferenc P, Solár P, Kleban J, Mikes J, Fedorocko P (2010) Down-regulation of Bcl-2 and Akt induced by combination of photoactivated hypericin and genistein in human breast cancer cells. J Photochem Photobiol B 98(1):25–34

Filomeni G, Graziani I, Rotilio G, Ciriolo MR (2007) Trans-resveratrol induces apoptosis in human breast cancer cells MCF-7 by the activation of MAP kinases pathways. Genes Nutr 2:295–305
Gartel AL, Tyner AL (2002) The role of the cyclin-dependent kinase inhibitor p21 in apoptosis. Mol Cancer Ther 1:639–649
Guo JM, Xiao BX, Liu DH, Grant M, Zhang S et al (2004) Biphasic effect of daidzein on cell growth of human colon cancer cells. Food Chem Toxicol 42(10):1641–1646
Gusman J, Malonne H, Atassi G (2001) A reappraisal of the potential chemopreventive and chemotherapeutic properties of resveratrol. Carcinogenesis 22(8):1111–1117
Hafeez BB, Siddiqui IA, Asim M, Malik A, Afaq F et al (2008) A dietary anthocyanidin delphinidin induces apoptosis of human prostate cancer PC3 cells in vitro and in vivo: involvement of nuclear factor-kappaB signaling. Cancer Res 68(20):8564–8572
Hakimuddin F, Paliyath G, Meckling K (2004) Selective cytotoxicity of a red grape wine flavonoid fraction against MCF-7 cells. Breast Cancer Res Treat 85(1):65–79
Han X, Shen T, Lou H (2007) Dietary polyphenols and their biological significance. Int J Mol Sci 8(9):950–988
Hastak K, Agarwal MK, Mukhtar H, Agarwal ML (2005) Ablation of either p21 or Bax prevents p53-dependent apoptosis induced by green tea polyphenol epigallocatechin-3-gallate. FASEB J 19(7):789–791
Hatipoglu A, Basaran A, Dikmen M, Turgut Cosan D, Degirmenci I et al (2010) Evaluation of effects of quercetin (3,3′,4′,5,7-pentohidroxyflavon) on apoptosis and telomerase enzyme activity in MCF-7 and NIH-3 T3 cell lines to compared with tamoxifen. Balkan Med J. doi:10.5174/tutfd.2010.03372.3
Hilchie AL, Furlong SJ, Sutton K, Richardson A, Robichaud MR et al (2010) Curcumin-induced apoptosis in PC3 prostate carcinoma cells is caspase-independent and involves cellular ceramide accumulation and damage to mitochondria. Nutr Cancer 62(3):379–389
Holdenrieder S, Stieber P (2004) Apoptotic markers in cancer. Clin Biochem 37(7):605–617
Hope C, Planutis K, Planutiene M, Moyer MP, Johal KS et al (2008) Low concentrations of resveratrol inhibit Wnt signal throughput in colon-derived cells: implications for colon cancer prevention. Mol Nutr Food Res 52(1):S52–S61
Hsieh TC (2009) Antiproliferative effects of resveratrol and the mediating role of resveratrol targeting protein NQO2 in androgen receptor-positive, hormone-non-responsive CWR22Rv1 cells. Anticancer Res 29(8):3011–3017
Hsieh TC, Wu JM (1999) Differential effects on growth, cell cycle arrest, and induction of apoptosis by resveratrol in human prostate cancer cell lines. Exp Cell Res 249:109–115
Hsu A, Bray TM, Helferich WG, Doerge DR, Ho E (2010) Differential effects of whole soy extract and soy isoflavones on apoptosis in prostate cancer cells. Exp Biol Med (Maywood) 235(1):90–97
Huang WU, Cai ZY, Zhang J (2010) Natural phenolic compounds from medicinal herbs and dietary plants: potential use for cancer prevention. Nutr Cancer 62(1):1–20
Hwang JT, Ha J, Park IJ, Lee SK, Baik HW et al (2007) Apoptotic effect of EGCG in HT-29 colon cancer cells via AMPK signal pathway. Cancer Lett 247(1):115–121
Ignatowicz E, Baer-Dubowska W (2001) Resveratrol, a natural chemopreventive agent against degenerative diseases. Pol J Pharmacol 53:557–569
Jeong JH, An JY, Kwon YT, Rhee JG, Lee YJ (2009) Effects of low dose quercetin: cancer cell-specific inhibition of cell cycle progression. J Cell Biochem 106(1):73–82
Jin S, Zhang QY, Kang XM, Wang JX, Zhao WH (2010) Daidzein induces MCF-7 breast cancer cell apoptosis via the mitochondrial pathway. Ann Oncol 21(2):263–268
Joe AK, Liu H, Suzui M, Vural ME, Xiao D et al (2002) Resveratrol induces growth inhibition, S-phase arrest, apoptosis, and changes in biomarker expression in several human cancer cell lines. Clin Cancer Res 8(3):893–903
Juan ME, Wenzel U, Daniel H, Planas JM (2008) Resveratrol induces apoptosis through ROS-dependent mitochondria pathway in HT-29 human colorectal carcinoma cells J. Agric Food Chem 56:4813–4818
Jung YH, Heo J, Lee YJ, Kwon TK, Kim YH (2010) Quercetin enhances TRAIL-induced apoptosis in prostate cancer cells via increased protein stability of death receptor 5. Life Sci 86(9–10):351–357

Kaur P, Shukla S, Gupta S (2008) Plant flavonoid apigenin inactivates Akt to trigger apoptosis in human prostate cancer: an in vitro and in vivo study. Carcinogenesis 29(11):2210–2217
Khan NS, Hadi SM (1998) Structural features of tannic acid important for DNA degradation in the presence of Cu(II). Mutagenesis 13(3):271–274
Khan NS, Ahmad A, Hadi SM (2000) Anti-oxidant, pro-oxidant properties of tannic acid and its binding to DNA. Chem Biol Interact 125(3):177–189
Kim YH, Lee YJ (2007) TRAIL apoptosis is enhanced by quercetin through Akt dephosphorylation. J Cell Biochem 100(4):998–1009
Kim YA, Choi BT, Lee YT, Park DI et al (2004) Resveratrol inhibits cell proliferation and induces apoptosis of human breast carcinoma MCF-7 cells. Oncol Rep 11:441–446
Kim WK, Bang MH, Kim ES, Kang NE, Jung KC et al (2005) Quercetin decreases the expression of ErbB2 and ErbB3 proteins in HT-29 human colon cancer cells. J Nutr Biochem 16(3):155–162
Kim YM, Hwang JT, Kwak DW, Lee YK, Park OJ (2007) Involvement of AMPK signaling cascade in capsaicin-induced apoptosis of HT-29 colon cancer cells. Ann N Y Acad Sci 1095:496–503
Kim YH, Lee DH, Jeong JH, Guo ZS, Lee YJ (2008) Quercetin augments TRAIL-induced apoptotic death: involvement of the ERK signal transduction pathway. Biochem Pharmacol 75(10): 1946–1958
Kim MY, Trudel LJ, Wogan GN (2009) Apoptosis induced by capsaicin and resveratrol in colon carcinoma cells requires nitric oxide production and caspase activation. Anticancer Res 29:3733–3740
Kim HJ, Kim SK, Kim BS, Lee SH, Park YS et al (2010) Apoptotic effect of quercetin on HT-29 colon cancer cells via the AMPK signaling pathway. J Agric Food Chem 58(15):8643–8650
Kotha A, Sekharam M, Cilenti L, Siddiquee K, Khaled A et al (2006) Resveratrol inhibits Src and Stat3 signaling and induces the apoptosis of malignant cells containing activated Stat3 protein. Mol Cancer Ther 5(3):621–629
Kralova J, Dvorak M, Koc M, Kral V (2008) p38 MAPK plays an essential role in apoptosis induced by photoactivation of a novel ethylene glycol porphyrin derivative. Oncogene 27:3010–3050
Lee SC, Chan J, Clement MV, Pervaiz S (2006) Functional proteomics of resveratrol-induced colon cancer cell apoptosis: caspase-6-mediated cleavage of lamin A is a major signaling loop. Proteomics 6:2386–2394
Lee DH, Szczepanski M, Lee YJ (2008) Role of Bax in quercetin-induced apoptosis in human prostate cancer cells. Biochem Pharmacol 75(12):2345–2355
Lee SC, Chan JY, Pervaiz S (2009a) Spontaneous and 5-fluorouracil-induced centrosome amplification lowers the threshold to resveratrol-evoked apoptosis in colon cancer cells. Cancer Lett 288(1):36–41
Lee YK, Park SY, Kim YM, Lee WS, Park OJ (2009b) AMP kinase/cyclooxygenase-2 pathway regulates proliferation and apoptosis of cancer cells treated with quercetin. Exp Mol Med 41(3):201–207
Lee YK, Park SY, Kim YM, Park OJ (2009c) Regulatory effect of the AMPK-COX-2 signaling pathway in curcumin-induced apoptosis in HT-29 colon cancer cells. Ann N Y Acad Sci 1171:489–494
Li Y, Liu J, Liu X, Xing K, Wang Y et al (2006) Resveratrol-induced cell inhibition of growth and apoptosis in MCF7 human breast cancer cells are associated with modulation of phosphorylated Akt and caspase-9. Appl Biochem Biotechnol 135:181–192
Li Z, Li J, Mo B, Hu C, Liu H et al (2008) Genistein induces cell apoptosis in MDA-MB-231 breast cancer cells via the mitogen-activated protein kinase pathway. Toxicol In Vitro 22(7):1749–1753
Liu Q, Loo WT, Sze SC, Tong Y (2009) Curcumin inhibits cell proliferation of MDA-MB-231 and BT-483 breast cancer cells mediated by down-regulation of NFkappaB, cyclinD and MMP-1 transcription. Phytomedicine 16(10):916–922
Lorenzo HK, Susin SA (2004) Mitochondrial effectors in caspase-independent cell death. FEBS Lett 557:14–20
Los M, Walczak H (2002) Caspases-their role in cell death and cell survival, Molecular biology intelligence, Unit 24. Kluwer Academic Press, Georgetown, pp 155–174, 221–235

Losso JN, Bansode RR, Trappey A 2nd, Bawadi HA, Truax R (2004) In vitro anti-proliferative activities of ellagic acid. J Nutr Biochem 15(11):672–678

Lu QJ, Yu ZL (2005) Effects of genistein on proliferation and apoptosis in HT-29 cells. Wei Sheng Yan Jiu 34(5):571–573

Mahyar-Roemer M, Katsen A, Mestres P, Roemer K (2001) Resveratrol induces colon tumor cell apoptosis independently of p53 and precede by epithelial differentiation, mitochondrial proliferation and membrane potential collapse. Int J Cancer 94:615–622

Mahyar-Roemer M, Kohler H, Roemer K (2002) Role of Bax in resveratrol-induced apoptosis of colorectal carcinoma cells. BMC Cancer 17:2–27

Marienfeld C, Tadlock L, Yamagiwa Y, Patel T (2003) Inhibition of cholangiocarcinoma growth by tannic acid. Hepatology 37:1097–1104

Mgbonyebi OP, Russo J, Russo IH (1998) Antiproliferative effect of synthetic resveratrol on human breast epithelial cells. Int J Oncol 12:865–869

Middleton E, Kandaswami C, Theoharides TC (2000) The effects of plant flavonoids on mammalian cells: implications for inflammation, heart disease, and cancer. Pharmacol Rev 52:673–751

Mohan J, Gandhi AA, Bhavya BC, Rashmi R, Karunagaran D et al (2006) Caspase-2 triggers Bax-Bak-dependent and -independent cell death in colon cancer cells treated with resveratrol. J Biol Chem 281(26):17599–17611

Nakagawa H, Kiyozuka Y, Uemura Y, Senzaki H, Shikata N et al (2001) Resveratrol inhibits human breast cancer cell growth and may mitigate the effect of linoleic acid, a potent breast cancer cell stimulator. J Cancer Res Clin Oncol 127:258–264

Nam S, Smith DM, Dou QP (2001) Tannic acid potently inhibits tumor cell proteasome activity, increases p27 and Bax expression, and induces G1 arrest and apoptosis. Cancer Epidemiol Biomarkers Prev 10:1083–1088

Narayanan BA, Narayanan NK, Re GG, Nixon DW (2003) Differential expression of genes induced by resveratrol in LNCaP cells: p53-mediated molecular targets. Int J Cancer 104:204–212

Naus PJ, Henson R, Bleeker G, Wehbe H, Meng F, Patel T (2007) Tannic acid synergizes the cytotoxicity of chemotherapeutic drugs in human cholangiocarcinoma by modulating drug efflux pathways. J Hepatol 46:222–229

Palozza P, Colangelo M, Simone R, Catalano A, Boninsegna A (2010) Lycopene induces cell growth inhibition by altering mevalonate pathway and Ras signaling in cancer cell lines. Carcinogenesis 31(10):1813–1821

Pan MH, Lin JH, Lin-Shiau SY, Lin JK (1999) Induction of apoptosis by penta-O-galloyl–D-glucose through activation of caspase-3 in human leukemia HL-60 cells. Eur J Pharmacol 381: 171–183

Perez-Vizcaino F, Duarte J, Jimenez R, Santos-Buelga C, Osuna A (2009) Antihypertensive effects of the flavonoid quercetin. Pharmacol Rep 61:67–75

Pervaiz S (2003) Resveratrol: from grapevines to mammalian biology. FASEB J 17:1975–1985

Pohland T, Wagner S, Mahyar-Roemer M, Roemer K (2006) Bax and Bak are the critical complementary effectors of colorectal cancer cell apoptosis by chemopreventive resveratrol. Anticancer Drugs 17:471–478

Pozo-Guisado E, Alvarez-Barrientos A, Mulero-Navarro S, Santiago-Josefat B, Fernandez-Salguero PM (2002) The antiproliferative activity of resveratrol results in apoptosis in MCF-7 but not in MDA-MB-231 human breast cancer cells: cell-specific alteration of the cell cycle. Biochem Pharmacol 64:1375–1386

Pozo-Guisado E, Merino JM, Mulero-Navarro S, Lorenzo-Benayas MJ, Centeno F et al (2005) Resveratrol-induced apoptosis in MCF-7 human breast cancer cells involves a caspase-independent mechanism with down-regulation of Bcl-2 and NF-κB. Int J Cancer 115:74–84

Psahoulia FH, Drosopoulos KG, Doubravska L, Andera L, Pintzas A (2007) Quercetin enhances TRAIL-mediated apoptosis in colon cancer cells by inducing the accumulation of death receptors in lipid rafts. Mol Cancer Ther 6(9):2591–2599

Ramanathan R, Tan CH, Das NP (1992) Cytotoxic effect of plant polyphenols and fat-soluble vitamins on malignant human cultured cells. Cancer Lett 62:217–224

Ramos S (2007) Effects of dietary flavonoids on apoptotic pathways related to cancer chemoprevention. J Nutr Biochem 18(7):427–442
Ramos S (2008) Cancer chemoprevention and chemotherapy: dietary polyphenols and signalling pathways. Mol Nutr Food Res 52:507–526
Reuter S, Eifes S, Dicato M, Aggarwal BB, Diederich M (2008) Modulation of anti-apoptotic and survival pathways by curcumin as a strategy to induce apoptosis in cancer cells. Biochem Pharmacol 76(11):1340–1351
Rodgers EH, Grant MH (1998) The effect of the flavonoids, quercetin, myricetin and epicatechin on the growth and enzyme activities of MCF7 human breast cancer cells. Chem Biol Interact 116(3):213–228
Romero I, Paez A, Ferruelo A, Lujan M, Berenguer A (2002) Polyphenols in red wine inhibit the proliferation and induce apoptosis of LNCaP cells. BJU Int 89:950–954
Sakagami H, Jiang Y, Kusama K, Atsumi T, Ueha T et al (2000) Cytotoxic activity of hydrolyzable tannins against human oral tumor cell lines - a possible mechanism. Phytomedicine 7:39–47
Sakamoto T, Horiguchi H, Oguma E, Kayama F (2010) Effects of diverse dietary phytoestrogens on cell growth, cell cycle and apoptosis in estrogen-receptor-positive breast cancer cells. J Nutr Biochem 21(9):856–864
Sala G, Minutolo F, Macchia M, Sacchi N, Ghidoni R (2003) Resveratrol structure and ceramide-associated growth inhibition in prostate cancer cells. Drugs Exp Clin Res 29(5–6):263–269
Salman H, Bergman M, Djaldetti M, Bessler H (2007) Lycopene affects proliferation and apoptosis of four malignant cell lines. Biomed Pharmacother 61(6):366–369
Sánchez AM, Malagarie-Cazenave S, Olea N, Vara D, Chiloeches A et al (2007) Apoptosis induced by capsaicin in prostate PC-3 cells involves ceramide accumulation, neutral sphingomyelinase, and JNK activation. Apoptosis 12(11):2013–2024
Sareen D, Darjatmoko SR, Albert DM, Polans AS (2007) Mitochondria, calcium, and calpain are key mediators of resveratrol-induced apoptosis in breast cancer. Mol Pharmacol 72(6):1466–1475
Saunders FR, Wallace HM (2010) On the natural chemoprevention of cancer. Plant Physiol Biochem 48(7):621–626
Scarlatti F, Sala G, Somenzi G, Signorelli P, Sacchi N et al (2003) Resveratrol induces growth inhibition and apoptosis in metastatic breast cancer cells via de novo ceramide signaling. FASEB J 17(15):2339–2341
Scarlatti F, Sala G, Ricci C, Maioli C, Milani F, et al. (2007) Resveratrol sensitization of DU145 prostate cancer cells to ionizing radiation is associated to ceramide increase. Cancer Lett 253(1): 124–130.
Schmitt E, Lehmann L, Metzler M, Stopper H (2002) Hormonal and genotoxic activity of resveratrol. Toxicol Lett 136(2):133–142
Schneider Y, Vincent F, Benoit D, Badolo L, Gosse F et al (2000) Anti-proliferative effect of resveratrol, a natural component of grapes and wine, on human colonic cancer cells. Cancer Lett 158:85–91
Seeram NP, Adams LS, Henning SM, Niu Y, Zhang Y et al (2005) In vitro antiproliferative, apoptotic and antioxidant activities of punicalagin, ellagic acid and a total pomegranate tannin extract are enhanced in combination with other polyphenols as found in pomegranate juice. J Nutr Biochem 16(6):360–367
Senthilkumar K, Elumalai P, Arunkumar R, Banudevi S, Gunadharini ND (2010) Quercetin regulates insulin like growth factor signaling and induces intrinsic and extrinsic pathway mediated apoptosis in androgen independent prostate cancer cells (PC-3). Mol Cell Biochem 344(1-2):173–184
Shan BE, Wang MX, Li RQ (2009) Quercetin inhibit human SW480 colon cancer growth in association with inhibition of cyclin D1 and survivin expression through Wnt/beta-catenin signaling pathway. Cancer Invest 27(6):604–612
Shankar S, Siddiqui I, Srivastava RK (2007a) Molecular mechanisms of resveratrol (3,4,5-trihydroxy-transstilbene) and its interaction with TNF-related apoptosis inducing ligand (TRAIL) in androgen-insensitive prostate cancer cells. Mol Cell Biochem 304:273–285
Shankar S, Chen Q, Siddiqui I, Sarva K, Srivastava RK (2007b) Sensitization of TRAIL-resistant LNCaP cells by resveratrol (3, 4′, 5 tri-hydroxystilbene): molecular mechanisms and therapeutic potential. J Mol Signal 2:7

Shankar S, Chen Q, Sarva K, Siddiqui I, Srivastava RK (2007c) Curcumin enhances the apoptosis-inducing potential of TRAIL in prostate cancer cells: molecular mechanisms of apoptosis, migration and angiogenesis. J Mol Signal 2:10

Shi RX, Ong CN, Shen HM (2004) Luteolin sensitizes tumor necrosis factor-alpha-induced apoptosis in human tumor cells. Oncogene 23(46):7712–7721

Shukla S, Gupta S (2008) Apigenin-induced prostate cancer cell death is initiated by reactive oxygen species and p53 activation. Free Radic Biol Med 44(10):1833–1845

Sprick MR, Walczak H (2004) The interplay between the Bcl-2 family and death receptor-mediated apoptosis. Biochim Biophys Acta 1644:125–132

Srivastava RC, Husain MM, Hasan SK, Athar M (2000) Green tea polyphenols and tannic acid act as potent inhibitors of phorbol ester-induced nitric oxide generation in rat hepatocytes independent of their antioxidant properties. Cancer Lett 153(1–2):1–5

Srivastava RK, Chen Q, Siddiqui I, Sarva K, Shankar S (2007) Linkage of curcumin-induced cell cycle arrest and apoptosis by cyclin-dependent kinase inhibitor p21(/WAF1/CIP1). Cell Cycle 6(23):2953–2961

Szendel B, Tyihák E, Király-Véghely Z (2000) Dose-dependent effect of resveratrol on proliferation and apoptosis in endothelial and tumor cell cultures. Exp Mol Med 32(2):88–92

Taffetani S, Ueno Y, Meng F, Venter J, Francis H et al (2005) Tannic acid inhibits cholangiocyte proliferation after bile duct ligation via a cyclic adenosine 5′,3′- monophosphate-dependent pathway. Am J Pathol 166(6):1671–1679

Tang Y, Zhao DY, Elliott S, Zhao W, Curiel TJ et al (2007) Epigallocatechin-3 gallate induces growth inhibition and apoptosis in human breast cancer cells through survivin suppression. Int J Oncol 31(4):705–711

Tang SN, Singh C, Nall D, Meeker D, Shankar S et al (2010) The dietary bioflavonoid quercetin synergizes with epigallocathechin gallate (EGCG) to inhibit prostate cancer stem cell characteristics, invasion, migration and epithelial-mesenchymal transition. J Mol Signal 18(5):14

Teiten MH, Gaascht F, Eifes S, Dicato M, Diederich M (2010) Chemopreventive potential of curcumin in prostate cancer. Genes Nutr 5(1):61–74

Thakur VS, Ruhul Amin AR, Paul RK, Gupta K, Hastak K et al (2010) p53-Dependent p21-mediated growth arrest pre-empts and protects HCT116 cells from PUMA-mediated apoptosis induced by EGCG. Cancer Lett 296(2):225–232

Thangapazham RL, Passi N, Maheshwari RK (2007) Green tea polyphenol and epigallocatechin gallate induce apoptosis and inhibit invasion in human breast cancer cells. Cancer Biol Ther 6(12):1938–1943

Thoennissen NH, O'Kelly J, Lu D, Iwanski GB, La DT et al (2010) Capsaicin causes cell-cycle arrest and apoptosis in ER-positive and -negative breast cancer cells by modulating the EGFR/HER-2 pathway. Oncogene 29(2):285–296

Tophkhane C, Yang S, Bales W, Archer L, Osunkoya A et al (2007) Bcl-2 overexpression sensitizes MCF-7 cells to genistein by multiple mechanisms. Int J Oncol 31(4):867–874

Trincheri NF, Nicotra G, Follo C, Castino R, Isidoro C (2007) Resveratrol induces cell death in colorectal cancer cells by a novel pathway involving lysosomal cathepsin D. Carcinogenesis 28(5):922–931

Twomey C, McCarthy JV (2005) Pathways of apoptosis and importance in development. J Cell Mol Med 9(2):345–359

Uchiumi F, Sato T, Tanuma S (1998) Identification and characterization of a tannic acid-responsive negative regulatory element in the mouse mammary tumor virus promoter. J Biol Chem 273:12499–12508

Van Erk MJ, Roepman P, van der Lende TR, Stierum RH, Aarts JM et al (2004) Integrated assessment by multiple gene expression analysis of quercetin bioactivity on anticancer-related mechanisms in colon cancer cells in vitro. Eur J Nutr 44(3):143–156

Van Erk MJ, Roepman P, van der Lende TR, Stierum RH, Aarts JM, et al (2005) Integrated assessment by multiple gene expression analysis of quercetin bioactivity on anticancer-related mechanisms in colon cancer in vitro. Eur J Nutr 44(3):143–156.

Vijayababu MR, Kanagaraj P, Arunkumar A, Ilangovan R, Aruldhas MM, Arunakaran J (2005) Quercetin-induced growth inhibition and cell death in prostatic carcinoma cells (PC-3) are associated with increase in p21 and hypophosphorylated retinoblastoma proteins expression. J Cancer Res Clin Oncol 131(11):765–771

Vijayababu MR, Arunkumar A, Kanagaraj P, Arunakaran J (2006a) Effects of quercetin on insulin-like growth factors (IGFs) and their binding protein-3 (IGFBP-3) secretion and induction of apoptosis in human prostate cancer cells. J Carcinog 6:5–10

Vijayababu MR, Kanagaraj P, Arunkumar A, Ilangovan R, Dharmarajan et al (2006b) Quercetin induces p53-independent apoptosis in human prostate cancer cells by modulating Bcl-2-related proteins: a possible mediation by IGFBP-3. Oncol Res 16(2):67–74

Wang AH, Zhang LS (2007a) Effect of lycopene on the proliferation of MCF-7 and MDA-MB-231 cells. Sichuan Da Xue Xue Bao Yi Xue Ban 38(6):958–960, 976

Wang A, Zhang L (2007b) Effect of lycopene on proliferation and cell cycle of hormone refractory prostate cancer PC-3 cell line. Wei Sheng Yan Jiu 36(5):575–578

Wang CC, Chen LG, Yang LL (2000) Cuphiin D1, the macrocyclic hydrolyzable tannin induced apoptosis in HL- 60 cell line. Cancer Lett 149:77–83

Wang HJ, Tashiro S, Onodera S, Ikejima T (2008) Inhibition of insulin-like growth factor 1 receptor signaling enhanced silibinin-induced activation of death receptor and mitochondrial apoptotic pathways in human breast cancer MCF-7 cells. J Pharmacol Sci 107(3):260–269

Wang Y-Z, Cao B, Li S-X, Zang Z-H, Zhang J-Z et al (2009a) Effect of proliferation, cell cycle, and Bcl-2s of MCF-7 cells by resveratrol. J Asian Nat Prod Res 11(4):380–390

Wang BF, Wang JS, Lu JF, Kao TH, Chen BH (2009b) Antiproliferation effect and mechanism of prostate cancer cell lines as affected by isoflavones from soybean cake. J Agric Food Chem 57(6):2221–2232

Watson JL, Hill R, Lee PW, Giacomantonio CA, Hoskin DW (2008) Curcumin induces apoptosis in HCT-116 human colon cancer cells in a p21-independent manner. Exp Mol Pathol 84(3):230–233

Wenzel U, Herzog A, Kuntz S, Daniel H (2004) Protein expression profiling identifies molecular targets of quercetin as a major dietary flavonoid in human colon cancer cells. Proteomics 4(7):2160–2174

Wolter F, Akoglu B, Clausnitzer A, Stein J (2001) Down-regulation of the cyclin D1/Cdk4 complex occurs during resveratrol-induced cell cycle arrest in colon cancer cell lines. J Nutr 131(8):2197–2203

Xavier CP, Lima CF, Preto A, Seruca R, Fernandes-Ferreira M et al (2009) Luteolin, quercetin and ursolic acid are potent inhibitors of proliferation and inducers of apoptosis in both KRAS and BRAF mutated human colorectal cancer cells. Cancer Lett 281(2):162–170

Yang QH, Church-Hajduk R, Ren J, Newton ML, Du C (2003) Omi/HtrA2 catalytic cleavage of inhibitor of apoptosis (IAP) irreversibly inactivates IAPs and facilitates caspase activity in apoptosis. Genes Dev 17(12):1487–1496

Yang KM, Pyo JO, Kim GY, Yu R, Han IS et al (2009) Capsaicin induces apoptosis by generating reactive oxygen species and disrupting mitochondrial transmembrane potential in human colon cancer cell lines. Cell Mol Biol Lett 14(3):497–510

Yoshida H, Kong YY, Yoshida R, Elia AJ, Hakem A, Hakem R, Penninger JM, Mak TW (1998) Apaf1 is required for mitochondrial pathways of apoptosis and brain development. Cell 94(6):739–750

Yun JM, Afaq F, Khan N, Mukhtar H (2009) Delphinidin, an anthocyanidin in pigmented fruits and vegetables, induces apoptosis and cell cycle arrest in human colon cancer HCT116 cells. Mol Carcinog 48(3):260–270

Zhang X, Anderson J, Kaushik RS, Dwivedi C (2009) Effects of resveratrol, an important component of red wine, on intestinal cancer development. Int J Wine Res 1:147–153

Chapter 9
Encapsulation of Natural Polyphenols with Antioxidant Properties in Polyelectrolyte Capsules and Nanoparticles

Tatsiana G. Shutava and Yuri M. Lvov

Abstract The chapter summarizes approaches to encase natural polyphenols with previously demonstrated anti-cancer potential, curcumin, (-)-epigallocatechin gallate, tannic acid, theaflavin, thearubigin, curcumin, etc. in polyelectrolyte microcapsules and nano/microparticles in order to modulate their biological activity, bioavailability and stability as an alternative to usage of free compounds. Taking into account the matrix-encapsulate interaction, the emphasis is made to the techniques based on reversible complex electrostatic interaction and hydrogen bonding of polyphenols with polymeric matrixes, stability and properties of the obtained microstructures as delivery vehicles, characteristics of polyphenol loading, and factors affecting their release from the nanocapsules. The controversies in manifesting biological and antioxidant activity by polyphenols encased in the aforementioned structures are discussed.

Keywords Encapsulation • Polyphenol • Polyelectrolyte • Microcapsules • Nanoparticles • Bioavailability • Antioxidant activity • ABTS cation-radical • Layer-by-layer assembly • Thin films • Delivery vehicles

---

T.G. Shutava (✉)
Institute for Micromanufacturing and Biomedical Engineering Program,
Louisiana Tech University, Ruston, LA, USA

Institute of Chemistry of New Materials, National Academy of Sciences of Belarus,
Minsk, Belarus
e-mail: tshutava@latech.edu

Y.M. Lvov
Institute for Micromanufacturing and Biomedical Engineering Program,
Louisiana Tech University, Ruston, LA, USA
e-mail: ylvov@latech.edu

M. Diederich and K. Noworyta (eds.), *Natural Compounds as Inducers of Cell Death: Volume 1*, DOI 10.1007/978-94-007-4575-9_9,

9.1 Introduction

Nanoparticulated compositions of polyphenolic compounds originated from plants are of great interest due to benefits of their usage in food, nutraceutical and pharmaceutical industries and high health implication. High antioxidant, antibacterial, antiviral, and other activities have been proven for a wide range of plant extracts and polymeric tannins including their isolated individual compounds (procyanidin B, (−)-epigallocatechin gallate (EGCG), tannic acid (TA), theaflavin, thearubigin, etc.) (Haslam 1996; Manach et al. 2004; Williamson and Manach 2005; Quideau and Feldman 1996; Bennick 2002). Green tea polyphenol complex has been recently demonstrated to be effective cancer chemopreventive agents in animal studies, and can slow the progression of prostate cancer or lower biological activities of proteins promoting cancer progression (Adhami and Mukhtar 2007; Bettuzzi et al. 2006). Other polyphenols such as curcumin, luteolin, resveratrol, and several others are under intensive investigation as possible anticancer agents (Ruby et al. 1995; Surh 2003; Lambert and Yang 2003). A large body of preclinical research and epidemiological data supports the hypothesis that plant phytochemicals can act as chemopreventive and anti-cancer agents in humans. Unfortunately, concentrations that appear effective in blocking tumor cell proliferation or inducing apoptosis *in vitro* are often an order of magnitude higher than levels measured *in vivo* (Manach et al. 2004; Williamson and Manach 2005). Polyphenol-loaded nanoparticles and sustained release compositions are alternatives to free compounds, which can optimally maintain circulating levels of the substances in the body at a certain threshold level over an extended time period or at target sites in the body, overcome the defense mechanisms of the gut and the liver, increase potentially low bioavailability and short half-life of polyphenols, influence their stability and bioactivity (Ravi Kumar et al. 2004; Vinogradov 2006; Al-Tahami and Singh 2007; Mozafari 2006; Zhang et al. 2010; Torchilin 2007; Scheepens et al. 2010). However, widely varying structures of natural polyphenols, their moderate solubility, and fast oxidation under basic conditions (Haslam 1996; Manach et al. 2004; Williamson and Manach 2005; Quideau and Feldman 1996; Bennick 2002; Calderon et al. 1968; Gámiz-Gracia and Luque de Castro 1997; Osawa and Walsho 1993; Barik et al. 2003; Yi et al. 2006) create additional challenges for encapsulation including choice of appropriate matrix material and encapsulation techniques.

In the last decade, evidences on biological affects caused by polymeric and metallic, oxide ultrafine and nanoparticles, carbon nanotubes, polymer nanostructured films, nanocomposite and dendrite structures have became available. Such effects as biocompatibility and biodegradability of encapsulating materials, cytotoxicity, genotoxicity and oxidative stress caused by matrix itself, as well as various type influence of matrix material on biological systems, etc. are often the reasons of observed controversies in manifesting biological properties of encapsulates (Ravi Kumar et al. 2004; Vinogradov 2006; Al-Tahami and Singh 2007; Mozafari 2006; Zhang et al. 2010; Torchilin 2007; Scheepens et al. 2010; Kreyling et al. 2006; Warheit et al. 2008; Kabanov 2006).

Despite steadily increasing interest to micro and nanoparticulated compositions containing polyphenols, there are limited number of publications devoted to different techniques of polyphenol encapsulation and summarizing the progress in the area (Fang and Bhandari 2010; Huang et al. 2010).

Taking into account the matrix-encapsulate interaction, numerous experimental methods of polyphenol-encased system preparation can be divided into few major groups. Among them, (1) systems comprising of polymeric nanoparticulated carrier with the release of active ingredient triggered by matrix degradation or physical diffusion out the inert core, (2) microemulsions, liposomes, nanosomes, as well as solid lipid micro/nanoparticles, (3) systems based on environmentally sensitive coacervation/complexation between functionalized, proteinaceous or polysaccharide, template and active ingredient, and (4) solid poorly soluble core comprising of the polyphenol to be encapsulated coated with layer-by-layer (LbL) shell of biocompatible, biodegradable polyelectrolytes.

9.2 Polymeric Nanoparticulated Carrier/Polyphenol Systems

Loading a substance with pharmaceutical, nutraceutical, or cosmetic activity into an inert matrix seems to be the most general encapsulation technique, widely used and applicable to high number of polyphenols (Fang and Bhandari 2010; Huang et al. 2010; Henry 1996). The size and form of the resulted encapsulated material is typically driven by step-by-step preparation sequences suitable for a given matrix. Such techniques can be expended over different substances providing their sustained delivery in the media of interest and allowing for tuning their cancer chemopreventive and therapeutic properties (Ravi Kumar et al. 2004; Vinogradov 2006; Al-Tahami and Singh 2007; Mozafari 2006; Zhang et al. 2010; Torchilin 2007; Scheepens et al. 2010; Kreyling et al. 2006; Warheit et al. 2008; Kabanov 2006; Fang and Bhandari 2010; Huang et al. 2010). At the present time, only relatively small number of polymeric materials are approved for administration in the human body (Kabanov 2006). Several considered as safe synthetic polymers when combined with the biological agents (low molecular weight drugs, DNA, and antigens) can alter genetically controlled cellular responses to these agents (Scheepens et al. 2010; Kabanov 2006).

Curcumin seems to be the most promising natural substance with anticancerogenic activity, but its extremely low solubility in different solvents limits the application (Henry 1996). Water-dispersible polymeric nanoparticle encapsulated formulation of curcumin utilizing the micellar aggregates of cross-linked and random copolymers of N-isopropylacrylamide (NIPAAM) with N-vinyl-2-pyrrolidone and poly(ethylene glycol)monoacrylate with a narrow size distribution in the 50 nm range has been reported (Bisht et al. 2007). These nanoparticles demonstrate comparable to free curcumin *in vitro* therapeutic efficacy against a panel of human pancreatic cancer cell lines; the mechanisms of the nanoparticles action mirror that of free curcumin (Ruby et al. 1995). Polymeric nanoparticle encapsulated curcumin formulation shows remarkably higher systemic bioavailability in plasma and tissues compared with free curcumin upon parenteral administration (Bisht et al. 2010).

(−)-Epigallocatechin-3-gallate in polylactic acid-polyethylene glycol copolymer nanoparticles retains its biological effectiveness with over tenfold dose advantage for exerting its proapoptotic and angiogenesis inhibitory effects in both *in vitro* and *in vivo* systems (Siddiqui et al. 2009).

In another research (Shao et al. 2009a), resveratrol-loaded methoxy polyethylene glycol and poly(ε-caprolactone) (mPEG-PC) diblock copolymer based nanoparticles at lower concentrations led to significantly higher cell death as compared with equivalent doses of free resveratrol and this difference of cytotoxicity was not quenched by a strong antioxidant. The effect was associated with significantly higher intracellular reactive oxygen species (ROS) level induced by resveratrol-loaded nanoparticles, as compared to free resveratrol (Shao et al. 2009a), probably due to matrix material induced cytotoxicity (Vinogradov 2006; Al-Tahami and Singh 2007; Mozafari 2006; Zhang et al. 2010; Torchilin 2007; Scheepens et al. 2010; Kreyling et al. 2006; Warheit et al. 2008; Kabanov 2006).

Biocompatible, biodegradable, and relatively inert substances such as poly (lactide) (PLA) or poly(lactide-co-glycolide) (PLGA) microspheres containing active agents to be administered are commonly utilized as sustained-release devices (Chasin 1995; Tamber et al. 2005). The PLGA nanoparticles embedded with curcumin with a size less than 300 nm have been reported (Nam et al. 2007; Shahani et al. 2010; Cartiera et al. 2010).

According to (Mulik et al. 2010), when injected subcut in mice, a single dose of PLGA microparticles sustained curcumin levels in the blood and other tissues for nearly a month. Curcumin levels in the lungs and brain, frequent sites of breast cancer metastases, were up to 30-fold higher than that in the blood. Curcumin microparticles also showed marked anticancer efficacy in nude mice bearing MDA-MB-231 xenografts compared with other controls, while repeated systemic injections of curcumin are not effective in inhibiting tumor growth (Shahani et al. 2010). Photostability, antioxidant, and antiamyloidogenic activities of curcumin were enhanced by loading into poly(butyl)cyanoacrylate nanoparticles coated with apolipoprotein E3 as compared to plain curcumin solution suggesting enhanced cell uptake due to the specific protein surface layer and a sustained drug release effect (Mulik et al. 2010).

Coating of drug eluting stents (DES) with PLGA nanoparticles containing curcumin (Nam et al. 2007) or polyisobutylene-polystyrene polymer nanoparticles with resveratrol and quercetin (Kleinedler et al. 2009) as antiproliferative agents has been proposed. The coatings release polyphenols within a therapeutic range and provide an extended release profile to inhibit cascades responsible for restenosis and thrombosis to prevent restenosis after angioplasty and stenting (Kleinedler et al. 2009).

Polymers of natural origin are often used as encapsulating matrixes because their biodegradability and biocompatibility. Chitosan appears to be the most popular for preparation of particulated systems polymer matrix (Ravi Kumar et al. 2004), clinically validated as safe for systemic administration in the body (Kabanov 2006). Chitosan-based micro (Kumar et al. 2002; Sowasod et al. 2005; Bao et al. 2009; Liang et al. 2011; Zhang and Kosaraju 2007) and nanoparticles (Das et al. 2010) containing curcumin (Kumar et al. 2002; Sowasod et al. 2005; Das et al. 2010), catechin (Zhang and Kosaraju 2007), tea polyphenol complex (Bao et al. 2009) have been obtained by various methods. Among them, glutaraldehyde (Kumar et al. 2002; Sowasod et al. 2005) and sodium tripolyphosphate (Zhang and Kosaraju 2007) crosslinking techniques coupled with emulsion-solvent evaporation methods and ionic gelation method using carboxymethyl chitosan and chitosan hydrochloride (Liang et al. 2011). More complicated systems, for example, curcumin-containing nanoparticles with an average size of 100 nm prepared from three biocompatible polymers, alginate, chitosan, and pluronic (for increase of curcumin contents), by ionotropic pre-gelation followed by polycationic cross-linking have been described (Kleinedler et al. 2009). These nanoparticles are readily internalized by HeLa cells being nontoxic to them in small concentrations (Das et al. 2010).

The entrapment efficacy of chitosan-based particulated systems ranges between 10% and 87% depending on the preparation conditions and polyphenols used, while different physical methods indicate minor structural interactions between polyphenol and chitosan matrix (Kumar et al. 2002; Sowasod et al. 2005; Bao et al. 2009; Liang et al. 2011; Zhang and Kosaraju 2007). Chitosan-based formulations show a sustain release of encapsulated polyphenols in aqueous buffers (Liang et al. 2011), oils (Bao et al. 2009), and enzyme-free simulated gastric and intestinal fluids (Zhang and Kosaraju 2007). Being affected by matrix nature and degree of its crosslinking, the release profile frequently shows a complex biphasic behaviour with an initial burst of loaded compound followed by a long-time slow period (Kumar et al. 2002). Being incorporated in chitosan nanoparticles, polyphenols significantly retain their antioxidant (Bao et al. 2009), as well as antitumor and antiflammatory activities, as shown in cell models (Kumar et al. 2002; Liang et al. 2011; Das et al. 2010).

Other potentially useful applications of particulated polyphenol-containing materials include colorants for cosmetic application (Sowasod et al. 2005) and edible systems suitable for preventing oxidation of food products (Bao et al. 2009).

9.3 Lipid-Based Systems

Lipid-based systems (microemulsions, liposomes, micelles, nanosomes, solid lipid micro/nanoparticles) have been identified as potential delivery preparations for lipophilic agents due to their transparent or translucent appearance, long time stability, large solubility capacity and simplicity of preparation (Mozafari 2006; Zhang et al. 2010; Torchilin 2007; Huang et al. 2010). They are highly promising for poorly water-soluble polyphenols, such as curcumin and resveratrol. Several microemulsion systems containing the polyphenols were prepared using natural oils, such as peppermint oil alone or mixed with common edible oils (soybean, peanut or rapeseed oil), different surfactants, such as lecithin, monoolein or Tween 20, and aqueous solutions (water or 20% solution of NaCl, sucrose, or citric acid) without or with ethanol as cosurfactant (Abd-El-Galeel 2002). Based on the mixtures of ethyl oleate with Tween 80 and lecithin surfactants (Lin et al. 2003) or palmitic acid, stearic acid and soya lecithin, with an optimized percentage of poloxamer 188 (Yadav et al. 2009), solid lipid nanoparticles containing polyphenols have been reported.

Lower degradation of curcumin (Abd-El-Galeel 2002) and ascorbic acid (Gallarate et al. 1999) in lipid-based systems than that in aqueous solutions was observed.

Ultrasound can be successfully employed to control the release of curcumin entrapped in micelles (Lin et al. 2003). According to (Lin et al. 2003), the initial curcumin release rate from Tween 80/lecithin micelles is also affected by pH, being low at acidic pH and increasing in a PBS buffer. Among newly developed techniques of liposomal target delivery of pharmaceutics is gold nanoparticles-assisted optically guided release with tunable plasmonic nanobubbles (Anderson et al. 2010).

Application of lipid-based nanoparticle delivery systems drastically increases solubility, stability and bioavailability of polyphenols (Manach et al. 2004; Williamson and Manach 2005; Huang et al. 2010; Yadav et al. 2009; Oganesyan et al. 2001; Teskac and Kristl 2010; Anand et al. 2007) and allows to achieve a site-specific delivery approach (Yadav et al. 2009). After oral administration of unmodified resveratrol to mice, only 19% of the dose was taken up into the blood, while the use of nanosomal resveratrol formulations based on Eudragit®RL and lecithin/chitosan with a resveratrol contents of 15–20% in lyophilized powder increased bioavailability to 39% and 61% respectively (Oganesyan et al. 2001). Increases in the peak plasma resveratrol concentration by factors of 4–5 were also seen in mice given nanoparticles (Oganesyan et al. 2001). Lecithin liposome encapsulation of curcumin enhances its gastrointestinal absorption in rat models (Yadav et al. 2009; Oganesyan et al. 2001; Takahashi et al. 2009). Orally given liposomes produce higher plasma antioxidant activity, higher C_{max}, and shorter T_{max} values, as well as a higher value for the area under the blood concentration-time curve, at all time points, as compared with free curcumin and its physical mixture with lecithin (Takahashi et al. 2009).

Loading resveratrol into solid lipid nanoparticles, which preserve cell morphology, overcame light cytotoxicity observed for the free substance in solution (Teskac and Kristl 2010) and polymeric nanoparticles containing resveratrol (Shao et al. 2009a). Solid lipid nanoparticles containing resveratrol with a size below 180 nm moved promptly through the cell membrane, distributed throughout the cytosol, moved successively among different cellular levels and localize in the perinuclear region without inducing cytotoxicity. The cytostatic effect of solid lipid nanoparticles containing resveratrol was much more expressed than that of resveratrol in solution (Teskac and Kristl 2010).

Recent studies show that exosomes (50–100 nm vesicles secreted by cells), but not lipid alone, are required for the enhanced activity of polyphenols and selected anticancer drugs *in vivo* (Andre et al. 2004; Iero et al. 2008). Exosomes provide a means for target delivery of anti-inflammatory agents, such as curcumin, to activated myeloid cells that play vital roles in inflammation-related autoimmune/inflammatory diseases and cancers and overcome unwanted off-target, toxic effects (Sun et al. 2010). Therapeutic relevance of this technique has been validated in a lipopolysaccharide induced septic shock mouse model. Curcumin delivered by exosomes is more stable and highly concentrated in the blood. Curcumin has been shown to reduce exosome immunosuppressive functions when administered to breast carcinoma cells (Zhang et al. 2007). The proposed mechanism includes modification of ubiquitinated proteins that help modulate exosome protein composition and thus its biological activity (Andre et al. 2004; Zhang et al. 2007).

Surfactant/polyelectrolyte aggregates (Thunemann 2002; Rinaudo et al. 2008; Buchhammer et al. 2000) is one more perspective, but narrowly used drug delivery system for phenols (Baumgart et al. 2005; Bai et al. 2010; Lee et al. 1991).

9.4 Polyphenol Containing System Based on Complexation

The systems based on complexation between matrix substances of high molecular weight and polyphenols to be delivered are of great interest because a higher solubility enhancement, better control over target substance release profile can be achieved (Baglole et al. 2005; Lumsden et al. 2001; Kalogeropoulos et al. 2010; Todd and Paul 1991; Paradkar et al. 2004; Xu et al. 2006; Zhang et al. 2005; Schranz 1983; Petyaev 2008; Sneharani et al. 2010; Morre et al. 2002; Robert et al. 2010). These routes mimic the dietary intake of polyphenols as a part of everyday consumed meals (Manach et al. 2004) or designed functional food (Williamson and Manach 2005) along with polysaccharide and/or protein-rich matrixes. Some of them, for example grapefruit juice, due to synergetic effect on the metabolic pathways can alter drug bioavailability (Scheepens et al. 2010) or cause unexpected cell response to the treatment (Kabanov 2006).

9.4.1 Water-Soluble Carriers

Cyclodextrins are widely used as water-soluble carriers for improving polyphenols bioavailability and dissolution rate. These cyclic polysaccharides form strong host/guest inclusion complexes with curcumin and some other polyphenols (Baglole et al. 2005; Lumsden et al. 2001; Kalogeropoulos et al. 2010; Todd and Paul 1991) releasing the encapsulated substance upon pH change, heating or enzymatic cleavage of the matrix. Up to a-500 fold increase in curcumin solubility with cyclodexrin as compared to free substance has been observed (Baglole et al. 2005). Enhancement of oral bioavailability and gastroprotective effects of curcumin and silybin delivered as water-soluble solid dispersions formulated with high molecular weight polyvinylpyrrolidones (PVP) has been reported (Paradkar et al. 2004; Xu et al. 2006; Zhang et al. 2005).

Among other substrates useful in water-dispersible preparations, which will not precipitate upon standing in water, are water-soluble or water-dispersible proline-rich proteins and peptides, such as albumines (Barik et al. 2003; Schranz 1983), gelatins (Schranz 1983), or lactoglobulins (Petyaev 2008; Sneharani et al. 2010). The formulations are prepared by contacting the substrate and polyphenol in an aqueous solution at a pH, at which the polyphenol is present in its water-soluble alkaline form, and then acidifying to drop the pH, thereby complexing the substance in its neutral form with the substrate (Todd and Paul 1991; Schranz 1983). An alternative way is to admix small aliquots of polyphenol solution in ethanol or another water-missible solvent with a water-soluble carrier (Petyaev 2008; Sneharani et al. 2010).

The preparation proposed for curcumin (Schranz 1983) comprises up to about 15% curcumin by weight. The stability of curcumin bound to beta-lactoglobulin in solution was enhanced 6.7 times, in comparison to curcumin alone (Sneharani et al. 2010). United States Patent Application 20080153921 (Petyaev 2008) discloses water-soluble lycopene formulations for the treatment of atherosclerotic conditions based on complex of lycopene with a solubilising agent, such as beta-lactoglobulin, alpha-lactalbumin, serum albumin, and whey protein. Lactolycopene preparations showed marked inhibition activity towards lipid oxidizing abzymes, or AtheroAbzyme™, *in vitro* and in a clinical trial, while free lycopene and other preparations did not.

US Patent 6410052 (Morre et al. 2002) discloses sustained release formulations of tea catechins as cancer specific proliferation inhibitors delivered as admixture to a slowly soluble pharmaceutically acceptable polymer (microcrystalline cellulose, maltodextrin, ethylcellulose, etc). Prepared by spray drying, maltodextrin matrix has enhanced encapsulating efficiency for anthocyanins extracted from Pomegranate (*Punica granatum*) and significant greater protective effect for all bioactive compounds, than soybean protein isolates (Robert et al. 2010).

9.4.2 Polyphenol/Polymer and Polyphenol/Protein Coacervates

Nano and microsized self-assembled complexes of gelatin/tannic acid, albumin/tannin, and casein/(−)-epigallocatechin gallate formed upon direct binding of protein and an excessive amount of the polyphenols have been previously reported (Yi et al. 2006; Jöbstl et al. 2004, 2006). Polyphenol/protein binding is a multistage reversible process, which is highly sensitive to pH, temperature, and reagent concentrations (Haslam 1996; Bennick 2002; Calderon et al. 1968; Gámiz-Gracia and Luque de Castro 1997; Osawa and Walsho 1993; Barik et al. 2003; Yi et al. 2006). The main advantages of such an approach are a high polyphenol holding capacity of the particulated material and sustained environmentally controlled release of the components; that, along with simple preparation techniques, compensates variable size and high aggregation of the particle in final suspensions.

Application of polyphenol/protein and polyphenol/polyelectrolyte composites for delivery both target proteins and polyphenols is highly patented (Goldenberg and Gu 2008; Levy and Andry 1998; Lerner et al. 1999). Thus, pharmaceutical compositions comprising a stable sustained release complex composed of a protein and/or peptide and a gallic acid ester or its salt that allow for sustained delivery of the protein or peptide *in vivo* upon administration of the complex, are disclosed in US Patent 7323169 (Goldenberg and Gu 2008). US Patent 5780060 (Levy and Andry 1998) covers microcapsules based on crosslinked plant polyphenols prepared by emulsification of an aqueous solution containing from 1% to 40% by weight of plant polyphenols of different structure, their mixtures, polyphenol-containing plant extracts, juices, and pharmaceutics of the polyphenol family in oil, followed by interfacial crosslinking with protein, polysaccharide, polyethylene glycol or their mixtures. International patent WO/1999/004764 (Lerner et al. 1999) reports application of complexes of tannic acid with cellulosic or proteinaceous polymer, for control release of pharmaceutical agents different from the polyphenol and polymer used, particularly in the oral cavity. Such poorly soluble in water complexes can be administered to a subject as a stable liquid suspension or semi-solid dispersion (Morre et al. 2002), in chewing gum, slow-release patches, sponges for release of pharmaceuticals, etc. (Lerner et al. 1999).

Self-assembled nanocomplexes of tannic acid with chitosan, a natural polycationic polysaccharide, possess better thermal stability, higher polyphenol content, and smaller nanoparticle size as compared with triple chitosan/Na-alginate/tannic acid and chitosan/carboxymethylcellulose/tannic acid coacervates (Aelenei et al. 2009). The *in vitro* release studies revealed two distinct periods in tannic acid delivery process from such complexes: an initial short period characterized by a high release rate with a delivered tannic acid amount of approximately 80% of the incorporated polyphenol and a second period when the release process takes place with a low and constant rate.

9.4.3 Polyphenol Encasing into Preformed Nano and Microparticles

Taking advantages of increased bioavailability, high loading capacity and environmentally triggered release of polyphenols from the complexed coacervates, adsorption of polyphenols into pre-formed protein and polysaccharide micro and nanoparticles allows to achieve better control over size distribution of particulated material in the nanometer region, increase colloidal stability of the obtained nanoparticles, and design surface-modified nanoparticles. Among techniques useful for bulk batch oil-free nanoparticle synthesis, there are desolvation of gelatin, albumin, or lactoglobulin with acetone or ethanol (Zwiorek et al. 2004; Zillies et al. 2007; Kommareddy and Amiji 2005; Das et al. 2005), pH (Takeoka et al. 2000; Zhang et al. 2004a) or sulphate salt (Shao et al. 2009b; Lu et al. 2004) driven precipitation of proteins and polysaccharides, thermally assisted denaturation of proteins (Sneharani et al. 2010; Livney 2010; Shpigelman et al. 2010; Liang et al. 2008; Woiszwillo et al. 1999), and polyelectrolyte/polyelectrolyte or polyelectrolyte/protein complexation (Aelenei et al. 2009; Muller et al. 2005; Yu et al. 2006). Biopolymer-based nanoparticles have been proven to be relatively safe and effective delivery vehicles with a prolonged *in vivo* circulation time and high accumulation at the tumor side (Ravi Kumar et al. 2004; Livney 2010; Kommareddy and Amiji 2007a, b; Kaul and Amiji 2005).

There are only few examples of polyphenol adsorption into nanoparticles of pre-determined size because the template material is supposed to possess a high affinity for polyphenols (Haslam 1996; Bennick 2002).

The preparation of highly porous 5–6 μm particles of kafirin, the sorghum grain prolamin storage protein, prepared by water desolvation of ethanol solution of the protein has been reported (Taylor et al. 2009). The microparticles were used for encapsulation of two bioactive polyphenols, catechin and sorghum condensed tannins.

Over a period of 4 h under simulated gastric conditions, the microparticles showed virtually no protein digestion but released approximately 70% and 50%, respectively, of total antioxidant activity.

Beta-lactoglobulin based nanoparticles of a 50 nm size were used for encapsulation of natural polyphenols, such as curcumin, (−)-epigallocatechin gallate, and resveratrol (Sneharani et al. 2010; Livney 2010; Shpigelman et al. 2010; Liang et al. 2008). The nanoparticles are found to encapsulate curcumin with more than 96% efficiency, significantly enhancing its bulk concentration in comparison with free curcumin aqueous solubility (625 μM vs. 30 nM) (Sneharani et al. 2010). The interaction of curcumin with beta-lactoglobulin occurs through the central calyx of the protein and does not affect its conformation or state of association (Sneharani et al. 2010). At the same time, binding mostly to the surface of beta-lactoglobulin globules was assumed for resveratrol taking into account partially disrupted tertiary structure of the protein (Liang et al. 2008). Livney (Shpigelman et al. 2010) reports that the initial degradation rate of (−)-epigallocatechin gallate complexed with 50 nm beta-lactoglobulin nanoparticles was 33-fold lower than that of unprotected polyphenol. Over the course of 8 days, the degradation rate was 3.2-fold slower. Complexing with beta-lactoglobulin provides slight increase in the photostability of resveratrol in addition to a significant increase in its hydrosolubility (Liang et al. 2008).

Modification of nanoparticle surfaces with polyelectrolyte layer-by-layer (LbL) shells (McShane and Lvov 2004; De Geest et al. 2007; Ai et al. 2003) allows for modulating nanoparticle cell uptake rate and ratio, providing a template for their modification with tumor-targeting agents, increasing nanoparticle colloidal stability, and controlling loading/release characteristics (Ai et al. 2003, 2005; Zahr and Pishko 2007; Zhou et al. 2009; Qiu et al. 2001). Gelatin-based 200 nm nanoparticles consisting of a soft gel-like interior with or without a surrounding LbL shell of polyelectrolytes (poly(styrene sulfonate)/poly(allylamine hydrochloride) (PSS/PAH), polyglutamic acid/poly-L-lysine, dextran sulfate/protamine sulfate, carboxymethyl cellulose/gelatin) assembled using the layer-by-layer technique (Shutava et al. 2009) have recently been proposed to produce nanoparticles containing a wide range of polyphenols with previously demonstrated anticancer potential (curcumin, EGCG, tannic acid, teaflavins). Loading of polyphenols with higher molecular weights and a larger number of phenolic -OH groups in the nanoparticles was found to be higher, reaching for theaflavin, the polyphenol with the highest molecular weight among those investigated, 70% of the mass of nanoparticulated solid material. The degree of tannic acid and EGCG encapsulation was lower, while it was almost negligible for curcumin. These regularities of polyphenol adsorption correspond to general features of polyphenol/protein interaction and binding (Haslam 1996; Bennick 2002; Calderon et al. 1968; Gámiz-Gracia and Luque de Castro 1997; Osawa and Walsho 1993; Barik et al. 2003; Yi et al. 2006). For EGCG, the initial rate of the polyphenol release from the nanoparticuled material, but not nanoparticle loading capacity was slightly decreased by selected polyelectrolyte coatings. All encapsulated polyphenols retained their antioxidant properties as proved with the ABTS cation-radical assay. After prolong exposure, nanoparticulated EGCG retained its biological activity and blocked hepatocyte growth factor (HGF)-induced intracellular signaling in the breast cancer cell line MBA-MD-231 as potently as free EGCG (Bigelow and Cardelli 2006).

Two examples of curcumin loading into the layer-by-layer assembled poly(styrene sulfonate)/poly(diallyldimethylammonium chloride) film (Kittitheeranun et al. 2010) or poly(styrene sulfonate)/polyethyleneimine shells (Manju and Sreenivasan 2011) through a partitioning mechanism probably due to specific inner polarity and high hydrophobicity of the polyelectrolyte film materials (Tedeschi et al. 2001) have been reported, with the curcumin level reaching 8 $\mu g/cm^2$ for a 20-layer film.

9.4.4 Polyphenol Based Layer-by-Layer Films and Microcapsules

Polyphenols adsorption in alternation with macromolecules (neutral and positively charged polymers, proteins and polysaccharides) via the layer-by-layer assembly technique that uses the macromolecules as structural blocks to build films on planar supports or shells around sacrificial cores is a promising way for polyphenol immobilization because a spatially localized network with a thickness of several nanometers and a high (up to 50–60 w %) content of target substance can be created (Wang et al. 2007; Liu et al. 2006; Chitpan et al. 2007; Shutava et al. 2005, 2008; Erel-Unal and Sukhishvili 2008; Shutava and Lvov 2006; Shutava and Agabekov 2008).

Quantitative parameters of (–)-epigallocatechin gallate, tannic acid, and black tea pigment thearubigin single layer adsorption on immobilized layer of bovine serum albumin (BSA) have been recently evaluated by quartz crystal microbalance technique with dissipation monitoring (QCM-D). From the analysis of the adsorption isotherms and data of other methods, a non-specific hydrophobic interaction was suggested for (–)-epigallocatechin gallate on albumin films, while for thearubigin, both electrostatic forces and hydrogen bonding were assumed (Wang et al. 2007; Liu et al. 2006; Chitpan et al. 2007). The thickness of a polyphenol layer formed upon a single adsorption step exceeds linear dimensions of corresponding molecules, indicating that hydrogen-bonded associates of polyphenol molecules are adsorbed (Shutava et al. 2005; Erel-Unal and Sukhishvili 2008; Shutava and Lvov 2006). Moreover, the thicknesses of polyphenol/polycation, polyphenol/proteins bilayers are somewhat higher than those of common polycation/polyanion LbL bilayers (Taylor et al. 2009; McShane and Lvov 2004; De Geest et al. 2007; Ai et al. 2003, 2005; Zahr and Pishko 2007; Zhou et al. 2009; Qiu et al. 2001). For polyphenol/protein assemblies, the buildup of multilayers displays an exponential growth probably related to multiple reversible binding of the components (Haslam 1996; Bennick 2002; Calderon et al. 1968; Gámiz-Gracia and Luque de Castro 1997; Osawa and Walsho 1993; Barik et al. 2003; Yi et al. 2006).

All the experimental data obtained allow to formulate main regularities in multilayer formation on the basis of polyphenols. Natural polyphenol compounds form multilayers with polymers bearing amine groups (Shutava et al. 2005; Erel-Unal and

Sukhishvili 2008), polysaccharides (Shutava and Lvov 2006) and proteins (Shutava et al. 2008; Shutava and Agabekov 2008). The complex interaction in the assemblies includes electrostatic and hydrophobic forces between polyphenols and polymeric components of the films. Upon complexation with strong polycation PDDA, tannic acid behaves as a typical polyanion with $pK_a = 2.3–3.2$ (Shutava et al. 2005), while properties of the multilayers formed on the basis of poly(allylamine hydrochloride) and chitosan indicate that both electrostatic interaction and hydrogen bonding contribute in the assembly process (Shutava et al. 2005; Shutava and Lvov 2006). In the LbL assembled multilayers of hydrophobic EGCG (apparent $pK_a = 3–4$ (Fang et al. 2006)) and thearubigin with gelatins, electrostatic interaction was minor (Shutava et al. 2008; Shutava and Agabekov 2008). The buildup of poly(4-vinylpyridine)/poly(4-vinylphenol) (PVPy/PVPh) multilayer film from ethanol/dimethylformamide solvents was completely identified as a hydrogen bonding directed (Zhang et al. 2004b). In general, it is impossible to associate the polyphenol/macromolecule interaction in the films with a specific structure because of multiplicity of reacting sites; however, for several neutral polymers and TA, simplified models taking into account a single type polyphenol/polymer interaction have been proposed (Erel-Unal and Sukhishvili 2008).

Possible application of multilayers formed by layer-by-layer assembly of tannic acid and typical polymeric electrolytes, such as poly(allylamine hydrochloride), poly(diallyldimethylammonium chloride) (Shutava et al. 2005), poly(N-vinylpiridine) (Erel-Unal and Sukhishvili 2008), chitosan (Shutava and Lvov 2006), and several neutral polymers, such as poly(N-vinylcaprolactam), poly(vinylpyrrolydone), poly(ethyleneoxide), poly(N-isopropylacrylamide) (Erel-Unal and Sukhishvili 2008), as potential materials with pH controlled solubility useful for prolonged release preparations has been shown. Moreover, similar films based on gelatins and EGCG (Shutava et al. 2008) or thearubigin (Shutava and Agabekov 2008) have been reported. The dissolution rate of the multilayers on the basis of natural polyphenols depends on pH of the medium and polyelectrolyte nature and directed by the balance of positive and negative charges of the components in the assemblies (Shutava et al. 2005; Erel-Unal and Sukhishvili 2008; Shutava and Lvov 2006). The minimum solubility of TA/polycation complexes was observed in the range of neutral pH (Shutava et al. 2005; Shutava and Lvov 2006), while films of TA with neutral polymers dissolved only in basic solutions after pH reaches a threshold value (Erel-Unal and Sukhishvili 2008).

By adsorbing polyphenols in alternation with positively charged polymers or proteins on the surface of sacrificial cores, microcapsules with a core-mimicking diameter and a 20–30 nm wall thickness have been obtained. Free-standing polyphenol/protein microcapsules retain their stability and wall integrity in aqueous solutions only if contribution of electrostatic attraction into the interaction between layered components is essential (Shutava et al. 2008). At the same time, the layers of polyphenols with proteins can be obtained on the surface of solid templates at pH values both below and above proteins' pI.

The permeability of polyphenol-based microcapsule walls selectively depends on pH and molecular weight of the permeating macromolecules that allow for using the capsules for encapsulation of polyelectrolytes, proteins, drug nanoparticles and their controllable release upon delivery (Shutava et al. 2005, 2008; Shutava and Lvov 2006).

9.5 LbL Coated Nanoparticles of Solid Poorly Soluble Polyphenols

A new method to prepare stable aqueous nanocolloids of poorly soluble materials having particle diameters in the range of 150–250 nm and very high holding capacity has emerged recently (Agarwal et al. 2008; Lvov et al. 2008; Zheng et al. 2010). This approach is based on the powerful sonication of powders of low soluble materials, curcumin and resveratrol are among them, in the presence of a polyelectrolyte which is adsorbing charging particles and preventing them from reaggregation. Multilayer polyelectrolyte shells of sophisticated architecture build on the surface of such nanoparticles provides a template for their further modification with specific targeting agents. The rate of nanocore dissolution under bath conditions increases in comparison with parent microcrystals and takes 4–10 h.

9.6 Controversies in Antioxidant Properties of Polyphenol Multilayered Film and Microcapsules

Despite the features of polyphenol-protein and polyphenol-amine interaction, as well as factors influenced stability, solubility and other characteristics of such complexes have been well-studied (Jöbstl et al. 2004, 2006; Charlton et al. 2002; Baxter et al. 1997; Pascal et al. 2007), the regularities of the interaction of oxidizing agents with nanostructured materials on the basis of polyphenols are still disputed.

Usually considered as inert, encapsulating matrix and products of its degradation play an important role in antioxidant activity exhibited by the systems by interfering with the antioxidant assays (Ravi Kumar et al. 2004; Moon and Shibamoto 2009; Li et al. 2010; Dehkharghanian et al. 2009). As measured by the *N,N*,-diethyl-*p*-phenylenediamine method, antioxidant activities of sodium or calcium caseinate protein beads containing encapsulated green tea polyphenols extract were principally caused by caseinate hydrolysates formed during beads dissolution. After removing the caseinate hydrolysates, the beads containing polyphenols did show the antioxidant activities higher than those of the same beads without the extract (Dehkharghanian et al. 2009).

Assembled in LbL films natural polyphenols retain their high ability to scavenge free radicals (Shutava and Agabekov 2008; Shutava et al. 2006a, 2007). For several polyphenols in LbL films, the maximum values of radical scavenging activity (RSA), which show how many 2,2′-azino-bis(3-ethylbenzthiazoline-6-sulphonic acid) cation-radicals ($ABTS^{+\bullet}$) are trapped by one polyphenol molecule after prolong time (Re et al. 1999; Riedl and Hagerman 2001; Campos et al. 2004; Hushpulian et al. 2003), are close to those found in solution. Both in solution and LbL films, all the investigated polyphenols show a biphasic scavenging activity toward $ABTS^{+\bullet}$, usually attributed to different kinetics of the reactions of polyphenol itself and its oxidation products formed on early stages of the reaction (Riedl and Hagerman 2001). The retaining of general reaction mechanism has been previously proven for different LbL assembled systems (Shutava et al. 2006b).

On the other hand, layered film architecture results in kinetic specificity of radical reactions with LbL-assembled films containing polyphenol (Shutava et al. 2006a, 2007). A single polyphenol layer in a LbL assemblies discolorates only a part of $ABTS^{+\bullet}$ diffused through it. It decreases the amount of the cation-radicals that can reach inner layers of the film brought into contact with an excessive amount of $ABTS^{+\bullet}$, as in case of polycation/TA multilayers, or that can leave the film and appear in surrounding solution, as in case of the cation-radicals formed in a horseradish peroxidase/PSS/PAH/TA film in a solution of ABTS and H_2O_2.

Immobilization of HRP and TA in LbL film spatially separates them and apparently excludes some of the reaction paths in which TA acts as a substrate for horseradish peroxidase (HRP) (Rodriguez-Lopez et al. 2001; Naumchik et al. 2004; Sang et al. 2004; Kobayashi et al. 2001). In LbL assemblies with polyelectrolytes, tannic acid behaves as an effective scavenger of the cation-radicals, whilst in HRP-ABTS-H_2O_2 solutions it does not show good inhibitor properties (Shutova et al. 2007).

In solutions at high pH, ionized forms of polyphenols (polygalloyl glucose, procyanidine, etc.) show higher RSA values and react faster with ABTS cation-radicals (Takebayashi et al. 2003; Jonson 2005). At the same time, the films with a PAH outermost layer, which shifts the local pH in the vicinity of the films to a high pH values, bleach less $ABTS^{+\bullet}$ with a lower reaction rate than TA-terminated films with the same number of TA layers. Deposition of a PAH layer on the top of a TA layer shifts the equilibrium to a reversible tannic acid/polycation complex, slowing down the reaction of tannic acid with the cation-radicals. Inhibition of the reaction of $ABTS^{+\bullet}$ with a polyphenol by a protein forming strong complexes with the compound has been previously reported (Riedl and Hagerman 2001).

The results suggest that polyphenol multilayers positioning as organized protective shells on the surface of biodevices or compacted drug forms may inhibit or diminish free-radical damage of encapsulated compound. The validity of a similar approach has been demonstrated by the examples of hemoglobin/polyelectrolyte LbL film (Shutava et al. 2006b) and albumin-containing microcapsules (Shchukin et al. 2004) protection by catalase layers under hydrogen peroxide treatment.

In conclusion, nanoparticulated compositions containing natural polyphenols can be a good alternative to free compounds in the fulfillment of their high potential as biologically active substances with a wide range of activities. Careful, well-design studies on the bioavailability, as well as mechanisms of action of these compounds in the presence of encapsulating matrixes *in vitro* and *in vivo* are needed to develop highly effective polyphenol-based formulations.

References

Abd-El-Galeel MAS (2002) Solubility and stability of natural food colourants in microemulsions. Dissertation, Rheinschen Friedrich-Wilhelms-Universität zu Bonn

Adhami VM, Mukhtar H (2007) Anti-oxidants from green tea and pomegranate for chemoprevention of prostate cancer. Mol Biotechnol 37:52–57. doi:10.1007/s12033-007-0047-8

Aelenei N, Popa MI, Novac O, Lisa G, Balaita L (2009) Tannic acid incorporation in chitosan-based microparticles and *in vitro* controlled release. J Mater Sci Mater Med 20(5):1095–1102. doi: 10.1007/s10856-008-3675-z

Agarwal A, Lvov Y, Sawant R, Torchilin V (2008) Stable nanocolloids of poorly soluble drugs with high drug content prepared using sonicated layer-by-layer technology. J Control Release 128:255–260. doi:10.1016/j.jconrel.2008.03.017

Ai H, Jones SA, Lvov YM (2003) Biomedical application of electrostatic layer-by-layer nano-assembly of polymers, enzymes, and nanoparticles. Cell Biochem Biophys 39:23–43. doi:10.1385/CBB:39:1:23

Ai H, Pink JJ, Shuai X, Boothman DA, Gao J (2005) Interactions between self-assembled polyelectrolyte shells and tumor cells. J Biomed Mater Res 73A:303–312. doi:10.1002/jbm.a.30289

Al-Tahami K, Singh J (2007) Smart polymer based delivery systems for peptides and proteins. Recent Pat Drug Deliv Formul 1:65–71

Anand P, Kunnumakkara AB, Newman RA, Aggarwal BB (2007) Bioavailability of curcumin: problems and promises. Mol Pharm 4(6):807–818. doi:10.1021/mp700113r

Anderson LJE, Hansen E, Lukianova-Hleb EY, Hafner JH, Lapotko DO (2010) Optically guided controlled release from liposemes with tunable plasmonic nanobubbles. J Control Release 144:151–158. doi:10.1016/j.jconrel.2010.02.012

Andre F, Escudier B, Angevin E, Tursz T, Zitvogel L (2004) Exosomes for cancer immunotherapy. Ann Oncol 15(4):iv141–iv144. doi:10.1093/annonc/mdh918

Baglole KN, Boland PG, Wagner BD (2005) Fluorescence enhancement of curcumin upon inclusion into parent and modified cyclodextrins. J Photochem Photobiol A Chem 173(3):230–237. doi:10.1016/j.jphotochem. 2005.04.002

Bai G, Nichifor M, Bastos M (2010) Cationic polyelectrolytes as drug delivery vectors: calorimetric and fluorescence study of rutin partitioning. J Phys Chem B Article ASAP. doi:10.1021/jp1071555

Bao S, Xu S, Wang Z (2009) Antioxidant activity and properties of gelatin films incorporated with tea polyphenol-loaded chitosan nanoparticles. J Sci Food Agric 89:2692–2700. doi:10.1002/jsfa.3775

Barik A, Priyadarsini KI, Mohan H (2003) Photophysical studies on binding of curcumin to bovine serum albumins. Photochem Photobiol 77:597–603. doi:10.1562/0031-8655

Baumgart M, Lindley M, Wright D, Anklam MR (2005) Solubilization of phenols in anionic polyelectrolyte gels with adsorbed cationic surfactant. Langmuir 21:4862–4867. doi:10.1021/la050155q

Baxter NJ, Lilley TH, Haslam E, Williamson MP (1997) Multiple interactions between polyphenols and a salivary proline-rich protein repeat result in complexation and precipitation. Biochemistry 36(17):5566–5577. doi:10.1021/bi9700328

Bennick A (2002) Interaction of plant polyphenols with salivary proteins. Crit Rev Oral Biol Med 13:184–196. doi:10.1177/154411130201300208

Bettuzzi S, Brausi M, Rizzi F, Castagnetti G, Peracchia G, Corti A (2006) Chemoprevention of human prostate cancer by oral administration of green tea catechins in volunteers with high-grade prostate intraepithelial neoplasia: a preliminary report from a one-year proof-of-principle study. Cancer Res 66(2):1234–1240. doi:10.1158/0008-5472.CAN-05-1145

Bigelow RLH, Cardelli JA (2006) The green tea catechins, (–)-Epigallocatechin-3-gallate (EGCG) and (–)-Epicatechin-3-gallate (ECG), inhibit HGF/Met signaling in immortalized and tumorigenic breast epithelial cellsGreen tea catechins inhibit HGF/Met signaling. Oncogene 25:1922–1930. doi:10.1038/sj.onc.1209227

Bisht S, Feldmann G, Soni S, Ravi R, Karikar C, Maitra A, Maitra A (2007) Polymeric nanoparticle-encapsulated curcumin ("nanocurcumin"): a novel strategy for human cancer therapy. J Nanobiotechnol 5:3. doi:10.1186/1477-3155-5-3

Bisht S, Mizuma M, Feldmann G, Ottenhof NA, Hong SM, Pramanik D, Chenna V, Karikari C, Sharma R, Goggins MG, Rudek MA, Ravi R, Maitra A, Maitra A (2010) Systemic administration of polymeric nanoparticle-encapsulated curcumin (NanoCurc) blocks tumor growth and metastases in preclinical models of pancreatic cancer. Mol Cancer Ther 9(8):2255–2264. doi:10.1158/1535-7163.MCT-10-0172

Buchhammer HM, Petzold G, Lunkwitz K (2000) Nanoparticles based on polyelectrolyte complexes: effect of structure and net charge on the sorption capatibily for solved organic molecules. Colloid Polym Sci 278(9):841–847. doi:10.1007/s003960000330

Calderon P, Van Buren J, Robinson WB (1968) Factors influencing the formation of precipitates and hazes by gelatine and condensed and hydrolysable tannins. J Agric Food Chem 16:479–482. doi:10.1021/jf60157a017

Campos AM, Sotomayor CP, Pino E, Lissi EA (2004) A pyranine based procedure for evaluation of the total antioxidant potential (TRAP) of polyphenols. A comparison with closely related methodologies. Biol Res 37:287–292. doi:10.4067/S0716-97602004000200015

Cartiera MS, Ferreira EC, Caputo C, Egan ME, Caplan MJ, Saltzman WM (2010) Partial correction of cystic fibrosis defects with PLGA nanoparticles encapsulating curcumin. Mol Pharm 7(1):86–93. doi:10.1021/mp900138a

Charlton AJ, Baxter NJ, Khan ML, Moir AJG, Haslam E, Davies AP, Williamson MP (2002) Polyphenol/peptide binding and precipitation. J Agric Food Chem 50:1593–1601. doi:10.1021/jf010897z

Chasin M (1995) Biodegradable polymers for controlled drug delivery. In: Hollinger JO (ed) Biomedical applications of synthetic biodegradable polymers. CRC Press, Boca Raton

Chitpan M, Wang X, Ho CT, Huang Q (2007) Monitoring the binding processes of black tea thearubigin to the bovine serum albumin surface using quartz crystal microbalance with dissipation monitoring. J Agric Food Chem 55:10110–10116. doi:10.1021/jf072236t

Das S, Banerjee R, Bellare J (2005) Aspirin loaded albumin nanoparticles by coacervation: implications in drug delivery. Trends Biomater Artif Organs 18(2):203–212

Das RK, Kasoju N, Bora U (2010) Encapsulation of curcumin in alginate-chitosan-pluronic composite nanoparticles for delivery to cancer cells. Nanomed Nanotechnol Biol Med 6:153–160. doi:10.1016/j.nano.2009.05.009

De Geest BG, Sanders NN, Sukhorukov GB, Demeestera J (2007) De Smedt SC Release mechanisms for polyelectrolyte capsules. Chem Soc Rev 36:636–649. doi:10.1002/chin.200724277

Dehkharghanian M, Lacroix M, Vijayalakshmi MA (2009) Antioxidant properties of green tea polyphenols encapsulated in caseinate beads. Dairy Sci Technol 89:485–499. doi:10.1051/dst/2009024

Erel-Unal I, Sukhishvili SA (2008) Hydrogen-bonded multilayers of a neutral polymer and a polyphenol. Macromolecules 41(11):3962–3970. doi:10.1021/ma800186q

Fang Z, Bhandari B (2010) Encapsulation of polyphenols – a review. Trends Food Sci Technol 21(10):510–523. doi:10.1016/j.tifs.2010.08.003

Fang JY, Hung CF, Hwang TL, Wong WW (2006) Transdermal delivery of tea catechins by electrically assisted methods. Skin Pharmacol Physiol 19(1):28–37. doi:10.1159/000089141

Gallarate M, Carlotti ME, Trotta M, Bovo S (1999) On the stability of ascorbic acid in emulsified systems for topical and cosmetic use. Int J Pharm 188:233–241. doi:10.1016/S0378-5173(99)00228-8

Gámiz-Gracia L, de Luque de Castro MD (1997) Development and validation of a flow-injection method for the determination of albumin tannate, the active component of a pharmaceutical preparation. J Pharm Biomed Anal 15:447–452. doi:10.1016/S0731-7085(96)01870-5

Goldenberg MS, Gu JH (2008) Sustained release formulations. US Patent 7323169

Haslam E (1996) Natural polyphenols (vegetable tannins) as drugs: possible modes of action. J Nat Prod 59:205–215. doi:10.1021/np960040+

Henry BS (1996) Natural food colours. In: Hendry GAF, Houghton JD (eds) Natural food colorants, 2nd edn. Blackie/Avi, Glasgow/New York

Huang Q, Yu Y, Ru Q (2010) Bioavailability and delivery of nutraceuticals using nanotechnology. J Food Sci 75(1):R50–R57. doi:10.1111/j.1750-3841.2009.01457.x

Hushpulian DM, Fechina VA, Kazakov SV, Sakharov IY, Gazaryan IG (2003) Non-enzymatic interaction of reaction products and substrates in peroxidase catalysis. Biochemistry (Moscow) 68(9):1006–1011. doi:10.1023/A:1026016730127

Iero M, Valenti R, Huber V, Filipazzi P, Parmiani G, Fais S, Rivoltini L (2008) Tumour-released exosomes and their implications in cancer immunity. Cell Death Differ 15:80–88. doi:10.1038/sj.cdd.4402237

Jöbstl E, O'Connell J, Fairclough JPA, Williamson MP (2004) Molecular model for astringency produced by polyphenol/protein interactions. Biomacromolecules 5(3):942–949. doi:10.1021/bm0345110

Jöbstl E, Howse JR, Fairclough JPA, Williamson MP (2006) Noncovalent cross-linking of casein by epigallocatechin gallate characterized by single molecule force microscopy. J Agric Food Chem 54(12):4077–4081. doi:10.1021/jf053259f

Jonson KS (2005) Plant phenolics behave as radical scavengers in the context of insect (*Manduca sexta*) hemolymph and midgut fluid. J Agric Food Chem 53(26):10120–10126. doi:10.1021/jf051942w

Kabanov AV (2006) Polymer genomics: an insight into pharmacology and toxicology of nanomedicines. Adv Drug Deliv Rev 58(15):1597–1621. doi:10.1016/j.addr.2006.09.019

Kalogeropoulos N, Yannakopoulou K, Gioxari A, Chiou A, Makris DP (2010) Polyphenol characterization and encapsulation in β-cyclodextrin of a flavonoid-rich *Hypericum perforatum* (St John's wort) extract. LWT- Food Sci Technol 43(6):882–889. doi:10.1016/j.lwt.2010.01.016

Kaul G, Amiji M (2005) Tumor-targeted gene delivery using poly(ethylene glycol)-modified gelatin nanoparticles: *in vitro* and *in vivo* studies. Pharm Res 22:951–961. doi:10.1007/s11095-005-4590-3

Kittitheeranun P, Sanchavanakit N, Sajomsang W, Dubas ST (2010) Loading of curcumin in polyelectrolyte multilayers. Langmuir 26(10):6869–6873. doi:10.1021/la1003676

Kleinedler J, Foley J, Dugas T (2009) Cytotoxicity and efficacy evaluation of polymeric nanoparticles containing resveratrol and quercetin for use on drug eluting stents. FASEB J 23:640.2

Kobayashi S, Uyama H, Kimura S (2001) Enzymatic polymerization. Chem Rev 101(12):3793–3818. doi:10.1021/cr990121l

Kommareddy S, Amiji M (2005) Preparation and evaluation of thiol-modified gelatin nanoparticles or intracellular DNA delivery in response to glutathione. Bioconjug Chem 16:1423–1432. doi:10.1021/bc050146t

Kommareddy S, Amiji M (2007a) Antiangiogenic gene therapy with systemically administered sFlt-1 plasmid DNA in engineered gelatin-based nanovectors. Cancer Gene Ther 14:488–498. doi:10.1038/sj.cgt.7701041

Kommareddy S, Amiji M (2007b) Biodistribution and pharmacokinetic analysis of long-circulating thiolated gelatin nanoparticles following systemic administration in breast cancer-bearing mice. J Pharm Sci 96:397–407. doi:10.1002/jps.20813

Kreyling WG, Semmler-Behnke M, Moeller W (2006) Health implications of nanoparticles. J Nanoparticle Res 8:543–562. doi:10.1007/s11051-005-9068-z

Kumar V, Lewis SA, Mutalik S, Shenoy DB, Venkatesh UN (2002) Biodegradable microspheres of curcumin for treatment of inflammation. Indian J Physiol Pharmacol 46:209–217

Lambert JD, Yang CS (2003) Cancer chemopreventive activity and bioavailability of tea and tea polyphenols. Mutat Res 523–524:201–208. doi:10.1016/s0027-5107(02)00336-6

Lee BH, Christian SD, Tucker EE, Scamehorn JF (1991) Effects of an anionic polyelectrolyte on the solubilization of mono- and dichlorophenols by aqueous solutions of N-hexadecylpyridinium chloride. Langmuir 7(7):1332–1335. doi:10.1021/la00055a007

Lerner EI, Rosenberger V, Flashner M (1999) Tannic acid-polymer compositions for controlled release of phermaceutical agents, particularly in the oral cavity. International Patent WO/1999/004764

Levy M, Andry M (1998) Microcapsules with a wall of crosslinked plant polyphenols and compositions containing them. U S Patent 5780060

Li R, Chen W, Wang W, Tian W, Zhang X (2010) Antioxidant activity of *Astragalus* polysaccharides and antitumour activity of the polysaccharides and siRNA. Carbohydr Polym 82(2):240–244. doi:10.1016/j.carbpol.2010.02.048

Liang L, Tajmir-Riahi HA, Subirade M (2008) Interaction of β-lactoglobulin with resveratrol and its biological implications. Biomacromolecules 9(1):50–56. doi:10.1021/bm700728k

Liang J, Li F, Fang Y, Yang W, An X, Zhao L, Xin Z, Cao L, Hu Q (2011) Synthesis, characterization and cytotoxicity studies of chitosan-coated tea polyphenols nanoparticles. Colloids Surf B Biointerfaces 82(2):297–301. doi:10.1016/j.colsurfb.2010.08.045

Lin HY, Thomas JL, Chen HC, Lee MH (2003) Control of the release of curcumin from micelles by ultrasound. Photochem Photobiol 77(6):597–603

Liu M, Zhang Y, Yang Q, Xie Q, Yao S (2006) Monitoring and estimation of the kinetics parameters in the binding process of tannic acid to bovine serum albumin with electrochemical quartz crystal impedance system. J Agric Food Chem 54:4087–4094. doi:10.1021/jf052489r

Livney YD (2010) Milk proteins as vehicles for bioactives. Current Opin Colloid Interface Sci 15:73–83. doi:10.1016/j.nano.2009.06.006

Lu Z, Yeh TK, Tsai M, Au JLS, Wientjes MG (2004) Paclitaxel-loaded gelatin nanoparticles for intravesical bladder cancer therapy. Clin Cancer Res 10:7677–7684. doi:10.1158/1078-0432.CCR-04-1443

Lumsden AB, Yao QZ, Chen CY, Literat A (2001) Regulation of pro-inflammatory cytokine expression by curcumin in hyaline membrane disease (HMD). Life Sci 70(3):253–267

Lvov Y, Agarwal A, Sawant R, Torchilin V (2008) Sonication assisted polyelectrolyte nanoencapsulation of paclitaxel and tamoxifen. Pharma Focus Asia 7:36–40

Manach C, Scalbert A, Morand C, Remesy C, Jimenez L (2004) Polyphenols: food sources and bioavailability. Am J Clin Nutr 79:727–747

Manju S, Sreenivasan K (2011) Hollow microcapsules built by layer by layer assembly for the encapsulation and sustained release of curcumin. Colloids Surf B Biointerfaces 82(2):588–593. doi:10.1016/j.colsurfb.2010.10.021

McShane M, Lvov Y (2004) Layer-by-layer electrostatic self-assembly. In: Schwartz J, Contescu C (eds) Dekker encyclopedia of nanoscience and nanotechnology. Marcel Dekker, New York

Moon JK, Shibamoto T (2009) Antioxidant assays for plant and food components. J Agric Food Chem 57(5):1655–1666. doi:10.1021/jf803537k

Morre DM, Morre DJ, Cooper R, Chang MN (2002) Tea catechins in sustained release formulations as cancer specific proliferation inhibitors. U S Patent 6410052

Mozafari MR (2006) Nanocarrier technologies: frontiers of nanotherapy. Springer, Dordrecht

Mulik RS, Monkkonen J, Juvonen RO, Mahadik KR, Paradkar AR (2010) ApoE3 Mediated poly(butyl) cyanoacrylate nanoparticles containing curcumin: study of enhanced activity of curcumin against beta amyloid induced cytotoxicity using *in vitro* cell culture model. Mol Pharm 7(3):815–825. doi:10.1021/mp900306x

Muller M, Kessler B, Richter S (2005) Preparation of monomodal polyelectrolyte comples nanoparticles of PDADMAC/poly(maleic acid-alt-α-methylstyrene) by consecutive centrifugation. Langmuir 21(15):7044–7051. doi:10.1021/la050716d

Nam SH, Nam HY, Joo JR, Baek IS, Park JS (2007) Curcumin-loaded PLGA nanoparticles coating onto metal stent by EPD. Bull Korean Chem Soc 28:397–402

Naumchik IV, Karasyova EI, Meteliza DI, Polozov GI, Shadyro OI (2004) Inhibition of the peroxidase-catalyzed oxidation of chromogenic substrates by alkyl-substituted diatomic phenols. Russ J Bioorg Chem 30(5):482–491. doi:10.1023/B:RUBI.0000043793.20541.85

Oganesyan EA, Miroshnichenko II, Vikhrieva NS, Lyashenko AA, Leshkov SY (2001) Use of nanoparticles to increase the systemic bioavailability of *trans*-resveratrol. Pharm Chem J 44(2): 74–76. doi:10.1007/s11094-010-0401-1

Osawa RSJ, Walsho TP (1993) Effects of acidic and alkaline treatments on tannic acid and its binding property to protein. J Agric Food Chem 41(5):704–707. doi:10.1021/jf00029a004

Paradkar A, Ambike AA, Jadhav BK, Mahadik KR (2004) Characterization of curcumin-PVP solid dispersion obtained by spray drying. Int J Pharm 271:281–286. doi:10.1016/j.ijpharm.2003.11.014

Pascal C, Poncet-Legrand CL, Imberty A, Gautier C, Sarni-Manchado P, Chenynier VR, Vernhet A (2007) Interactions between a non glycosylated human proline-rich protein and flavan-3-ols are affected by protein concentration and polyphenol/protein ratio. J Agric Food Chem 55(12):4895–4901. doi:10.1021/jf0704108

Petyaev I (2008) Lycopene Formulations For the Treatment of Atherosclerotic Conditions U S Patent Application 20080153921

Qiu X, Leporatti S, Donath E, Mohwald H (2001) Studies on the drug release properties of polysaccharide multilayers encapsulated ibuprofen microparticles. Langmuir 17:5375–5380. doi:10.1021/la010201w

Quideau S, Feldman KS (1996) Ellagitannin chemistry. Chem Rev 96:475–503. doi:10.1021/cr940716a

Ravi Kumar MNV, Muzzarelli RAA, Muzzarelli C, Sashiwa H, Domb AJ (2004) Chitosan chemistry and pharmaceutical perspectives. Chem Rev 104:6017–6084. doi:10.1021/cr030441b

Re R, Pellegrini A, Proteggente A, Pannala A, Yang M, Rice-Evans C (1999) Antioxidant activity applying an improved ABTS radical-cation decolorization assay. Free Radic Biol Med 26: 1231–1237. doi:10.1016/S0891-5849(98)00315-3

Riedl KM, Hagerman AE (2001) Tannin – protein complexes as radical scavengers and radical sinks. J Agric Food Chem 49(10):4917–4923. doi:10.1021/jf010683h

Rinaudo M, Kil'deeva NR, Babak VG (2008) Surfactant-polyelectrolyte complexes on the basis of chitin. Russ J Gen Chem 78(11):2239–2246. doi:10.1134/S1070363208110455

Robert P, Gorena T, Romero N, Sepulveda E, Chavez J, Saenz C (2010) Encapsulation of polyphenols and anthocyanins from pomegranate (*Punica granatum*) by spray drying. Int J Food Sci Technol 45(7):1386–1394. doi:10.1111/j.1365-2621.2010.02270.x

Rodriguez-Lopez JN, Lowe DJ, Hernandez-Ruiz J, Hiner ANP, Garcia-Canovas F, Thorneley RNF (2001) Mechanism of reaction of hydrogen peroxide with horseradish peroxidase: identification of intermediates in the catalytic cycle. J Am Chem Soc 123(48):11838–11847. doi:10.1021/ja011853+

Ruby AJ, Kuttan G, Dinesh Babu KV, Rajasekharan KN, Kuttan R (1995) Antitumor and atioxidant activity of natural curcuminoids. Cancer Lett 94:79–83. doi:10.1016/0304-3835(95)03827-J

Sang S, Lambert JD, Tian S, Hong J, Hou Z, Ryu JH, Stark RE, Rosen RT, Huang MT, Yang CS, Ho CT (2004) Enzymatic synthesis of tea theaflavin derivatives and their anti-inflammatory and cytotoxic activities. Bioorg Med Chem 12(2):459–467. doi:10.1016/j.bmc.2003.10.024

Scheepens A, Tan K, Paxton JW (2010) Improving the oral bioavailability of beneficial polyphenols through designed synergies. Genes Nutr 5:75–87. doi:10.1007/s12263-009-0148-z

Schranz JL (1983) Water-soluble curcumin complex. U S Patent 4368208

Shahani K, Swaminathan SK, Freeman D, Blum A, Ma L, Panyam J (2010) Injectable sustained release microparticles of curcumin: a new concept for cancer chemoprevention. Cancer Res 70:4443–4452. doi:10.1158/0008-5472.CAN-09-4362

Shao J, Li X, Lu X, Jiang C, Hu Y, Li Q, You Y, Fu Z (2009a) Enhanced growth inhibition effect of resveratrol incorporated into biodegradable nanoparticles against glioma cells is mediated by the induction of intracellular reactive oxygen species levels. Colloids Surf B Biointerfaces 72(1):40–47. doi:10.1016/j.colsurfb.2009.03.010

Shao Y, Zhu B, Li J, Liu X, Tan X, Yang X (2009b) Novel chitosan microsphere-templated microcapsules suitable for spontaneous loading of heparin. Mater Sci Eng C 29:936–941. doi:10.1016/j.msec.2008.08.017

Shchukin DG, Shutava T, Shchukina E, Sukhorukov GB, Lvov YM (2004) Modified polyelectrolyte microcapsules as smart defense systems. Chem Mater 16(18):3446–3451. doi:10.1021/cm049506x

Shpigelman A, Israeli G, Livney YD (2010) Thermally-induced protein–polyphenol co-assemblies: beta-lactoglobulin-based nanocomplexes as protective nanovehicles for EGCG. Food Hydrocolloids 24(8):735–743. doi:10.1016/j.foodhyd.2010.03.015

Shutava TG, Agabekov VE (2008) Multilayer film structures based on polyphenols, and their antioxidant properties. Proc Natl Acad Sci Belarus Ser Chem Sci 1:28–40

Shutava TG, Lvov YM (2006) Nano-engineered microcapsules of tannic acid and chitosan for protein encapsulation. J Nanosci Nanotechnol 6(6):1655–1661. doi:10.1166/jnn.2006.225

Shutava T, Prouty M, Kommirredy D, Lvov Y (2005) pH responsive decomposable layer-by-layer nanofilms and capsules on the basis of tannic acid. Macromolecules 38(7):2850–2858. doi:10.1021/ma047629x

Shutava TG, Prouty MD, Agabekov VE, Lvov YM (2006a) Antioxidant properties of layer-by-layer films on the basis of tannic acid. Chem Lett 35(10):1144–1145. doi:10.1246/cl.2006.1144

Shutava T, Kommirredy D, Lvov Y (2006b) Layer-by-layer enzyme/polyelectrolyte films as a functional protective barrier in oxidizing media. J Am Chem Soc 128:9926–9934. doi:10.1021/ja062318i

Shutava TG, Balkundi SS, Lvov YM (2008) (−)-Epigallocatechin gallate/gelatin layer-by-layer assembled films and microcapsules. J Colloid Interface Sci 330(2):276–283. doi:10.1016/j.jcis.2008.10.082

Shutava TG, Balkundi SS, Vangala P, Steffan JJ, Bigelow RL, Cardelli JA, O'Neal DP, Lvov YM (2009) Layer-by-layer-coated gelatin nanoparticles as a vehicle for delivery of natural polyphenols. ACS Nano 3(7):1877–1885. doi:10.1021/nn900451a

Shutova TG, Agabekov VE, Lvov YM (2007) Reaction of radical-cations with multilayers of tannic acid and polyelectrolytes. Russ J Gen Chem 77(9):1494–1501. doi:10.1134/S1070363207090034

Siddiqui IA, Adhami VM, Bharali DJ, Hafeez BB, Asim M, Khwaja SI, Ahmad N, Cui H, Mousa SA, Mukhtar H (2009) Introducing nanochemoprevention as a novel approach for cancer control: proof of principle with green tea polyphenol epigallocatechin-3-gallate. Cancer Res 69(5):1712–1716. doi:10.1158/0008-5472.CAN-08-3978

Sneharani AH, Karakkat JV, Singh SA, Rao AGA (2010) Interaction of curcumin with β-lactoglobulin – stability, spectroscopic analysis, and molecular modeling of the complex. J Agric Food Chem 58(20):11130–11139. doi:10.1021/jf102826q

Sowasod N, Charinpanitkul T, Tanthapanichakoon W (2005) Encapsulation of curcumin in chitosan nanospheres for cosmetic application. MaDParT 2005 Proceedings

Sun D, Zhuang X, Xiang X, Liu Y, Zhang S, Liu C, Barnes S, Grizzle W, Miller D, Zhang HG (2010) A novel nanoparticle drug delivery system: the anti-inflammatory activity of curcumin is enhanced when encapsulated in exosomes. Mol Ther 18:1606–1614. doi:10.1038/mt.2010.105

Surh YJ (2003) Cancer chemoprevention with dietary phytochemicals. Nat Rev Cancer 3:768–780. doi:10.1038/nrc1189

Takahashi M, Uechi S, Takara K, Asikin Y, Wada K (2009) Evaluation of an oral carrier system in rats: bioavailability and antioxidant properties of liposome-encapsulated curcunim. J Agric Food Chem 57(19):9141–9146. doi:10.1021/jf9013923

Takebayashi J, Tai A, Yamamoto I (2003) pH-dependent long-term radical scavenging activity of AA-2G and 6-octa-AA-2G against 2,2′-azinobis(3-ethylbenzothiazoline-6-sulfonic acid) radical cation. Biol Pharm Bull 26:1368–1370. doi:10.1248/bpb.26.1368

Takeoka S, Teramura Y, Ohkawa H, Ikeda Y, Tsuchida E (2000) Conjugation of Von Willebrand factor-binding domain of platelet glycoprotein Ibr to size-controlled albumin microspheres. Biomacromolecules 1:290–295. doi:10.1021/bm0055293

Tamber H, Johansen P, Merkle HP, Gander B (2005) Formulation aspects of biodegradable polymeric microspheres for antigen delivery. Adv Drug Deliv Rev 57(3):357–376. doi:10.1016/j.addr.2004.09.002

Taylor J, Taylor JRN, Belton PS, Minnaar A (2009) Kafirin microparticle encapsulation of catechin and sorghum condensed tannins. J Agric Food Chem 57(16):7523–7528. doi:10.1021/jf901592q

Tedeschi C, Mohwald H, Kirstein S (2001) Polarity of layer-by-layer deposited polyelectrolyte films as determined by pyrene fluorescence. J Am Chem Soc 123(5):954–960. doi:10.1021/ja0031974

Teskac K, Kristl J (2010) The evidence for solid lipid nanoparticles mediated cell uptake of resveratrol. Int J Pharm 390(1):61–69. doi:10.1016/j.ijpharm.2009.10.01

Thunemann AE (2002) Polyelectrolyte-surfactant complexes (synthesis, structure and materials aspects). Prog Polym Sci 27(8):1473–1572

Todd Jr, Paul H (1991) Curcumin complexed on water-dispersible substrates. U S Patent 4999205
Torchilin VP (2007) Micellar nanocarriers: pharmaceutical perspectives. Pharm Res 24:1–16. doi:10.1007/s11095-006-9132-0
Vinogradov SV (2006) Colloidal microgels in drug delivery applications. Curr Pharm Des 12:4703–4712. doi:10.2174/138161206779026254
Wang X, Ho CT, Huang Q (2007) Investigation of adsorption behavior of (–)-epigallocatechin gallate on bovine serum albumin surface using quartz crystal microbalance with dissipation monitoring. J Agric Food Chem 55:4987–4992. doi:10.1021/jf070590l
Warheit DB, Sayes CM, Reed KL, Swain KA (2008) Health effects related to nanoparticle exposures: environmental, health and safety considerations for assessing hazards and risks. Pharmacol Ther 120(1):35–42
Williamson G, Manach C (2005) Bioavailability and bioefficacy of polyphenols in himans. II. Review of 93 intervantion studies. Am J Clin Nutr 81:243S–255S
Woiszwillo JE, Brown LR, Scott TL, Di J, Sudhalter J, Blizzard CD, Riske FJ (1999) Macromolecular microparticles and methods of production and use. U S Patent 5981719
Xu DH, Wang S, Jin J, Mei XT, Xu SB (2006) Dissolution and absorption researches of curcumin in solid dispersions with the polymers PVP. Asian J Pharmacodyn Pharmacokinet 6(4):343–349
Yadav VR, Suresh S, Devi K, Yadav S (2009) Novel formulation of solid lipid microparticles of curcumin for anti-angiogenic and anti-inflammatory activity for optimization of therapy of inflammatory bowel disease. J Pharm Pharmacol 61(3):311–321. doi:10.1211/jpp. 61.03.0005
Yi K, Cheng G, Xing F (2006) Gelatin/tannin complex nanospheres via molecular assembly. J Appl Polym Sci 101:3125–3125. doi:10.1002/app. 22416
Yu S, Hu J, Pan X, Yao P, Jiang M (2006) Stable and pH-sensitive nanogels prepared by self-assembly of chitosan and ovalbumin. Langmuir 22(6):2754–2759. doi:10.1021/la053158b
Zahr AS, Pishko MV (2007) Encapsulation of paclitaxel in macromolecular nanoshells. Biomacromolecules 8:2004–2010. doi:10.1021/bm070177m
Zhang L, Kosaraju SL (2007) Biopolymeric delivery system for controlled release of polyphenolic antioxidants. EurPolym J 43:2956–2966. doi:10.1016/j.eurpolymj.2007.04.033
Zhang H, Oh M, Allen C, Kumacheva E (2004a) Monodisperse chitosan nanoparticles for mucosal drug delivery. Biomacromolecules 5:2461–2468. doi:10.1021/bm0496211
Zhang H, Wang Z, Zhang Y, Zhang X (2004b) Hydrogen-bonding-directed layer-by-layer assembly of poly(4-vinylpyridine) and poly(4-vinylphenol): effect of solvent composition on multilayer buildup. Langmuir 20:9366–9370. doi:10.1021/la048685u
Zhang HL, Bai TC, Yan GB, Hu YJ (2005) Solubility of silybin in aqueous poly (vinylpyrrolidone) solution. Fluid Phase Equilibria 238:186–192. doi:10.1016/j.fluid.2005.10.004
Zhang HG, Kim H, Liu C, Yu S, Wang J, Grizzle WE (2007) Curcumin reverses breast tumor exosomes mediated immune suppression of NK cell tumor cytotoxicity. Biochim Biophys Acta 1773:1116–11123. doi:10.1016/j.bbamer.2007.04.015
Zhang L, Pornpattananangkul D, Hu CMJ, Huang CM (2010) Development of nanoparticles for antimicrobial drug delivery. Curr Med Chem 17:585–594
Zheng Z, Zhang X, Carbo D, Clark C, Nathan CA, Lvov Y (2010) Sonication assisted synthesis of polyelectrolyte coated curcumin nanoparticles. Langmuir 26:7679–7681. doi:10.1021/la101246a
Zhou J, Moya S, Ma L, Gao C, Shen J (2009) Polyelectrolyte coated PLGA nanoparticles: templation and release behavior. Macromol Biosci 4:326–335. doi:10.1002/mabi.200800188
Zillies JC, Zwiorek K, Winter G, Coester C (2007) Method for quantifying the PEGylation of gelatin nanoparticle drug carrier systems using asymmetrical flow field-flow fractionation and refractive index detection. Anal Chem 79:4574–4580. doi:10.1021/ac062135e
Zwiorek K, Klockner J, Wanger E, Coester C (2004) Gelatin nanoparticles as a new and simple gene delivery system. J Pharm Pharm Sci 7:22–28

Chapter 10
Induction of Autophagy by Polyphenolic Compounds in Cancer: A Novel Strategy to induce cell death and to Treat Cancer

Bulent Ozpolat, Kevin Dalby, and Gabriel Lopez-Berestein

Abstract Apoptosis (type I) and autophagy-associated cell death (type II) are both highly regulated forms of programmed cell death and play crucial roles in physiological processes such as the development, homeostasis and selective elimination of cells. Autophagy is an evolutionarily conserved lysosomal pathway for degrading cytoplasmic proteins, macromolecules, and organelles and functions as a survival pathway in response to nutrient and growth factor deprivation. If the process is induced excessively, autophagy leads to cell death. In contrast to apoptosis, cell death occurring with autophagy is caspase-independent and does not involve classic DNA laddering. Accumulating evidence suggests that cancer cells that are resistant to apoptosis can be killed by death associated with autophagy, providing an alternative cell death pathway to eliminate cancer cells. We and others found that natural polyphenolic compounds, such as rottlerin, resveratrol, curcumin, genistein, and quercetin can induce cell death associated with autophagy in a variety of cancer cells, including pancreatic, breast, glioma, colon, ovarian cancers and acute myeloid leukemia. More importantly, these compounds can enhance the effects of chemotherapy and reduce the required dose to induce cell death in cancer cells. In this chapter we will discuss the polyphenolic compounds and the mechanism by which they induce cell death occurring with autophagy in cancer cells and their potential as a novel strategy for the treatment of cancer.

B. Ozpolat (✉) • G. Lopez-Berestein
Department of Experimental Therapeutics, M.D. Anderson Cancer Center, The University of Texas, Houston, TX 77030, USA
e-mail: bozpoldt@mddnderson.org

K. Dalby
Division of Medicinal Chemistry, College of Pharmacy, The University of Texas at Austin, Austin, TX 78712, USA

M. Diederich and K. Noworyta (eds.), *Natural Compounds as Inducers of Cell Death: Volume 1*, DOI 10.1007/978-94-007-4575-9_10,

10.1 Introduction

Autophagy is an evolutionarily conserved and highly regulated process of large-scale lysosomal degradation of long-lived proteins, macromolecules, ribosomes, and organelles, such as the endoplasmic reticulum, Golgi apparatus, and mitochondria. The term authophagy is derived from the Greek roots "auto" (self) and "phagy" (to eat) and means self-digestion. It is considered to be a physiological mechanism that may serve as a means of temporary survival, and is triggered by starvation (amino acid and nutrient deprivation), hypoxia, and metabolic stress. Self-digestion provides a means of recycling macromolecules as an alternative energy source; however, if the cellular stress leads to continuous or excessively induced autophagy, cell death may ensue. Autophagy requires the sequestration of cytoplasmic content through the formation of double-membrane vesicles, mediated by a highly organized and hierarchical team of ATG proteins (Klionsky and Emr 2000) (Fig. 10.1). The initial phagophores are formed from the endoplasmic reticulum and surround and pack organelles to form autophagosomes (Klionsky and Emr 2000; Levine and Klionsky 2004). Subsequently, autophagosomes merge with lysosomes and digest the contents (i.e., misfolded proteins and organelles), generating building blocks for the synthesis of macromolecules and metabolites for use as an energy source, eventually leading

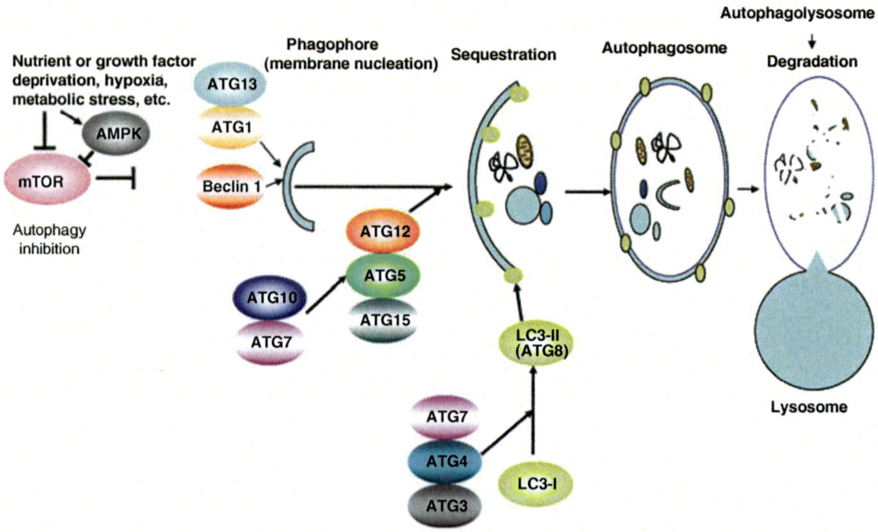

Fig. 10.1 Regulation of autophagic process in cells. Autophagy is induced in response to nutrient or growth factor deprivation, hypoxia and cellular stress. PI3K/mTOR pathway suppresses induction of autophagy under normal conditions. Starvation and reduced ATP/ADP ratio lead to inhibition of mTOR, which function as a energy sensor, leading to induction of autophagy. The process requires involvement of ATG proteins and eventually formation of double-layer membrane and engulfment of cellular component that are digested by merging with lysosomes following formation of autophagolysosomes

to either cell survival or cell death depending on the duration and severity of the process (Klionsky and Emr 2000; Levine and Klionsky 2004).

Autophagy associated cell – death occurs during tissue and organ development to eliminate unnecessary cells (Clarke 1990; Klionsky and Emr 2000). Depending on cell type and context, macroautophagy (autophagy from here on) seems to have different roles. For example, in fully transformed or cancer cells it appears to function as a tumor suppressor as defective autophagy is associated with malignant transformation and carcinogenesis. However, in normal cells and in some cancer cells it appears to function as a protective mechanism against cellular stress and yet the induction of autophagy by some natural compounds is associated with cell death in some type of cancers.

10.2 Cell Death Occurring with Autophagy

Apoptosis (programmed cell death-PCD-type I) and necrosis are well known mechanisms of cell death induced by anticancer therapies. Recent studies have demonstrated the existence of a non-apoptotic form of programmed death called cell death associated with autophagy, which is now considered as a PCD-type II. In contrast to apoptosis, this type of cell death is caspase-independent and does not involve classic DNA laddering and is believed to be a result of an extensive autophagic degradation of intracellular content (Kirisako et al. 1999).

Studies showed that cytotoxic signals can induce autophagy in cells that are resistant to apoptosis (apoptosis defective), such as those expressing high levels of Bcl-2 or Bcl-XL, those lacking Bax and Bak, or those being exposed to pan-caspase inhibitors, such as zVAD-fmk (Shimizu et al. 2004). Pro-apoptotic Bcl-2 family member proteins, Bak and Bax, regulate an intrinsic apoptotic pathway by causing mitochondrial outer membrane permeabilization and cyctochrome c release. Bax and Bak (–/–) knockout fibroblast cells have been shown to be resistant to apoptosis and undergo an autophagy associated cell death, following starvation, growth factor withdrawal, chemotherapy (etoposide) or radiation (Moretti et al. 2007; Shimizu et al. 2004). The evidence suggests that autophagy leads to cell death in response to several compounds, including polyphenols such as rottlerin, (Akar et al. 2007) (Fig. 10.2), curcumin (Shinojima et al. 2007), resveratrol, genistein and quercetin (Singletary and Milner 2008), and some chemotherapeutics (cytosine arabinoside (Xue et al. 1999), etoposide) and staurosporine (Shimizu et al. 2004) as well as growth factor deprivation (Xue et al. 1999). A link between autophagy and related cell death has been demonstrated using pharmacological (e.g. 3-MA) and genetic (silencing of *ATG5, ATG7 and Beclin-1*) approaches for suppression of autophagy. For example, the knockdown of ATG5 or Beclin-1 in cancer cells containing defects in apoptosis lead to a marked reduction in cell death and autophagic response in response to cell death stimuli with no sign of apoptosis (Akar et al. 2007, 2008). Studies also suggest that apoptosis and autophagy are linked by effector proteins (e.g., Bcl-2, Bcl-XL, Mcl-1, ATG5, p53) and common pathways (e.g., PI3K/Akt/mTOR,

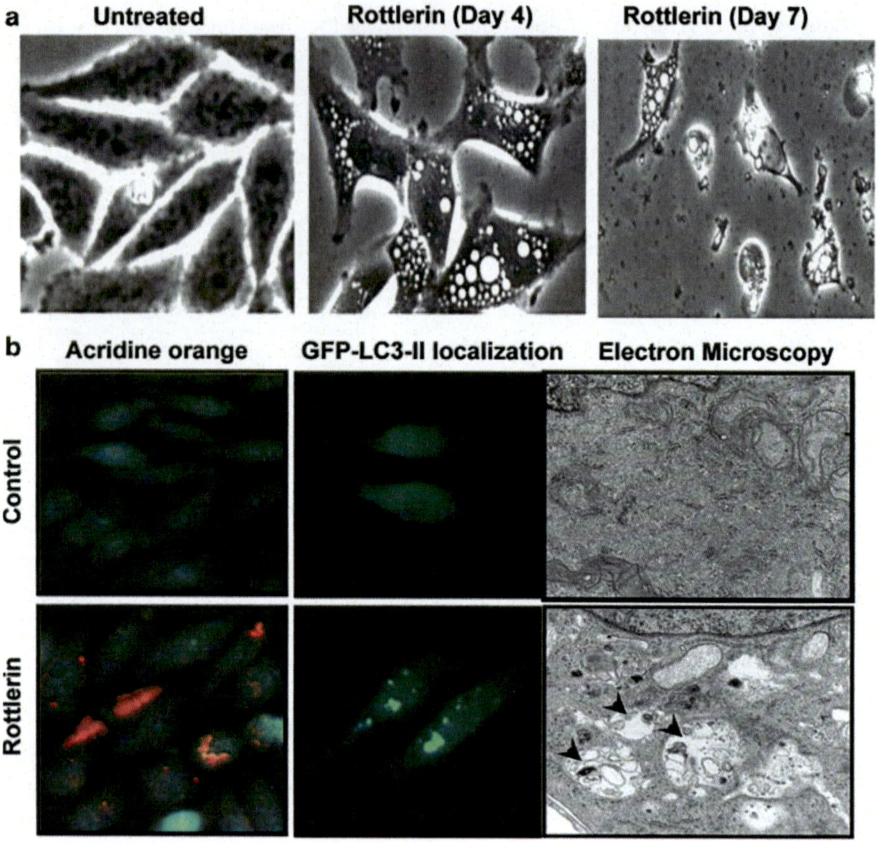

Fig. 10.2 Rottlerin induced autophagy and detection of autophagolysosomes; (**a**) MDA-Panc28 cells were treated with Rottlerin for 48 h. acridine orange staining of the acidic vesicular organelles by fluorescent microscopy (*left panels*) and the localization LC3- II at autophagosomes in cells after transfection with GFP-LC3 plasmid (*middle panels*). Green fluorescence intensity indicates cytoplasm and nucleus, while *red color* intensity shows acidic vesicular organelles. Electron micrographs showing the ultrastructure of panc28 cells treated with Rottlerin (4 μM). Numerous autophagic vacuoles pointed by *arrows* were observed in the rottlerin treated cells. (**b**). Morphological changes and formation of autophagic vacuoles observed after rottlerin treatment of Panc28 cells that were treated with 4 μM rottlerin. Microphotographs were taken using a phase-contrast microscope (300× magnification). *Left panel*, untreated cells at 48 h of treatment; *center panel*, cells treated for 96 h; and *right panel*, cells treated for 7 days (168 h)

NF-kB, ERK1/2) (Akar et al. 2008; Lockshin and Zakeri 2007; Pattingre et al. 2005; Shimizu et al. 2004; Yousefi et al. 2006). Overall, there is evidence that autophagy may function as a type II PCD in cancer cells in which apoptosis is defective or hard to induce. Therefore it is reasonable to propose the notion that the induction of cell death occurring with autophagy may be used as a novel therapeutic strategy to treat cancer.

10.2.1 Autophagy as a Tumor Suppressor Mechanism

Cancer cells often display a reduced autophagic capacity compared to their normal counterparts. Studies have shown that cancer cells express lower levels of the autophagy-related proteins LC3-II and Beclin-1 (BECN1) when compared to normal epithelial cells (Kondo et al. 2005; Qu et al. 2003), and that while heterozygous disruption of *BECN1* promotes tumorigenesis (Qu et al. 2003) the overexpression inhibits tumorigenesis (Liang et al. 1999), supporting the contention that defective autophagy or the inhibition of autophagy plays a role in malignant transformation. The Beclin-1 gene is deleted in about 40% of prostate, 50% of breast, and 75% of ovarian cancers (Aita et al. 1999; Liang et al. 1999; Shen et al. 2008). In addition, reduced expression of *Beclin-1* has been reported in other types of cancers, including human colon cancer (Koneri et al. 2007), brain tumors (Miracco et al. 2007) hepatocellular carcinomas (Daniel et al. 2007), and cervical cancers (Wang et al. 2006). Overall, data suggest that a defective autophagic process is linked to cancer development.

The most important evidence linking dysfunctional autophagy and cancer come from studies demonstrating that the inhibition of autophagy in mice, by disruption of *BECN1*, increases cellular proliferation, increases the frequency of spontaneous malignancies (i.e., lung cancer, liver cancer, and lymphomas) as well as mammary hyperplasia and accelerates the development of carcinogen (i.e., hepatitis B virus)-induced pre-malignant lesions. In addition, transfection of MCF-7 breast cancer cells (which express low levels of Beclin-1) with Beclin-1 inhibits growth and tumor formation (Liang et al. 1999), further suggesting that Beclin-1 is a haploinsufficient tumor suppressor and that defective autophagy may be critical for the malignant transformation of cells (Qu et al. 2003; Yue et al. 2003; Edinger and Thompson 2003). Furthermore, defects in autophagy (e.g., reduced beclin-1 expression) have not only been shown to be associated with a malignant phenotype, but also poor prognosis of cancer patients with hepatocellular carcinoma (Ding et al. 2008).

Overall, the available evidence suggests that the expression of autophagic genes and their corresponding autophagic activities are frequently suppressed in cancer cells and that autophagy plays a critical role in carcinogenesis as a tumor suppressor, which impacts patient response to therapy. Therefore, the induction of autophagy may help to reverse the malignant phenotype.

10.2.2 Autophagy as a Survival Pathway

The physiological function of autophagy is related to the maintenance of cellular homeostasis in response to nutrient and growth factor deprivation and under cellular and metabolic stress, such as hypoxia. Starvation or nutrient deprivation-induced autophagy is mediated by mTOR and AMPK. mTOR has been reported to functions as a suppressor of autophagy in response to an increased ADP/ATP ratio. Reduction of ATP during starvation activates AMP-activated protein kinase (AMPK), an evolutionarily conserved serine/threonine protein kinase, serves as an energy sensor in all eukaryotic cells and inhibits mTOR (Klionsky and Emr 2000). While a number of protein kinases have been reported to regulate the induction of autophagy following nutrient deprivation or other cell stresses, to date, only the following protein kinases have been reported to induce 'protective' autophagy in cancer cells in response to cytotoxic agents: AMP-activated protein kinase (AMPK) (Harhaji-Trajkovic et al. 2009; Herrero-Martin et al. 2009; Liang et al. 2007; Meijer and Codogno 2007), jun *N*-terminal kinase (JNK) (Zhang et al. 2008, 2009b), eukaryotic elongation factor-2 kinase (eEF2K) (Wu et al. 2009), extracellular signal-regulated kinases 1 and 2 (ERK1/2) (Shinojima et al. 2007; Sivaprasad and Basu 2008), protein kinase C (Zhang et al. 2009a), PKR-like endoplasmic reticulum kinase (PERK) (Park et al. 2008a, b), and glycogen synthase kinase 3 (GSK3) beta (Wang et al. 2009).

In some cases (e.g., AMPK and JNK), there is mechanistic evidence linking the kinases to known regulators of autophagy. For example, AMPK inhibits the phosphatidylinositol kinase homolog mammalian target of rapamycin (mTOR) under conditions of energy stress (Meijer and Codogno 2007). mTOR is activated by nutrients and amino acids, as well as mitogenic signaling molecules such as insulin, and is an important negative regulator of autophagy (Meijer and Codogno 2004). Inhibition of mTOR by AMPK is, therefore, believed to be the mechanism by which AMPK induces protective autophagy (Papandreou et al. 2008). JNK has been shown to promote the expression of the pro-autophagy protein BECN-1 in a c-Jun-dependent manner following ceramide treatment (Li et al. 2009a). BECN-1 is an important autophagy protein, which is recruited to a multi-protein complex containing the lipid kinase Vps34, which induces nucleation of autophagosomes (Liang et al. 2006; Takahashi et al. 2007). JNK has also been shown to promote autophagy by inducing the release of BECN-1 from an inhibitory Bcl-2–BECN-1 complex (Wei et al. 2008). The protein serine/threonine kinase eEF2K is negatively regulated by mTOR and promotes autophagy in several tumor cells in response to cell stress (Hait et al. 2006; Wu et al. 2006, 2009), suggesting a possible link between the inhibition of global protein synthesis and the induction of autophagy. The mechanisms underlying the activity of ERK2, PKC, GSK3, and PERK are presently unknown. Other protein kinases implicated in the promotion of autophagy include death-associated protein kinase (DAPK) (Gozuacik and Kimchi 2006) and Unc-51-like kinase 1 (ULK-1) (Ganley et al. 2009; Hara and Mizushima 2009). DAPK interacts with and is activated by the microtubule-associated protein MAP1B, which also binds the autophagy protein LC3. DAPK is reported to promote Vps34 activation by promoting the release of BECN-1 from inhibitory complexes (Zalckvar et al. 2009). ULK-1 appears to be a major downstream effector of mTOR and may be essential for the induction of autophagy (Chan et al. 2009).

Autophagy is upregulated at advanced stages of tumor progression. Utilizing autophagy as a survival mechanism in the harsh tumor microenvironment, which is highly hypoxic and acidic, works in favor of cancer cells as a survival pathway. Indeed, some types of cancer cells may exploit autophagy as a means to adapt to the hypoxic, nutrient-limiting, and metabolically stressful tumor microenvironment and to therapeutically induced cell stress or damage (Rouschop and Wouters 2009).

A number of antineoplastic therapies, including, radiation therapy, chemotherapy (e.g., doxorubicin, temozolomide, etoposide), histone deaceltylase inhibitors, arsenic trioxide, TNF-α, IFN-γ, imatinib, rapamycin, and anti-estrogen hormonal therapy (e.g., tamoxifen), have been observed to induce autophagy as a protective and pro-survival mechanism in human cancer cell lines (Lavieu et al. 2007). In fact, the therapeutic efficacy of these agents can be increased if autophagy is inhibited (Abedin et al. 2007; Amaravadi et al. 2007; Apel et al. 2008; Boya et al. 2005; Carew et al. 2007; Hayashi et al. 2007; Kanzawa et al. 2004; Katayama et al. 2007; Paglin et al. 2001; Qadir et al. 2008; Sotelo et al. 2006).

Hypoxia is one of the most important factors in tumor microenvironment that induces autophagy through a HIF1-α-dependent and independent mechanisms, suggesting that autophagy is involved in cancer cell survival by increasing resistance to hypoxic stress in the tumor microenvironment (Zhang et al. 2008a, b; Bellot et al. 2009) . Overall, data suggest that anti-cancer therapies induce a type of protective orpro-survival autophagy, which increases the cancer cells' resistance to therapies, and that inhibition of autophagy may lead to increased cell death and inhibition of tumor growth.

10.3 Monitoring Autophagy in Eukaryotic Cells

Recently guidelines and methods for the use and interpretation of assays for monitoring autophagy in higher eukaryotic cells were published (Klionsky et al. 2008). There are many useful and convenient methods to monitor macroautophagy in yeast, but relatively few acceptable methods are available for higher eukaryotic model systems. Briefly, autophagy is evidenced nonspecifically by acridine orange (AO) (Fig. 10.2a, left panel) or monodansylcadaverine (MDC) staining that reveal the presence of acidic vacuoles (Akar et al. 2007). The number of AO or MDC-stained cells can be quantitatively determined by fluorescence-activated cell sorting (FACS) analysis. More specifically, autophagic vacuoles or autophagosomes are demonstrated by increased expression of microtubule-associated protein light chain 3-II (LC3-II), a hallmark of autophagy, by Western blot analysis LC3, the homologue of the yeast *Atg8/Aut7p* gene, localizes to the autophagosomal membrane during autophagy. During autophagy LC3-I (16 kDa) is cleaved at the *C*-terminus and becomes attached covalently to phosphatidyl ethanolamine (PE), generating LC3-II (18 kDa). This specifically localizes to autophagosome membranes and is indicative of autophagy induction. Similarly, the translocation or accumulation of GFP-LC3-II into autophagosomes of GFP-LC3-transfected cells provides evidence for autophagy as seen during the course of rottlerin treatment(Fig. 10.2a, middle panel and b) (Akar et al. 2007). A gold standard for assessing the presence of autophagy is transmission electron microscopy (TEM), which can clearly demonstrate the presence of autophagosomes in cells (Fig.10.2a right panel). Assessment of the half-life of long-lived proteins, co-localization with lysosomal markers overlapping detection signals with the mitochondrion and endoplasmic reticulum provide alternative methods for detecting autophagy that are explained in detail in a recent review

(Tasdemir et al. 2008). The key point is that there is a difference between measurements that monitor the numbers of autophagosomes versus those that measure flux through the autophagy pathway; thus, a block in macroautophagy that results in autophagosome accumulation needs to be differentiated from fully functional autophagy that includes delivery to, and degradation within, lysosomes (in most higher eukaryotes) or the vacuole (in plants and fungi) (Galluzzi et al. 2009). Usually, several of the assays described above are used to demonstrate autophagy, because no individual assay is guaranteed to be the most appropriate one in every situation. Thus, the use of multiple assays to verify an autophagic response is recommended.

Cell death occurring with autophagy is considered caspase independent cell death and does not show the classical DNA laddering associated with apoptosis. However membrane blebbing is observed in both types of cell death (Kondo et al. 2005). Most studies first demonstrate induction of autophagy following insult using some of the assays mentioned above. Later the induction of apoptosis is ruled out as a mechanism of cell death using a pan-caspase inhibitor (e.g. zVAD-fms) and evaluating whether cell death is inhibited. If cell death is not inhibited then the inhibition of the autophagic process is affected either by using chemical inhibitors, such as 3-methyladenine (3-MA), bafilomycin A1, hydroxychloroquine or chloroquine, or by genetically knocking down autophagy genes, such as ATG6 (Beclin-1), ATG7, ATG8, or ATG5 using siRNA. If inhibition of cell death after treatment with a drug being tested is blocked by chemical or genetic methods (siRNA) the mechanism of cell death is most likely through autophagy.

10.4 Polyphenolic Compounds and Cell Death Occurring with Autophagy

Polyphenols are a group of chemical substances found in plants, characterized by the presence of more than one phenol unit or building block per molecule (Fig. 10.3). A variety of natural polyphenolic compounds found in food possess anticancer activity against different cancer types. The flavonoid polyphenols genistein, and quercetin, the flavonoid-like rottlerin, the stilbene resveratrol and the curcuminoid curcumin have been shown to induce cell death occurring with autophagy in a variety of cancer cells, including pancreatic, breast, glioma and ovarian cancers and acute myeloid leukemia (Table 10.1). More importantly, these compounds can enhance the effects of chemotherapy and reduce the required dose to induce cell death in cancer cells.

10.4.1 Rottlerin

Rottlerin, isolated from Mallotus Philippinensis, has been used as a selective inhibitor of PKC delta. However, recent studies suggest that rottlerin can inhibit many kinases and exerts many biological effects, such as autophagic, apoptotic cell death and mitochondrial uncoupling (Akar et al. 2007; Lim et al. 2008; Soltoff 2007; Song et al. 2008).

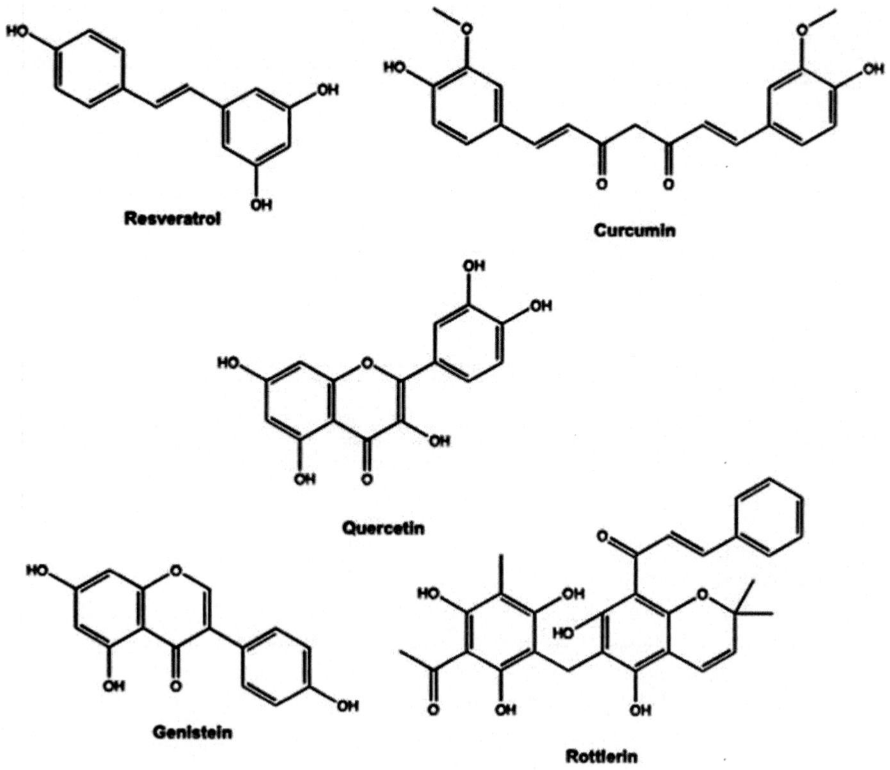

Fig. 10.3 Structure of polyphenolic compounds that induce cell death occurring with autophagy in various cancer cells

Our recent study provided the first evidence that Rottlerin induces significant cell death occurring with autophagy in pancreatic cancer cells (Akar et al. 2007). Pancreatic ductal adenocarcinomas are one of the most aggressive human malignancies with a 2–3% 5-year survival rate. The major reason for poor prognosis is that pancreatic cancer cells are frequently insensitive to the induction of apoptosis by standard chemotherapeutic agents. Therefore induction of cell death occurring with autophagy provides an alternative mechanism, which could potentially be used as a novel therapeutic strategy to kill apoptosis-defective or resistant cancer cells.

Rottlerin inhibits PKCδ, PI3K/Akt and NF-κB at doses of 2–4 μM and induces autophagy in pancreatic cancer cells (Akar et al. 2007). We found that at this dose it induced significant autophagic changes, including vacuole formation and eventually cell death occurring with autophagy with no sign of apoptosis (Fig. 10.2a, b). Rottlerin and inhibition of TG2 induced significant vacuolization at day 1 and a marked cell death at days 4–7 (Fig. 10.2a). We found no evidence of apoptosis (examined by three different assays, data not shown) (Akar et al. 2007). Rottlerin inhibits the expression of PKCδ at both the protein and message level detected by RT-PCR, as well as tissue transglutaminase 2 (TG2) at the protein level. It was also

Table 10.1 Induction of autophagic death by polyphenolic compounds (Modified from Singletary and Milner 2008)

Treatment	Cell/tissue	Mechanism	Dose μM	Reference
Rottlerin	Pancreatic cancer	PKCδ/TG2	4	Akar et al. (2007)
Resveratrol	Ovarian cancer	Akt, mTOR, glycolysis	50	Opipari et al. (2004)
Resveratrol	Colorectal cancer	Vps34, AMPK	100	Hwang et al. (2007)
Resveratrol	Salivary gland cancer	PELP1	50–100	Ohshiro et al. (2007)
Resveratrol	Lung cancer	PELP1	50–100	Ohshiro et al. (2007)
Resveratrol	CML	AMPK		Puissant et al. (2010)
Curcumin	Brain cancer	Akt/mTOR/S6 kinase, ERK1/2	40	Aoki et al. (2007) and Shinojima et al. (2007)
Curcumin	CML	Bcl-2, SIRT1		Jia et al. (2009)
Genistein	Ovarian cancer	Akt	50	Gossner et al. (2007)
Quacertin	Colon cancer	Ras	20	Psahoulia et al. (2007)

demonstrated that a specific inhibition of PKCδ by siRNA leads to inhibition of TG2 expression suggesting that PKCδ plays a critical role in the regulation of TG2 expression in pancreatic cancer cells (Akar et al. 2007). Inhibition of PKCδ and TG2 expression by rottlerin treatment induced expression of LC-3-II, a hallmark of autophagy, in all pancreatic cancer cell lines tested, including Panc28, Capan-2, Bx-PC3, Panc1 and MIAPaCA (Ozpolat et al. 2007). Rottlerin-induced autophagy was demonstrated by acridine orange staining, punctuate patterning of GFP-LC3 transfected cells and the formation of autophagosomes in Panc28 pancreatic cancer cells (detected by electron microscopy, Fig. 10.2a). The knocking down of TG2 by siRNA also result in the induction of autophagy in Panc28 cells. These results suggest that rottlerin induces cell death occurring with autophagy by the inhibition of PKCδ and its downstream target TG2 in pancreatic cancer cells. Knockdown of Beclin-1 by siRNA in the panc28 pancreatic cancer cell line does not reduce the number of cells undergoing autophagy (as detected by acridine orange staining and inhibition of LC3-II expression), suggesting that Beclin-1 mediates cell death occurring with autophagy induced by the inhibition of PKCδ and/or TG2.

The protein kinase C family is associated with the development of many types of cancers, and have emerged as well-defined targets for directed cancer chemotherapy (Koivunen et al. 2006). PKCδ can function as an anti-apoptotic or pro-apoptotic factor and can regulate cell proliferation and cell survival functions and metastatic phenotype depending on the cell type (Jackson and Foster 2004; La Porta and Comolli 2000). In pancreatic cancer cells, PKCδ expression promotes anchorage-independent growth and activation of NF-κB (Satoh et al. 2004). More importantly, it was previously reported that TG2 expression induces activation of the transcription factor NF-κB (Mann et al. 2006), suggesting that PKCδ-induced NF-κB may be mediated by TG2. Recent findings of Fabre et al. (Fabre et al. 2007) showed that NF-κB inhibition could lead to an inhibition of cell death occurring with autophagy. Rottlerin has been shown to inhibits the NF-κB pathway (Ozpolat et al. 2007), of which inhibition leads to autophagy in glioma cells however it remains to be tested whether the inhibition of NF-κB induces cell death occurring with autophagy in pancreatic cancer cells.

Thus, further investigation is required to show whether rottlerin-induced inhibition of NF-κB also plays a role in the induction of cell death occurring with autophagy in pancreatic cancers. In addition to Beclin-1, ATG5 may also be involved in PKCδ/TG2-mediated suppression of autophagy. Down-regulation of Bcl-2 (anti-apoptotic and anti-autophagic protein) leads to autophagy in breast and leukemia cells. Rottlerin also induces the down-regulation of Bcl-2, which suggests it may participate in autophagy induction following down-regulation of Bcl-2 in the pancreatic cancer cells (B. Ozpolat unpublished observations). mTOR (mammalian target of rapamycin) has been shown to regulate autophagy. Although rottlerin induced-authophagy is associated with inhibition the activity of mTOR (p-mTOR) and p-p70S6K, a downstream target of mTOR in Panc28 cells, rapamycin, a specific inhibitor of mTOR, fails to induce autophagy, indicating that rottlerin-induced autophagy is not mediated by inhibition of mTOR alone (Akar et al. 2007).

Rottlerin inhibits the expression of TG2, which is a highly important survival protein in cancer cells. Tissue transglutaminase (TG2, EC 2.3.2.13) catalyzes Ca^{2+}-dependent post-translational modifications of proteins (Lorand and Graham 2003; Mhaouty-Kodja 2004). Transamidation by TG2 can both facilitate and inhibit apoptosis, while the GTP-bound form of the enzyme generally protects cells against death (Fesus and Szondy 2005). We and others found that TG2 is over-expressed not only in pancreatic cancer cell lines and primary cancer cells but also in other solid tumors such as breast cancer and melanoma (Herman et al. 2006; Mehta et al. 2004) (Elsasser et al. 1993; Iacobuzio-Donahue et al. 2003; Verma et al. 2006). More importantly, our recent findings suggest that TG2 expression plays a role in the development of drug resistance, metastatic phenotypes and poor prognosis in pancreatic cancer cells (Verma et al. 2006). However, the regulation of TG2 is still not well understood. Our current data shed some light on the regulation, a novel function of TG2 in autophagy and its possible role in tumorigenesis and in reducing chemosensitivity of pancreatic cancer cells, which is virtually resistant to standard chemotherapy and radiation. These observations suggest that rottlerin inhibits PKCδ/TG2 signaling which may serve as an excellent therapeutic target for the induction of cell death occurring with autophagy in pancreatic cancer and possibly other solid tumors over-expressing TG2. Whether targeting TG2 can induce *in vivo* cell death occurring with autophagy and inhibit tumor growth remains to be tested.

Rottlerin was also shown to induce autophagy and apoptotic cell death through a PKC-delta-independent pathway in HT1080 human fibrosarcoma cells. However, in this case rottlerin induced-autophagy did not lead to cell death, rather it functioned as a protective survival pathway (Song et al. 2008). In HT1080 human fibrosarcoma cells, rottlerin treatment induced a dose- and time-dependent inhibition of cell growth and formation of autophagic vacuoles that were associated with the induction of the LC3-II autophagy marker protein level. Prolonged exposure to rottlerin eventually caused apoptosis via loss of mitochondrial membrane potential and translocation of AIF from mitochondria to the nucleus. However, the activities of caspase-3, -8, and -9 were not changed, and PARP did not show signs of cleavage. The pretreatment of cells with an inhibitor of autophagy (3-methyladenine) accelerated rottlerin-induced apoptosis as revealed by an analysis of the subdiploid fraction (sub G1 DNA contents) and TUNEL assay, indicating that rottlerin-induced early autophagy may act as a survival mechanism against late apoptosis in HT1080 human fibrosarcoma cells. Song et al., found that the knockdown of PKC-δ by RNA interference neither affected cell growth nor acidic vacuole formation. Similarly, rottlerin-induced cell death was not prevented by PKCδ over-expression. Taken together, these findings suggest that rottlerin induces early autophagy and late apoptosis in a PKCδ-independent manner in the fibroblastoma cell line (Song et al. 2008).

In conclusion, elucidating molecular mechanisms by which rottlerin induces autophagy is invaluable to identifying effective strategies for the development of novel agents against different cancer types.

10.4.2 Resveratrol

Resveratrol (3,5,4-trihydroxystilbene), a polyphenol stilbene found in the skins of red grapes, red wine, berries, and nuts, has been shown to induce apoptosis, necrosis and autophagy in cancer cells. Resveratrol also exhibits a wide range of biological activities, including anti-inflammatory, anticancer, antimutagenic, antiplatelet, and antifungal properties (Jang et al. 1997). Resveratrol induces cell death by different mechanisms. These include the activation of caspases through CD95/CD95L, the up-regulation of the cyclin-dependent kinase (CDK) inhibitor $p21^{Waf1/Cip1}$, and the up-regulation of cytokines such as TNFα. It also leads to the down-regulation of cell survival proteins such as survivin, cFLIP, cIAPs, XIAP, Bcl-2, and Bcl-XL as well as the up-regulation of bax and bak. Resveratrol is also known to inhibit cell survival pathways related kinases (e.g., p38 MAPK, ERK1/2, IκBα kinase, JNK, PKD, AKT/Phosphoinositide 3-Kinase (PI3K), PKC, EGFR kinase) and HIF-1α, (Shakibaei et al. 2009). Resveratrol can suppress the activation of several transcription factors, including STAT3, NF-κB, activating protein 1 (AP-1), and Egr-1 and it can down-regulate products of genes such as COX-2, 5-LOX, VEGF, IL-1, IL-6, IL-8, AR and PSA. These activities may account for the suppression of angiogenesis by resveratrol. Resveratrol has also been shown to potentiate the apoptotic effects of cytokines (e.g., TRAIL), chemotherapeutic agents and gamma-radiation (Aggarwal et al. 2004).

In A2780 ovarian cancer cells, resveratrol exhibited antineoplastic activity and caused mitochondrial release of cytochrome c, apoptosome formation, and caspase activation (Opipari et al. 2004). Resveratrol inhibits growth and induces death in five different ovarian carcinoma cell lines. Interestingly, resveratrol-induced death is caspase independent and is accompanied by formation of monodansylcadaverine-positive autophagocytic granules containing extensively degraded organelles (Opipari et al. 2004). Consistent with resveratrol's ability to kill cells via non-apoptotic or cell death occurring with autophagy, cells transfected to express high levels of the anti-apoptotic proteins Bcl-x(L) and Bcl-2 are found to be equally sensitive to resveratrol. In A2780 cells resveratrol-induced autophagocytosis involves inhibition of glucose uptake and glycolysis and is associated with the down-regulation of p-Akt and mTOR (Kueck et al. 2007). Thus, the relative contribution of each pathway to resveratrol-induced cell death seems to be dose dependent. Resveratrol causes Tyr-15 phosphorylation of cdc2 via the ATM/ATR-Chk1/2-Cdc25C pathway as a central mechanism for S phase arrest in human ovarian carcinoma Ovcar-3 cells. More importantly, resveratrol suppresses growth of human ovarian cancer tumors in murine xenograft models (Lee et al. 2009), suggesting that this compound is effective in *in vivo* settings and has potential to be used as a mono therapy or in combination with conventional therapies against ovarian cancer.

Resveratrol have also been shown to activate SIRT1 directly or indirectly in a variety of models (Chung et al. 2010). However, resveratrol induces cell survival by stimulating SIRT1-dependent deacetylation of p53, leading to protective or pro-survival type of autophagy rather than autophagy associated cell death in yeast. In the same system, resveratrol mimics calorie restriction by stimulating Sir2, increasing DNA stability and extending lifespan by 70% (Howitz et al. 2003). Resveratrol-induced SIRT1 seems to be responsible not only for autophagy also for apoptosis and exerts multiple effects such as in the regulation of metabolism, cellular survival and longevity. SIRT1 regulates autophagic vacuole formation and degradation of toxic debris, misfolded proteins and damaged organelles, either directly or indirectly suggesting that autophagy may play a key role of in survival and the regulation of longevity.

Resveratrol triggers autophagy associated cell death in imatinib-sensitive and imatinib-resistant chronic myelogenous leukemia cells (CML) K562, via JNK-mediated p62/SQSTM1 expression and AMPK activation (Puissant et al. 2010). It inhibits both mTOR and S6 kinase and activates AMP-activated protein kinase (AMPK); an evolutionarily conserved serine/threonine protein kinase that serves as an energy sensor in all eukaryotic cells. Recent studies suggest that AMPK activation strongly suppresses cell proliferation and induces cell apoptosis and autophagy in a variety of cancer cells (Kourelis and Siegel 2012).

Resveratrol has been shown to strongly activate AMPK in a ROS-dependent manner in chemoresistant (etoposide) HT-29 colon cancer cells and enhances etoposide-induced apoptosis, suggesting that AMPK is an important downstream target that contributes to the effects of resveratrol in colon cancer cells (Hwang et al. 2007).

Resveratrol has been shown to inhibit proliferation and induce autophagy in lung cancer and salivary adenocarcinoma cell lines, at doses ranging from 50 to 100 μM (Ohshiro et al. 2007). Furthermore, resveratrol has gained much attention because it can act as both an estrogen receptor agonist and antagonist, depending on dosage and cellular context. Resveratrol was shown to induce the accumulation of the proline-, glutamic acid, and leucine-rich protein-1 (PELP1), a novel estrogen receptor (ER) coactivator that plays an important role in transcriptional functions of ER. PELP1 accumulates in autophagosomes after resveratrol treatment, providing a link between the actions of PELP1 and autophagy (Ohshiro et al. 2007).

In human U251 glioma and colorectal cancer cells, resveratrol rapidly stimulates autophagy as part of a prosurvival stress response (Trincheri et al. 2008; Li et al. 2009b). However, chronic exposure to resveratrol ultimately leads to autophagy- and caspase-dependent cell death in colorectal cancer cells (Trincheri et al. 2008), suggesting that the length of exposure to resveratrol may also determine type of cell death and its cytotoxic potential. In addition, resveratrol was shown to induce cell death in colorectal cancer cells by a novel pathway involving lysosomal cathepsin D (Trincheri et al. 2007). Resveratrol-induced cell death of U251 glioma was associated with a collapse of the mitochondrial membrane potential (Li et al. 2009b). Li et al. found that pan-caspase inhibitor Z-VAD-fmk suppressed resveratrol-induced U251 cell death. Autophagy inhibitors 3-methylademine (3-MA) and bafilomycin A1 sensitized the cytotoxicity of resveratrol. Together, these findings indicate that resveratrol induces autophagy in human U251 glioma cells and autophagy suppressed resveratrol-induced apoptosis. This study thus suggests that autophagy inhibitors can increase the cytotoxicity of resveratrol to glioma cells. In contrast, in other types of cancer cells such as U937 leukemia cells, resveratrol has been observed to induce only apoptosis (Park et al. 2001). The relative importance of autophagy and apoptosis associated with these cell specific differences needs to be characterized for resveratrol.

In conclusion, resveratrol is an attractive candidate for cancer therapy because of its ability to intervene in different signaling pathways and cellular proteins for the induction of cell death occurring with autophagy, which may be highly useful in triggering cell death in advance cancers and those cancer cells resistant to apoptosis. More importantly resveratrol has potential to go into clinical trials as a monotherapy or in combination with conventional therapies against some cancers.

10.4.3 Curcumin

Curcumin, a nonflavonoid polyphenolic constituent of the spice turmeric, possess a broad spectrum of chemopreventive and therapeutic properties against various tumors in both *in vitro* and *in vivo* models (Thangapazham et al. 2006). It is considered as a promising new therapeutic strategy in cancer because of its potent anticancer activity (Aoki et al. 2007). Currently, curcumin is being tested in phase I and II clinical trials in multiple myeloma and advanced pancreatic cancer, myleodysplastic syndrome and colon cancers. Shinojima et al., demonstrated that curcumin induced non-apoptotic autophagy associated cell death in malignant glioma cells in *in vitro* and *in vivo* models (Shinojima et al. 2007). Curcumin treatment at a dose of 40 μM stimulated G2-M arrest and autophagic death in U87-MG and U373-MG malignant glioma. Curcumin inhibited the Akt/mammalian target of rapamycin (mTOR)/p70 ribosomal protein S6 kinase (p70S6K) pathway and activated the extracellular signal-regulated kinases 1/2 (ERK1/2) thereby inducing autophagy (Aoki et al. 2007). Activation of the Akt/mTOR pathway inhibits curcumin-induced autophagy and cytotoxicity, whereas inhibition of the ERK1/2 pathway inhibits curcumin-induced autophagy and induces apoptosis, thus enhancing the cytotoxicity of curcumin. These results imply that these two autophagic pathways have opposite effects on curcumin's cytotoxicity. However, inhibition of nuclear factor kappaB (NF-κB), which is the main target of curcumin for its anticancer effect, was not observed in malignant glioma cells. These results suggest that autophagy plays a major role in curcumin anticancer therapy. Furthermore, in the subcutaneous xenograft model of U87-MG cells, curcumin inhibited *in vivo* tumor growth significantly and induced autophagy as measured by substantially increased expression of LC-II. These results suggest that curcumin has high anticancer efficacy *in vitro* and *in vivo* by inducing autophagy and warrants further investigation towards possible clinical application in patients with malignant glioma (Aoki et al. 2007).

Curcumin inhibited the viability of K562 CML cells in a dose- and time-dependent manner (Jia et al. 2009). Furthermore, curcumin-induced cell death was associated with the formation of the apoptosome complex, the collapse of the mitochondrial membrane potential, and caspase-3 activation. Curcumin treatment also induced Bid cleavage and down-regulated the expression of Bcl-2, which inhibits autophagy by binding to beclin-1 an autophagy promoting protein. Curcumin also increases the protein levels of beclin 1 as well as levels of membrane LC3-II. The autophagy inhibitor bafilomycin A1 and the pan-caspase inhibitor Z-VAD-fms suppress curcumin-induced K562 cell death, suggesting that curcumin induces autophagic and apoptotic death of K562 leukemia cells and that both apoptotic and autophagic mechanisms contribute to the curcumin-induced cell death. Not only curcumin but also polyphenols such as resveratrol have also been shown to activate SIRT1 directly or indirectly in a variety of models (Chung et al. 2010). Therefore, activation of SIRT1 by these polyphenols is required not only for regulation of autophagy/apoptosis, but also for regulation of oxidative stress, inflammation, cellular senescence, metabolism, adipogenesis, and mitochondria biogenesis, indicating these compounds exerts multiple effects.

Curcumin strongly activates AMPK signaling in a p38-dependent manner in CaOV3 ovarian cancer cells (Pan et al. 2008). Pretreatment of cells with compound C (AMPK inhibitor) and SB203580 (p38 inhibitor) attenuates curcumin-induced cell death, suggesting AMPK and p38 signaling pathways are involved. Curcumin induces p53 phosphorylation (Ser 15) and both compound C and SB203580 pretreatment inhibit p53 phosphorylation. Collectively, data suggest that AMPK, which is a well-established inducer of autophagy, is a molecular effector of curcumin and its activation partially contributes to the cytotoxic effect of curcumin in ovarian cancer cells. Surprisingly, the induction of autophagy and related cell death has not been investigated in this model. However, it is expected that autophagy is induced by curcumin due to strong AMPK induction in ovarian cancer cells.

Overall, curcumin is being evaluated in clinical trials due to its effects on multiple signaling pathways and potent anticancer effects. It not only causes autophagy associated cell death, but also apoptosis depending on the cancer cell type. This compound may be highly useful in triggering cell death in cancers that are resistant to therapy induced apoptosis.

10.4.4 Genistein

Genistein (4′, 5, 7-trihydroxyisoflavone), a naturally occurring isoflavenoid found abundantly in soy products and cruciferous vegetables, has anti-neoplastic activity against various cancer types. Genistein has been shown to induce both apoptotic and cell death occurring with autophagy in cancer cells. Genistein enhances the induction of apoptosis by chemotherapeutic agents, and radiotherapy in cancer cell lines (Banerjee et al. 2008). Genistein is best known for its ability to inhibit cancer progression (Pavese et al. 2010). In particular, genistein has emerged as an important inhibitor of cancer metastasis. Based on a number of population-based studies, consumption of genistein in the diet has been linked to decreased rates of metastatic cancer. Genistein has multiple biochemical effects, including the alteration of cell cycle-regulatory kinase activities (Banerjee et al. 2008). Genistein has been shown to act as an antagonist for estrogen receptor (ER), and inhibits the proliferation of breast cancer cells induced by estradiol (Peterson and Barnes 1996). Because ER receptor antagonists induce protective/pro-survival type autophagy, genistein induced autophagic death may be mediated by another mechanism. In fact, most transcription activation bioassays were not able to show estrogen receptor antagonism of genistein. It is therefore controversial whether the anti-proliferative effect of genistein is ER-dependent or not. There are several mechanisms reported for genistein's anti-neoplastic activity. In ovarian cancer cells, genistein treatment results in apoptosis and a caspase-independent cell death with hallmarks of autophagy (translocation of GFP-LC3 autophagosomes) (Gossner et al. 2007). Genistein treatment was shown to dramatically inhibit glucose uptake in ovarian cancer cells, suggesting that it mimics starvation, which is known to induce autophagy. Methyl pyruvate, a cell-permeable 3-carbon substrate for oxidative phosphorylation and fatty acid synthesis rescues cells from genistein-induced autophagy. In addition, genistein treatment results in reduced levels of phosphorylated Akt, which may contribute towards a mechanism of limiting glucose utilization and reducing activity of mTOR, leading to induction of autophagy (Gossner et al. 2007). A combination of indol-3-carbinol and genistein synergistically induces apoptosis in human colon cancer HT-29 cells by inhibiting Akt phosphorylation and induction of autophagy (Nakamura et al. 2009). Although *in vivo* studies are further required to evaluate efficacy and toxicity of the combination treatment, these findings provide new insight into the development of novel combination therapies against malignant tumors using genistein. Interestingly, genistein just like other polyphenolic compounds (i.e., resveratrol and curcumin) was shown to induce activity of AMP kinase, which may be the major factor contributing to its autophagy-inducing effect (Park et al. 2010).

In summary, genistein is capable of inducing both apoptotic and autophagy associated cell death depending on the cancer cell type and currently is being evaluated in clinical trials. More importantly, it enhances the induction of cell death by chemotherapeutic agents, and radiotherapy in cancer cell lines. It also acts as an chemopreventive agent, making this compound a highly attractive for further testing as single therapeutic agent, co-therapy with conventional agents and chemeopreventive agent in new studies.

10.4.5 Quercetin

Quercetin (3, 3′, 4′, 5, 7-pentahydroxyflavone), a polyphenolic flavonoid found in onions, apples and red wine, has been shown to have anti-proliferative activity *in vitro* and is known to inhibit signal transduction targets including tyrosine kinases, protein kinase C, and PI3 kinase (Matter et al. 1992). It can down-regulate mutant p53 levels (Avila et al. 1994), and as mutant p53 can block apoptosis this is a potential mechanism through which quercetin could facilitate cell death. Interestingly, many studies have provided evidence that quercetin occasionally induces apoptosis in high concentrations in colon cancer cells. Psahoulia et al., provided the first evidence that quercetin induces autophagy in Ha-Ras–transformed human Caco-2 colon cancer cells (Psahoulia et al. 2007), suggesting that quercetin induces cell death occurring with autophagy in colon cancers. In Caco-2, DLD-1 and HT-29 human colon cells, exposure to 5 and 10 μM of quercetin reduced their ability to form colonies in semisolid agar. Quercetin treatment also results in cell cycle arrest and a reduction of Ras protein levels in cell lines expressing oncogenic Ras proteins but not in wild-type Ras-expressing cells (Psahoulia et al. 2007). Interestingly, in cells that only express wild-type Ras or in those where the oncogenic Ras allele is knocked out, quercetin does not induce reduction of Ras levels. However, expression of wild-type Ras or the Ki-Ras proto-oncogene resisted quercetin-induced autophagy, suggesting that activity of specific oncogenes may determine the cellular sensitivity to autophagy (Psahoulia et al. 2007). Moreover, in Ha-*RAS*-transformed cells, quercetin induces autophagic processes.

Overall, in contrast to the polyphenolic compound mentioned earlier quecertin induce predominantly autophagy associated cell death. It needs to determined that when used as co-therapy whether it enhances induction of cell death by chemotherapeutic agents. The data suggest that the quercetin flavonoid may be useful as a chemopreventive agent for cancers expressing frequent mutations of *RAS* genes.

10.5 Concluding Remarks

10.5.1 Targeting Autophagy as a Novel Cancer Therapy

Current data suggest that depending on the context, the induction of autophagy associated cell death may provide therapeutic benefits to patients whose tumors are resistant to apoptosis and that the identification of natural compounds and the design of autophagy-inducing agents may provide novel therapeutic tools and may ultimately lead to new therapeutic strategies in cancer (Figs. 10.4 and 10.5) (Table 10.1). However, precaution must be taken before designing therapies based on induction of autophagy as an anti-cancer therapy because of the role of autophagy, which is complex and may promote survival. It should be kept in mind that the role of autophagy should be carefully evaluated since it may vary between tumor types with regard to their genetic background, mutations, and activated or dominant signaling pathways.

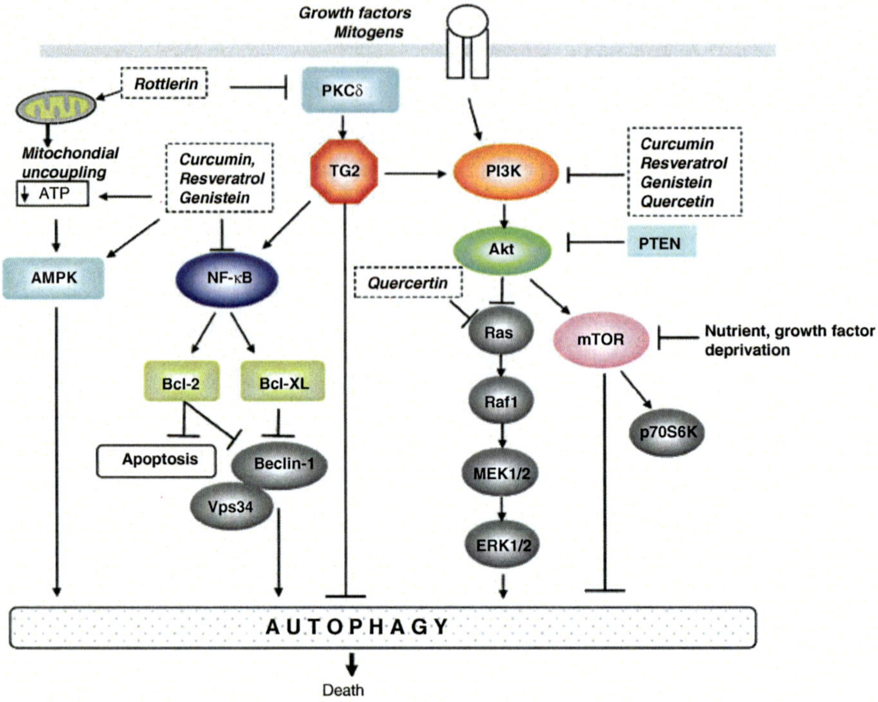

Fig. 10.4 Polyphenolic compounds, including rottlerin, curcumin, resveratrol, genistein, and quercetin, induce cell death occurring with autophagy through inhibition or activation of different signaling pathways and cellular targets in cancer cells. Identification of the molecular targets and the mechanisms by which these compounds induce cell death occurring with autophagy may lead to development of molecularly targeted strategies

Defects in apoptosis leads to increased resistance to chemotherapy, radiotherapy, some anticancer agents and targeted therapies. Therefore, induction of cell death occurring with autophagy may be an ideal approach in those cancers that are resistant to apoptosis by anticancer therapies (e.g., chemotherapy, radiation) (Fig. 10.5). As explained in previous sections cancer cells can undergo cell death occurring with autophagy when apoptotic pathways are defective, or when they are resistant to therapy-induced apoptosis (e.g. in response to DNA-damaging agents such as etoposide). This suggest that autophagic cell death can be induced as an alternative cell death mechanism when cancer cells fail to undergo apoptosis. Therefore, induction of cell death occurring with autophagy may serve as a novel therapeutic tool to eliminate cancer cells with defective apoptosis, which is the case in many advanced, drug resistant and metastatic cancers. We and others have recently demonstrated that the inhibition of some protein kinases (e.g., PKCδ in pancreatic cancer, PI3K/mTOR) or the targeting of key proteins that are involved in the suppression of autophagy (e.g. Bcl-2, TG2, oncogenic Ras and NF-κB) by polyphenolic compounds such as rottlerin, curcumin, resveratrol and quercetin can trigger cell death occurring with autophagy in a variety of cancer cells. On the other hand,

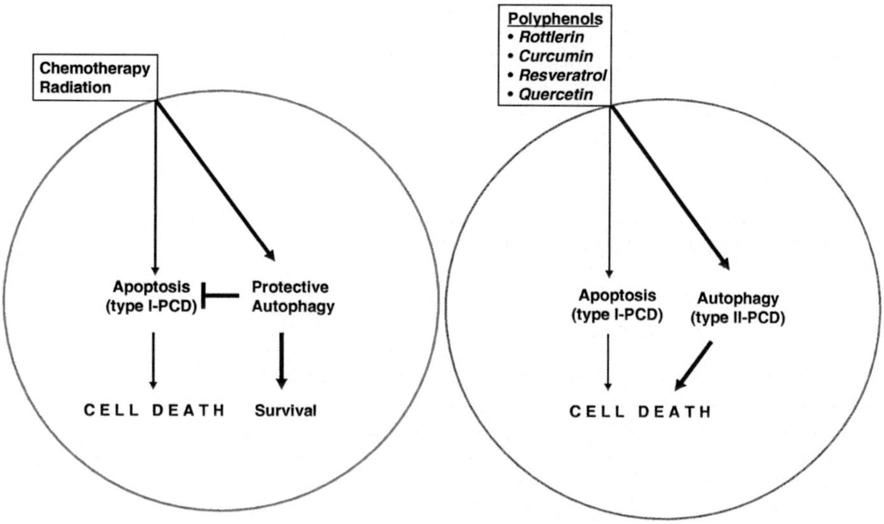

Fig. 10.5 Current hypothesis for eliminating cancer cells through the induction of autophagic cell death. Resistance to induction of apoptosis in response to conventional threrapies, such as chemotherapy, radiotherapy, some anticancer agents and targeted therapies prevent successful elimination cancer cells. Therefore, induction of cell death occurring with autophagy by polyphenolic compounds may be used as an alternative approach to kill cancer cells that are resistant to apoptosis by anticancer therapies (e.g., chemotherapy, radiation)

because a number of cancer therapies, such as radiation therapy, chemotherapy and targeted therapies (e.g. imatinib) induce autophagy as a protective resistance mechanism against anticancer therapies for cancer cell survival, the inhibition of autophagy can be used to enhance the efficacy of anticancer therapies. Future studies need to determine the *in vivo* efficacy of these compounds in preclinical human cancer models in animals. Also, further understanding of the mechanisms by which these compounds induce cell death occurring with autophagy may help in the identification of novel molecules for the development of new molecularly targeted therapies against cancer.

References

Abedin MJ, Wang D, McDonnell MA, Lehmann U, Kelekar A (2007) Autophagy delays apoptotic death in breast cancer cells following DNA damage. Cell Death Differ 14:500–510

Aggarwal BB, Bhardwaj A, Aggarwal RS, Seeram NP, Shishodia S, Takada Y (2004) Role of resveratrol in prevention and therapy of cancer: preclinical and clinical studies. Anticancer Res 24:2783–2840

Aita VM, Liang XH, Murty VV, Pincus DL, Yu W, Cayanis E, Kalachikov S, Gilliam TC, Levine B (1999) Cloning and genomic organization of beclin 1, a candidate tumor suppressor gene on chromosome 17q21. Genomics 59:59–65

Akar U, Chaves-Reyez A, Barria M, Tari A, Sanguino A, Kondo Y, Kondo S, Arun B, Lopez-Berestein G, Ozpolat B (2008) Silencing of Bcl-2 expression by small interfering RNA induces autophagic cell death in MCF-7 breast cancer cells. Autophagy 4:669–679

Akar U, Ozpolat B, Mehta K, Fok J, Kondo Y, Lopez-Berestein G (2007) Tissue transglutaminase inhibits autophagy in pancreatic cancer cells. Mol Cancer Res 5:241–249

Amaravadi RK, Yu D, Lum JJ, Bui T, Christophorou MA, Evan GI, Thomas-Tikhonenko A, Thompson CB (2007) Autophagy inhibition enhances therapy-induced apoptosis in a Myc-induced model of lymphoma. J Clin Invest 117:326–336

Aoki H, Takada Y, Kondo S, Sawaya R, Aggarwal BB, Kondo Y (2007) Evidence that curcumin suppresses the growth of malignant gliomas in vitro and in vivo through induction of autophagy: role of Akt and extracellular signal-regulated kinase signaling pathways. Mol Pharmacol 72:29–39

Apel A, Herr I, Schwarz H, Rodemann HP, Mayer A (2008) Blocked autophagy sensitizes resistant carcinoma cells to radiation therapy. Cancer Res 68:1485–1494

Avila MA, Velasco JA, Cansado J, Notario V (1994) Quercetin mediates the down-regulation of mutant p53 in the human breast cancer cell line MDA-MB468. Cancer Res 54:2424–2428

Banerjee S, Li Y, Wang Z, Sarkar FH (2008) Multi-targeted therapy of cancer by genistein. Cancer Lett 269:226–242

Bellot G, Garcia-Medina R, Gounon P, Chiche J, Roux D, Pouysségur J, Mazure NM (2009) Hypoxia-induced autophagy is mediated through hypoxia-inducible factor induction of BNIP3 and BNIP3L via their BH3 domains. Mol Cell Biol 29(10):2570–2581

Boya P, Gonzalez-Polo RA, Casares N, Perfettini JL, Dessen P, Larochette N, Metivier D, Meley D, Souquere S, Yoshimori T et al (2005) Inhibition of macroautophagy triggers apoptosis. Mol Cell Biol 25:1025–1040

Carew JS, Nawrocki ST, Kahue CN, Zhang H, Yang C, Chung L, Houghton JA, Huang P, Giles FJ, Cleveland JL (2007) Targeting autophagy augments the anticancer activity of the histone deacetylase inhibitor SAHA to overcome Bcr-Abl-mediated drug resistance. Blood 110:313–322

Chan EY, Longatti A, McKnight NC, Tooze SA (2009) Kinase-inactivated ULK proteins inhibit autophagy via their conserved C-terminal domains using an Atg13-independent mechanism. Mol Cell Biol 29:157–171

Chung S, Yao H, Caito S, Hwang JW, Arunachalam G, Rahman I (2010) Regulation of SIRT1 in cellular functions: role of polyphenols. Arch Biochem Biophys 501:79–90

Clarke PG (1990) Developmental cell death: morphological diversity and multiple mechanisms. Anat Embryol (Berl) 181:195–213

Daniel F, Legrand A, Pessayre D, Borrega-Pires F, Mbida L, Lardeux B, Degott C, van Nhieu JT, Bernuau D (2007) Beclin 1 mRNA strongly correlates with Bcl-XLmRNA expression in human hepatocellular carcinoma. Cancer Invest 25:226–231

Ding ZB, Shi YH, Zhou J, Qiu SJ, Xu Y, Dai Z, Shi GM, Wang XY, Ke AW, Wu B et al (2008) Association of autophagy defect with a malignant phenotype and poor prognosis of hepatocellular carcinoma. Cancer Res 68:9167–9175

Edinger AL, Thompson CB (2003) Defective autophagy leads to cancer. Cancer Cell 4:422–424

Elsasser HP, MacDonald R, Dienst M, Kern HF (1993) Characterization of a transglutaminase expressed in human pancreatic adenocarcinoma cells. Eur J Cell Biol 61:321–328

Fabre C, Carvalho G, Tasdemir E, Braun T, Ades L, Grosjean J, Boehrer S, Metivier D, Souquere S, Pierron G et al (2007) NF-kappaB inhibition sensitizes to starvation-induced cell death in high-risk myelodysplastic syndrome and acute myeloid leukemia. Oncogene 26:4071–4083

Fesus L, Szondy Z (2005) Transglutaminase 2 in the balance of cell death and survival. FEBS Lett 579:3297–3302

Galluzzi L, Aaronson SA, Abrams J, Alnemri ES, Andrews DW, Baehrecke EH, Bazan NG, Blagosklonny MV, Blomgren K, Borner C et al (2009) Guidelines for the use and interpretation of assays for monitoring cell death in higher eukaryotes. Cell Death Differ 16:1093–1107

Ganley IG, Lam DH, Wang J, Ding X, Chen S, Jiang X (2009) ULK1-ATG13-FIP200 complex mediates mTOR signaling and is essential for autophagy. J Biol Chem 284(18):12297–12305

Gossner G, Choi M, Tan L, Fogoros S, Griffith KA, Kuenker M, Liu JR (2007) Genistein-induced apoptosis and autophagocytosis in ovarian cancer cells. Gynecol Oncol 105:23–30

Gozuacik D, Kimchi A (2006) DAPk protein family and cancer. Autophagy 2:74–79

Hait WN, Wu H, Jin S, Yang JM (2006) Elongation factor-2 kinase: its role in protein synthesis and autophagy. Autophagy 2:294–296

Hara T, Mizushima N (2009) Role of ULK-FIP200 complex in mammalian autophagy: FIP200, a counterpart of yeast Atg17? Autophagy 5:85–87

Harhaji-Trajkovic L, Vilimanovich U, Kravic-Stevovic T, Bumbasirevic V, Trajkovic V (2009) AMPK-mediated autophagy inhibits apoptosis in cisplatin-treated tumor cells. J Cell Mol Med 13(9B):3644–3654

Hayashi M, Ikezawa K, Ono A, Okabayashi S, Hayashi Y, Shimizu S, Mizuno T, Maeda K, Akasaka T, Naito M et al (2007) Evaluation of the effects of combination therapy with branched-chain amino acid and zinc supplements on nitrogen metabolism in liver cirrhosis. Hepatol Res 37:615–619

Herman JF, Mangala LS, Mehta K (2006) Implications of increased tissue transglutaminase (TG2) expression in drug-resistant breast cancer (MCF-7) cells. Oncogene 25:3049–3058

Herrero-Martin G, Hoyer-Hansen M, Garcia-Garcia C, Fumarola C, Farkas T, Lopez-Rivas A, Jaattela M (2009) TAK1 activates AMPK-dependent cytoprotective autophagy in TRAIL-treated epithelial cells. EMBO J 28:677–685

Howitz KT, Bitterman KJ, Cohen HY, Lamming DW, Lavu S, Wood JG, Zipkin RE, Chung P, Kisielewski A, Zhang LL et al (2003) Small molecule activators of sirtuins extend Saccharomyces cerevisiae lifespan. Nature 425:191–196

Hwang JT, Kwak DW, Lin SK, Kim HM, Kim YM, Park OJ (2007) Resveratrol induces apoptosis in chemoresistant cancer cells via modulation of AMPK signaling pathway. Ann N Y Acad Sci 1095:441–448

Iacobuzio-Donahue CA, Ashfaq R, Maitra A, Adsay NV, Shen-Ong GL, Berg K, Hollingsworth MA, Cameron JL, Yeo CJ, Kern SE et al (2003) Highly expressed genes in pancreatic ductal adenocarcinomas: a comprehensive characterization and comparison of the transcription profiles obtained from three major technologies. Cancer Res 63:8614–8622

Jackson DN, Foster DA (2004) The enigmatic protein kinase Cdelta: complex roles in cell proliferation and survival. FASEB J 18:627–636

Jang M, Cai L, Udeani GO, Slowing KV, Thomas CF, Beecher CW, Fong HH, Farnsworth NR, Kinghorn AD, Mehta RG et al (1997) Cancer chemopreventive activity of resveratrol, a natural product derived from grapes. Science 275:218–220

Jia YL, Li J, Qin ZH, Liang ZQ (2009) Autophagic and apoptotic mechanisms of curcumin-induced death in K562 cells. J Asian Nat Prod Res 11:918–928

Kanzawa T, Germano IM, Komata T, Ito H, Kondo Y, Kondo S (2004) Role of autophagy in temozolomide-induced cytotoxicity for malignant glioma cells. Cell Death Differ 11:448–457

Katayama M, Kawaguchi T, Berger MS, Pieper RO (2007) DNA damaging agent-induced autophagy produces a cytoprotective adenosine triphosphate surge in malignant glioma cells. Cell Death Differ 14:548–558

Kirisako T, Baba M, Ishihara N, Miyazawa K, Ohsumi M, Yoshimori T, Noda T, Ohsumi Y (1999) Formation process of autophagosome is traced with Apg8/Aut7p in yeast. J Cell Biol 147:435–446

Klionsky DJ, Abeliovich H, Agostinis P, Agrawal DK, Aliev G, Askew DS, Baba M, Baehrecke EH, Bahr BA, Ballabio A et al (2008) Guidelines for the use and interpretation of assays for monitoring autophagy in higher eukaryotes. Autophagy 4:151–175

Klionsky DJ, Emr SD (2000) Autophagy as a regulated pathway of cellular degradation. Science 290:1717–1721

Koivunen J, Aaltonen V, Peltonen J (2006) Protein kinase C (PKC) family in cancer progression. Cancer Lett 235:1–10

Kondo Y, Kanzawa T, Sawaya R, Kondo S (2005) The role of autophagy in cancer development and response to therapy. Nat Rev Cancer 5:726–734

Koneri K, Goi T, Hirono Y, Katayama K, Yamaguchi A (2007) Beclin 1 gene inhibits tumor growth in colon cancer cell lines. Anticancer Res 27:1453–1457

Kourelis TV, Siegel RD (2012) Metformin and cancer: new applications for an old drug. Med Oncol 29(2):1314–1327

Kueck A, Opipari AW Jr, Griffith KA, Tan L, Choi M, Huang J, Wahl H, Liu JR (2007) Resveratrol inhibits glucose metabolism in human ovarian cancer cells. Gynecol Oncol 107:450–457
La Porta CA, Comolli R (2000) Overexpression of nPKCdelta in BL6 murine melanoma cells enhances TGFbeta1 release into the plasma of metastasized animals. Melanoma Res 10:527–534
Lavieu G, Scarlatti F, Sala G, Levade T, Ghidoni R, Botti J, Codogno P (2007) Is autophagy the key mechanism by which the sphingolipid rheostat controls the cell fate decision? Autophagy 3:45–47
Lee MH, Choi BY, Kundu JK, Shin YK, Na HK, Surh YJ (2009) Resveratrol suppresses growth of human ovarian cancer cells in culture and in a murine xenograft model: eukaryotic elongation factor 1A2 as a potential target. Cancer Res 69:7449–7458
Levine B, Klionsky DJ (2004) Development by self-digestion: molecular mechanisms and biological functions of autophagy. Dev Cell 6:463–477
Li DD, Wang LL, Deng R, Tang J, Shen Y, Guo JF, Wang Y, Xia LP, Feng GK, Liu QQ et al (2009a) The pivotal role of c-Jun NH2-terminal kinase-mediated Beclin 1 expression during anticancer agents-induced autophagy in cancer cells. Oncogene 28:886–898
Li J, Qin Z, Liang Z (2009b) The prosurvival role of autophagy in Resveratrol-induced cytotoxicity in human U251 glioma cells. BMC Cancer 9:215
Liang C, Feng P, Ku B, Dotan I, Canaani D, Oh BH, Jung JU (2006) Autophagic and tumour suppressor activity of a novel Beclin1-binding protein UVRAG. Nat Cell Biol 8:688–699
Liang J, Shao SH, Xu ZX, Hennessy B, Ding Z, Larrea M, Kondo S, Dumont DJ, Gutterman JU, Walker CL et al (2007) The energy sensing LKB1-AMPK pathway regulates p27(kip1) phosphorylation mediating the decision to enter autophagy or apoptosis. Nat Cell Biol 9:218–224
Liang XH, Jackson S, Seaman M, Brown K, Kempkes B, Hibshoosh H, Levine B (1999) Induction of autophagy and inhibition of tumorigenesis by beclin 1. Nature 402:672–676
Lim JH, Park JW, Kim SH, Choi YH, Choi KS, Kwon TK (2008) Rottlerin induces pro-apoptotic endoplasmic reticulum stress through the protein kinase C-delta-independent pathway in human colon cancer cells. Apoptosis 13:1378–1385
Lockshin RA, Zakeri Z (2007) Cell death in health and disease. J Cell Mol Med 11:1214–1224
Lorand L, Graham RM (2003) Transglutaminases: crosslinking enzymes with pleiotropic functions. Nat Rev Mol Cell Biol 4:140–156
Mann AP, Verma A, Sethi G, Manavathi B, Wang H, Fok JY, Kunnumakkara AB, Kumar R, Aggarwal BB, Mehta K (2006) Overexpression of tissue transglutaminase leads to constitutive activation of nuclear factor-kappaB in cancer cells: delineation of a novel pathway. Cancer Res 66:8788–8795
Matter WF, Brown RF, Vlahos CJ (1992) The inhibition of phosphatidylinositol 3-kinase by quercetin and analogs. Biochem Biophys Res Commun 186:624–631
Mehta K, Fok J, Miller FR, Koul D, Sahin AA (2004) Prognostic significance of tissue transglutaminase in drug resistant and metastatic breast cancer. Clin Cancer Res 10:8068–8076
Meijer AJ, Codogno P (2004) Regulation and role of autophagy in mammalian cells. Int J Biochem Cell Biol 36:2445–2462
Meijer AJ, Codogno P (2007) AMP-activated protein kinase and autophagy. Autophagy 3:238–240
Mhaouty-Kodja S (2004) Ghalpha/tissue transglutaminase 2: an emerging G protein in signal transduction. Biol Cell 96:363–367
Miracco C, Cosci E, Oliveri G, Luzi P, Pacenti L, Monciatti I, Mannucci S, De Nisi MC, Toscano M, Malagnino V et al (2007) Protein and mRNA expression of autophagy gene Beclin 1 in human brain tumours. Int J Oncol 30:429–436
Moretti L, Attia A, Kim KW, Lu B (2007) Crosstalk between Bak/Bax and mTOR signaling regulates radiation-induced autophagy. Autophagy 3:142–144
Nakamura Y, Yogosawa S, Izutani Y, Watanabe H, Otsuji E, Sakai T (2009) A combination of indol-3-carbinol and genistein synergistically induces apoptosis in human colon cancer HT-29 cells by inhibiting Akt phosphorylation and progression of autophagy. Mol Cancer 8:100
Ohshiro K, Rayala SK, Kondo S, Gaur A, Vadlamudi RK, El-Naggar AK, Kumar R (2007) Identifying the estrogen receptor coactivator PELP1 in autophagosomes. Cancer Res 67:8164–8171

Opipari AW Jr, Tan L, Boitano AE, Sorenson DR, Aurora A, Liu JR (2004) Resveratrol-induced autophagocytosis in ovarian cancer cells. Cancer Res 64:696–703

Ozpolat B, Akar U, Mehta K, Lopez-Berestein G (2007) PKC delta and tissue transglutaminase are novel inhibitors of autophagy in pancreatic cancer cells. Autophagy 3(5):480–483

Paglin S, Hollister T, Delohery T, Hackett N, McMahill M, Sphicas E, Domingo D, Yahalom J (2001) A novel response of cancer cells to radiation involves autophagy and formation of acidic vesicles. Cancer Res 61:439–444

Pan W, Yang H, Cao C, Song X, Wallin B, Kivlin R, Lu S, Hu G, Di W, Wan Y (2008) AMPK mediates curcumin-induced cell death in CaOV3 ovarian cancer cells. Oncol Rep 20:1553–1559

Papandreou I, Lim AL, Laderoute K, Denko NC (2008) Hypoxia signals autophagy in tumor cells via AMPK activity, independent of HIF-1, BNIP3, and BNIP3L. Cell Death Differ 15:1572–1581

Park CE, Yun H, Lee EB, Min BI, Bae H, Choe W, Kang I, Kim SS, Ha J (2010) The antioxidant effects of genistein are associated with AMP-activated protein kinase activation and PTEN induction in prostate cancer cells. J Med Food 13:815–820

Park JW, Choi YJ, Suh SI, Baek WK, Suh MH, Jin IN, Min DS, Woo JH, Chang JS, Passaniti A et al (2001) Bcl-2 overexpression attenuates resveratrol-induced apoptosis in U937 cells by inhibition of caspase-3 activity. Carcinogenesis 22:1633–1639

Park MA, Curiel DT, Koumenis C, Graf M, Chen CS, Fisher PB, Grant S, Dent P (2008a) PERK-dependent regulation of HSP70 expression and the regulation of autophagy. Autophagy 4:364–367

Park MA, Zhang G, Norris J, Hylemon PB, Fisher PB, Grant S, Dent P (2008b) Regulation of autophagy by ceramide-CD95-PERK signaling. Autophagy 4:929–931

Pattingre S, Tassa A, Qu X, Garuti R, Liang XH, Mizushima N, Packer M, Schneider MD, Levine B (2005) Bcl-2 antiapoptotic proteins inhibit Beclin 1-dependent autophagy. Cell 122:927–939

Pavese JM, Farmer RL, Bergan RC (2010) Inhibition of cancer cell invasion and metastasis by genistein. Cancer Metastasis Rev 29:465–482

Peterson G, Barnes S (1996) Genistein inhibits both estrogen and growth factor-stimulated proliferation of human breast cancer cells. Cell Growth Differ 7:1345–1351

Psahoulia FH, Moumtzi S, Roberts ML, Sasazuki T, Shirasawa S, Pintzas A (2007) Quercetin mediates preferential degradation of oncogenic Ras and causes autophagy in Ha-RAS-transformed human colon cells. Carcinogenesis 28:1021–1031

Puissant A, Robert G, Fenouille N, Luciano F, Cassuto JP, Raynaud S, Auberger P (2010) Resveratrol promotes cell death occurring with autophagy in chronic myelogenous leukemia cells via JNK-mediated p62/SQSTM1 expression and AMPK activation. Cancer Res 70:1042–1052

Qadir MA, Kwok B, Dragowska WH, To KH, Le D, Bally MB, Gorski SM (2008) Macroautophagy inhibition sensitizes tamoxifen-resistant breast cancer cells and enhances mitochondrial depolarization. Breast Cancer Res Treat 112:389–403

Qu X, Yu J, Bhagat G, Furuya N, Hibshoosh H, Troxel A, Rosen J, Eskelinen EL, Mizushima N, Ohsumi Y et al (2003) Promotion of tumorigenesis by heterozygous disruption of the beclin 1 autophagy gene. J Clin Invest 112:1809–1820

Rouschop KM, Wouters BG (2009) Regulation of autophagy through multiple independent hypoxic signaling pathways. Curr Mol Med 9:417–424

Satoh A, Gukovskaya AS, Nieto JM, Cheng JH, Gukovsky I, Reeve JR Jr, Shimosegawa T, Pandol SJ (2004) PKC-delta and -epsilon regulate NF-kappaB activation induced by cholecystokinin and TNF-alpha in pancreatic acinar cells. Am J Physiol Gastrointest Liver Physiol 287:G582–G591

Shakibaei M, Harikumar KB, Aggarwal BB (2009) Resveratrol addiction: to die or not to die. Mol Nutr Food Res 53:115–128

Shen Y, Li DD, Wang LL, Deng R, Zhu XF (2008) Decreased expression of autophagy-related proteins in malignant epithelial ovarian cancer. Autophagy 4:1067–1068

Shimizu S, Kanaseki T, Mizushima N, Mizuta T, Arakawa-Kobayashi S, Thompson CB, Tsujimoto Y (2004) Role of Bcl-2 family proteins in a non-apoptotic programmed cell death dependent on autophagy genes. Nat Cell Biol 6:1221–1228

Shinojima N, Yokoyama T, Kondo Y, Kondo S (2007) Roles of the Akt/mTOR/p70S6K and ERK1/2 signaling pathways in curcumin-induced autophagy. Autophagy 3:635–637

Singletary K, Milner J (2008) Diet, autophagy, and cancer: a review. Cancer Epidemiol Biomarkers Prev 17:1596–1610

Sivaprasad U, Basu A (2008) Inhibition of ERK attenuates autophagy and potentiates tumour necrosis factor-alpha-induced cell death in MCF-7 cells. J Cell Mol Med 12:1265–1271

Soltoff SP (2007) Rottlerin: an inappropriate and ineffective inhibitor of PKCdelta. Trends Pharmacol Sci 28:453–458

Song KS, Kim JS, Yun EJ, Kim YR, Seo KS, Park JH, Jung YJ, Park JI, Kweon GR, Yoon WH et al (2008) Rottlerin induces autophagy and apoptotic cell death through a PKC-delta-independent pathway in HT1080 human fibrosarcoma cells: the protective role of autophagy in apoptosis. Autophagy 4:650–658

Sotelo J, Briceno E, Lopez-Gonzalez MA (2006) Adding chloroquine to conventional treatment for glioblastoma multiforme: a randomized, double-blind, placebo-controlled trial. Ann Intern Med 144:337–343

Takahashi Y, Coppola D, Matsushita N, Cualing HD, Sun M, Sato Y, Liang C, Jung JU, Cheng JQ, Mul JJ et al (2007) Bif-1 interacts with Beclin 1 through UVRAG and regulates autophagy and tumorigenesis. Nat Cell Biol 9:1142–1151

Tasdemir E, Galluzzi L, Maiuri MC, Criollo A, Vitale I, Hangen E, Modjtahedi N, Kroemer G (2008) Methods for assessing autophagy and cell death occurring with autophagy. Methods Mol Biol 445:29–76

Thangapazham RL, Sharma A, Maheshwari RK (2006) Multiple molecular targets in cancer chemoprevention by curcumin. AAPS J 8:E443–E449

Trincheri NF, Follo C, Nicotra G, Peracchio C, Castino R, Isidoro C (2008) Resveratrol-induced apoptosis depends on the lipid kinase activity of Vps34 and on the formation of autophagolysosomes. Carcinogenesis 29:381–389

Trincheri NF, Nicotra G, Follo C, Castino R, Isidoro C (2007) Resveratrol induces cell death in colorectal cancer cells by a novel pathway involving lysosomal cathepsin D. Carcinogenesis 28:922–931

Verma A, Wang H, Manavathi B, Fok JY, Mann AP, Kumar R, Mehta K (2006) Increased expression of tissue transglutaminase in pancreatic ductal adenocarcinoma and its implications in drug resistance and metastasis. Cancer Res 66:10525–10533

Wang SH, Shih YL, Kuo TC, Ko WC, Shih CM (2009) Cadmium toxicity toward autophagy through ROS-activated GSK-3beta in mesangial cells. Toxicol Sci 108:124–131

Wang ZH, Peng ZL, Duan ZL, Liu H (2006) Expression and clinical significance of autophagy gene Beclin 1 in cervical squamous cell carcinoma. Sichuan Da Xue Xue Bao Yi Xue Ban 37:860–863

Wei Y, Sinha S, Levine B (2008) Dual role of JNK1-mediated phosphorylation of Bcl-2 in autophagy and apoptosis regulation. Autophagy 4:949–951

Wu H, Yang JM, Jin S, Zhang H, Hait WN (2006) Elongation factor-2 kinase regulates autophagy in human glioblastoma cells. Cancer Res 66:3015–3023

Wu H, Zhu H, Liu DX, Niu TK, Ren X, Patel R, Hait WN, Yang JM (2009) Silencing of elongation factor-2 kinase potentiates the effect of 2-deoxy-D-glucose against human glioma cells through blunting of autophagy. Cancer Res 69:2453–2460

Xue L, Fletcher GC, Tolkovsky AM (1999) Autophagy is activated by apoptotic signalling in sympathetic neurons: an alternative mechanism of death execution. Mol Cell Neurosci 14:180–198

Yousefi S, Perozzo R, Schmid I, Ziemiecki A, Schaffner T, Scapozza L, Brunner T, Simon HU (2006) Calpain-mediated cleavage of Atg5 switches autophagy to apoptosis. Nat Cell Biol 8:1124–1132

Yue Z, Jin S, Yang C, Levine AJ, Heintz N (2003) Beclin 1, an autophagy gene essential for early embryonic development, is a haploinsufficient tumor suppressor. Proc Natl Acad Sci USA 100:15077–15082

Zalckvar E, Berissi H, Mizrachy L, Idelchuk Y, Koren I, Eisenstein M, Sabanay H, Pinkas-Kramarski R, Kimchi A (2009) DAP-kinase-mediated phosphorylation on the BH3 domain of

beclin 1 promotes dissociation of beclin 1 from Bcl-XL and induction of autophagy. EMBO Rep 10:285–292
Zhang H, Bosch-Marce M, Shimoda LA, Tan YS, Baek JH (2008) Mitochondrial autophagy is an HIF-1-dependent adaptive metabolic response to hypoxia. J Biol Chem 283:10892–10903
Zhang Y, Wu Y, Tashiro S, Onodera S, Ikejima T (2009a) Involvement of PKC signal pathways in oridonin-induced autophagy in HeLa cells: a protective mechanism against apoptosis. Biochem Biophys Res Commun 378:273–278
Zhang Y, Wu Y, Cheng Y, Zhao Z, Tashiro S, Onodera S, Ikejima T (2009b) Fas-mediated autophagy requires JNK activation in HeLa cells. Biochem Biophys Res Commun 377:1205–1210

Part IV
Redox Active Natural Compounds

Chapter 11
Total Antioxidant Capacity: A Useful Tool in Assessing Antioxidant Intake Status

Ying Wang, Meng Yang, Sang-Gil Lee, Catherine Davis, Christopher Masterjohn, Anne Kenny, Richard S. Bruno, and Ock K. Chun

Abstract Total antioxidant capacity (TAC) considering the cumulative protective activities of all the antioxidants present in food was inversely associated with cardiovascular disease (CVD) risk factors, suggesting a great potential of dietary TAC as a useful dietary assessment tool in human clinical and intervention studies for assessing dietary antioxidant status and predicting plasma antioxidant defense. However, none of these factors has been successfully validated for relevance under different physiological conditions, or for reliability and predictability for in vivo antioxidant status. The objective of this study is to validate TAC as a useful dietary tool in assessing dietary antioxidant status. Forty postmenopausal, overweight and healthy women were recruited for an observational study. Seven day diet recalls and 12-h fasting blood samples were collected for dietary and plasma antioxidant assessments. Results: After multivariate adjustment, TAC from foods and TAC from foods and supplements were both positively associated with intakes of dietary antioxidants, including α-tocopherol ($p<0.001$), vitamin C ($p<0.01$), flavonoids ($p<0.001$) and proanthocyanidins ($p<0.01$); they were also positively associated with plasma TAC assayed by VCEAC, FRAP and ORAC methods ($p<0.05$), and with plasma α-tocopherol ($p<0.0001$), and β-cryptoxanthin ($p<0.01$) concentrations. Fruits and fruit juices were the primary contributor to dietary TAC (from foods/foods and supplement) followed by tea and vegetable and vegetable juices. Conclusion: Dietary TAC could be used as a useful tool in predicting dietary and plasma antioxidant status.

Y. Wang • M. Yang • S.-G. Lee • C. Davis • C. Masterjohn • R.S. Bruno
• O.K. Chun, Ph.D., M.P.H (✉)
Department of Nutritional Sciences, University of Connecticut,
3624 Horsebarn Road Extension Unit, 4017 Storrs, CT, USA
e-mail: ock.chun@uconn.edu

A. Kenny
School of Medicine, University of Connecticut Health Center, Farmington, CT, USA

M. Diederich and K. Noworyta (eds.), *Natural Compounds as Inducers of Cell Death: Volume 1*, DOI 10.1007/978-94-007-4575-9_11,

Keywords Total antioxidant capacity (TAC) • Diet • Vitamin C equivalent (VCE) • Obese • Postmenopausal women

Abbreviations

AAPH	2,2′-azobis (2-amidinopropane) dihydrochloride
ABAP	2,2′-diazobis (2-amidinopropane) dihydrochloride
ABTS	2,2′-azino-bis (3-ethylbenzthiazoline-6-sulphonic acid)
BODIPY	4,4-difluoro-5-(4-phenyl-1,3-butadienyl)-4-bora-3a,4a-diaza-s-indacene-3-undecanoic acid
BHT	butylated hydroxytoluene
CRP	C-reactive protein
CVD	cardiovascular disease
DR	diet recall
FFQ	food frequency questionnaire
FRAP	ferric reducing ability of plasma
HPLC	high performance liquid chromatography
KOH	potassium hydroxide
MeO-AMVN	2,2′-azobis(4-methoxy-2,4-dimethylvaleronitrile)
ORAC	oxygen radical absorbance capacity
ROS	reactive oxygen species
TAC	total antioxidant capacity
TAP	total antioxidant performance
TEAC	trolox equivalent antioxidant capacity
TG	triglyceride
TRAP	total radical-trapping antioxidant parameters
HDL-C	high density lipoprotein cholesterol
LDL-C	low density lipoprotein cholesterol
VCE	vitamin C equivalent
VCEAC	vitamin C equivalent antioxidant capacity

11.1 Introduction

Oxidative stress has been identified as a key factor in the pathogenesis of many degenerative diseases such as cardiovascular disease (CVD), cancer, and immune dysfunction (Ames et al. 1993) via the oxidation of lipid, nucleic acid and protein by reactive oxygen species (ROS). Oxidative stress is defined as an imbalance between pro-oxidants and antioxidants in favor of the former (Sies 1985). Dietary antioxidants, then, have been thought to reverse this imbalance (Prior 2003). Several epidemiological studies have observed that high consumption of fruits and vegetables are associated with a lower incidence and mortality rate of these diseases (Doll 1990;

Hertog et al. 1995; Liu et al. 2000; Bazzano et al. 2002). However, it is still inconclusive which dietary antioxidants are responsible for this association (Reaven et al. 1993; Knekt et al. 1994).

Some randomized controlled trials focusing on antioxidants from food extract failed to observe any beneficial effects on the risk of chronic diseases (Drieling et al. 2010); also, numerous studies documented that antioxidant vitamins failed to improve health status (Bjelakovic et al. 2008; Neuhouser et al. 2009). Furthermore, supplements are drawing safety concern recently due to their adverse health effects (Bjelakovic et al. 2004; Soni et al. 2010). In contrast, in a recent randomized controlled trial, a diet high in antioxidants improved endothelial function (Franzini et al. 2010), suggesting that combined multiple antioxidants in the diet might exert more beneficial effects on oxidative stress than a single antioxidant does. Plant foods contain a variety of compounds with antioxidant activity, including ascorbic acid, tocopherols, carotenoids, and antioxidant phytochemicals such as simple phenolics, flavonoids and procyanidins. Since no single antioxidant may reflect the total antioxidant power of food, the concept of total antioxidant capacity (TAC) was introduced (Serafini and Del Rio 2004).

TAC represents the cumulative protective activities of all the antioxidants present in food, plasma, or body fluids, thus providing an integrated parameter rather than the simple sum of measurable antioxidants (Serafini and Del Rio 2004). Although TAC provides a new tool to assess the antioxidant quality of the diet or antioxidant status in vivo, recently the applicability and scientific appropriateness of the TAC concept have been debated due to the fact that plasma TAC may be affected by plasma protein, uric acid, and antioxidant enzymes rather than antioxidant nutrients/compounds and their metabolites directly originating from the diet (Day and Stansbie 1995). Also, dietary TAC does not reflect bioavailability as determined by absorption and excretion. Furthermore, the successful application of this tool is highly dependent on the completeness and validity of dietary intake data as well as the accuracy of food composition data. Nevertheless, dietary TAC still has a great potential for clinical and public health applications since it exclusively provides the sum of protective activities of dietary antioxidants. At present, a critical need exists to validate this dietary tool by examining the association with antioxidant intake levels and plasma antioxidant defense status.

Studies may have provided inconsistent findings on the ability of enhanced antioxidant intake to improve plasma antioxidant defense and reduce oxidative stress because they lacked information on subjects' cumulative antioxidant intake and physiological antioxidant and inflammatory status, and were therefore unable to consider changes in these parameters. To our knowledge, no prior studies have estimated the predictive value of cumulative intakes of dietary antioxidants, specifically those functioning as reactive oxygen species (ROS) scavengers. Thus, we conducted an observational study with overweight/obese postmenopausal women to document the associations of dietary TAC with intakes of individual antioxidants and biomarkers of plasma antioxidant defense. In this study, if not pointed out specifically, dietary TAC refers to both TAC from diet and TAC from diet and supplements.

11.2 Participants and Methods

11.2.1 Study Population

A cross-sectional study was conducted in 40–70 year old, overweight/obese (BMI 25–39.9 kg/m^2), non-smoking postmenopausal women ($n=40$) without CVD and other inflammatory diseases. This population was specifically chosen for the following reasons: (1) obesity is a significant risk factor toward oxidative stress-mediated CVD (Billington et al. 2000); (2) obese individuals have a greater degree of chronic inflammation (Weyer et al. 2002); and (3) obese individuals are more likely to have lower antioxidant status, likely due to their less frequent consumption of fruits and vegetables (Ford et al. 2003); and (4) risk of CVD in women is significantly increased after menopause. Exclusion criteria included a diagnosis of CVD, diabetes, or arthritis (excluding osteoarthritis), currently being treated for cancer (i.e., chemotherapy, radiation therapy), estrogen replacement therapy, slimming diets, or alcohol consumption exceeding 2 drinks/day or total of 12 drinks/week.

11.2.2 Study Design

Potential participants were recruited in the Hartford, Connecticut area through printed flyers, email and newspaper advertisements. The potential subjects who were qualified for this study through a telephone interview were immediately invited to the General Clinical Research Center located in the University of Connecticut Health Center (UCHC) in Farmington, CT, and completed the written informed consent form. Prior to the initiation of the project, its protocols and procedures was reviewed and approved by the Human Investigation Review Committees of the UCHC and University of Connecticut Storrs Campus. At the first screening visit, the subjects were given a brief physical examination by a nurse, including measured weight, height, and blood pressures (systolic blood pressure; diastolic blood pressure), followed by an interview regarding their medical, dietary, smoking, and alcohol consumption histories, and a fasting blood collection. The eligible participants were instructed to follow their usual dietary habits and how to record 24-h diet recall (DR) by an experienced research staff and then asked to bring a completed 7-day DR when they visit the center 7 days after the initial screening.

11.2.3 Dietary Assessment

Each subject's dietary data of all food sources from 7-day DR were input into Nutrition Data System for Research (NDSR) software (Nutrition Coordinating Center, Minneapolis, MN) for food composition analyses. Flavonoid and proanthocyanidin intakes were estimated by matching food consumption data with the nutrients in flavonoids and proanthocyanidins databases as described in our previous study (Chun et al. 2007). The subject's individual antioxidant intake was estimated by multiplying the content of the individual antioxidants (flavonoid, proanthocyanidins, carotenoids, vitamins C and E) by the daily consumption of each selected food item. Individual antioxidant capacity was then determined by multiplying the individual amount of each antioxidant compound by their respective antioxidant capacities expressed as vitamin C equivalent antioxidant capacity (VCEAC) (Floegel et al. 2010). Dietary TAC was determined by summating the individual antioxidant capacities as described in our previous publication. In this study, the TAC values of the subjects' diet were reported as mg VCE per day.

11.2.4 Anthropometrics

Subjects' height, weight, and blood pressure were recorded. After a 5-min rest period, subjects' blood pressure was measured with a Welch Allyn, Tycos cuff. The mean of 2 blood pressure readings was used to ensure accuracy. Physical activity levels were measured using the Health and Nutrition Survey Form.

11.2.5 Blood Collection and Plasma Antioxidant Analyses

Twelve-hour fasting blood samples were collected in evacuated containers with EDTA or heparin. Samples were centrifuged immediately in a dark room at 500 × g for 15 min at 4°C. After plasma samples were isolated, they were immediately separated in small portions, and stored at –80°C until analyzed after specific pretreatments for each assay.

The outcome measures included plasma TAC, glucose, lipid profiles (total cholesterol, TG, HDL-C, LDL-C), plasma antioxidant nutrients and enzymes. Plasma TAC was determined by the VCEAC, FRAP and ORAC assays, respectively. VCEAC assay, which was developed by Miller et al. (Miller et al. 1993) and modified by Kim et al. (2002), measures the ABTS radical chromogen at 734 nm, using AAPH as a thermolabile water-soluble radical initiator. The reduction of ABTS radical chromogen is proportional to the TAC in plasma. The results were expressed as mg vitamin C equivalent (VCE) per liter plasma. The FRAP assay determines the ability of the sample to reduce ferric iron to ferrous iron in a low-pH environment. A colored ferrous-tripyridyltriazine complex is formed during this process and has a maximum absorbance at 593 nm (Benzie and Strain 1996). The results are expressed as μmol trolox per liter plasma. ORAC assay determines the antioxidant capacity of plasma by measuring the oxidative degradation of a fluorescent molecule after being mixed and heated with AAPH; it was first developed by Cao et al. (1993) and further developed by Huang et al. using microplate fluorescence reader for analyses of large number of samples (Huang et al. 2002). The results are expressed as μmol trolox per liter plasma. Plasma total phenolics were analyzed using Folin-Ciocalteu method described by another study (Singleton and Rossi 1965).

Plasma vitamin C and uric acid were determined as described (Ross 1994) using high-performance liquid chromatography (HPLC, Agilent Technology 1200, Santa Clara, CA) with a UV detector, separated with an Eclipse XDB-C18 column (5 μm;250 mm × 4.6 mm, Agilent Technology, Santa Clara, CA) and Zorbax C18 guard column (5 μm; 12 mm × 4.6 mm, Agilent Technology, Santa Clara, CA). The analytical conditions were modified in the present study. In order to preserve vitamin C, an aliquot of plasma was deproteinized with 10% perchloric acid. This sample was then centrifuged (15,000 × g, 5 min, 4°C) and the supernatant was kept at −80°C until analysis. All plasma samples were pretreated within an hour of blood collection. The mobile phase was 25 mM myristyltrimethylammonium bromide, 0.05 M sodium hydroxide, 0.06 M acetic acid, 7.5% (v/v) acetonitrile in pH 5.5. Samples and standards were prepared with mobile phase and then analyzed by UV at 262 nm with a flow rate of 0.45 mL/min.

Vitamin E (as α- and γ-tocopherol) was measured by HPLC-Coularrary (ESA Inc., Chelmsford, MA), as described previously (Bruno et al. 2008) with minor modifications. In brief, 350 μL plasma was mixed with 2 mL 1% ascorbic acid prepared in ethanol (w/v), 1 mL purified water, and 500 μL saturated KOH (79.2 g KOH dissolved in 74.2 mL water). Following saponification (30 min, 70°C), samples were rapidly chilled, and mixed with water (1 mL) and 4.54 mM BHT (25 μL) prepared in reagent alcohol. Tocopherols were extracted with hexane (2 mL), the extract was dried under nitrogen, and dissolved in a known volume of 1:1 methanol:ethanol. The injected sample was separated isocratically (0.6 mL/min) on a Luna C18(2) column (150 mm × 3 mm i.d., 3 μ; Phenomenex, Torrence, CA) and detected at potential settings of 350, 450, 525 and 600 mV. The mobile phase was 98:2 methanol:water containing 10 mmol/L lithium perchlorate.

The slightly modified method described by Karppia et al. (2008) was used for carotenoid analyses. Briefly, 200 μL sample was mixed with 300 μL distilled deionized water, 500 μL ethanol (containing 0.1% BHT and 0.1 mg/L of rac-tocol as an internal standard) and 1 mL of hexane (containing 0.1% BHT). After 3 min vortexing and 5 min ultra sonication samples were centrifuged for 5 min (15,000 × g, 4°C) and the supernatant was transferred. This extract step was repeated twice. Transferred supernatants were evaporated by nitrogen and dissolved in 200 μL of mobile phase. One hundred microlitre of sample was injected and detected at 450 nm for carotenoids and 290 nm for the internal standard. An HPLC system (Agilent 1100, Hewlett Packard, Palo Alto, CA) with a photodiode array detector and a C18 RP Symmetry analytical column (5 μm, 250 mm × 4.6 mm, Agilent Technology, Santa Clara, CA) was used for the analysis. The solvent gradient conditions of binary mobile phases (solvent A, acetonitrile; solvent B, methanol, THF, and methylene chloride (85:5:10)) for the HPLC analysis was as follows: 93% A/7% B from 0 to 7 min, 88.6% A/11.4% B from 8 to 15 min, 21% A/79% B from 16 to 17 min, 16% A/84% B from 18 to 50 min, and 93% A/7% B from 51 to 55 min. The flow rate was set at 1 mL/min and changed to 1.8 mL/min at 16 min until 50 min.

Superoxide dismutase (SOD), catalase (CAT), and glutathione peroxidase (GPx) activities in plasma were determined by using commercially available kits (Cayman Chemical Company, Ann Arbor, MI, US). One unit of SOD in plasma is defined as the amount of enzyme needed to exhibit 50% dismutation of the superoxide radical. One unit CAT in plasma is defined as the amount of enzyme that will cause the formation of 1.0 nmol of formaldehyde per minute at 25°C. One unit GPx in plasma is defined the amount of enzyme that will cause the oxidation of 1.0 nmol of NADPH to $NADP^+$ per minute at 25°C.

11.2.6 *Statistical Analysis*

Statistical Analysis System (SAS) software, release 9.2, 2009 (SAS Institute Inc., Cary, NC) was used for statistical calculation. To test the distribution of dietary TAC estimates and plasma antioxidant nutrients, residual and goodness-of-fit analyses were used. If these analyses showed any evidence of departure from normality, we used log-transformed variables in the analysis. To evaluate the association between dietary or plasma antioxidants and dietary TAC, subjects were divided into two groups according to TAC intakes. P values were tested across the median values of dietary TAC in each group by analysis of covariance using the General Linear Model procedure. To investigate the association between dietary TAC intakes and plasma levels, data was analyzed by two regression models. The simple model was adjusted for age, ethnicity, and plasma cholesterol (except ascorbic acid and uric acid). To test the sensitivity of dietary TAC as a predicting tool, the simple model was further adjusted for fruit and fruit juices, vegetable and vegetable juices and supplement use, which are the major contributors of dietary TAC. Data were reported as geometric least square means and 95% CIs if strongly skewed. In addition, to evaluate relative validity, the associations between antioxidant nutrient intakes estimated by 7-day DR and their plasma profiles were analyzed. The level of statistical significance was set at $p<0.05$.

11.3 Results

11.3.1 *Dietary and Clinical Characteristics of Study Population*

In this study population, the average TAC from diet was 686.6 mg VCE/day and the average TAC from both diet and supplements was 832.6 mg. Table 11.1 describes the general characteristics of the study population according to the intake of dietary TAC in two groups. Subjects in the high TAC intake groups were more likely to report hypertension but less likely to report hypercholesterolemia and had lower total-and LDL-cholesterol. Meanwhile they consumed more tea, wine and less beer; they consumed more fruit and vegetable products, especially berries and apples, as compared with those in the low TAC intake groups.

Table 11.1 Demographic, clinical, and dietary characteristics according to the total antioxidant capacity levels of the study subjects[a]

Total antioxidant capacity (TAC)	TAC from diet		TAC from diet and supplement	
(mg VCE/day)	Low ($n=20$)	High ($n=20$)	Low ($n=20$)	High ($n=20$)
Ranges[b]	54.4–524	559–2608	54.4–721	729–2608
Median	[329]	[846]	[365]	[1182]
Mean	303.2 ± 159.0	1069.9 ± 592.5	378.5 ± 216.1	1286.6 ± 534.8
Age (y)	57 ± 6	60 ± 6	57 ± 7	59 ± 5
BMI (kg/m^2)	30.3 ± 3.6	30.2 ± 2.5	30.1 ± 3.4	30.4 ± 2.8
Fasting glucose (mg/dL)	98.4 ± 11.2	96.1 ± 7.7	100.9 ± 10.5	93.6 ± 7.1
Triglycerides (mg/dL)	91.0 ± 29.0	101.5 ± 50.9	96.9 ± 37.9	95.6 ± 45.4
LDL cholesterol (mg/dL)	137.9 ± 35.3	134.65 ± 32.0	136.8 ± 37.1	135.7 ± 30.0
HDL cholesterol (mg/dL)	69.0 ± 11.7	65.4 ± 16.3	67.4 ± 12.1	67.0 ± 16.2
Total:HDL cholesterol ratio	3.1 ± 0.7	3.2 ± 0.8	3.1 ± 0.7	3.2 ± 0.7
Albumin (mg/dL)	4.1 ± 0.2	4.1 ± 0.2	4.1 ± 0.2	4.1 ± 0.2
Bilirubin, total (mg/dL)	0.35 ± 0.12	0.43 ± 0.19	0.37 ± 0.21	0.41 ± 0.11
Cholesterol, total (mg/dL)	206.8 ± 31.9	199.9 ± 34.8	204.1 ± 36.1	202.6 ± 30.8
Hypertension (self reported) (%)	15	35	15	35
Hypercholesterolemia (self reported) (%)	30	25	35	20
Anti-hypertensive (%)	10	15	5	20
Aspirin (%)	30	50	25	55
NSAID (%)	5	5	5	5
Supplement use (%)	35	55	30	60
Energy intake (kcal/d)	1531 ± 369	1788 ± 335	1512 ± 317	1812 ± 373
Food intake				
Tea (g/day)	24.9 ± 48.5	233.9 ± 199.9	32.7 ± 52.5	226.0 ± 207.0
Wine (g/day)	27.0 ± 50.0	54.4 ± 71.7	31.3 ± 56.2	50.1 ± 67.8

Beer (g/day)	35.5 ± 128.3	22.8 ± 50.5	33.1 ± 125.0	24.7 ± 52.1
Onions (g/day)	12.0 ± 11.4	10.7 ± 9.6	12.5 ± 10.9	10.2 ± 10.0
Berries (g/day)	20.7 ± 25.6	70.2 ± 52.1	31.4 ± 32.1	63.2 ± 55.9
Apples (g/day)	16.5 ± 27.3	34.3 ± 57.8	19.9 ± 41.4	30.9 ± 49.8
Legumes (g/day)	22.8 ± 23.0	28.9 ± 42.1	23.8 ± 22.9	27.9 ± 422
Fruits and fruit juices (serving/day)	2.5 ± 2.0	3.6 ± 1.3	2.8 ± 2.0	3.4 ± 1.4
Vegetables and vegetable juices (serving/day)	3.1 ± 1.4	4.0 ± 2.1	3.5 ± 2.2	3.7 ± 1.5

[a]Values are mean ± SD
[b]Values within brackets are the medians

11.3.2 Major Food Sources

Main food sources for TAC were tea, wine, vegetables and vegetable juices, fruits and fruit juices (Fig. 11.1). Fruits and fruit juices contributed the most to dietary TAC, accounting for 44.3% of TAC from diet and 36.6% of TAC from diet and supplements, followed by tea (33.1% and 27.3%, respectively).

11.3.3 Associations Between Individual Antioxidant Intakes and TAC from Diet/Diet and Supplements

After adjustment for total energy intake, higher intake of TAC from diet was associated with higher intakes of α-tocopherol ($p<0.001$), vitamin C ($p<0.001$), flavonoids ($p<0.001$) and proanthocyanidins ($p<0.001$) (Table 11.2). However, it was negatively associated with intakes of γ-tocopherol ($p<0.001$) and total tocopherols (including α, β, γ and δ-tocopherols) ($p<0.001$). For TAC from both diet and supplements, those positive associations still existed. Further, total tocopherol ($p<0.001$) and total carotenoids ($p<0.01$) became significantly associated with TAC from diet and supplements, which could be attributed to the large amount and high prevalence of α-tocopherol and β-carotene supplement use in this study population (Table 11.3). Indeed, 48% of the participants used α-tocopherol supplements and 42.5% used β-carotene supplements in this study.

11.3.4 Associations Between Plasma Antioxidant Status and TAC from Diet/Diet and Supplements

After adjustment for basic characteristics in the simple model, TAC from diet was positively associated with plasma TAC determined by VCEAC ($p<0.01$), FRAP (<0.0001) and ORAC ($p<0.05$); it was positively associated with catalase ($p<0.05$), α-tocopherol ($p<0.0001$) and β-cryptoxanthin concentrations ($p<0.01$) and it was negatively correlated with total phenolics ($p<0.01$) and lycopene ($p<0.05$) (Table 11.4). After further adjustment for fruit and fruit juices, vegetable and vegetable juices and supplement use, the association with ORAC, catalase and lycopene disappeared; total phenolics became positively correlated with TAC from diet ($p<0.05$) and others stayed the same (Table 11.4). As for TAC from diet and supplements, it was also positively associated with plasma TAC determined by VCEAC ($p<0.001$), FRAP ($p<0.0001$) and ORAC ($p<0.05$); it was positively associated with α-tocopherol ($p<0.001$), β-cryptoxanthin ($p<0.05$) and negatively associated with total phenolics ($p<0.01$) in the simple model (Table 11.5). After further adjustment, except ORAC, all of these variables remained significant.

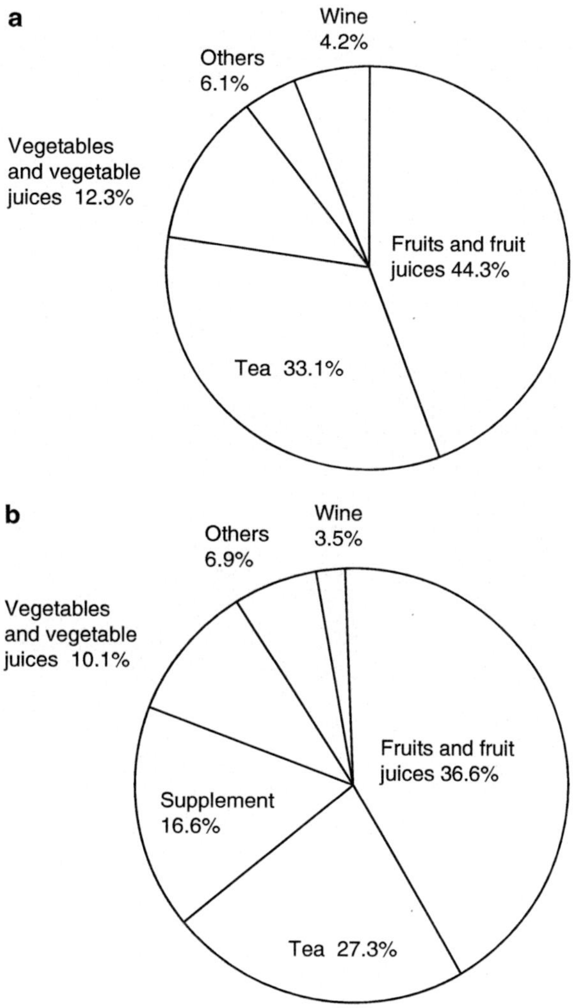

Fig. 11.1 Contributions of major food sources to dietary total antioxidant capacity (*TAC*). Contribution of major food sources to TAC from diet (**a**); contribution of major sources to TAC from diet and supplements (**b**)

11.3.5 Dietary Antioxidants and the Corresponding Concentrations in Plasma

To further confirm that dietary TAC parallels dietary antioxidants in predicting the corresponding plasma antioxidant concentrations, the correlation between dietary antioxidants and their concentrations in plasma was examined. After multivariable adjustment, α-tocopherol ($p<0.001$), β-carotene ($p<0.05$) and β-cryptoxanthin ($p<0.05$) concentrations in plasma were positively correlated with their intakes from diet (Table 11.6). Taking the supplement use into account, β-carotene became not significant. Although Vitamin C and β-carotene supplement uses tremendously

Table 11.2 Comparison of dietary intakes of individual antioxidants according to the levels of total antioxidant capacity from diet in the study subjects[a]

Total antioxidant capacity (TAC)	Model	Low TAC ($n=20$)	95% CIs	High TAC ($n=20$)	95% CIs	P value[b]
Ranges[c] (mg VCE/day)		54.4–524		559–2608		
Median (mg VCE/day)		[329]		[846]		
Tocopherol intake[c] (mg/day)	Basic	19.0	[16.2 22.4]	22.1	[18.8 25.9]	0.20
	Energy-adjusted	20.9	[18.7 23.4]	20.1	[18.0 22.5]	<0.001
α-Tocopherol (mg/day)	Basic	7.3	[6.0 8.9]	9.2	[7.5 11.3]	0.11
	Energy-adjusted	8.0	[6.6 9.5]	8.5	[7.1 10.1]	<0.001
γ-Tocopherol (mg/day)	Basic	9.1	[7.6 10.9]	10.0	[8.3 12.0]	0.48
	Energy-adjusted	10.0	[8.7 11.5]	9.0	[7.9 10.4]	<0.001
Ascorbic acid (mg/day)	Basic	78.9	[66.9 93.0]	95.4	[80.9 112.5]	<0.001
	Energy-adjusted	70.2	[56.9 86.6]	107.2	[86.9 132.2]	<0.001
Carotenoid intake (mg/day)	Basic	10.4	[7.9 13.8]	12.3	[9.3 16.3]	0.40
	Energy-adjusted	10.9	[8.2 14.5]	11.8	[8.9 15.6]	0.30
β-Carotene (mg/day)	Basic	2.7	[1.9 3.8]	4.0	[2.8 5.6]	0.10
	Energy-adjusted	2.8	[2.0 4.0]	3.8	[2.7 5.4]	0.10
α-Carotene (mg/day)	Basic	0.18	[0.10 0.33]	0.33	[0.18 0.61]	0.18
	Energy-adjusted	0.20	[0.10 0.37]	0.30	[0.16 0.57]	0.25
β-Cryptoxanthin (mg/day)	Basic	0.07	[0.05 0.10]	0.13	[0.09 0.18]	<0.05
	Energy-adjusted	0.07	[0.05 0.11]	0.12	[0.09 0.18]	0.10
Lutein + zeaxanthin (mg/day)	Basic	1.7	[1.24 2.42]	2.5	[1.8 3.5]	0.14
	Energy-adjusted	1.9	[1.34 2.62]	2.3	[1.6 3.2]	0.07
Lycopene (mg/day)	Basic	4.2	[1.7 10.1]	2.5	[1.0 6.0]	0.41
	Energy-adjusted	4.5	[1.8 11.3]	2.3	[0.9 5.7]	0.55
Flavonoid intake (mg/day)	Basic	64.3	[46.1 89.6]	320.9	[230.2 447.5]	<0.001
	Energy-adjusted	66.5	[47.1 93.9]	310.2	[219.7 438.0]	<0.001
Isoflavones (mg/day)	Basic	0.8	[0.4 1.4]	1.9	[1.1 3.5]	<0.05
	Energy-adjusted	0.8	[0.4 1.5]	1.9	[1.0 3.5]	0.12

Anthocyanidins (mg/day)	Basic	10.6	[4.6	24.7]	77.9	[33.4	181.3]	<0.01
	Energy-adjusted	11.6	[4.8	27.9]	71.1	[29.6	170.7]	<0.01
Flavan-3-ols (mg/day)	Basic	12.0	[6.6	22.0]	153.2	[83.8	280.2]	<0.001
	Energy-adjusted	13.2	[7.1	24.6]	139.0	[74.9	258.0]	<0.001
Flavanones (mg/day)	Basic	2.6	[1.2	5.5]	7.0	[3.3	15.1]	0.07
	Energy-adjusted	2.3	[1.1	5.1]	7.8	[3.5	17.1]	0.11
Flavones (mg/day)	Basic	0.7	[0.5	1.2]	2.2	[1.4	3.5]	<0.01
	Energy-adjusted	0.8	[0.5	1.3]	2.0	[1.2	3.2]	<0.01
Flavonols (mg/day)	Basic	10.2	[8.2	12.8]	24.0	[19.1	30.1]	<0.001
	Energy-adjusted	10.5	[8.3	13.3]	23.2	[18.4	29.4]	<0.001
Proanthocyanidins (mg/day)	Basic	12.6	[8.1	19.6]	47.7	[30.7	73.9]	<0.001
	Energy-adjusted	14.1	[9.1	21.8]	42.8	[27.7	66.3]	<0.001

[a]Values are geometric means [and 95% CIs]

[b]Antioxidant intake data were log transformed for test for trend. P value was calculated across the median value of intake of TAC from diet in each tertile using general linear model

[c]Tocopherol includes α, β, γ and δ-tocopherols

Table 11.3 Comparison of dietary intakes of individual antioxidants according to the levels of total antioxidant capacity from diet and supplements in the study subjects[a]

Total antioxidant capacity (TAC)	Model	Low TAC (*n*=20)	95% CIs		High TAC (*n*=20)	95% CIs		P value[b]
Ranges (mg VCE/day)		54.4–721			729–2608			
Median (mg VCE/day)		[365]			[1182]			
Tocopherol (mg/day)[c]	Basic	18.2	[11.6	28.6]	64.0	[40.8	100.5]	<0.001
	Energy-adjusted	21.5	[13.7	34.1]	54.1	[34.1	84.8]	<0.001
α-Tocopherol (mg/day)	Basic	8.5	[4.9	14.8]	44.5	[25.6	77.5]	<0.001
	Energy-adjusted	10.1	[5.6	18.0]	37.7	[21.1	66.7]	<0.001
γ-Tocopherol (mg/day)	Basic	8.8	[7.3	10.5]	10.3	[8.6	12.4]	0.21
	Energy-adjusted	10.1	[8.8	11.6]	9.0	[7.8	10.4]	<0.001
Ascorbic acid (mg/day)	Basic	80.9	[59.5	109.9]	205.8	[151.5	279.6]	<0.001
Carotenoid intake (mg/day)	Basic	18.6	[9.2	37.8]	106.4	[52.4	216.1]	<0.01
	Energy-adjusted	21.8	[10.3	46.1]	90.9	[42.9	192.5]	<0.01
β-Carotene (mg/day)	Basic	6.2	[2.5	15.4]	68.9	[27.5	172.6]	<0.001
	Energy-adjusted	7.6	[2.9	20.3]	55.7	[21.1	146.9]	<0.05
α-Carotene (mg/day)	Basic	0.20	[0.11	0.37]	0.30	[0.16	0.56]	0.36
	Energy-adjusted	0.23	[0.12	0.44]	0.26	[0.14	0.51]	0.37
β-Cryptoxanthin (mg/day)	Basic	0.09	[0.06	0.13]	0.10	[0.07	0.15]	0.55
	Energy-adjusted	0.09	[0.06	0.14]	0.10	[0.07	0.15]	0.64
Lutein + zeaxanthin (mg/day)	Basic	2.0	[1.2	3.4]	3.0	[1.8	5.0]	0.31
	Energy-adjusted	2.4	[1.4	4.1]	2.5	[1.5	4.3]	0.11
Lycopene (mg/day)	Basic	4.9	[1.9	12.5]	2.5	[1.0	6.3]	0.31
	Energy-adjusted	5.9	[2.2	16.1]	2.1	[0.8	5.6]	0.32
Flavonoid intake (mg/day)	Basic	77.8	[51.6	117.4]	265.1	[175.8	399.8]	<0.001
	Energy-adjusted	81.5	[52.5	126.5]	252.1	[162.4	395.4]	<0.001
Isoflavones (mg/day)	Basic	0.7	[0.4	1.3]	2.1	[1.2	3.9]	<0.01
	Energy-adjusted	0.7	[0.4	1.3]	2.2	[1.2	4.1]	<0.05

Anthocyanidins (mg/day)	Basic	14.9	[6.0	37.2]	55.4	[22.2	138.2]	<0.05
	Energy-adjusted	17.5	[6.6	46.5]	47.0	[17.8	125.2]	0.09
Flavan-3-ols (mg/day)	Basic	14.6	[7.4	28.9]	125.9	[63.7	248.7]	<0.0001
	Energy-adjusted	16.3	[7.8	33.8]	113.3	[54.6	232.8]	<0.001
Flavanones (mg/day)	Basic	4.5	[2.0	9.9]	4.0	[1.8	8.9]	0.85
	Energy-adjusted	4.3	[1.8	10.2]	4.1	[1.8	9.9]	0.95
Flavones (mg/day)	Basic	0.8	[0.5	1.3]	2.0	[1.2	3.2]	<0.05
	Energy-adjusted	0.9	[0.5	1.5]	1.8	[1.0	2.9]	<0.05
Flavonols (mg/day)	Basic	11.5	[8.8	15.0]	21.3	[16.3	27.7]	<0.01
	Energy-adjusted	12.1	[9.1	16.0]	20.3	[15.3	26.8]	<0.01
Proanthocyanidins (mg/day)	Basic	15.2	[9.3	24.7]	39.7	[24.4	64.7]	<0.01
	Energy-adjusted	18.0	[10.8	29.7]	33.8	[20.3	55.7]	<0.01

[a]Values are geometric means [and 95% CIs]
[b]Antioxidant intake data were log transformed for test for trend. P value was calculated across the median value of intake of TAC from diet in each tertile using general linear model
[c]Tocopherols include α, β, γ and δ-tocopherols

Table 11.4 Plasma antioxidant profiles according to intake of TAC from diet in the study subjects[a]

Total antioxidant capacity (TAC)	Model	Low TAC ($n=20$)	95% CIs		High TAC ($n=20$)	95% CIs		P-trend[b]
Ranges[c] (mg VCE/d)		54.4–524			559–2608			
Median (mg VCE/d)		[329]			[846]			
Antioxidant enzymes								
Superoxide Dismutase (U/ml)	Adjusted[d]	13.5	[11.7	15.7]	13.0	[11.2	15.1]	0.44
	Adjusted[e]	13.4	[11.4	15.8]	13.1	[11.1	15.4]	0.78
Catalase (nmol formaldehyde	Adjusted[d]	21.3	[16.9	27.0]	35.0	[27.7	44.3]	<0.05
/min/ml)	Adjusted[e]	20.9	[16.2	26.9]	35.8	[27.7	46.2]	0.13
Glutathione peroxidase	Adjusted[d]	109	[103	116]	114	[108	120]	0.26
(nmol NADPH/min/ml)	Adjusted[e]	109	[102	116]	115	[108	121]	0.59
Antioxidant nutrients								
Ascorbic acid (μmol/L)	Adjusted[f]	42.8	[35.2	50.4]	47.4	[40.0	54.7]	0.56
	Adjusted[g]	44.8	[37.0	52.6]	45.4	[37.8	53.0]	0.36
Total phenolics (mg GE/L)	Adjusted[d]	2156	[2112	2200]	2149	[2105	2193]	<0.01
	Adjusted[e]	2146	[2099	2192]	2159	[2113	2206]	<0.05
α-Tocopherol (μmol/L)	Adjusted[d]	30.7	[27.5	33.9]	33.8	[30.6	37.0]	<0.0001
	Adjusted[e]	31.1	[28.2	34.0]	33.4	[30.5	36.3]	<0.0001
γ-tocopherol (μmol/L)	Adjusted[d]	2.50	[1.89	3.31]	1.73	[1.31	2.30]	0.45
	Adjusted[e]	2.37	[1.78	3.17]	1.83	[1.37	2.44]	0.27
β-Carotene (μmol/L)	Adjusted[d]	0.091	[0.061	0.134]	0.200	[0.135	0.297]	0.07
	Adjusted[e]	0.091	[0.059	0.140]	0.200	[0.130	0.307]	0.19
α-Carotene (μmol/L)	Adjusted[d]	0.074	[0.016	0.133]	0.133	[0.075	0.192]	0.66
	Adjusted[e]	0.071	[0.007	0.135]	0.136	[0.072	0.200]	0.80
β-Cryptoxanthin (μmol/L)	Adjusted[d]	0.225	[0.164	0.285]	0.303	[0.242	0.363]	<0.0001
	Adjusted[e]	0.215	[0.152	0.278]	0.312	[0.250	0.375]	<0.001
Lutein (μmol/L)	Adjusted[d]	0.118	[0.069	0.202]	0.206	[0.121	0.353]	0.47
	Adjusted [e]	0.121	[0.067	0.219]	0.202	[0.111	0.365]	0.78

Zeaxanthin (μmol/L)	Adjusted[d]	0.024	[0.021	0.028]	0.025	[0.022	0.029]	0.78
	Adjusted[e]	0.023	[0.020	0.027]	0.026	[0.022	0.030]	0.5
Lycopene (μmol/L)	Adjusted[d]	0.122	[0.099	0.146]	0.097	[0.073	0.120]	<0.05
	Adjusted[e]	0.122	[0.097	0.148]	0.097	[0.071	0.122]	0.09
Uric acid (μmol/L)	Adjusted[f]	292	[256	328]	241	[205	277]	0.21
	Adjusted[g]	302	[265	339]	231	[194	268]	0.17
TAC by VCEAC (mg VCE/L)	Adjusted[h]	299	[290	308]	303	[294	313]	<0.001
	Adjusted[i]	297	[287	307]	305	[296	316]	<0.001
TAC by FRAP (μmolTrolox/L)	Adjusted[h]	489	[459	521]	522	[489	558]	<0.0001
	Adjusted[i]	490	[457	525]	522	[485	561]	<0.001
TAC by ORAC (μmolTrolox/L)	Adjusted[h]	3796	[3292	4299]	4284	[3781	4787]	<0.05
	Adjusted[i]	3796	[3210	4382]	4284	[3698	4870]	0.19

[a]Values are geometric means [and 95% CIs]
[b]Plasma antioxidant data were log transformed for test for trend. P value was calculated across the median value of intake of TAC from diet in each tertile using general linear model
[c]Values within brackets are the medians
[d]Model was adjusted for age, ethnicity, plasma cholesterol
[e]Model was adjusted for age, ethnicity, plasma cholesterol, fruit and fruit juice intake, vegetable and vegetable juice intake and supplement use
[f]Model was adjusted for age, ethnicity
[g]Model was adjusted for age, ethnicity, fruit and fruit juice intake, vegetable and vegetable juice intake and supplement use
[h]Model was adjusted for age, ethnicity, plasma cholesterol, uric acid
[i]Model was adjusted for age, ethnicity, plasma cholesterol, uric acid, fruit and fruit juice intake, vegetable and vegetable juice intake and supplement use

Table 11.5 Plasma antioxidant profiles according to intake of TAC from diet and supplement in the study subjects[a]

Total antioxidant capacity (TAC)	Model	Low TAC (n = 20)	95% CIs		High TAC (n = 20)	95% CIs		P-trend[b]
Ranges[c] (mg VCE/day)		54.4–721			729–2608			
Median (mg VCE/day)		[365]			[1182]			
Antioxidant enzymes								
Superoxide Dismutase (U/ml)	Adjusted[d]	13.9	[12.0	16.2]	12.6	[10.8	14.6]	0.35
	Adjusted[e]	13.9	[11.8	16.3]	12.6	[10.8	14.8]	0.72
Catalase (nmol formaldehyde	Adjusted[d]	25.6	[19.6	33.5]	29.2	[22.3	38.1]	0.55
/min/ml)	Adjusted[e]	25.7	[19.4	34.0]	29.1	[22.0	38.5]	0.70
Glutathione peroxidase	Adjusted[d]	110	[104	117]	113	[107	120]	0.31
(nmol NADPH/min/ml)	Adjusted[e]	110	[103	117]	113	[106	120]	0.68
Antioxidant nutrients								
Ascorbic acid (μmol/L)	Adjusted[f]	44.5	[36.5	52.4]	45.8	[38.1	53.5]	0.68
	Adjusted[g]	45.4	[37.6	53.2]	44.9	[37.3	52.5]	0.36
Total phenolics (mg GE/L)	Adjusted[d]	2164	[211	92209]	2141	[2096	2186]	<0.01
	Adjusted[e]	2159	[2113	2205]	2146	[2100	2192]	<0.05
α-Tocopherol (μmol/L)	Adjusted[d]	29.5	[26.4	32.6]	35.0	[31.9	38.1]	<0.0001
	Adjusted[e]	30.4	[27.6	33.2]	34.1	[31.3	36.9]	<0.0001
γ-tocopherol (μmol/L)	Adjusted[d]	0.985	[0.708	1.262]	0.483	[0.205	0.760]	0.21
	Adjusted[e]	0.923	[0.645	1.200]	0.545	[0.268	0.822]	0.16
β-Carotene (μmol/L)	Adjusted[d]	0.104	[0.067	0.159]	0.175	[0.114	0.269]	0.33
	Adjusted[e]	0.109	[0.070	0.172]	0.166	[0.106	0.261]	0.54
α-Carotene (μmol/L)	Adjusted[d]	0.089	[0.028	0.151]	0.118	[0.057	0.179]	0.89
	Adjusted[e]	0.087	[0.023	0.152]	0.120	[0.056	0.184]	0.92
β-Cryptoxanthin (μmol/L)	Adjusted[d]	0.247	[0.183	0.311]	0.280	[0.216	0.344]	<0.001
	Adjusted[e]	0.235	[0.171	0.299]	0.292	[0.228	0.357]	<0.001
Lutein (μmol/L)	Adjusted[d]	0.112	[0.065	0.193]	0.218	[0.127	0.375]	0.39
	Adjusted[e]	0.116	[0.065	0.207]	0.211	[0.118	0.377]	0.71

Zeaxanthin (μmol/L)	Adjusted[d]	0.026	[0.022	0.030]	0.023	[0.020	0.027]	0.63
	Adjusted[e]	0.025	[0.022	0.029]	0.024	[0.021	0.027]	0.58
Lycopene (μmol/L)	Adjusted[d]	0.117	[0.093	0.142]	0.101	[0.077	0.126]	0.05
	Adjusted[e]	0.117	[0.092	0.143]	0.102	[0.076	0.127]	0.19
Uric acid (μmol/L)	Adjusted[f]	268	[230	307]	265	[226	304]	0.73
	Adjusted[g]	273	[233	314]	260	[219	300]	0.74
TAC by VCEAC (mg VCE/L)	Adjusted[h]	300.9	[291.8	310.3]	301.3	[292.1	310.7]	<0.001
	Adjusted[i]	300.7	[291.6	310.1]	301.5	[292.4	310.9]	<0.001
TAC by FRAP (μmolTrolox/L)	Adjusted[h]	495	[465	528]	515	[483	550]	<0.0001
	Adjusted[i]	496	[465	528]	515	[482	550]	<0.001
TAC by ORAC (μmolTrolox/L)	Adjusted[h]	3742	[3251	4233]	4338	[38474829]		<0.05
	Adjusted[i]	3744	[3213	4275]	4336	[3805	4866]	0.14

[a]Values are geometric means [and 95% CIs]
[b]Plasma antioxidant data were log transformed for test for trend. P value was calculated across the median value of intake of TAC from diet in each tertile using general linear model
[c]Values within brackets are the medians
[d]Model was adjusted for age, ethnicity, plasma cholesterol
[e] Model was adjusted for age, ethnicity, plasma cholesterol, fruit and fruit juice intake, vegetable and vegetable juice intake and supplement use
[f]Model was adjusted for age, ethnicity
[g]Model was adjusted for age, ethnicity, fruit and fruit juice intake, vegetable and vegetable juice intake and supplement use
[h]Model was adjusted for age, ethnicity, plasma cholesterol, uric acid
[i]Model was adjusted for age, ethnicity, plasma cholesterol, uric acid, fruit and fruit juice intake, vegetable and vegetable juice intake and supplement use

Table 11.6 Plasma antioxidant concentrations according to the intakes of individual antioxidants from diet in the study subjects[a]

	Model	Low intake ($n=20$)	95% CIs		High intake ($n=20$)	95% CIs		P value[b]
Ascorbic acid (μmol/L)	Basic	40.78	[34.44	48.30]	44.19	[37.48	52.11]	0.45
	Adjusted[c]	43.37	[36.17	52.01]	41.68	[34.95	49.71]	0.17
α-Tocopherol (μmol/L)	Basic	28.41	[25.22	32.00]	33.99	[30.18	38.29]	<0.05
	Adjusted[d]	30.07	[27.71	32.63]	32.11	[29.59	34.85]	<0.001
γ-tocopherol (μmol/L)	Basic	2.10	[1.61	2.74]	2.07	[1.59	2.70]	0.95
	Adjusted[d]	2.09	[1.58	2.75]	2.08	[1.58	2.74]	0.34
β-Carotene (μmol/L)	Basic	0.10	[0.07	0.14]	0.18	[0.13	0.27]	<0.05
	Adjusted[d]	0.09	[0.06	0.13]	0.20	[0.14	0.29]	<0.05
α-Carotene (μmol/L)	Basic	0.04	[0.02	0.06]	0.08	[0.05	0.15]	<0.05
	Adjusted[d]	0.03	[0.02	0.06]	0.09	[0.05	0.17]	0.14
β-Cryptoxanthin (μmol/L)	Basic	0.23	[0.18	0.30]	0.21	[0.17	0.28]	0.61
	Adjusted[d]	0.25	[0.20	0.32]	0.20	[0.16	0.25]	<0.05
Lutein + Zeaxanthin (μmol/L)	Basic	0.07	[0.04	0.11]	0.13	[0.08	0.20]	0.08
	Adjusted[d]	0.06	[0.04	0.11]	0.14	[0.08	0.24]	0.49
Lycopene (μmol/L)	Basic	0.08	[0.07	0.11]	0.11	[0.08	0.14]	0.16
	Adjusted[d]	0.08	[0.06	0.10]	0.11	[0.09	0.15]	0.15

[a]Values are geometric means [and 95% CIs]

[b]Plasma antioxidant data were log transformed for test for trend. P value was calculated across the median value of intake of antioxidant from diet and supplement in each tertile using general linear model

[c]Model was adjusted for age, BMI, ethnicity, fruit and fruit juice intake, vegetable and vegetable juice intake and supplement use

[d]Model was adjusted for age, BMI, ethnicity, plasma cholesterol, fruit and fruit juice intake, vegetable and vegetable juice intake and supplement use

contributed to their intake levels, their contribution to the plasma ascorbic acid and β-carotene concentrations were not significant (Table 11.7). In general, dietary TAC was in accordance with dietary antioxidants in predicting their concentrations in plasma.

11.4 Discussion

In the present study, dietary TAC (from diet/diet and supplement) was positively associated with intakes of dietary antioxidants, including α-tocopherol, ascorbic acid, flavonoids and proanthocyanidins. In addition, higher dietary TAC was associated with increased plasma TAC determined by VCEAC, FRAP and ORAC after adjusting for uric acid and other confounders and was also associated with increased plasma concentrations of individual antioxidants, including α-tocopherol, and β-Cryptoxanthin. The participants in high dietary TAC groups reported more hypertension and medication use than those in low dietary TAC groups. The associations did not necessarily reflect causal relationships, for this is a cross-sectional study. It is plausible that those participants who self-reported hypertension tended to consume more fruits and vegetables and lived a healthier life style as an attempt to improve their condition.

11.4.1 Dietary TAC Assessments

To estimate TAC from the entire diet is a novel concept that characterizes the sum of antioxidant properties of nutrients known and unknown. It considers the additive and synergistic effects of dietary antioxidants rather than simple sum of single antioxidants' actions. A few studies have estimated dietary TAC (Halvorsen et al. 2002; Serafini et al. 2002; Pellegrini et al. 2007; Rautiainen et al. 2008; Mekary et al. 2010). Rautiainen et al. (2008) showed a correlation of theoretical TAC assessed by a food frequency questionnaire (FFQ) and plasma TAC determined by ORAC, the total radical-trapping antioxidant parameters (TRAP) and ferric reducing ability of plasma (FRAP) assays in Swedish women. An Italian research group (Serafini et al. 2002) developed the first TAC database. Although their FFQ was limited to 12 food items, they found that non-smoking subjects with the highest antioxidant intake had a reduced risk of developing gastric cancer compared to non-smoking subjects with the lowest TAC of the diet. However, when they tried to validate their method against plasma TAC, there was no relationship. TAC estimated by either 3-day weighted food record or an FFQ that included 150 foods had no correlation with plasma TAC determined by TEAC as documented by Pellegrini et al. (2007). Most of the studies used TAC food composition database for the FFQ to assess dietary TAC (Mekary et al. 2010). The food database was limited by the number of foods that have been measured, the differences in growing

Table 11.7 Plasma antioxidant concentrations according to the intakes of individual antioxidants from diet and supplements in the study subjects[a]

	Model	Low intake ($n=20$)	95% CIs		High intake ($n=20$)	95% CIs		P value[b]
Ascorbic acid (μmol/L)	Basic	39.78	[33.64	47.03]	45.26	[38.44	53.28]	0.27
	Adjusted[c]	39.76	[32.54	48.59]	45.27	[37.30	54.95]	0.14
α-Tocopherol (μmol/L)	Basic	27.14	[24.33	30.27]	35.58	[31.90	39.69]	<0.01
	Adjusted[d]	29.66	[26.91	32.69]	32.56	[29.54	35.88]	< 0.001
γ-Tocopherol (μmol/L)	Basic	2.48	[1.93	3.20]	1.75	[1.36	2.25]	0.05
	Adjusted[d]	2.30	[1.66	3.19]	1.89	[1.36	2.61]	0.30
β-Carotene (μmol/L)	Basic	0.11	[0.08	0.17]	0.16	[0.11	0.24]	0.21
	Adjusted[d]	0.11	[0.07	0.19]	0.16	[0.09	0.27]	0.25
α-Carotene (μmol/L)	Basic	0.04	[0.02	0.06]	0.08	[0.05	0.15]	<0.05
	Adjusted[d]	0.03	[0.02	0.06]	0.09	[0.05	0.17]	0.14
β-Cryptoxanthin (μmol/L)	Basic	0.23	[0.18	0.30]	0.21	[0.17	0.28]	0.61
	Adjusted[d]	0.25	[0.20	0.32]	0.20	[0.16	0.25]	<0.05
Lutein + Zeaxanthin (μmol/L)	Basic	0.07	[0.04	0.11]	0.13	[0.08	0.21]	<0.05
	Adjusted[d]	0.06	[0.03	0.10]	0.15	[0.09	0.26]	0.37
Lycopene (μmol/L)	Basic	0.08	[0.07	0.11]	0.11	[0.08	0.14]	0.16
	Adjusted[d]	0.08	[0.06	0.10]	0.11	[0.09	0.15]	0.15

[a]Values are geometric means [and 95% CIs]

[b]Plasma antioxidant data were log transformed for test for trend. P value was calculated across the median value of intake of antioxidant from diet and supplement in each tertile using general linear model

[c]Model was adjusted for age, BMI, ethnicity, fruit and fruit juice intake, vegetable and vegetable juice intake and supplement use

[d]Model was adjusted for age, BMI, ethnicity, plasma cholesterol, fruit and fruit juice intake, vegetable and vegetable juice intake and supplement use

seasons, and geographical locations. The present study's advantage in assessing dietary TAC is using the TAC nutrient database instead of a food database, thus avoiding the loss of TAC in the process of food analyses and not being restricted by number of food items. Consequently, the different results from previous studies could be partly attributed to different methodologies in dietary data collection and plasma TAC measurement. TAC from the diet of the U.S. population is yet to be determined.

11.4.2 TAC Measurements

As each antioxidant compound yields a varying degree of antioxidant capacity, researchers have tried to standardize antioxidant capacity, which is the ability to scavenge various kinds of free radicals, in reference to a known compound. A variety of assays have been developed to measure TAC in foods and plasma, as summarized in Table 11.8. Trolox equivalent antioxidant capacity (TEAC) is one of the most commonly reported methods. Trolox is a water-soluble analogue of vitamin E and a Trolox antioxidant activity unit is equivalent to one mole of Trolox. TEAC was originally introduced for the clinical investigation of premature infants' low serum antioxidant concentrations due to vitamin E deficiency (Miller et al. 1993). This method was modified by Kim et al. (2002). They used vitamin C as standard, thus making the value of this method more straightforward for the public. Others have reported antioxidant capacity by total radical-trapping antioxidant parameters (TRAP) (Ghiselli et al. 1995), ORAC (Cao et al. 1993), FRAP (Benzie and Strain 1996), total antioxidant performance (TAP) (Beretta et al. 2006). Of these methods, the VCEAC method developed by Kim et al. offers several strengths: (1) it expresses antioxidant capacity as a vitamin C equivalent, which represents a leading natural nutrient and antioxidant; (2) hydrophilic (vitamin C) and lipophilic antioxidants (carotenes and tocopherols) can be expressed as VCEAC; and (3) its weight-based expression can be used with consumption data that are usually weight-based, allowing for quantitative measurement.

11.4.3 Dietary Modulation of Plasma TAC and Pitfall of Uric Acid

One method for determining the validity of a dietary assessment is to compare dietary intake with a nutrient's plasma value. The plasma value of a nutrient can reflect its intake in a more meaningful way, as it is considered to be independent from the respondent bias (Resnicow et al. 2000). In the present study, dietary TAC had significantly positive association with plasma TAC after adjustment for uric acid and other confounders. Also, TAC from diet was a good predictor of plasma

Table 11.8 Experimental characteristics of some methods for measuring plasma or serum TAC

Method[a]	Principle[b]	Free Radical	Standard	pH	Measurement	Solubility	References
TEAC	Decolorization of $ABTS^{+}$	$ABTS^{+}$	Trolox	7.4	Absorbance (734 nm)	Hydrophilic	Miller et al. (1993)
VCEAC	Decolorization of $ABTS^{+}$	$ABTS^{+}$	Vitamin C	7.4	Absorbance (734 nm)	Hydrophilic	Kim et al. (2002)
FRAP	Reduction of Fe^{3+} to Fe^{2+}	–	Trolox	3.6	Absorbance (593 nm)	Hydrophilic	Benzie and Strain (1996)
ORAC	Degradation of a florescent molecule (Fluorescein) after being mixed with a free radical generator (AAPH)	ROO·	Trolox	7.4	Fluorescence (ex 485 nm, em 520 nm)	Hydrophilic	Cao et al. (1993)
TRAP	Degradation of a florescent molecule (R-hycoerythin) after being mixed with a free radical generator (ABAP)	ROO·	Trolox	7.4	Fluorescence (ex 495 nm, em 575 nm)	Hydrophilic	Ghiselli et al. (1995)
TAP	Degradation of a lipid-soluble florescentmolecule (BODIPY) after being mixed with a lipophilic radical generator (Meo-AMVN)	ROO·	–	7.4	Fluorescence (ex 502 nm, em 520 nm)	Hydrophilic and lipophilic	Beretta et al. (2006).

[a]*TEAC* trolox equivalent antioxidant capacity, *VCEAC* vitamin C equivalent antioxidant capacity, *FRAP* ferric reducing ability of plasma, *ORAC* oxygen radical absorbance capacity, *TRAP* total radical-trapping antioxidant parameter, *TAP* total antioxidant performance

[b]*ABTS*$^{·+}$ 2,2′-azino-bis (3-ethylbenzthiazoline-6-sulphonic acid), *AAPH* 2,2′-azobis (2-amidinopropane) dihydrochloride, *ABAP* 2,2′-diazobis (2-amidinopropane) dihydrochloride, *BODIPY* 4,4-difluoro-5-(4-phenyl-1,3-butadienyl)-4-bora-3a,4a-diaza-s-indacene-3-undecanoic acid, *MeO-AMVN* 2,2′-azobis(4-methoxy-2,4-dimethylvaleronitrile)

catalase, total α-tocopherol and β-cryptoxanthin after other confounders were adjusted. Many studies reported plasma TAC increased immediately after a diet rich in fruits and vegetables (Cao et al. 1998a, b). Since some studies also found the increase in plasma TAC paralleled increase in uric acid concentration (Day and Stansbie 1995; Cao et al. 1998b; Natella et al. 2002), Lotito and Frei (2006) reviewed numerous studies of this kind and pointed out that uric acid accounted for the primary increase in plasma TAC due to relatively higher concentrations as compared with the concentrations of flavonoids, which have limited bioavailability. Although the present observational study also found uric acid was highly correlated with plasma TAC ($r = 0.56$), this association lost significance after adjustment. This suggests that the positive correlation between dietary TAC and plasma TAC could not be attributed to uric acid. Also, uric acid and plasma TAC went back down to the normal level a few hours after the acute increase induced by red wine consumption (Day and Stansbie 1995), thus 12-h fasting blood samples in the present study excluded the acute action of uric acid to plasma TAC. Obviously the present study does not support Lotito and Frei's viewpoint that it is the uric acid induced by consumption of flavonoid-rich food. We unexpectedly observed that dietary TAC was negatively associated with plasma total phenolics. Several studies have reported an acute increase of total phenolics and total antioxidant capacity a few hours after consuming a phenolic-rich food (Serafini et al. 1998; Price et al. 2008; Torabian et al. 2009). Nevertheless, similarly with uric acid, most of the phenolics only remain in plasma for a few hours after consumption (Manach et al. 2005). Therefore, the total phenolics concentration in 12-h fasting blood samples may not accurately reflect the intake of phenolics. Still, some studies observed increased fasting plasma total phenolics after consumption of a phenolic-rich diet or supplement (Devaraj et al. 2002; Tsang et al. 2005). Clearly, further investigation is warranted to confirm the long-term effects of consumption of fruits and vegetables on plasma TAC and total phenolics.

11.4.4 Limitations

The study has the following limitations: (1) participants in this study were from the Hartford area in Connecticut; therefore, the foods they consumed may vary from nationally representative foods in NDSR software. (2) it focused on the total antioxidant intakes including flavonoids and antioxidant vitamins, and did not consider individual bioavailability and metabolism in the human body; (3) health outcomes resulting from interactions among food components were not examined in the present study (i.e. synergic antioxidant effects of flavonoids and/or vitamins); (4) although many confounders have been adjusted, the positive correlation of TAC from diet with plasma TAC could be attributed to a healthy lifestyle or other beneficial compounds present in the foods; (5) this is a cross-sectional study, no cause and effect conclusion can be drawn.

11.4.5 Conclusion

Our findings supported an association between TAC intake and individual antioxidant intakes as well as plasma TAC, indicating that dietary TAC may be a useful tool in predicting dietary antioxidant status. The role of dietary TAC in predicting plasma antioxidant status needs further investigation. For future studies, TAC of the U.S. diet can be estimated and linked to biomarkers of oxidative stress and chronic diseases. Further studies need to be conducted in order to determine an adjusting factor for the bioavailability of each antioxidant nutrient. The TAC database of the U.S. population can then be modified considering the bioavailability of individual antioxidants in the human body. Polyphenolics have different bioactive or functional properties, intake levels, and antioxidant capacities (Institute of Medicine 1998; Williamson and Holst 2008), thus obstructing the progress in establishing the recommendations for optimal antioxidant intake levels. TAC considering not only individual polyphenolics or antioxidant vitamins but also all antioxidants exerting similar antioxidant activities can be applied to establish recommendations for the optimal level of dietary antioxidant intake and lifestyle modifications, and for a long-term strategy of chronic disease prevention.

Conflict of Interest The authors bear no conflict of interest regarding this article manuscript submitted to the Springer Publisher;

Supported by the Donaghue Research Foundation Nutrition Research Grant.

References

Ames BN, Shigenaga MK, Hagen TM (1993) Oxidants, antioxidants, and the degenerative diseases of aging. Proc Natl Acad Sci USA 90:7915–7922

Bazzano LA, He J, Ogden LG, Loria CM, Vupputuri S, Myers L, Whelton PK (2002) Fruit and vegetable intake and risk of cardiovascular disease in US adults: the first National Health and Nutrition Examination Survey Epidemiologic Follow-up Study. Am J Clin Nutr 76:93–99

Benzie IFF, Strain JJ (1996) The ferric reducing ability of plasma (FRAP) as a measure of "antioxidant power": the FRAP assay. Anal Biochem 239:70–76

Beretta G, Aldini G, Facino RM, Russell RM, Krinsky NI, Yeum KJ (2006) Total antioxidant performance: a validated fluorescence assay for the measurement of plasma oxidizability. Anal Biochem 354(2):290–298

Billington C, Epstein LH, Goodwin NJ, Hill JO, Pi-Sunyer FX, Rolls BJ (2000) Overweight, obesity, and health risk. Arch Intern Med 160:898–904

Bjelakovic G, Nikolova D, Simonetti RG, Gluud C (2004) Antioxidant supplements for prevention of gastrointestinal cancers: a systematic review and meta-analysis. Lancet 364(9441):1219–1228

Bjelakovic G, Nikolova D, Gluud LL, Simonetti RG, Gluud C (2008) Antioxidant supplements for prevention of mortality in healthy participants and patients with various diseases. Cochrane Database Syst Rev 2:CD007176

Bruno RS, Dugan CE, Smyth JA, DiNatale DA, Koo SI (2008) Green tea extract protects leptin-deficient, spontaneously obese mice from hepatic steatosis and injury. J Nutr 138:323–331

Cao GH, Alessio HM, Cutler RG (1993) Oxygen-radical absorbance capacity assay for antioxidants. Free Radic Biol Med 14:303–311

Cao G, Booth SL, Sadowski JA, Prior RL (1998a) Increases in human plasma antioxidant capacity after consumption of controlled diets high in fruit and vegetables. Am J Clin Nutr 68:1081–1087

Cao G, Russell RM, Lischner N, Prior RL (1998b) Serum antioxidant capacity is increased by consumption of strawberries, spinach, red wine or vitamin C in elderly women. J Nutr 128:2383–2390

Chun OK, Chung S, Song W (2007) Estimated dietary flavonoid intakes and major food sources of U.S. adults. J Nutr 137:1244–1252

Day A, Stansbie D (1995) Cardioprotective effect of red wine may be mediated by urate. Clin Chem 41:1319–1320

Devaraj S, Vega-López S, Kaul N, Schönlau F, Rohdewald P, Jialal I (2002) Supplementation with a pine bark extract rich in polyphenols increases plasma antioxidant capacity and alters the plasma lipoprotein profile. Lipids 37(10):931–934

Doll R (1990) An overview of the epidemiological evidence linking diet and cancer. Proc Nutr Soc 49:119–131

Drieling RL, Gardner CD, Ma J, Ahn DK, Stafford RS (2010) No beneficial effects of pine bark extract on cardiovascular disease risk factors. Arch Intern Med 170(17):1541–1547

Floegel A, Kim D-O, Chung S-J, Song WO, Fernandez ML, Bruno RS, Koo SI, Chun OK (2010) Development and validation of an algorithm to establish a total antioxidant capacity database of the US diet. Int J Food Sci Nutr 61(6):600–623

Ford E, Mokdad A, Giles W, Brown D (2003) The metabolic syndrome and antioxidant concentrations: findings from the Third National Health and Nutrition Examination Survey. Diabetes 52:2346–2352

Franzini L, Ardigò D, Valtueña S, Pellegrini N, Del Rio D, Bianchi MA, Scazzina FPP, Brighenti F, Zavaroni I (2010) Food selection based on high total antioxidant capacity improves endothelial function in a low cardiovascular risk population. Nutr Metab Cardiovasc Dis. doi:10.1016/j.numecd.2010.04.001

Ghiselli A, Serafini M, Maiani G, Azzini E, Ferro-Luzzi A (1995) A fluorescence-based method for measuring total plasma antioxidant capability. Free Radic Biol Med 18(1):29–36

Halvorsen BL, Holte K, Myhrstad MCW, Barikmo I, Hvattum E, Remberg SF, Wold A-B, Haffner K, Baugerod H (2002) A systematic screening of total antioxidants in dietary plants. J Nutr 132:461–471

Hertog MGL, Kromhout D, Aravanis C, Blackburn H, Buzina R, Fidanza F, Giampaoli S, Jansen A, Menotti A, Nedeljkovic S, Pekkarinen M, Simic BS, Toshima H, Feskens EJM, Hollman PCH, Katan MB (1995) Flavonoid intake and long-term risk of coronary heart disease and cancer in the seven countries study. Arch Intern Med 155:381–386

Huang D, Ou B, Hampsch-Woodill M, Flanagan JA, Prior RL (2002) High-throughput assay of oxygen radical absorbance capacity (ORAC) using a multichannel liquid handling system coupled with a microplate fluorescence reader in 96-Well format. J Agric Food Chem 50:4437–4444

Institute of Medicine (1998) Dietary reference intakes: proposed definition and plan for review of dietary antioxidants and related compounds. National Academies Press, Washington, DC

Karppia J, Nurmia T, Olmedilla-Alonsob B, Granado-Lorenciob F, Nyyssönen K (2008) Simultaneous measurement of retinol, α-tocopherol and six carotenoids in human plasma by using an isocratic reversed-phase HPLC method. J Chromatogr B 867:226–232

Kim DO, Lee KW, Lee HJ, Lee CY (2002) Vitamin C equivalent antioxidant capacity (VCEAC) of phenolic phytochemicals. J Agric Food Chem 50:3713–3717

Knekt P, Reunanen A, Järvinen R, Seppänen R, Heliövaara M, Aromaa A (1994) Antioxidant vitamin intake and coronary mortality in a longitudinal population study. Am J Epidemiol 139:1180–1189

Liu S, Manson JE, Lee IM, Cole SR, Hennekens CH, Willett WC, Buring JE (2000) Fruit and vegetable intake and risk of cardiovascular disease: the Women's Health Study. Am J Clin Nutr 72:922–928

Lotito SB, Frei B (2006) Consumption of flavonoid-rich foods and increased plasma antioxidant capacity in humans: cause, consequence, or epiphenomenon? Free Radic Biol Med 41(12):1727–1746

Manach C, Williamson G, Morand C, Scalbert A, Rémésy C (2005) Bioavailability and bioefficacy of polyphenols in humans. I. Review of 97 bioavailability studies. Am J Clin Nutr 81:230S–242S
Mekary RA, Wu K, Giovannucci E, Sampson L, Fuchs C, Spiegelman D, Willett WC, Smith-Warner SA (2010) Total antioxidant capacity intake and colorectal cancer risk in the Health Professionals Follow-up Study. Cancer Causes Control 21(8):1315–1321
Miller NJ, Rice-Evans C, Davies MJ, Gopinathan V, Milner A (1993) A novel method for measuring antioxidant capacity and its application to monitoring the antioxidant status in premature neonates. Clin Sci 84(4):407–412
Natella F, Nardini M, Giannetti I, Dattilo C, Scaccini C (2002) Coffee drinking influences plasma antioxidant capacity in humans. J Agric Food Chem 50(21):6211–6216
Neuhouser ML, Wassertheil-Smoller S, Thomson C, Aragaki A, Anderson GL, Manson JE, Patterson RE, Rohan TE, van Horn L, Shikany JM, Thomas A, LaCroix A, Prentice RL (2009) Multivitamin use and risk of cancer and cardiovascular disease in the Women's Health Initiative cohorts. Arch Intern Med 169(3):294–304
Pellegrini N, Salvatore S, Valtuena S, Bedogni G, Porrini M, Pala V, Del Rio D, Sieri S, Miglio C, Krogh V, Zavaroni I, Brighenti F (2007) Development and validation of a food frequency questionnaire for the assessment of dietary total antioxidant capacity. J Nutr 137(1):93–98
Price RK, Welch RW, Lee-Manion AM, Bradbury I, Strain JJ (2008) Total phenolics and antioxidant potential in plasma and urine of humans after consumption of wheat bran. Cereal Chem 85:152–157
Prior RL (2003) Fruits and vegetables in the prevention of cellular oxidative damage. Am J Clin Nutr 78:570S–578S
Rautiainen S, Serafini M, Morgenstern R, Prior RL, Wolk A (2008) The validity and reproducibility of food-frequency questionnaire-based total antioxidant capacity estimates in Swedish women. Am J Clin Nutr 87:1247–1253
Reaven PD, Khouw A, Beltz WF, Parthasarathy S, Witztum JL (1993) Effect of dietary antioxidant combinations in humans. Protection of LDL by vitamin E but not by beta-carotene. Arterioscler Thromb 13:590–600
Resnicow K, Odom E, Wang T, Dudley W, Mitchell D, Vaughan R, Jackson A, Baranowski T (2000) Validation of three food frequency questionnaires and 24-hour recalls with serum carotenoid levels in a sample of African-American adults. Am J Epidemiol 152:1072–1080
Ross MA (1994) Determination of ascorbic acid and uric acid in plasma by high-performance liquid chromatography. J Chromatogr B 657:197–200
Serafini M, Del Rio D (2004) Understanding the association between dietary antioxidants, redox status and disease: is the Total Antioxidant Capacity the right tool? Redox Rep 9:145–152
Serafini M, Maiani G, Ferro-Luzzi A (1998) Alcohol-free red wine enhances plasma antioxidant capacity in humans. J Nutr 128(6):1003–1007
Serafini M, Bellocco R, Wolk A, Ekstrom AM (2002) Total antioxidant potential of fruit and vegetables and risk of gastric cancer. Gastroenterology 123(4):985–991
Sies H (1985) Oxidative stress: introductory remarks. Academic, London
Singleton VL, Rossi JA Jr (1965) Colorimetry of total phenolics with phosphomolybdic-phosphotungstic acid reagents. Am J Enol Vitic 16:144–158
Soni M, Thurmond TS, Miller ER 3rd, Spriggs T, Bendich A, Omaye ST (2010) Safety of vitamins and minerals: controversies and perspective. Toxicol Sci. doi:10.1093/toxsci/kfq293
Torabian S, Haddad E, Rajaram S, Banta J, Sabaté J (2009) Acute effect of nut consumption on plasma total polyphenols, antioxidant capacity and lipid peroxidation. J Hum Nutr Diet 22(1):64–71
Tsang C, Higgins S, Duthie GG, Duthie SJ, Howie M, Mullen W, Lean ME, Crozier A (2005) The influence of moderate red wine consumption on antioxidant status and indices of oxidative stress associated with CHD in healthy volunteers. Br J Nutr 93(2):233–240
Weyer C, Yudkin J, Stehouwer C, Schalkwijk C, Pratley R, Tataranni P (2002) Humoral markers of inflammation and endothelial dysfunction in relation to adiposity and in vivo insulin action in Pima Indians. Atherosclerosis 161:233–242
Williamson G, Holst B (2008) Dietary reference intake (DRI) value for dietary polyphenols: are we heading in the right direction? Br J Nutr 99:S55–S58

Chapter 12
Natural Sulfur Products as Redox Modulators and Selective Inducers of Cell Death

Brigitte Czepukojc, Thomas Schneider, Torsten Burkholz, Vincent Jamier, and Claus Jacob

Abstract Numerous plants, fungi and microorganisms contain organic sulfur compounds (OSCs), which during the last couple of decades have been associated increasingly with chemoprevention, antibacterial and anticancer activity. These compounds also play a particular role as intracellular redox modulators and inducers of apoptosis. Among the various OSCs, redox-active, reactive sulfur species, such as allicin and polysulfanes (RS_xR, $R \neq H$, $x \geq 3$) from garlic and onion, show particularly interesting properties. These compounds are able to S-thiolate or oxidize a wide range of peptides and proteins, and hence modulate intracellular redox processes, either directly or by oxidizing GSH to GSSG, which shifts the intracellular redox balance to more oxidizing potentials. Such interference with the intracellular 'thiolstat' has widespread consequences, ranging from an activation of antioxidant defenses to induction of apoptosis. While S-thiolation may be the most prominent mode of action associated with OSCs, the chemistry of these compounds has many facets, including superoxide radical generation, binding to metal centres of metallo-proteins and hydrophobic interactions with various cellular membranes and proteins. Ultimately, many of these reactions also have the potential to trigger apoptotic pathways.

Keywords Cysteine • Oxidation • Perthiol • S-thiolation • Thiolstat

Abbreviations

AIF	apoptosis-inducing factor
ALA	α-lipoic acid
AM	allylmercaptan

B. Czepukojc • T. Schneider • T. Burkholz • V. Jamier • C. Jacob (✉)
Division of Bioorganic Chemistry, School of Pharmacy,
Saarland University, Campus, D-66123, Saarbruecken, Germany
e-mail: c.jacob@mx.uni-saarland.de

M. Diederich and K. Noworyta (eds.), *Natural Compounds as Inducers of Cell Death: Volume 1*, DOI 10.1007/978-94-007-4575-9_12,

ANT	adenine nucleotide translocase
AP-1	activator protein-1
AR	androgen receptor
ATC	Human anaplastic thyroid carcinoma
Bad	B-cell lymphoma protein 2 associated death promoter
Bak	B-cell lymphoma protein 2 homologous antagonist/killer
Bax	B-cell lymphoma protein 2 associated X protein
Bcl-2	B-cell lymphoma protein 2
Bcl-xL	B-cell lymphoma protein 2-extra large
cdk1	cyclin dependent kinase 1
DADS	diallyldisulfide
DAS	diallylsulfide
DATS	diallyltrisulfide
DATTS	diallyltetrasulfide
DHLA	dihydrolipoic acid
DPTTS	dipropyltetrasulfide
1,2-DT	3-vinyl-4*H*-1,2-dithiin
1,3-DT	2-vinyl-4*H*-1,3-dithiin
ERK	extracellular signal-regulated kinases
FACS	Fluorescence activated cell sorting
ERK	extracellular signal-regulated kinases
GSH	glutathione
GSSG	glutathione disulfide
HDACs	histone deacetylases
HMG-CoA	3-hydroxy-3-methyl-glutaryl coenzyme A
H_2S	hydrogen sulfide
JNK	c-Jun N-terminal kinase
MAPKs	mitogen-activated protein kinases
MCF-7	human mammary carcinoma cells
MPTP	mitochondrial permeability transition pore
NHE	normal hydrogen electrode
OSCs	organic sulfur compounds
OS	oxidative stress
PARP-1	poly(ADT-ribose) polymerase 1
PC-3	human prostate cancer cells
PDIs	protein disulfide isomerases
PFTase	protein FTase
PKA	protein kinase A
PKB	protein kinase B
PrSH	protein thiol
PrSSG	S-glutathiolated protein thiol
PrSSPr	protein disulfides
Rb	human retinoblastoma protein
ROS	reactive oxygen species.

12.1 Introduction

Many plants, fungi, bacteria and algae are rich in organic sulfur compounds (OSCs). These natural products are chemically highly diverse, yet often exhibit a characteristic sulfur chemistry, which combines redox activity, catalysis, metal binding and hydrophobic interactions. Figure 12.1 illustrates various physical and chemical properties associated with natural sulfur products. The last decade has witnessed a surge in interest in OSCs, fuelled in part by new insights into intracellular redox control mechanisms and their importance for cell proliferation, differentiation and apoptosis. Here, a landmark publication by Freya Schafer and Garry R. Buettner, published in 2001, links the intracellular redox state, expressed as electrochemical potential *E*' of the glutathione disulfide/glutathione (GSSG/GSH) redox pair, to major cellular events (Schafer and Buettner 2001). Considering that natural OSCs are well suited to modulate such thiol-based intracellular redox states, the huge impact such compounds may potentially have on cellular processes becomes apparent. It is therefore hardly surprising that many OSCs have been considered as part of novel chemopreventive and possibly even therapeutic strategies.

As part of this chapter, we will briefly consider the emerging concept of the intracellular 'thiolstat'. The latter represents a complex network of numerous intracellular thiol-based redox systems, which enables the mammalian cell to respond

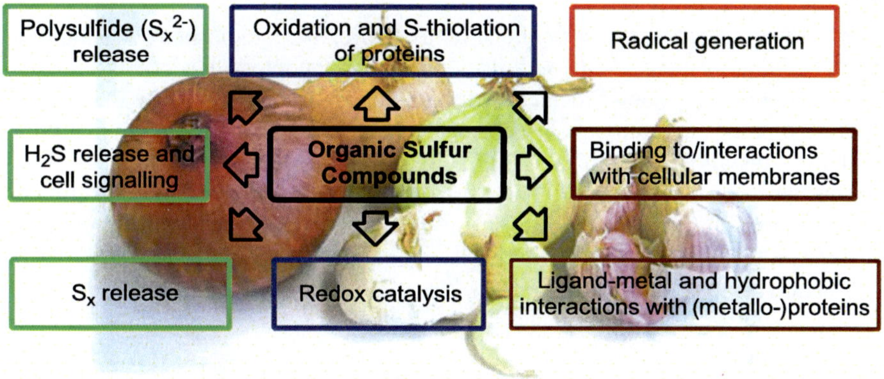

Fig .12.1 A brief overview of the various physical properties and chemical reactivities associated with organic sulfur compounds (*OSCs*). Some of these processes may explain certain aspects of the different biological activities associated with individual natural sulfur products. One should notice, however, that the list of properties and reactivities is necessarily incomplete and that some of these actions are still speculative at the time. Furthermore, different OSCs may react differently, and even their individual reactivities may depend on the respective concentrations they are applied at and the specific cellular environment they are placed into

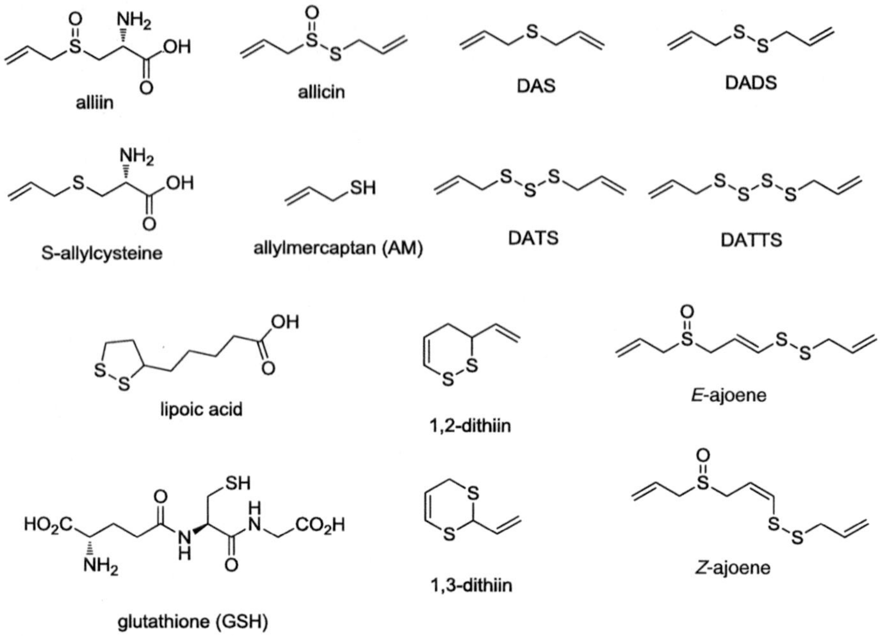

Fig. 12.2 Summary of the chemical structures of the various OSCs referred to in the text

gradually to changes in the intracellular redox environment, for instance by mounting an antioxidant response or by cell cycle arrest and apoptosis (Jacob et al. 2010). Numerous OSCs are known to interfere with cellular redox systems. We will therefore take a closer look at a number of selected – and in many ways representative – OSCs, including disulfides, allicin, and polysulfanes (Fig. 12.2). While most of these agents appear to develop their characteristic biological activity *via* S-thiolation of cysteine proteins, others seem to act *via* different mechanisms which do not primarily involve redox reactions. Aspects of these compounds, and their emerging modes of action, are being explored as part of a more speculative discussion.

12.2 Aspects of the Intracellular Thiolstat

The original picture proposed by Schafer and Buettner in 2001 links the intracellular redox potential, represented by the potential of the GSSG/GSH redox pair, to essential cellular processes, such as cell proliferation, differentiation and apoptosis (Schafer and Buettner 2001). From today's perspective, this model may appear somewhat crude, yet its basic ideas are still valid today. Since then, a range of additional aspects of intracellular redox signaling have been emerging which essentially support and refine the original concept.

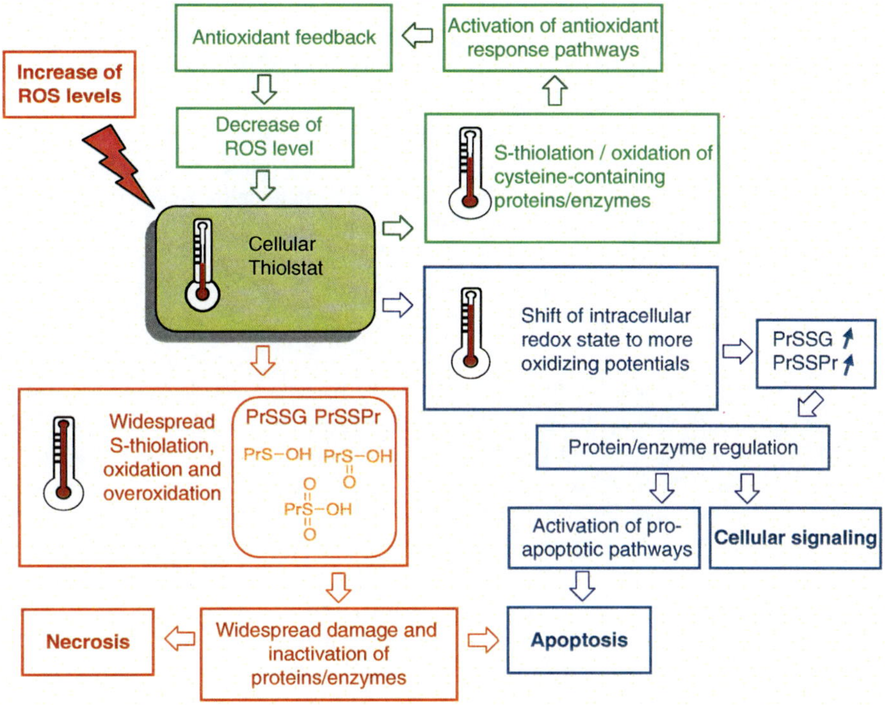

Fig. 12.3 The cellular thiolstat as a central element allowing the cell to respond fast and efficiently to concentration- and time-dependent changes of the intracellular redox state. The multitude of cellular proteins and enzymes involved in the thiolstat enables a measured and often rapidly reversible response to gradual changes of the intracellular redox state, either by mounting an antioxidant response, widespread cellular signaling and/or induction of apoptosis and necrosis. One of the key elements of the thiolstat is the diversity of the thiol oxidation potentials which exists among cellular cysteine proteins and the reversibility of some – but not all – of the oxidative cysteine modifications (Jacob et al. 2004)

It has become evident, for instance, that reversible disulfide formation, including processes such as S-thiolation and dethiolation, but also irreversible overoxidation of cysteine residues to sulfinic and sulfonic acids, are important intracellular events involved in the posttranslational modification and hence control of many cysteine-containing proteins and enzymes (Mieyal et al. 2008). These processes are to a large extent themselves controlled by the intracellular redox environment which over time may vary considerably in the same cell.

Under normal non-stress conditions, the intracellular cytosolic redox environment, dominated by GSH, is rather reducing (Fig. 12.3). A potential of −240 mV vs. NHE, for instance, has recently been estimated by Talia Miron and colleagues for human promyelocytic leukemia-derived HL-60 and human myelomonocytic U937 cells, which is in line with Schafer and Buettner's initial proposal. Under those conditions, most of the intracellular thiols are present in the reduced state (PrSH)

(Miron et al. 2008). The dominance of intracellular thiols over disulfides is reflected in the ratio of GSH over GSSG, but also when considering the amount of intracellular protein thiols (PrSH) versus protein disulfides (PrSSPr) or S-glutathiolated cysteine residues in proteins (PrSSG). A recent landmark study by Jakob Winther and colleagues on the 'global cellular thiol-disulfide status' has demonstrated that the content of total disulfide in cells is rather low under normal conditions (Hansen et al. 2009). In human embryonic kidney HEK cells, for instance, only around 8.5% of total glutathione is present as GSSG, and only around 5.8% of protein thiols are present as protein disulfides, PrSSPr. Importantly, virtually no protein S-glutathiolation occurs under those conditions, with a cellular PrSSG content as low as 0.037% of protein thiols. Similar results were also obtained for immortalized human cervical HeLa cells.

This situation changes dramatically, however, when (external) oxidative stress (OS) is applied. A shift in intracellular redox potential from −240 to −170 mV has been observed in HL-60 cells treated with the thiosulfinate allicin, which is accompanied by a significant increase in disulfide bond formation (see also later on) (Miron et al. 2008). The latter may occur directly, for instance by interactions with oxidizing and/or thiolating agents, or indirectly via shifts in the GSSG/GSH ratio to more oxidizing potentials. In HEK cells, the use of the oxidant diamide results in widespread oxidation of thiols to disulfides, which ultimately account for more than 50% of the total thiol/disulfide content (*i.e.* 47% of thiols reduced in RSH, 53% oxidized in RSSR). Importantly, most of the thiols oxidized by diamide are actually part of cysteine residues in proteins, and not in GSH (56% of disulfides in proteins *vs.* 44% in GSSG in HEK cells, 67% *vs.* 33% in HeLa cells) (Hansen et al. 2009).

Overall, these findings by Winther and colleagues have a number of serious implications for our understanding of intracellular redox processes. Firstly, they firmly reject the 'myth' that S-thiolation or disulfide formation in proteins is not possible within the human cell due to the presence of a large excess of GSH. Neither is GSH present in excess over PrSH (quite the opposite actually seems to be the case: the total thiol pool in HEK and HeLa cells consists of around two-thirds of PrSH and just one-third of GSH), nor is GSH more reactive than most PrSH. Secondly, the numbers confirm that PrSH are major targets of oxidative modifications and ultimately provide the basis for widespread redox sensing, signaling and control via disulfide formation (either as PrSSPr or PrSSG). Upon treatment of HEK cells with diamide, for instance, the cellular content of PrSSG increased by around 300-fold, while the content of GSSG increased 'just' sixfold and the content of PrSSPr just 3.5-fold (similar results were obtained in HeLa cells). Thirdly, such redox processes (in response to diamide) are reversible, with full recovery of PrSH within 20 or 30 min after removal of the stressor. A similar, yet slightly slower 'recovery' of intracellular thiols was also found by Miron and colleagues in HL-60 and U937 cells (Miron et al. 2008). Nonetheless, it should be emphasized that oxidation of cysteine residues may also result in irreversible modifications, such as cysteine sulfinic and sulfonic acids, as demonstrated by Philip Eaton and colleagues (Saurin et al. 2004).

Importantly, intracellular cysteine modifying processes are not random or of an 'all or nothing' Nature but rather occur *gradually*, in line with the different 'sensitivities' of cysteine proteins towards oxidation. Redox sensitivity is a property specific for each individual cysteine protein, in essence controlled by the microenvironment the cysteine residue in question is placed in. Thiol oxidation potentials associated with proteins found in the human cell therefore vary significantly, often by more than 145 mV. Thioredoxin (Trx) proteins, for instance, contain active site residues with a formal redox potential[1] of –270 mV, while protein disulfide isomerases (PDIs) are considerably more oxidizing, with a potential of –125 mV *vs.* NHE (Lundstrom and Holmgren 1993; Nishinaka et al. 2001; Giles et al. 2003). Glutathione itself has a standard redox potential between –230 and –240 mV (although some sources provide slightly different values depending on the techniques used to measure it). As the intracellular redox environment shifts towards more oxidizing potentials, individual cysteine proteins therefore *gradually* become targets of oxidative modifications, in line with their individual $E^{0\prime}$ values. Interestingly, the most reactive cysteine residues in proteins are often active site residues, since these residues are activated in order to carry out particular transformations. Hence catalytic activity generally goes hand in hand with sensitivity towards oxidation, and those cysteine proteins and enzymes are prime targets for oxidative modifications and also thiol-based redox regulation.

Besides the gradual Nature of changes in response to a particular shift in the intracellular redox state, another important aspect of intracellular redox regulation is the *time-dependence* of these changes. It is possible, for instance, that an oxidative assault initially results in loss of GSH and widespread formation of S-thiolated or oxidized proteins, while in the longer term, the antioxidant defense system takes over and GSH levels actually rise above normal levels. The apparent 'recovery' of the normal thiol status after a couple of minutes or hours, which has been observed independently by Miron, Winther and colleagues in various cells lines (see above), underlines the time-dependence of such intracellular changes. The fact that ROS cause a depletion or an increase of GSH in some cells, which is sometimes discussed as a paradox, is therefore easily explained when considering the time-dependence of these changes and bearing in mind that the cell has various avenues available to respond to OS, including the activation of a sophisticated antioxidant defense system (Fig. 12.3).

A more refined picture of the intracellular 'thiolstat' is therefore emerging, whereby gradual oxidation of key (regulatory, signaling) cysteine proteins and enzymes enables the cell to sense the severity of OS and to respond accordingly (Fig. 12.3). This ability to respond in different ways, yet quite appropriately to *gradual* changes

---

[1] In the biochemical literature, the use of electrochemical potentials attributed to cysteine residues is sometimes confusing. In essence, the oxidation potential E_{ox} reflects the ease of oxidation of the cysteine thiol to an oxidized form, usually the disulfide. The reduction potential E_{red}, on the other hand, reflects the ease of reduction of the disulfide to the thiol. The redox potential $E^{0\prime}$ is calculated mathematically as the midpoint between these potentials (essentially the 'average'). Importantly, $E^{0\prime}$ requires full reversibility of the oxidation and reduction processes, and can only be used to describe the thiol/disulfide pair, but not processes involving other sulfur oxidation states, such as sulfenic or sulfinic acids. It may therefore be more adequate to discuss redox sensitivity of the thiol groups of cysteine proteins in terms of E_{ox} rather than $E^{0\prime}$.

to the intracellular redox state is crucial for the cell. It may answer an oxidative stimulus either by mounting an antioxidant defense, arrest the cell cycle, or induce apoptosis or even necrosis (Fig. 12.3). This decision, its execution and its rapid reversal upon the removal of the oxidative stimulus, ultimately depend in large parts on the cellular thiolstat. As already mentioned, the latter represents not just one or a few proteins but a complex medley of different proteins and enzymes. When searching the existing literature for aspects of intracellular redox regulation via protein thiols, one ends up with a seemingly endless list of individual cysteine proteins which may be affected by redox events, ranging from proteins of the cytoskeleton, such as β-tubulin and actin, to proteins involved in antioxidant defense, such as Keap-1. Which of these proteins are the prime targets for oxidizing species remains unclear. In fact, it is unlikely that an oxidative stimulus attacks just one single target protein. Various cellular signaling and response pathways are probably activated/deactivated at the same time, resulting in a more effective, yet also more complex cellular response. We now know, for instance, that many of the enzymes involved in cell cycle control and apoptosis are redox sensitive cysteine proteins, whose activity can be controlled by thiol modifications (Table 12.1). These enzymes include cdc25 C, a protein essential for dephosphorylation and activation of cyclin dependent kinase 1 (cdk1), (Cunat et al. 2008) Bcl-2 and certain caspases. During the last couple of years, other important potential players of redox signaling and control have emerged, such as the microtubulin network, the histone deacetylases (HDACs, see Sect.12.6), various transcription factors (*e.g.* NFκ-B), the 20S proteasome, the mitochondrial permeability transition pore and certain telomerases. These proteins are either directly or indirectly affected by redox agents, especially by thiol-specific reagents, which, of course, include many naturally occurring OSCs.

12.3 Disulfides and Apoptosis

Among the various OSCs found in Nature, we find a number of substances able to react highly selectively, yet also effectively with thiol groups in proteins and enzymes. Most of these thiol-specific OSCs are based on the disulfide-motif RSSR and react with PrSH in reactions resembling thiol/disulfide exchange reactions. Here, we will focus on two selected disulfides, namely α-lipoic acid (ALA, thioctic acid or 5-(1,2-dithiolan-3-yl)pentanoic acid) and diallyldisulfide (DADS) (for chemical structures see Fig. 12.2).

α-Lipoic acid is a natural antioxidant occurring in plants and animals including humans, where it serves as a cofactor of several mitochondrial enzymes. ALA is redox active with a comparably low thiol/disulfide redox potential of $E^{0\prime}=-290$ mV *vs.* NHE for lipoate/dihydrolipoate compared to $E^{0\prime}=-230$ mV for GSSG/GSH (Bilska and Wlodek 2005). *In vivo*, ALA is reduced to dihydrolipoic acid (DHLA) by dihydrolipoyl dehydrogenase in the presence of NADH (other enzymes such as glutathione reductase or thioredoxine reductase are also able to reduce ALA but at a lower rate) (Roy and Packer 1998). DHLA is able to scavenge various reactive

Table 12.1 A brief and necessarily preliminary and incomplete list of redox-sensitive cysteine proteins and enzymes which are involved in redox signaling, antioxidant defense, the regulation of the cell cycle and processes inducing apoptosis

	Redox sensitive human protein	Cys residue position to modification	*E* (mV)[a] *vs.* NHE	Modifying agents	Function	References
Cell cycle	**cdc25 family**					
	cdc25 C	330, 377	–	H_2O_2 (*in vitro*)	Dephosphorylation of cyclin B	Savitsky and Finkel (2002)
	cip/kip family					
	p53	275, 277 (redox regulation + DNA-binding) 141, 124, 182 (glutathiolation)	–	ROS GSH UV-radiation H_2O_2	G1 regulator (p21)	Rainwater et al. (1995), Buzek et al. (2002), Velu et al. (2007), and Menon and Goswami (2007)
	INK4a/ARF family					
	TGF β	7, 15, 16, 44, 48, 78, 109, 111 (disulfide pairs), 77	–	Radiation ROS Iron	Regulation of proliferation, differentiation and apoptosis	Daopin et al. (1992), Kraaij et al. (2010), and Pociask et al. (2004)
	TNF α	Cys in the 4 domains	–	Inflammatory cells; B cells	Regulation of immune cells	Vilcek and Lee (1991)
	NF-κB	38, 120 (p65 subunit), 62 (DNA binding)	–	H_2O_2 Cytokines Free radicals UV irradiation	Transcription regulator	Trachootham et al. (2008) and Meyer et al. (1993)
	Cyclin D1	285	–	Redox modifications (H_2O_2)	Cell cycle progression factor	Menon and Goswami (2007)
	Tubulin	20 Cys residus	–	Redox state, alkylating agents; $^{\bullet}NO$, $ONOO^-$	Cell division	Stamatakis et al. (2006), Landino et al. (2007), Huber et al. (2008), and Filomeni et al. (2008)

(continued)

Table 12.1 (continued)

	Redox sensitive human protein	Cys residue position to modification	*E* (mV)[a] *vs.* NHE	Modifying agents	Function	References
Apoptosis	**Bcl-2 family**					
	Bcl-2	155 (α5 domain) 226 (anchoring domain), 158,229	–	NO, ERK ½	Contribution to apoptosis pathway	Maser et al. (2000) and Adams and Cory (1998)
	Bax family					
	Bax	62	–	H_2O_2	Anti- or pro-apoptotic regulators	Nie et al. (2008) and Adams and Cory (1998)
	Caspase 9	403	–	ROS H_2O_2	Mitochondrial apoptotic cascade	Zuo et al. (2009)
Redox signalling/ Antioxidant defense	**Peroxiredoxin**					
	Prx 1	47, 83, 170, 52, 173, Cys [47] to RSOH	–288	Antioxidant enzymes, which reduce H_2O_2 and alkyl hydroperoxides	Antioxidant enzyme Activation of CD8(+) T-cells	Cox et al. (2009) and Lee et al. (2007)
	Prx 2	51,172	–325	H_2O_2 peroxides	Antioxidant enzyme Activation of CD8(+) T-cells	Cox et al. (2009), Lee et al. (2007), and Peskin et al. (2007)
	Prx 3	107, 229	–290	H_2O_2, apoptotic inducers, Trx reductase inhibitors	Decomposition of H_2O_2	Cox et al. (2009)

Thioredoxin					
Trx 1	32, 35	−230	Oxidative stress	Protein reduction	Cox et al. (2009) and Watson et al. (2003)
Trx 2	31, 34	−292	Oxidative stress	Mitochondrial apoptosis	Cox et al. (2009) and Tanaka et al. (2002)
Glutathione peroxidase	Seleno-protein	–	Peroxides	Antioxidant enzyme	Ren et al. (1997)
Glutathione S-transferase	47, 101	–	Toxines, lipophilic molecules	Detoxification	Ricci et al. (1995) and Lo Bello et al. (1995)
Keap-1	151(ox.stress); 273, 288	–	H_2O_2, ·NO, HOCl	Inhibitor of Nrf2 (a master regulator of antioxidant response)	Brandes et al. (2009), Hong et al. (2005) and Fourquet et al. (2010)

Where available, the redox-sensitive cysteine residue in the protein/enzyme is provided, together with its (estimated) redox potential and known modifying (*i.e.* S-thiolating, oxidizing) agents. Since these proteins/enzymes may represent important constituents of the intracellular thiolstat, their respective functions inside the cell are highlighted

[a]For comparison, glutathione has a redox potential of around −230 to −240 mV *vs.* NHE

oxygen species (ROS). DHLA is also capable of regenerating certain antioxidants (*e.g.* vitamin C and E), and can elevate the level of GSH in certain tissues (Bilska and Wlodek 2005; Roy and Packer 1998). Because of its exceptional redox properties, ALA is used in diseases where OS is involved, such as diabetes, neurodegenerative diseases, ischemia-reperfusion injury, hypertension and liver cirrhosis.

While lipoate is often considered as "an antioxidant of antioxidants" (Bilska and Wlodek 2005), some authors speculate that ALA has a dual Nature, which also includes a more sinister, pro-oxidant side. At high concentrations of 100 μmol/L of ALA (and DHLA), the compound inhibits the proliferation of a wide variety of cancer cells and induces apoptosis without affecting normal cells (Bilska and Wlodek 2005). This anti-proliferative effect may be linked to apoptosis. Recently, Hyeyoung Kim and colleagues could demonstrate that ALA, mediated by intracellular Ca^{2+}, induces apoptosis in A549 lung cancer cells through caspase-dependent and caspase-independent pathways (Choi et al. 2009). In the case of caspase-dependent apoptosis, ALA caused cytochrome *c* release from mitochondria and thus triggered the formation of apoptosomes, which in turn activated the caspase cascade and resulted in poly(ADT-ribose) polymerase 1 (PARP-1) cleavage. In the caspase-independent apoptotic pathway, ALA caused activation and over-expression of PARP-1. This process subsequently resulted in nuclear translocation of the apoptosis-inducing factor (AIF) from the mitochondria to the nucleus and cell death through DNA fragmentation initiated by chromatin condensation (Choi et al. 2009; Hong et al. 2004). In other studies, it was shown that the cleavage of PARP-1 could also be responsible for the activation of the apoptotic endonuclease DNAS1L3, with subsequent cleavage of DNA (Yakovlev et al. 2000; Soldani and Scovassi 2002).

The pro-apoptotic effects of high concentrations of ALA have been confirmed independently in a range of different cells lines. In human HL-60 cells, for instance, ALA induced apoptosis using the mitochondrial machinery, whereby AIF and cytochrome *c* were translocated to the nucleus and caused caspase-independent cell death. In these cells, ALA was also able to inhibit cell proliferation by cell cycle arrest at G1/S and G2/M phases, an effect which correlated with the down-regulation of human retinoblastoma protein (Rb) phosphorylation (Selvakumar and Hsieh 2008).

To date, it is still not entirely clear how ALA exerts this kind of pro-apoptotic biological activity, *i.e.* how its physical properties and chemical reactivity induce these processes. Some studies point toward changes to the intracellular redox homeostasis. High concentrations of ALA seem to trigger a redox imbalance in cells, due to an increase in ROS generation. This effect has been observed, for instance, by Amedeo Columbano and colleagues in the FaO rat hepatoma cell line treated with 500 μM of ALA (Simbula et al. 2007). In human and in rat hepatoma cells, increased ROS generation leads to a cascade of events which involves p53 activation, up-regulation of $p21^{Cip1}$ and $p27^{Kip1}$ (cyclin/CDKs inhibitors), induction of Bax, release of cytochrome *c* into the cytosol, activation of the caspase cascade and induction of pro-apoptotic signals (c-Jun N-terminal kinase (JNK)) with concomitant inhibition of anti-apoptotic signals (protein kinase B (PKB/Akt)).

ALA-induced ROS-formation therefore may primarily be responsible for activation of pro-apoptotic pathways in these cells. ROS generation (in particular $O_2^{\bullet-}$ and H_2O_2)

along with Bcl-2 down-regulation in human lung epithelial cell line H460 treated with 100 μM of ALA supports the pro-oxidant role of ALA in the induction of apoptosis (Moungjaroen et al. 2006). Similar links between ALA, ROS generation and apoptosis were observed in human colon cancer cell line HT-29 (with a higher dose of 1 mM of ALA) (Wenzel et al. 2005) and in human breast cancer cells MCF-7, where down-regulation of Akt appeared to be one of the critical down-stream signals of ALA and its effects on those cells (Dozio et al. 2010).

This emerging redox hypothesis explaining the cytotoxicity of ALA is not entirely unreasonable. Oxidized ALA, when applied in high concentrations, may react with certain cysteine-containing proteins and enzymes via thiol/disulfide exchange reactions, hence depleting levels of GSH and shifting the intracellular redox environment to more oxidizing potentials. In line with this hypothesis, pretreatment of cells with *N*-acetylcysteine (NAC) or vitamin C generally inhibits ALA-induced apoptosis (Simbula et al. 2007).

Similar effects have also been observed for other disulfides, which further corroborates this redox hypothesis. Apoptotic and anti-proliferative effects, for instance, were found in cancer cells treated with diallyldisulfide (DADS), a major sulfur-containing constituent of garlic oils and extracts which is formed by decomposition of allicin. In a recent study by Young Chul Park and colleagues, DADS (200–400 μM) treated HCT-116 colon cancer cells showed a p53-independent cell cycle arrest in G2/M phase in combination with a time dependent increase of cyclin B1. At the same time, a dose- and time-dependent increase in ROS production was observed (Song et al. 2009). The molecular mechanism of cell cycle arrest caused by DADS was studied in human prostate cancer cells (PC-3). At 25 and 40 μM concentrations of DADS, levels of the pro-apoptotic B proteins Bax and Bad increased whereas the level of anti-apoptotic Bcl-2 protein decreased, and a significant increase in the expression of caspases 3, 9 and 10 occurred (Gayathri et al. 2009).

While increased intracellular ROS production is frequently being associated with OSCs, and may indeed explain some of the biological effects these compounds exert on cells, matters are often more complicated. Diallylsulfide (DAS), for instance, is a redox-inactive homolog of DADS which is unable to form ROS directly. Nonetheless, DAS exhibits anti-proliferative properties in many cell culture models (Sparnins et al. 1988; Wargovich et al. 1988; Brady et al. 1991; Powolny and Singh 2008). Human anaplastic thyroid carcinoma (ATC) cells treated with DAS, for instance, show a concentration-dependent accumulation of cells in the G2/M phase and an increase in sub-G1 DNA. In ATC cells, DAS also causes apoptosis, which is linked to a decrease in Bcl-2 expression and an increase in Bax expression (the latter triggers the mitochondrial pathway of apoptosis, with cytochrome *c* release from the mitochondria into the cytosol and caspase 3 and 9 activation followed by PARP cleavage) (Truong et al. 2009; Shin et al. 2010; Nagaraj et al. 2010).

How DAS initially acts and interacts in these cells is still a bit of a mystery. One may speculate that DAS binds to certain metallo-proteins. Michael J. Wargovich and colleagues, for instance, have recently shown that DAS inhibits cytochrome P450 2E1 (CYP 2E1) (Wargovich 2006). Alternatively, David W. Kraus and colleagues have postulated that DAS (and other diallylsulfides) release H_2S (Benavides et al. 2007). It is possible that hydrogen sulfide, which is able to bind strongly to metal sites in proteins and enzymes, is actually an or even the active form of DAS – and possibly also of other sulfides (see later on).

12.4 Direct S-thiolation by Allicin

From a chemical perspective, 'normal' disulfides such as GSSG, ALA and DADS are not particularly reactive. These disulfides are either weak oxidants, such as GSSG and ALA, or react with thiols very slowly. Hypothetical modifications on the disulfide motif, such as the ones summarized in Fig. 12.4, however, would increase this reactivity dramatically. This kind of 'disulfide activation' is either due to changes in thermodynamic stability or reaction kinetics. Interestingly, these more reactive sulfur chemotypes also occur in Nature. Let's briefly compare diallyldisulfide (DADS) and allicin, two chemically closely related natural products from garlic. While DADS is

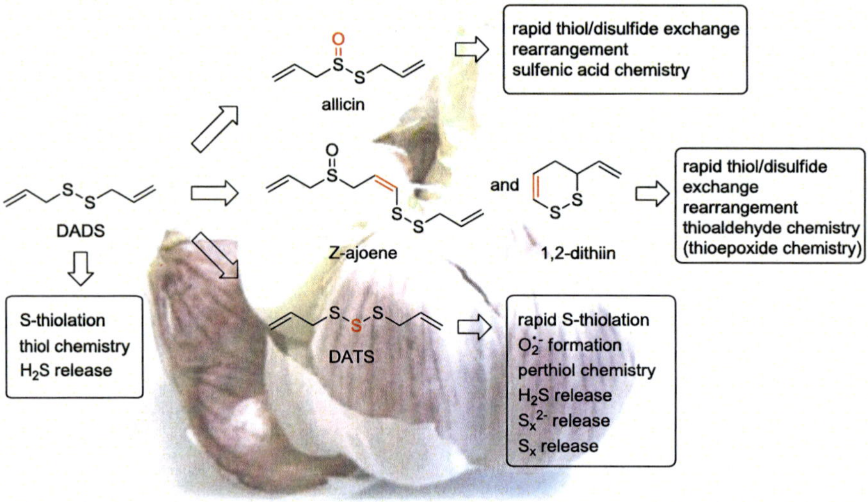

Fig. 12.4 While simple disulfides, such as ALA and DADS, may react with peptide and protein thiols *via* S-thiolation, these reactions are usually slow and often incomplete. Hence those disulfides only react and show biological activity at rather high (sometimes millimolar) concentrations. Nonetheless, several motifs may be derived from the disulfide bond, which are chemically related yet considerable more (re-)active. These chemotypes include thiosulfinates, α,β-unsaturated disulfides and polysulfanes, all of which can be found in natural sulfur compounds. These substances are frequently not only more reactive than the (related) disulfide, but also open up a considerable variety of chemical transformations and biochemical actions which are not accessible to the simple disulfide. Please note that the arrows used to highlight the chemical 'activation' of *DADS* are of a purely logical Nature and do under no circumstances indicate that compounds such as allicin, Z-ajoene or DATS are actually formed from DADS. In garlic oils and extracts, quite the opposite is often the case

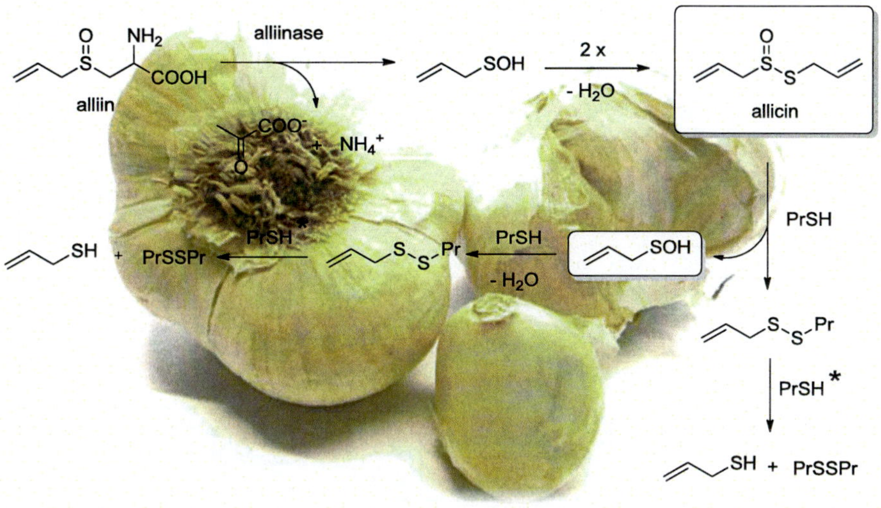

Scheme 12.1 Enzymatic formation of allicin from alliin in the presence of the enzyme alliinase and subsequent reactions of this highly reactive and cytotoxic thiosulfinate with protein thiols. Please note that one allicin molecule is able to S-thiolate up to four cysteine residues depending on the stability and reactivity of the mixed allylSSPr intermediate. *The reaction of allylSSPr with *PrSH* is a possible yet not a necessary conversion which depends on a range of factors, such as the availability and reactivity of PrSH and the stability of allylSSPr in comparison to PrSSPr

a 'simple' disulfide, allicin, the corresponding disulfide-S-oxide, is a thiosulfinate orders of magnitude more reactive towards thiols when compared to DADS.

In garlic (*Allium sativum*), allicin is not stored but formed on demand (Scheme 12.1). In intact garlic bulbs, a range of biologically active OSCs are found, primarily *S*-allyl-L-cysteine sulfoxide (alliin) and γ-glutamyl-*S*-allyl-L-cysteine, but also *S*-methylcysteine sulfoxide, *S*-*trans*-1-propenylcysteine sulfoxide, *S*-2-carboxypropylglutathione and *S*-allylcysteine (Amagase 2006). Upon crushing or cutting garlic bulbs, alliin is transformed within seconds by an enzymatic reaction involving the vacuolar glyco-enzyme alliinase to allicin, the main sulfur compound of freshly prepared garlic and the source of its pungent flavour.

During the last couple of decades, there has been mounting evidence of chemopreventive and anticancer activities associated with allicin. The anti-proliferative effect of allicin has been observed in different cancer cell lines, including MCF-7, endometrial (Ishikawa) and colon (HT-29) cancer cells. Notably, cytotoxicity has also been found in primary skin fibroblasts, yet with a higher IC_{50} value: After incubation of MCF-7, Ishikawa and HT-29 cells with allicin (10–40 μM) for 2–3 days, allicin inhibited cell proliferation with an IC_{50} of 10–25 μM, whereas the cell growth of a normal fibroblast line was inhibited with an IC_{50} of 16 and 40 μM (Hirsch et al. 2000). Further investigations with MCF-7 cells have indicated that allicin transiently decreases intracellular levels of GSH and slows down cell cycle progression. Growth inhibition is accompanied by accumulation of cells at the regulatory checkpoints, in G1 or in the G1 and G2/M phases of the cell cycle (Hirsch et al. 2000).

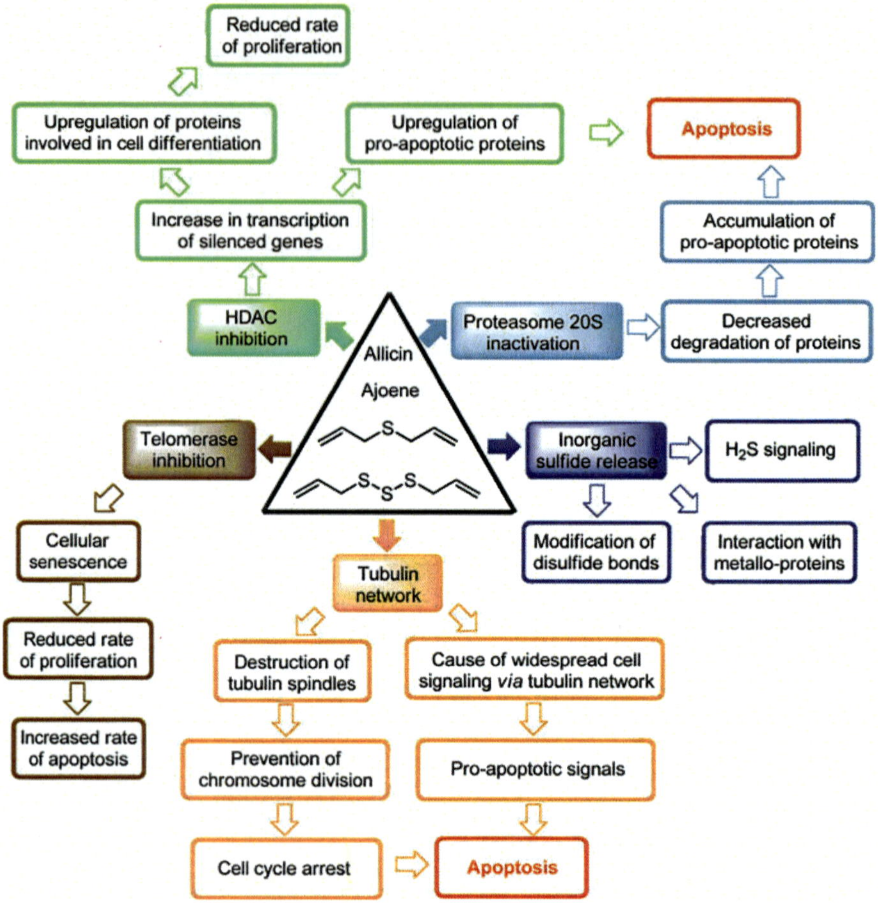

Fig. 12.5 During the last couple of years, a range of new and highly exciting cellular targets of natural OSCs have emerged, including the intracellular β-tubulin network, the 20S proteasome, various HDAC enzymes and telomerases. Some of these targets are currently attracting massive interest in the field of anticancer drug development. This places several of the naturally occurring sulfur compounds right at the centre of cutting-edge research. Nonetheless, one must emphasize that some of the underlying mechanisms responsible for these effects are still not fully understood, while others are highly speculative and sometimes even based primarily on *in vitro* evidence

As part of a similar study in gastric cancer SGC-7901 cells, Li Sun and colleagues have confirmed the ability of allicin to inhibit cell proliferation in a dose-dependent manner. In this study, the ability of allicin to arrest SGC-9701 cells in the G2/M phase and to induce apoptosis has been linked directly to the ability of allicin to inhibit telomerase activity (Sun and Wang 2003). This finding is of particular significance, since telomerases represent a new target for innovative, selective anticancer therapies, which may in part rely on natural products (Fig. 12.5). How allicin, or one of its follow-on reaction products, inhibits telomerase activity, however, is still little understood.

In other cell lines, the initial targets of allicin responsible for the induction of apoptosis have partially been emerging. In human cervical cancer SiHa cells and mouse fibroblast-like L-929 cells, for instance, allicin causes characteristic apoptotic morphological changes in apoptotic bodies, through DNA fragmentation and activation of caspases 3, 8 and 9 (Oommen et al. 2004). In human epithelial carcinoma cells, however, allicin acts through a caspase-independent apoptotic pathway, mediated by the mitochondrial release of AIF and protein kinase A (PKA) activation (Park et al. 2005).

An association with the mitochondrial pathway of apoptosis has also been postulated on several occasions. In HL-60 and U937 cells, for instance, allicin induces cell death by bebbling, mitochondrial release of cytrochrome *c*, activation of caspases 3 and 9 and DNA fragmentation (Miron et al. 2008). The initial target of allicin in this study actually appears to be GSH, which is depleted by allicin (Scheme 12.1). GSH depletion subsequently results in the widespread formation of intracellular disulfides and a general shift of the intracellular redox state to more oxidizing values, *e.g.* from −240 to −170 mV in HL-60 cells (see Sect. 12.2). The value of −170 mV is typical of the apoptotic state (Miron et al. 2008).

Nonetheless, it still remains unclear if allicin acts *via* a specific (cysteine protein) target or *via* a more general shift in intracellular redox potential followed by widespread S-thiolation. In line with the findings by Miron and colleagues, such a mechanism of widespread redox changes has been postulated recently by Alan Slusarenko and colleagues to occur in yeast (Gruhlke et al. 2010). In contrast, possible, more singular targets of allicin involve the apoptotic repair system, various components of which are redox sensitive; and possibly adenine nucleotide translocase (ANT), an enzyme involved in the opening of the mitochondrial permeability transition pore (MPTP). ANT contains two cysteine residues (Cys^{160} and Cys^{257}), which can be cross-linked by oxidative disulfide formation (McStay et al. 2002).

Ultimately, the induction of apoptosis by allicin is still not fully understood. It may proceed *via* different mechanisms and may also differ from one cell type to another. Furthermore, allicin is not particularly stable chemically, and some of the biological effects associated with this compound may in fact be due to its follow-on products, such as DATS, DATTS and allylmercaptan (AM).

12.5 S-thiolation and Induction of Apoptosis by Reactive Disulfides

Ajoene (4,5,9-trithiadodeca-1,6,11-triene-9-oxide) is one of the main compounds formed when crushed garlic is heated, and, together with the various diallylsulfanes, represents one of the major follow-on decomposition products of allicin (Scheme 12.2) (Amagase 2006). Ajoene is more stable than allicin itself and exists as *cis*(*Z*)-ajoene and *trans*(*Z*)-ajoene, whereby the *Z*-isomer appears to be generally biologically more active (Scharfenberg et al. 1990; Yoshida et al. 1998; Li et al. 2002a). The compound exhibits a broad spectrum of biological activities, including

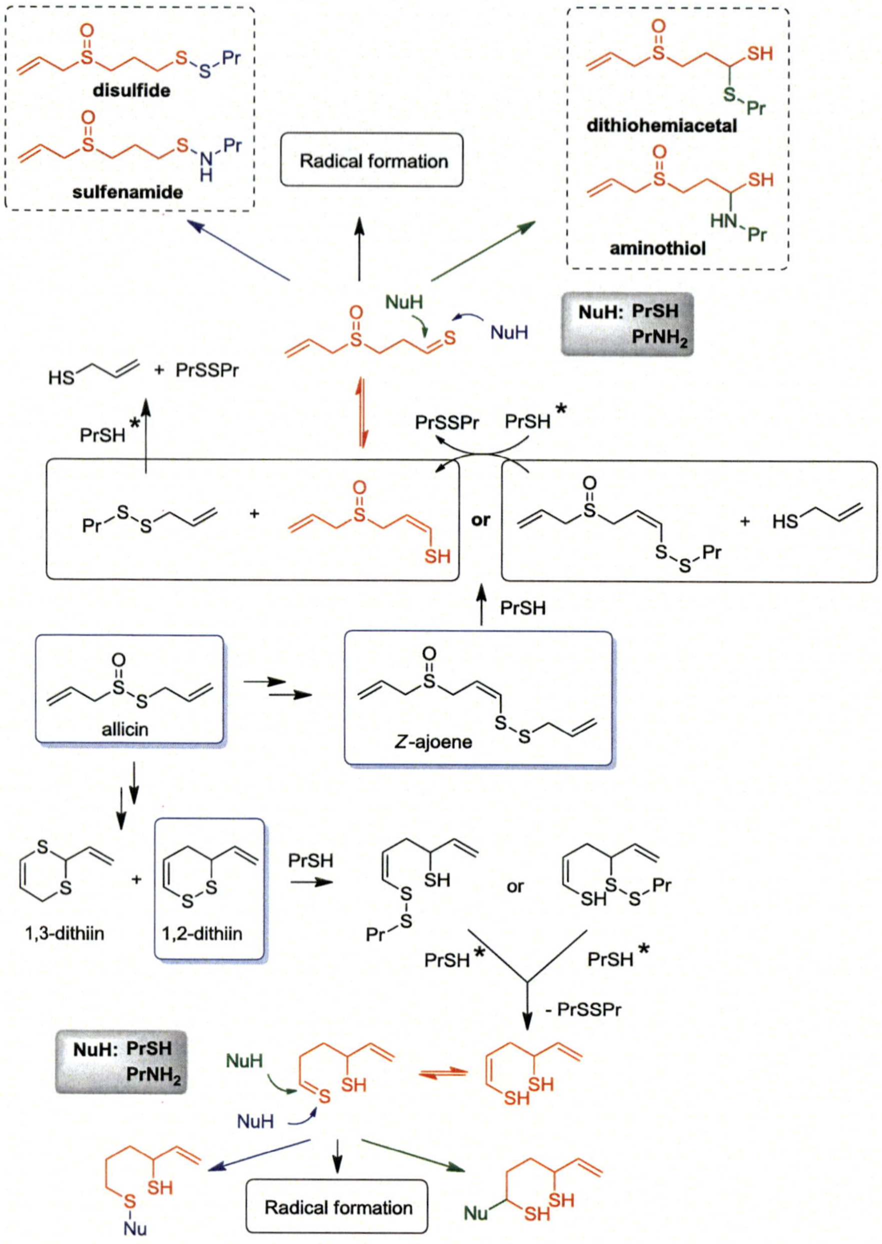

Scheme 12.2 Although *Z*-ajoene and 1,2-DT chemically at first sight resemble typical disulfides, their chemical reactivities differ vastly from the ones of simple disulfides, such as ALA or DADS. In the case of *Z*-ajoene and 1,2-DT, thiol/disulfide reactions not only result in S-thiolation of cysteines, but also in the liberation of a thioaldehyde. The latter in itself is a highly reactive species which triggers a cascade of follow-on chemical reactions, some of which may involve the reversible or irreversible modification of protein residues (*e.g.* lysine, cysteine). It should be emphasized that several of these transformations are speculative at this time and their occurrence *in vivo* is uncertain. Ultimately, some of the species formed, such as the sulfonamide, disulfide and dithiohemiacetals may react further or decompose to other, in part reactive species. *The reaction of allylSSPr with PrSH is a possible yet not a necessary conversion which depends on a range of factors, such as the availability and reactivity of PrSH and the stability of allylSSPr in comparison to PrSSPr

antimicrobial,(Naganawa et al. 1996) anti-thrombotic,(Rendu et al. 1989) antidiabetic (Hattori et al. 2005) and cholesterol lowering actions. It also interferes with HIV-1 replication (Walder et al. 1997) and shows beneficial effects in the context of atherosclerosis (Dirsch et al. 1998a). In the context of cancer cells, ajoene exhibits antitumour activity both *in vitro* (*e.g.* against breast cancer, hepatocellular, gastric and colon carcinoma cells), and *in vivo* on hepatocarcinoma and sarcoma. Here, ajoene causes cell cycle blockage (usually in the G2/M phase) and apoptosis of tumour cells (Li et al. 2002a).

From a chemist's point of view, ajoene is a reactive disulfide which undergoes thiol/disulfide exchange reactions. Its particularly high reactivity appears to be due to an increased reactivity of the disulfide bond due to the presence of a vinylic carbon-carbon double bond and the stabilisation of the reaction products, such as 3-(allylsulfinyl)prop-1-ene-1-thiol, which is in tautomeric equilibrium with the thioaldehyde 3-(allylsulfinyl)propanethial (Scheme 12.2). Interestingly, the thioaldehyde is in itself rather reactive both at the carbon atom and at the sulfur atom. It is a potent electrophile able to react with various nucleophilic residues in proteins and enzymes to form either dithiohemiacetal and aminothiol species or disulfide and sulfenamide species. In proteins, these modifications may be reversible or irreversible, and the sulfur species formed may themselves react further under physiological conditions. This 'special chemistry' of ajoene and related disulfides is highlighted in Scheme 12.2. Although some parts of the scheme are clearly still speculative, it illustrates the extraordinary ability of such disulfides to react with biomolecules and to cause widespread modifications, especially in proteins and enzymes.

Not surprisingly, the apoptotic processes triggered by ajoene seem to involve various proteins and enzymes. In 2001, Angelika Vollmar's group has published a key paper on the molecular events leading to ajoene-triggered apoptosis in a leukemia cell line. Here, ajoene triggered the generation of ROS and the activation of NF-κB (Dirsch et al. 1998b, 2002). There is also evidence that ajoene causes a time-dependent activation of caspase 3(Ledezma et al. 2004) and induces proteolytic processing of procaspases 3 and 8 (Dirsch et al. 2002). Since activation of caspases is induced by the release of cytochrome *c* from mitochondria, these findings point towards the involvement of the mitochondrial pathway of apoptosis. Indeed, the apoptotic effect of ajoene in these leukemia cells diminishes in cells over-expressing Bcl-xL and Bcl-2, which is evidence that a mitochondrial-dependent caspase cascade is involved (Dirsch et al. 2002; Li et al. 2002b).

Subsequent investigations with HL-60 cells have shown that ajoene induces the activation of a range of proteins and enzymes, including mitogen-activated protein kinases (MAPKs) such as c-Jun NH_2-terminal kinase (JNK), p38 and extracellular signal-regulated kinases (ERK) ½ as well as the survival kinase Akt. Some of these proteins are associated with the pro-apoptotic effects of ajoene (Antlsperger et al. 2003)

Despite the fact that most studies on the pro-apoptotic effects of allicin to date have focussed on a direct reaction with subsequent inhibition of cysteine proteins, or the control of protein expression (*e.g. via* transcription factors, HDACs), another possible mode of action has recently been emerging, which considers the cellular proteasome as potential and potent target (Fig. 12.5) (Yu et al. 2010).

The proteasome is responsible for the degradation of a variety of intracellular proteins and plays a key role in the regulation of many cellular processes. Inhibition of (some of) its activity obviously has far reaching consequences, including a build-up of (undesired) signaling proteins. A few years ago, Elisabeth Girbal-Neuhauser's group has shown that ajoene interacts with the human 20S proteasome *in vitro* and in HL-60 cells (Xu et al. 2004). The compound inhibits the trypsin-like activity of the proteasome *in vitro*, and affects both, its trypsin- and chymotrypsin-like activities in HL-60 cells. In this particular study, the HL-60 cells subsequently arrested in G2/M phase and the total amount of cytosolic proteasome increased due to the auto-regulatory feedback of its inhibition. In a subsequent study, Christian Davrinche and colleagues have also observed a significant accumulation of p53-family products in *Z*-ajoene-treated cells, which may explain the cytotoxic, pro-apoptotic activity of this compound in various cell lines (Terrasson et al. 2007). This increase in p53-familiy proteins is likely to be due to an increase in gene transcription *and* an inhibition of proteolysis of these proteins by the proteasome.

In an idealistic scenario, *Z*-ajoene in appropriate concentrations may therefore act as an anticancer agent, exerting its effects for instance through activation and stabilization of p53-family members, a process which subsequently leads to the permeabilization of the mitochondria and activation of caspases. The anti-proteasomal activity of *Z*-ajoene could also have other interesting effects in the context of fighting cancer, such as a decreased expression of cell surface major histocompatibility complex (MHC)-class I molecules, without impairing the recognition of target cells by $CD8^+$ T cells (Terrasson et al. 2007).

It should be mentioned, however, that the biological chemistry of ajoene is still not fully understood. Other cellular events associated with this compound include the generation of H_2O_2, which leads to the activation of MAPKs, degradation of PARP-1, translocation of AIF and fragmentation of DNA (Yang et al. 2006). It has also been shown that ajoene inhibits 3-hydroxy-3-methyl-glutaryl coenzyme A (HMG-CoA) reductase, a key enzyme involved in mevalonate (MVA) synthesis. Covalent attachment of MVA-derived isoprenoid groups (*i.e.* prenylation) is a required activation step for several proteins that regulate cell proliferation (Liu and Yeh 2002; Ferri et al. 2003). Recently, Jose Cardier's group has investigated the possible use of ajoene and statins as synergic antitumour agents targeting HMG-CoA (Ledezma et al. 2009).

Apart from ajoene, garlic extracts, in particular macerated garlic oil, also contain 3-vinyl-4*H*-1,2-dithiin (1,2-DT), another α,β-unsaturated disulfide and chemical breakdown product of allicin (Scheme 12.2). 1,2-DT exhibits characteristic disulfide redox behaviour and usually appears in samples together with its isomer 2-vinyl-4*H*-1,3-dithiin (1,3-DT), which is not redox active. Although 1,2-DT forms a major constituent of garlic preparations, little is known about its chemical reactivity and biological activity. Previous pharmacokinetic studies in mice have detected orally administered 1,2-DT in the serum, kidney and fat tissue (Egen-Schwind et al. 1992), hence confirming a certain stability and bioavailability of this compound in mammals. The high lipophilicity of 1,2-DT may explain its accumulation in fat tissue. Indeed, some studies even point towards an effect of 1,2-DT on the differentiation and inflammation of human preadipocytes. The underlying (bio)chemical processes are still largely unknown, but may involve the reduction of PPARγ2 activity and a reduced expression and secretion of leptin and adiponectin (Keophiphath et al. 2009). If and how these effects are related to the redox activity of 1,2-DT is unclear. Our own studies involving this natural product point towards considerable toxicity in the nematode model and also a rather reducing redox behaviour of its reduced form (Sarakbi 2009).

To the best of our knowledge, there are no studies yet on the possible pro-apoptotic effects of 1,2-DT and 1,3-DT in human cells. Since the reactivity of the disulfide bond in 1,2-DT seems to be enhanced in part by the presence of the carbon-carbon double bond, it nonetheless represents another interesting 'activated' natural disulfide worth investigating in more detail.

12.6 Polysulfanes: S-thiolation, Persulfide Chemistry and Radical Generation

Besides allicin, diallylsulfide, diallyldisulfide, ajoene and dithiins, garlic is also rich in a couple of sulfur compounds with a rather unusual chemical structure and reactivity. Polysulfanes,[2] such as diallyltrisulfide (DATS) and diallyltetrasulfide (DATTS), but also corresponding penta- and hexasulfanes have been isolated from garlic extracts. While these compounds at first sight seem to resemble sulfides and disulfides chemically, their reactivity *in vitro* and *in vivo* is vastly different (Jacob and Anwar 2008; Anwar et al. 2008; Cerella et al. 2009; Busch et al. 2010; Viry et al. 2010). Polysulfanes, like disulfides, react with thiols to form mixed disulfides. Hence compounds such as DATS and DATTS can also S-thiolate and oxidize cysteine residues in proteins and enzymes and interfere with various cellular processes. In stark contrast to a simple thiol/disulfide exchange reaction, however, the thiol/polysulfane exchange also liberates perthiols (RSSH) and even hydrogenpolysulfanes (RS_xH, $x \geq 3$). The latter are highly reactive sulfur species, whose biological chemistry is only just emerging.

Figure 12.6 provides a brief and necessarily incomplete overview of the chemistry associated with such species to date. Of particular interest is the ability of RS_xH to induce protein modifications, interfere with cellular signaling and induce apoptosis. Within this context, perthiols and other RS_xH species are electron rich reducing agents

[2] Polysulfanes have the chemical formula RS_xR' ($R,R' \neq H$ and $x \geq 3$). They should not be confused with polysulfides, which, strictly speaking, are charged, often inorganic species of the type RS_xH or S_x^{2-} ($R \neq H$ and $x \geq 2$). In the case of DATS and DATTS, the widely used 'trisulfide' and 'tetrasulfide' terminology is therefore somewhat misleading.

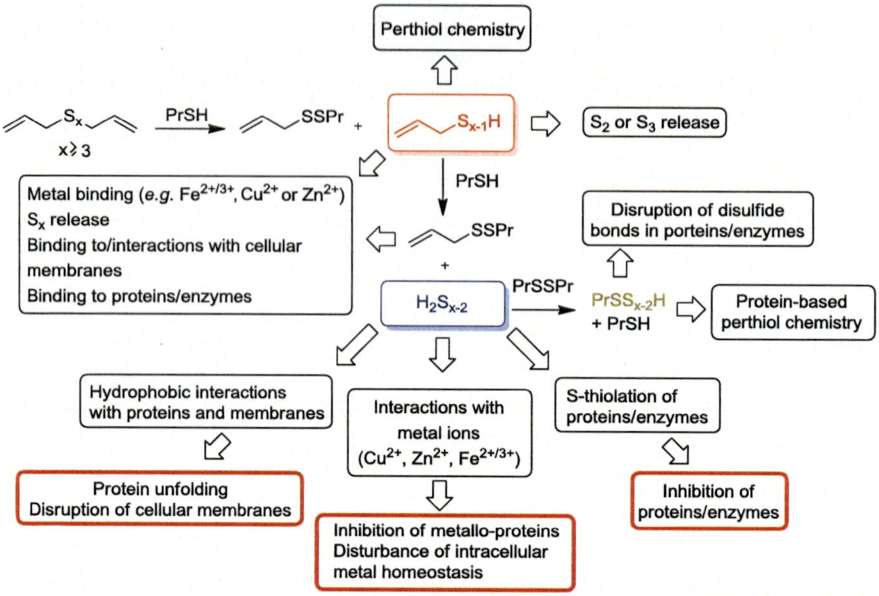

Fig. 12.6 During the last decade, numerous studies have investigated the different chemical and biochemical processes associated with polysulfanes, such as DATS and DATTS. In contrast, there are virtually no reliable studies to date dealing with the biological activity (*e.g.* cytotoxicity) and possible mode(s) of action of inorganic polysulfides. From a chemical perspective, the latter form an interesting and clearly underexplored group of agents, which may exert a significant biological activity *via* a range of rather specific chemical transformations. This chemistry, although highly speculative at this time, is likely to involve a range of fairly unusual reactions, which may involve oxidation and reduction of proteins, the release of S_2 or S_3 and the formation of various sulfur- and oxygen centred radicals

which can break disulfide bonds in proteins and react with metal ions and dioxygen to generate superoxide radicals ($O_2^{\bullet-}$). Ultimately, this leads to a build-up of ROS and OS, causing widespread protein oxidation and activation apoptotic pathways.

Interestingly, disulfide reduction and $O_2^{\bullet-}$ radical generation is not the only chemistry open to RS_xH. These compounds can also decompose by expulsion of elemental S_x species, some of which are highly damaging reactive electrophiles (*e.g.* S_2 or S_3). Furthermore, RS_xH still contains one or more sulfur-sulfur bonds and therefore – in addition to its reducing capacity – can also act as oxidant. Such a reaction would ultimately result in S-thiolation or other, rather unusual peptide or protein disulfide modifications (*e.g.* in form of $PrSS_xH$) – accompanied by the liberation of hydrogen sulfide (H_2S) or indeed longer chain inorganic polysulfides (H_2S_x, in equilibrium with HS_x^- and S_x^{2-}). Hydrogen sulfide is a cellular signaling molecule in its own right, which may interfere with certain apoptotic pathways, especially when generated in higher concentrations.

Unfortunately, very little is known to date about the impact of inorganic polysulfides on cells. It is likely that such species will exhibit their very own redox behavior, possibly as S-thiolating agents (Fig. 12.6). Highly reducing S_x^{2-} species may also form $O_2^{\bullet -}$ from dioxygen and attack disulfide bonds in proteins, hence interfering with protein function and enzyme activity.

It should be mentioned that species such as RS_xH or H_2S_x are also excellent ligands for metal ions, such as zinc, copper and iron ions. These sulfur species may bind adventitiously to metallo-proteins and enzymes, activating or inhibiting the latter as a result. Such ligands may even liberate metal ions from metallo-proteins, which would not only inactivate the protein but also increase the pool of labile, adventitious metal ions. In the case of copper and iron, such effects may ultimately cause Fenton-type redox processes and a significant build-up of intracellular levels of ROS (Bhat et al. 2007; Hadi et al. 2007). The ability of such sulfide-metal complexes to perform Fenton-type chemistry largely depends on their specific redox properties, which may vary considerably from the ones of the corresponding unchelated metal ions.

Finally, longer chain RS_x^- or S_x^{2-} molecules are likely to exhibit amphiphilic properties, paired with a rather interesting helical molecular geometry, which again could promote interactions with (hydrophobic parts of) proteins and membranes.

Together, the rather diverse properties and chemical reactivities of polysulfanes and their follow-on products enable these molecules to interfere with various cellular processes. Not surprisingly, there is considerable and largely consistent evidence in the literature that such natural sulfur compounds, especially DATS and DATTS, also induce apoptosis in a range of cells.

In essence, DATS and DATTS exhibit a wide spectrum of antibiotic, antibacterial, antiviral, antifungal and also antimicrobial properties[3] (Munchberg et al. 2007). They seem to interact with multiple molecular targets, such as proteins involved in the cell cycle arrest and/or apoptosis (Dirsch et al. 1998b; Cerella et al. 2009; Herman-Antosiewicz and Singh 2004; Wu et al. 2005; Chung 2006; Herman-Antosiewicz et al. 2007a, b; Karmakar et al. 2007). The exact mode of action of polysulfanes leading to apoptosis, however, is not yet completely understood (Cerella et al. 2009; Jacob 2006; Jacob et al. 2006; Munchberg et al. 2007). Here, we will briefly consider emerging links between polysulfanes and their chemistry on the one hand and the induction of apoptosis on the other, focusing on a selection of the most recent developments, some of which are still speculative at this time.

One of the first comprehensive studies concerning the intracellular targets of DATS was published by Taiichiro Seki and colleagues in 2005. In this study, DATS induced apoptosis in human colon cancer cell lines HCT-15 (IC_{50} = 11.5 μM) and DLD-1 (IC_{50} = 13.3 μM), whereas DADS and DAS showed no significant effect on the growth of these cells. FACS analysis performed on the cells arrested at the G1/S boundary revealed cell cycle-dependent induction of apoptosis through initial cell cycle arrest in the G2/M phase. Interestingly, in this study, DATS inhibited tubulin

[3] It is likely that other diallylpolysulfanes, such as the penta- and hexasulfane, exhibit similar biological activities. Those longer-chain analogues have hardly been studied so far, mostly due to their inherent chemical instability.

polymerization, and microtubule fragments could be observed at the interphase. β-Tubulin may therefore represent an initial target for DATS and related polysulfanes. Indeed, LC-MS/MS analysis of DATS treated β-tubulin *in vitro* confirmed specific oxidative modifications of cysteine residues $Cys^{12\beta}$ and $Cys^{354\beta}$, which were modified to S-allylmercaptocysteine (Hosono et al. 2005). This finding is of paramount importance, since it strongly points towards direct S-thiolation of β-tubulin by DATS rather than an indirect oxidative process *via* GSSG or up-regulation of ROS (see below).

While β-tubulin may be affected by DATS, this does not mean that this protein necessarily is the only protein target of these polysulfanes (Fig. 12.5). Marc Diederich and colleagues have recently studied the effect of different polysulfanes on U937 leukemia cells. Compounds tested in this study, which included DATS and DATTS, frequently induced apoptosis in U937 cells, with efficiency depending on the length of the sulfur-sulfur chain present in the molecule. In line with various earlier studies, the most effective polysulfane with the highest biological activity was DATTS. Ten micromolar of the compound induced an accumulation of cells in early mitosis (G2/M phase), followed by the activation of caspase-dependent apoptosis. Interestingly, DATTS was counteracting different anti-apoptotic Bcl-2 family members, such as Bcl-xL, phospho-Bad and Bcl-2. Furthermore, the polysulfane was promoting the activation of Bax and Bak and induced the release of cytochrome *c* into the cytoplasm (Cerella et al. 2009). While these studies could not yet completely answer the question how compounds such as DATTS initially trigger apoptotic events, one may speculate that cysteine residues in some of the proteins involved may form an initial target for S-thiolation. Alternatively, DATTS may cause widespread cysteine oxidation by raising the intracellular level of ROS, as has been postulated for a range of other OSCs (see above) and would be in agreement with the distinct polysulfane/perthiol chemistry associated with DATS and DATTS.

Within this context, Mathias Montenarh and colleagues have recently conducted a series of experiments with colorectal carcinoma HCT116 cells, in which DATS and DATTS (at 40 μM) led to reduced cell viability, cell cycle arrest and apoptosis. As could be shown, the induction of apoptosis was indeed dependent on the redox-state of the cell, with certain anti-oxidants being able to prevent polysulfane-induced apoptosis. Growth arrest and induction of apoptosis were also closely related to a reduction in the level of cdc25 C (Busch et al. 2010). In fact, DATTS and also its propyl analogue DPTTS inhibit the cdc25 isoforms A and C *in vitro*, possibly by S-thiolating the active site catalytic cysteine residue present in these enzymes (Viry et al. 2010).

A link between DATS, cdc25 C, the induction of pro-apoptotic proteins and apoptosis has also been observed by Dong Xiao and his colleagues, in human prostate cancer cells as well as in a PC-3 human prostate cancer xenograft in male athymic mice implanted with PC-3 cells. In these studies, DATS reduced significantly the growth of PC-3 xenografts when administered orally, and without causing weight loss in the animals. In this study, DATS-mediated suppression of PC-3 xenograft growth correlated with the induction of pro-apoptotic proteins Bax and Bak (Xiao et al. 2005, 2006; Xiao 2005).

To elucidate the biochemical mechanisms behind this observation in more detail, the group also studied the effects of DATS on PC-3 and DU145 human prostate cancer cells. Application of DATS (20–40 μM) in DU145 cells resulted in a concentration- and time-dependent accumulation of cells in the G2/M phase, which correlated with delayed nuclear translocation of cdk I. As already observed in previous studies, cell cycle arrest was accompanied by the down-regulation and increased Ser^{216} phosphorylation of cdc25 C (Busch et al. 2010; Viry et al. 2010; Herman-Antosiewicz et al. 2010).

While cdc25 C levels and activity may be affected by DATS, the protein itself may not be the initial or indeed the only target of such polysulfanes. In related studies, other possible targets have emerged, including the protein Akt, a serine/threonine protein kinase which plays a key role in multiple cellular processes such as cell proliferation or apoptosis and even the androgen receptor (AR), a member of the nuclear receptor superfamily and a ligand-activated transcription factor. Xiao and colleagues, for instance, could show that DATS (40 μM) led to a fast increase in Ser^{473} and Thr^{308} phosphorylation of Akt followed by an inhibition of its kinase activity. Inactivation of Akt was related to the down-regulation of insulin-like growth factor receptor 1 protein levels and inhibition of its autophosphorylation. In this study, DATS was also responsible for a decrease in Ser^{155} and Ser^{136} phosphorylation of Bad (Xiao 2005). Then again, Shivendra V. Singh and colleagues could show a concentration-dependent decrease in protein levels of AR in DATS treated human prostate cancer cells (LNCaP, C4-2 and TRAMP-C1) and a suppression of AR protein function (Xiao et al. 2005). Indeed, quantitative reverse transcription-PCR showed a dose-dependent reduction of the AR mRNA level, which correlated with the inhibition of AR promoter activity (Stan and Singh 2009).

This data is of particular interest since it points towards a regulatory event triggered by DATS *at the level of DNA transcription* rather than a direct inhibition of enzymes involved in cell cycle control or apoptosis, some of which do not contain crucial cysteine residues and hence cannot be affected directly by S-thiolation or oxidation. This raises the question if the biochemical effects associated with DATS and DATTS are actually due to a modification and inhibition of existing proteins, such as *β*-tubulin and cdc25 C, or rather the result of events at the level of DNA transcription, which subsequently cause a genuine up- or down-regulation of various key signaling proteins. Indeed, there is some evidence which points towards regulation of protein synthesis as the crucial step in the pro-apoptotic activity of polysulfanes. Xiao and colleagues, for instance, could show that DATS causes the generation of ROS and an increase in the protein level of cdk inhibitor p21 in prostate cancer cells. At the same time, apoptosis in these cells was linked to a decrease in the protein level of Bcl-2 (as well as kinase-mediated phosphorylation of Bcl-2 leading to reduced interaction between Bcl-2 and Bax) (Xiao et al. 2004, 2005).

The involvement of ROS in DATS-mediated apoptosis is another, recurrent theme confirmed by various groups in various cancer cell lines. As discussed already for various disulfides and allicin, an involvement of ROS has a certain logical attraction, since it allows us to link the sulfur chemistry of OSCs to a wide range of cellular (signaling) events. In this model, DATS (and DATTS) may initially cause a sharp increase of the intracellular level of ROS, which subsequently leads to a widespread cellular response, including the activation of antioxidant defense mechanisms or the induction of pro-apoptotic pathways (Fig. 12.3).

A ROS-mediated activity would also explain a range of other observations, such as changes in DNA transcription, which may be due to transcription factor (de)-activation. Even a certain selectivity of polysulfane activity against cancer cells could be accounted for, since many cancer cells – unlike normal cells – are suffering from OS, and agents able to increase ROS levels in these cells have a particularly damaging effect.

There is mounting evidence that the biochemical action of DATS and DATTS involves S-thiolation of proteins and subsequent formation of ROS, probably *via* the radical generating chemistry of RS_xH or S_x^{2-}. Nonetheless, one must be very cautious when considering processes such as S-thiolation and ROS formation in the same context. While S-thiolation and ROS formation are both processes which ultimately result in similar, oxidative cysteine modifications in proteins and enzymes, they do not necessarily have to occur together. It is entirely possible that DATS and DATTS cause widespread S-thiolation of proteins and enzymes in cells *without* the formation of ROS. Indeed, several studies have noticed a protective effect of NAC against DATS-induced cell death, while the vitamin E analogue trolox was inactive (Xiao et al. 2005). This apparent paradox is easily explained. While both, NAC and trolox are antioxidants, NAC reacts fairly efficiently with thiol-modifying agents undergoing thiol/disulfide exchange reactions, while trolox, as an electron donor and radical quencher, acts preferably against ROS (Forrest et al. 1994).

Nonetheless, the chemistry of polysulfanes provides several avenues which simultaneously lead to both, thiol/polysulfane exchange reactions *and* sulfur and oxygen radical generation. Recent studies by Lee-Yan Sheen and colleagues in A375 and BCC skin cancer cells, for instance, have shown that DATS increases intracellular ROS levels, induces cytosolic Ca^{2+} mobilization and decreases the mitochondrial membrane potential ($\Delta\Psi m$) (Wang et al. 2010). Furthermore, activation of the p53 pathway in response to the oxidative DNA damage was observed, which clearly cannot be caused by polysulfanes such as DATS and DATTS directly. Such DNA damage is most likely due to the presence of highly aggressive ROS. p53 in turn induces the expression of p21 and affects G2/M modulators such as Wee I kinase, cdc25 C and cdc2. It also triggers the mitochondrial pathway of apoptosis that induces the activation of caspase 3, caspase 9 and PARP cleavage (Wang et al. 2010). One should note, however, that the role of p53 in polysulfane-mediated cell death is still a matter of debate, and p53-dependent apoptotic pathways may not be the only ones triggered by DATS and DATTS (Busch et al. 2010).

Further support for an involvement of ROS, DNA damage and altered protein expression comes from studies considering the antioxidant effects of DATS. From a chemical point of view, DATS is clearly not a good reducing agent. Its apparent antioxidant activity observed in various cell lines is more likely due to an indirect effect which involves the activation of certain antioxidant defense systems (Fig. 12.3). This antioxidant response appears to be mostly due to the *de novo* synthesis of antioxidant proteins and enzymes. In this scenario, DATS acts similar to a vaccine: it causes a mild form of OS, probably mostly by reversible S-thiolation – which subsequently arms the cell against a more severe (oxidative) insult, for instance by ROS or other toxic agents. The chemopreventive properties of natural polysulfanes from garlic, for instance, are related to the induction of phase II detoxification enzymes, such as glutathione S-transferase, which is induced *via* the GPE I enhancer element (Tsai et al. 2007). Similarly, the DNA binding activity of nuclear activator protein-1 (AP-1) is increased in the presence of DADS and DATS[4] (Tsai et al. 2007). In mice intoxicated with ethanol, pretreatment with DATS was able to prevent decreases of hepatic GSH levels and actually increased mitochondrial levels of GSH as well as the activity of antioxidant enzymes, a protective effect which subsequently attenuated acute ethanol-induced liver injury and mitochondrial dysfunction (Zeng et al. 2008).

While there is considerable evidence supporting a connection between polysulfanes, S-thiolation and increased ROS levels on the one hand, and altered gene expression, cell cycle control and apoptosis on the other, there are also other possible mechanisms which may explain the biological activity of compounds such as DATS and DATTS. Recently, Roderick H. Dashwood and colleagues could show that OSCs are rapidly metabolized to AM, which in turn is a competitive inhibitor of certain HDAC enzymes. This is not particularly surprising, since HDAC enzymes contain Zn^{2+} ions at their active site and AM is an excellent ligand for such metal ions. In this particular study, AM induced fast and sustained histone hyperacetylation in human colon cancer cells, which is linked to Sp3 transcription factor binding to the promoter region of the *P21WAF1* gene and finally to cell cycle arrest (Nian et al. 2008, 2009).

12.7 Outlook

While numerous studies support a general redox hypothesis, whereby redox active OSCs S-thiolate and oxidize key signaling proteins and enzymes and/or generate ROS, there are some indications that compounds such as DATS or DATTS may also act by alternative pathways, without the need of extensive redox regulation. As part of this final section, we will therefore briefly consider some of these less obvious modes of action associated with polysulfanes.

As mentioned in Sect.12.3, various diallylsulfides are able to release hydrogen sulfide under physiological conditions. While H_2S release in itself may be the result

[4] Most of these studies have been conducted with DAS, DADS and DATS. DATTS is chemically more unstable and, at least in the past, has been more difficult to obtain. As a consequence, less is known about the various activities of DATTS and higher polysulfanes. Nonetheless, it is likely that these agents will exhibit a similar biochemical behavior.

of certain redox transformations, the subsequent biological activity of H_2S is mostly due to interactions with metal ions present in metallo-proteins. Although experimental evidence is still limited, interactions of hydrogen sulfide with iron and zinc containing proteins (*e.g.* cytochromes, HDACs) may also play an important role in cell cycle control and apoptosis. Furthermore, H_2S is a fairly good reducing agent able to reduce and hence break disulfide bonds in proteins and enzymes. If and how such disulfide reduction processes interfere with apoptotic pathways is still unclear.

Similar considerations apply to inorganic polysulfides and AM. AM, in particular, is known to bind fairly strongly to metal ions, including the active site Zn^{2+} ions in various HDACs (see Sect. 12.6). It has therefore been speculated that AM is the biologically active form of DADS, DATS and DATTS, and that the key event associated with the biological activity of these OSCs after liberation of AM is the binding of this thiol to regulatory metallo-proteins. Indeed, some – but not all – studies confirm a reasonable cytotoxicity of AM and its ability to induce apoptosis in certain cells (Xu and Simon Cho 1999).

There has also been some speculation that the lipophilicity of DATS and DATTS, and their ability to interact with (hydrophobic parts of) proteins and membranes may explain some of the biological activity associated with these compounds. Indeed, there is some evidence that such polysulfanes, which are partly helical in structure, are able to interact rather strongly with proteins and cellular membranes (Tsuchiya and Nagayama 2008). If such interactions are strong enough to inhibit enzymes or even to disrupt membranes needs to be studied in the future. At the same time, polysulfanes exhibit a high 'density' of sulfur atoms right next to each other, an arrangement which may facilitate binding to metal ions and interference with metallo-proteins. If such interactions occur inside the cell, and if they have any major influence on cell proliferation, differentiation or apoptosis needs to be studied in the future.

In summary, there are numerous, chemically vastly different OSCs which interact strongly with mammalian cells, often causing cell cycle arrest and inducing apoptosis. In most cases, the precise mode(s) of action are still not fully understood. In the future, this area of research provides ample opportunities for interdisciplinary investigations involving a wide range of different scientific disciplines.

References

Adams JM, Cory S (1998) The Bcl-2 protein family: arbiters of cell survival. Science 281(5381):1322–1326

Amagase H (2006) Clarifying the real bioactive constituents of garlic. J Nutr 136(3):716s–725s

Antlsperger DS, Dirsch VM, Ferreira D, Su JL, Kuo ML, Vollmar AM (2003) Ajoene-induced cell death in human promyeloleukemic cells does not require JNK but is amplified by the inhibition of ERK. Oncogene 22(4):582–589. doi:10.1038/sj.onc.1206161 1206161 [pii]

Anwar A, Burkholz T, Scherer C, Abbas M, Lehr CM, Diederich M, Jacob C, Daum N (2008) Naturally occurring reactive sulfur species, their activity against Caco-2 cells, and possible modes of biochemical action. J Sulfur Chem 29(5):573–573. doi:10.1080/17415990802519103

Benavides GA, Squadrito GL, Mills RW, Patel HD, Isbell TS, Patel RP, Darley-Usmar VM, Doeller JE, Kraus DW (2007) Hydrogen sulfide mediates the vasoactivity of garlic. Proc Natl Acad Sci USA 104(46):17977–17982. doi:0705710104 [pii] 10.1073/pnas.0705710104

Bhat SH, Azmi AS, Hadi SM (2007) Prooxidant DNA breakage induced by caffeic acid in human peripheral lymphocytes: involvement of endogenous copper and a putative mechanism for anticancer properties. Toxicol Appl Pharmacol 218(3):249–255. doi:S0041-008X(06)00450-9 [pii] 10.1016/j.taap. 2006.11.022

Bilska A, Wlodek L (2005) Lipoic acid - the drug of the future? Pharmacol Rep 57(5):570–577

Brady JF, Ishizaki H, Fukuto JM, Lin MC, Fadel A, Gapac JM, Yang CS (1991) Inhibition of cytochrome P-450 2E1 by diallyl sulfide and its metabolites. Chem Res Toxicol 4(6):642–647. doi:10.1021/tx00024a008

Brandes N, Schmitt S, Jakob U (2009) Thiol-based redox switches in eukaryotic proteins. Antioxid Redox Signal 11(5):997–1014. doi:10.1089/ARS.2008.2285

Busch C, Jacob C, Anwar A, Burkholz T, Aicha Ba L, Cerella C, Diederich M, Brandt W, Wessjohann L, Montenarh M (2010) Diallylpolysulfides induce growth arrest and apoptosis. Int J Oncol 36(3):743–749. doi:10.3892/ijo_00000550

Buzek J, Latonen L, Kurki S, Peltonen K, Laiho M (2002) Redox state of tumor suppressor p53 regulates its sequence-specific DNA binding in DNA-damaged cells by cysteine 277. Nucleic Acids Res 30(11):2340–2348

Cerella C, Scherer C, Cristofanon S, Henry E, Anwar A, Busch C, Montenarh M, Dicato M, Jacob C, Diederich M (2009) Cell cycle arrest in early mitosis and induction of caspase-dependent apoptosis in U937 cells by diallyltetrasulfide (Al2S4). Apoptosis 14(5):641–654. doi:10.1007/s10495-009-0328-8

Choi SY, Yu JH, Kim H (2009) Mechanism of alpha-lipoic acid-induced apoptosis of lung cancer cells involvement of Ca2+. Ann N Y Acad Sci 1171:149–155. doi:10.1111/j.1749-6632.2009.04708.x

Chung LY (2006) The antioxidant properties of garlic compounds: allyl cysteine, alliin, allicin, and allyl disulfide. J Med Food 9(2):205–213. doi:10.1089/jmf.2006.9.205

Cox AG, Peskin AV, Paton LN, Winterbourn CC, Hampton MB (2009) Redox potential and peroxide reactivity of human peroxiredoxin 3. Biochemistry 48(27):6495–6501. doi:10.1021/bi900558g

Cunat S, Anahory T, Berthenet C, Hedon B, Franckhauser C, Fernandez A, Hamamah S, Lamb NJ (2008) The cell cycle control protein cdc25C is present, and phosphorylated on serine 214 in the transition from germinal vesicle to metaphase II in human oocyte meiosis. Mol Reprod Dev 75(7):1176–1184. doi:10.1002/mrd.20853

Daopin S, Piez KA, Ogawa Y, Davies DR (1992) Crystal structure of transforming growth factor-beta 2: an unusual fold for the superfamily. Science 257(5068):369–373

Dirsch VM, Kiemer AK, Wagner H, Vollmar AM (1998a) Effect of allicin and ajoene, two compounds of garlic, on inducible nitric oxide synthase. Atherosclerosis 139(2):333–339. doi:S002191509800094X [pii]

Dirsch VM, Gerbes AL, Vollmar AM (1998b) Ajoene, a compound of garlic, induces apoptosis in human promyeloleukemic cells, accompanied by generation of reactive oxygen species and activation of nuclear factor kappaB. Mol Pharmacol 53(3):402–407

Dirsch VM, Antlsperger DS, Hentze H, Vollmar AM (2002) Ajoene, an experimental anti-leukemic drug: mechanism of cell death. Leukemia 16(1):74–83. doi:10.1038/sj.leu.2402337

Dozio E, Ruscica M, Passafaro L, Dogliotti G, Steffani L, Pagani A, Demartini G, Esposti D, Fraschini F, Magni P (2010) The natural antioxidant alpha-lipoic acid induces p27(Kip1)-dependent cell cycle arrest and apoptosis in MCF-7 human breast cancer cells. Eur J Pharmacol 641(1):29–34. doi:S0014-2999(10)00425-5 [pii] 10.1016/j.ejphar.2010.05.009

Egen-Schwind C, Eckard R, Jekat FW, Winterhoff H (1992) Pharmacokinetics of vinyldithiins, transformation products of allicin. Planta Med 58(1):8–13. doi:10.1055/s-2006-961379

Ferri N, Yokoyama K, Sadilek M, Paoletti R, Apitz-Castro R, Gelb MH, Corsini A (2003) Ajoene, a garlic compound, inhibits protein prenylation and arterial smooth muscle cell proliferation. Br J Pharmacol 138(5):811–818. doi:10.1038/sj.bjp. 0705126

Filomeni G, Rotilio G, Ciriolo MR (2008) Molecular transduction mechanisms of the redox network underlying the antiproliferative effects of allyl compounds from garlic. J Nutr 138(11): 2053–2057. doi:138/11/2053 [pii]

Forrest VJ, Kang YH, McClain DE, Robinson DH, Ramakrishnan N (1994) Oxidative stress-induced apoptosis prevented by Trolox. Free Radic Biol Med 16(6):675–684

Fourquet S, Guerois R, Biard D, Toledano MB (2010) Activation of NRF2 by nitrosative agents and H2O2 involves KEAP1 disulfide formation. J Biol Chem 285(11):8463–8471. doi:M109.051714 [pii] 10.1074/jbc.M109.051714

Gayathri R, Gunadharini DN, Arunkumar A, Senthilkumar K, Krishnamoorthy G, Banudevi S, Vignesh RC, Arunakaran J (2009) Effects of diallyl disulfide (DADS) on expression of apoptosis associated proteins in androgen independent human prostate cancer cells (PC-3). Mol Cell Biochem 320(1–2):197–203. doi:10.1007/s11010-008-9903-5

Giles NM, Watts AB, Giles GI, Fry FH, Littlechild JA, Jacob C (2003) Metal and redox modulation of cysteine protein function. Chem Biol 10(8):677–693. doi:S1074552103001741 [pii]

Gruhlke MC, Portz D, Stitz M, Anwar A, Schneider T, Jacob C, Schlaich NL, Slusarenko AJ (2010) Allicin disrupts the cell's electrochemical potential and induces apoptosis in yeast. Free Radic Biol Med. doi:S0891-5849(10)00565-4 [pii] 10.1016/j.freeradbiomed.2010.09.019

Hadi SM, Bhat SH, Azmi AS, Hanif S, Shamim U, Ullah MF (2007) Oxidative breakage of cellular DNA by plant polyphenols: a putative mechanism for anticancer properties. Semin Cancer Biol 17(5):370–376. doi:S1044-579X(07)00025-9 [pii] 10.1016/j.semcancer.2007.04.002

Hansen RE, Roth D, Winther JR (2009) Quantifying the global cellular thiol-disulfide status. Proc Natl Acad Sci USA 106(2):422–427. doi:10.1073/pnas.0812149106

Hattori A, Yamada N, Nishikawa T, Fukuda H, Fujino T (2005) Antidiabetic effects of ajoene in genetically diabetic KK-A(y) mice. J Nutr Sci Vitaminol (Tokyo) 51(5):382–384

Herman-Antosiewicz A, Singh SV (2004) Signal transduction pathways leading to cell cycle arrest and apoptosis induction in cancer cells by Allium vegetable-derived organosulfur compounds: a review. Mutat Res 555(1–2):121–131. doi:S0027-5107(04)00287-8 [pii] 10.1016/j.mrfmmm.2004.04.016

Herman-Antosiewicz A, Powolny AA, Singh SV (2007a) Molecular targets of cancer chemoprevention by garlic-derived organosulfides. Acta Pharmacol Sin 28(9):1355–1364. doi:10.1111/j.1745-7254.2007.00682.x

Herman-Antosiewicz A, Stan SD, Hahm ER, Xiao D, Singh SV (2007b) Activation of a novel ataxia-telangiectasia mutated and Rad3 related/checkpoint kinase 1-dependent prometaphase checkpoint in cancer cells by diallyl trisulfide, a promising cancer chemopreventive constituent of processed garlic. Mol Cancer Ther 6(4):1249–1261. doi:1535-7163.MCT-06-0477 [pii] 10.1158/1535-7163.MCT-06-0477

Herman-Antosiewicz A, Kim YA, Kim SH, Xiao D, Singh SV (2010) Diallyl trisulfide-induced G2/M phase cell cycle arrest in DU145 cells is associated with delayed nuclear translocation of cyclin-dependent kinase 1. Pharm Res 27(6):1072–1079. doi:10.1007/s11095-010-0060-7

Hirsch K, Danilenko M, Giat J, Miron T, Rabinkov A, Wilchek M, Mirelman D, Levy J, Sharoni Y (2000) Effect of purified allicin, the major ingredient of freshly crushed garlic, on cancer cell proliferation. Nutr Cancer 38(2):245–254

Hong SJ, Dawson TM, Dawson VL (2004) Nuclear and mitochondrial conversations in cell death: PARP-1 and AIF signaling. Trends Pharmacol Sci 25(5):259–264. doi:10.1016/j.tips.2004.03.005

Hong F, Freeman ML, Liebler DC (2005) Identification of sensor cysteines in human Keap1 modified by the cancer chemopreventive agent sulforaphane. Chem Res Toxicol 18(12):1917–1926. doi:10.1021/tx0502138

Hosono T, Fukao T, Ogihara J, Ito Y, Shiba H, Seki T, Ariga T (2005) Diallyl trisulfide suppresses the proliferation and induces apoptosis of human colon cancer cells through oxidative modification of beta-tubulin. J Biol Chem 280(50):41487–41493. doi:M507127200 [pii] 10.1074/jbc.M507127200

Huber K, Patel P, Zhang L, Evans H, Westwell AD, Fischer PM, Chan S, Martin S (2008) 2-[(1-methylpropyl)dithio]-1 H-imidazole inhibits tubulin polymerization through cysteine oxidation. Mol Cancer Ther 7(1):143–151. doi:7/1/143 [pii] 10.1158/1535-7163.MCT-07-0486

Jacob C (2006) A scent of therapy: pharmacological implications of natural products containing redox-active sulfur atoms. Nat Prod Rep 23(6):851–863. doi:10.1039/b609523m

Jacob C, Anwar A (2008) The chemistry behind redox regulation with a focus on sulphur redox systems. Physiol Plant 133(3):469–480. doi:10.1111/j.1399-3054.2008.01080.x

Jacob C, Holme AL, Fry FH (2004) The sulfinic acid switch in proteins. Org Biomol Chem 2(14):1953–1956. doi:10.1039/b406180b

Jacob C, Knight I, Winyard PG (2006) Aspects of the biological redox chemistry of cysteine: from simple redox responses to sophisticated signalling pathways. Biol Chem 387(10–11):1385–1397. doi:10.1515/BC.2006.174

Jacob C, Jamier V, Ba LA (2010) Redox active secondary metabolites. Current Opin Chem Biol. doi:10.1016/j.cbpa.2010.10.015

Karmakar S, Banik NL, Patel SJ, Ray SK (2007) Garlic compounds induced calpain and intrinsic caspase cascade for apoptosis in human malignant neuroblastoma SH-SY5Y cells. Apoptosis 12(4):671–684. doi:10.1007/s10495-006-0024-x

Keophiphath M, Priem F, Jacquemond-Collet I, Clement K, Lacasa D (2009) 1,2-vinyldithiin from garlic inhibits differentiation and inflammation of human preadipocytes. J Nutr 139(11):2055–2060. doi:jn.109.105452 [pii] 10.3945/jn.109.105452

Kraaij MD, Savage ND, van der Kooij SW, Koekkoek K, Wang J, van den Berg JM, Ottenhoff TH, Kuijpers TW, Holmdahl R, van Kooten C, Gelderman KA (2010) Induction of regulatory T cells by macrophages is dependent on production of reactive oxygen species. Proc Natl Acad Sci USA 107(41):17686–17691. doi:1012016107 [pii] 10.1073/pnas.1012016107

Landino LM, Koumas MT, Mason CE, Alston JA (2007) Modification of tubulin cysteines by nitric oxide and nitroxyl donors alters tubulin polymerization activity. Chem Res Toxicol 20(11):1693–1700. doi:10.1021/tx7001492

Ledezma E, Apitz-Castro R, Cardier J (2004) Apoptotic and anti-adhesion effect of ajoene, a garlic derived compound, on the murine melanoma B16F10 cells: possible role of caspase-3 and the alpha(4)beta(1) integrin. Cancer Lett 206(1):35–41. doi:10.1016/j.canlet.2003.10.031 S0304383503007729 [pii]

Ledezma E, Wittig O, Alonso J, Cardier JE (2009) Potentiated cytotoxic effects of statins and ajoene in murine melanoma cells. Melanoma Res 19(2):69–74. doi:10.1097/CMR.0b013e32831bc45a

Lee W, Choi KS, Riddell J, Ip C, Ghosh D, Park JH, Park YM (2007) Human peroxiredoxin 1 and 2 are not duplicate proteins: the unique presence of CYS83 in Prx1 underscores the structural and functional differences between Prx1 and Prx2. J Biol Chem 282(30):22011–22022. doi:M610330200 [pii] 10.1074/jbc.M610330200

Li M, Ciu JR, Ye Y, Min JM, Zhang LH, Wang K, Gares M, Cros J, Wright M, Leung-Tack J (2002a) Antitumor activity of Z-ajoene, a natural compound purified from garlic: antimitotic and microtubule-interaction properties. Carcinogenesis 23(4):573–579. doi:10.1093/carcin/23.4.573

Li M, Min JM, Cui JR, Zhang LH, Wang K, Valette A, Davrinche C, Wright M, Leung-Tack J (2002b) Z-ajoene induces apoptosis of HL-60 cells: involvement of Bcl-2 cleavage. Nutr Cancer 42(2):241–247

Liu L, Yeh YY (2002) S-alk(en)yl cysteines of garlic inhibit cholesterol synthesis by deactivating HMG-CoA reductase in cultured rat hepatocytes. J Nutr 132(6):1129–1134

Lo Bello M, Battistoni A, Mazzetti AP, Board PG, Muramatsu M, Federici G, Ricci G (1995) Site-directed mutagenesis of human glutathione transferase P1-1. Spectral, kinetic, and structural properties of Cys-47 and Lys-54 mutants. J Biol Chem 270(3):1249–1253

Lundstrom J, Holmgren A (1993) Determination of the reduction-oxidation potential of the thioredoxin-like domains of protein disulfide-isomerase from the equilibrium with glutathione and thioredoxin. Biochemistry 32(26):6649–6655. doi:10.1021/bi00077a018

Maser RS, Antoku K, Scully WJ Jr, Cho RL, Johnson DE (2000) Analysis of the role of conserved cysteine residues in the bcl-2 oncoprotein. Biochem Biophys Res Commun 277(1):171–178. doi:10.1006/bbrc.2000.3652 S0006-291X(00)93652-0 [pii]

McStay GP, Clarke SJ, Halestrap AP (2002) Role of critical thiol groups on the matrix surface of the adenine nucleotide translocase in the mechanism of the mitochondrial permeability transition pore. Biochem J 367(Pt 2):541–548. doi:10.1042/BJ20011672 BJ20011672 [pii]

Menon SG, Goswami PC (2007) A redox cycle within the cell cycle: ring in the old with the new. Oncogene 26(8):1101–1109. doi:1209895 [pii] 10.1038/sj.onc.1209895

Meyer M, Schreck R, Baeuerle PA (1993) H2O2 and antioxidants have opposite effects on activation of NF-kappa B and AP-1 in intact cells: AP-1 as secondary antioxidant-responsive factor. EMBO J 12(5):2005–2015

Mieyal JJ, Gallogly MM, Qanungo S, Sabens EA, Shelton MD (2008) Molecular mechanisms and clinical implications of reversible protein S-glutathionylation. Antioxid Redox Signal 10(11):1941–1988. doi:10.1089/ars.2008.2089

Miron T, Wilchek M, Sharp A, Nakagawa Y, Naoi M, Nozawa Y, Akao Y (2008) Allicin inhibits cell growth and induces apoptosis through the mitochondrial pathway in HL60 and U937 cells. J Nutr Biochem 19(8):524–535. doi:S0955-2863(07)00179-9 [pii] 10.1016/j.jnutbio.2007.06.009

Moungjaroen J, Nimmannit U, Callery PS, Wang L, Azad N, Lipipun V, Chanvorachote P, Rojanasakul Y (2006) Reactive oxygen species mediate caspase activation and apoptosis induced by lipoic acid in human lung epithelial cancer cells through Bcl-2 down-regulation. J Pharmacol Exp Ther 319(3):1062–1069. doi:jpet.106.110965 [pii] 10.1124/jpet.106.110965

Munchberg U, Anwar A, Mecklenburg S, Jacob C (2007) Polysulfides as biologically active ingredients of garlic. Org Biomol Chem 5(10):1505–1518. doi:10.1039/b703832a

Naganawa R, Iwata N, Ishikawa K, Fukuda H, Fujino T, Suzuki A (1996) Inhibition of microbial growth by ajoene, a sulfur-containing compound derived from garlic. Appl Environ Microbiol 62(11):4238–4242

Nagaraj NS, Anilakumar KR, Singh OV (2010) Diallyl disulfide causes caspase-dependent apoptosis in human cancer cells through a Bax-triggered mitochondrial pathway. J Nutr Biochem 21(5):405–412. doi:10.1016/j.jnutbio.2009.01.015

Nian H, Delage B, Pinto JT, Dashwood RH (2008) Allyl mercaptan, a garlic-derived organosulfur compound, inhibits histone deacetylase and enhances Sp3 binding on the P21WAF1 promoter. Carcinogenesis 29(9):1816–1824. doi:bgn165 [pii] 10.1093/carcin/bgn165

Nian H, Delage B, Ho E, Dashwood RH (2009) Modulation of histone deacetylase activity by dietary isothiocyanates and allyl sulfides: studies with sulforaphane and garlic organosulfur compounds. Environ Mol Mutagen 50(3):213–221. doi:10.1002/em.20454

Nie C, Tian C, Zhao L, Petit PX, Mehrpour M, Chen Q (2008) Cysteine 62 of Bax is critical for its conformational activation and its proapoptotic activity in response to H2O2-induced apoptosis. J Biol Chem 283(22):15359–15369. doi:M800847200 [pii] 10.1074/jbc.M800847200

Nishinaka Y, Masutani H, Nakamura H, Yodoi J (2001) Regulatory roles of thioredoxin in oxidative stress-induced cellular responses. Redox Rep 6(5):289–295

Oommen S, Anto RJ, Srinivas G, Karunagaran D (2004) Allicin (from garlic) induces caspase-mediated apoptosis in cancer cells. Eur J Pharmacol 485(1–3):97–103. doi:S0014299903027262 [pii]

Park SY, Cho SJ, Kwon HC, Lee KR, Rhee DK, Pyo S (2005) Caspase-independent cell death by allicin in human epithelial carcinoma cells: involvement of PKA. Cancer Lett 224(1):123–132. doi:S0304-3835(04)00804-3 [pii] 10.1016/j.canlet.2004.10.009

Peskin AV, Low FM, Paton LN, Maghzal GJ, Hampton MB, Winterbourn CC (2007) The high reactivity of peroxiredoxin 2 with H(2)O(2) is not reflected in its reaction with other oxidants and thiol reagents. J Biol Chem 282(16):11885–11892. doi:M700339200 [pii] 10.1074/jbc.M700339200

Pociask DA, Sime PJ, Brody AR (2004) Asbestos-derived reactive oxygen species activate TGF-beta1. Lab Invest 84(8):1013–1023. doi:10.1038/labinvest.3700109 3700109 [pii]

Powolny AA, Singh SV (2008) Multitargeted prevention and therapy of cancer by diallyl trisulfide and related Allium vegetable-derived organosulfur compounds. Cancer Lett 269(2):305–314. doi:S0304-3835(08)00397-2 [pii] 10.1016/j.canlet.2008.05.027

Rainwater R, Parks D, Anderson ME, Tegtmeyer P, Mann K (1995) Role of cysteine residues in regulation of p53 function. Mol Cell Biol 15(7):3892–3903

Ren B, Huang W, Akesson B, Ladenstein R (1997) The crystal structure of seleno-glutathione peroxidase from human plasma at 2.9 A resolution. J Mol Biol 268(5):869–885. doi:S0022-2836(97)91005-6 [pii] 10.1006/jmbi.1997.1005

Rendu F, Daveloose D, Debouzy JC, Bourdeau N, Levy-Toledano S, Jain MK, Apitz-Castro R (1989) Ajoene, the antiplatelet compound derived from garlic, specifically inhibits platelet release reaction by affecting the plasma membrane internal microviscosity. Biochem Pharmacol 38(8):1321–1328

Ricci G, Lo Bello M, Caccurri AM, Pastore A, Nuccetelli M, Parker MW, Federici G (1995) Site-directed mutagenesis of human glutathione transferase P1-1. Mutation of Cys-47 induces a positive cooperativity in glutathione transferase P1-1. J Biol Chem 270(3):1243–1248

Roy S, Packer L (1998) Redox regulation of cell functions by alpha-lipoate: biochemical and molecular aspects. Biofactors 8(1–2):17–21

Sarakbi M-B (2009) Natural products and related compounds as promising antioxidants and antimicrobial agents. Universitaet des Saarlandes, Saarbruecken

Saurin AT, Neubert H, Brennan JP, Eaton P (2004) Widespread sulfenic acid formation in tissues in response to hydrogen peroxide. Proc Natl Acad Sci USA 101(52):17982–17987. doi:0404762101 [pii] 10.1073/pnas.0404762101

Savitsky PA, Finkel T (2002) Redox regulation of Cdc25C. J Biol Chem 277(23):20535–20540. doi:10.1074/jbc.M201589200 M201589200 [pii]

Schafer FQ, Buettner GR (2001) Redox environment of the cell as viewed through the redox state of the glutathione disulfide/glutathione couple. Free Radic Biol Med 30(11):1191–1212. doi:10.1016/S0891-5849(01)00480-4

Scharfenberg K, Wagner R, Wagner KG (1990) The cytotoxic effect of ajoene, a natural product from garlic, investigated with different cell lines. Cancer Lett 53(2–3):103–108

Selvakumar E, Hsieh TC (2008) Regulation of cell cycle transition and induction of apoptosis in HL-60 leukemia cells by lipoic acid: role in cancer prevention and therapy. J Hematol Oncol 1:4. doi:1756-8722-1-4 [pii] 10.1186/1756-8722-1-4

Shin HA, Cha YY, Park MS, Kim JM, Lim YC (2010) Diallyl sulfide induces growth inhibition and apoptosis of anaplastic thyroid cancer cells by mitochondrial signaling pathway. Oral Oncol 46(4):E15–E18. doi:10.1016/j.oraloncology.2009.10.012

Simbula G, Columbano A, Ledda-Columbano GM, Sanna L, Deidda M, Diana A, Pibiri M (2007) Increased ROS generation and p53 activation in alpha-lipoic acid-induced apoptosis of hepatoma cells. Apoptosis 12(1):113–123. doi:10.1007/s10495-006-0487-9

Soldani C, Scovassi AI (2002) Poly(ADP-ribose) polymerase-1 cleavage during apoptosis: an update. Apoptosis 7(4):321–328. doi:10.1023/A:1016119328968

Song JD, Lee SK, Kim KM, Park SE, Park SJ, Kim KH, Ahn SC, Park YC (2009) Molecular mechanism of diallyl disulfide in cell cycle arrest and apoptosis in HCT-116 colon cancer cells. J Biochem Mol Toxicol 23(1):71–79. doi:10.1002/jbt.20266

Sparnins VL, Barany G, Wattenberg LW (1988) Effects of organosulfur compounds from garlic and onions on benzo[a]pyrene-induced neoplasia and glutathione S-transferase activity in the mouse. Carcinogenesis 9(1):131–134. doi:10.1093/carcin/9.1.131

Stamatakis K, Sanchez-Gomez FJ, Perez-Sala D (2006) Identification of novel protein targets for modification by 15-deoxy-Delta12,14-prostaglandin J2 in mesangial cells reveals multiple interactions with the cytoskeleton. J Am Soc Nephrol 17(1):89–98. doi:ASN.2005030329 [pii] 10.1681/ASN.2005030329

Stan SD, Singh SV (2009) Transcriptional repression and inhibition of nuclear translocation of androgen receptor by diallyl trisulfide in human prostate cancer cells. Clin Cancer Res 15(15):4895–4903. doi:1078-0432.CCR-09-0512 [pii] 10.1158/1078-0432.CCR-09-0512

Sun L, Wang X (2003) Effects of allicin on both telomerase activity and apoptosis in gastric cancer SGC-7901 cells. World J Gastroenterol 9(9):1930–1934

Tanaka T, Hosoi F, Yamaguchi-Iwai Y, Nakamura H, Masutani H, Ueda S, Nishiyama A, Takeda S, Wada H, Spyrou G, Yodoi J (2002) Thioredoxin-2 (TRX-2) is an essential gene regulating mitochondria-dependent apoptosis. EMBO J 21(7):1695–1703. doi:10.1093/emboj/21.7.1695

Terrasson J, Xu B, Li M, Allart S, Davignon JL, Zhang LH, Wang K, Davrinche C (2007) Activities of Z-ajoene against tumour and viral spreading in vitro. Fundam Clin Pharmacol 21(3):281–289. doi:FCP470 [pii] 10.1111/j.1472-8206.2007.00470.x

Trachootham D, Lu W, Ogasawara MA, Nilsa RD, Huang P (2008) Redox regulation of cell survival. Antioxid Redox Signal 10(8):1343–1374. doi:10.1089/ars.2007.1957

Truong D, Hindmarsh W, O'Brien PJ (2009) The molecular mechanisms of diallyl disulfide and diallyl sulfide induced hepatocyte cytotoxicity. Chem Biol Interact 180(1):79–88. doi:S0009-2797(09)00075-1 [pii] 10.1016/j.cbi.2009.02.008

Tsai CW, Chen HW, Yang JJ, Sheen LY, Lii CK (2007) Diallyl disulfide and diallyl trisulfide up-regulate the expression of the pi class of glutathione S-transferase via an AP-1-dependent pathway. J Agric Food Chem 55(3):1019–1026. doi:10.1021/jf061874t

Tsuchiya H, Nagayama M (2008) Garlic allyl derivatives interact with membrane lipids to modify the membrane fluidity. J Biomed Sci 15(5):653–660. doi:10.1007/s11373-008-9257-8

Velu CS, Niture SK, Doneanu CE, Pattabiraman N, Srivenugopal KS (2007) Human p53 is inhibited by glutathionylation of cysteines present in the proximal DNA-binding domain during oxidative stress. Biochemistry 46(26):7765–7780. doi:10.1021/bi700425y

Vilcek J, Lee TH (1991) Tumor necrosis factor. New insights into the molecular mechanisms of its multiple actions. J Biol Chem 266(12):7313–7316

Viry E, Anwar A, Kirsch G, Jacob C, Diederich M, Bagrel D (2010) Antiproliferative effect of natural tetrasulfides in human breast cancer cells is mediated through the inhibition of the cell division cycle 25 phosphatase. Int J Oncol. doi:10.3892/ijo_xxxxxxxx

Walder R, Kalvatchev Z, Garzaro D, Barrios M, Apitz-Castro R (1997) In vitro suppression of HIV-1 replication by ajoene [(e)-(z)-4,5,9-trithiadodeca-1,6,11-triene-9 oxide]. Biomed Pharmacother 51(9):397–403. doi:S0753332297894334 [pii]

Wang HC, Yang JH, Hsieh SC, Sheen LY (2010) Allyl sulfides inhibit cell growth of skin cancer cells through induction of DNA damage mediated G2/M arrest and apoptosis. J Agric Food Chem 58(11):7096–7103. doi:10.1021/jf100613x

Wargovich MJ (2006) Diallylsulfide and allylmethylsulfide are uniquely effective among organosulfur compounds in inhibiting CYP2E1 protein in animal models. J Nutr 136(3 Suppl):832S–834S. doi:136/3/832S [pii]

Wargovich MJ, Woods C, Eng VW, Stephens LC, Gray K (1988) Chemoprevention of N-nitrosomethylbenzylamine-induced esophageal cancer in rats by the naturally occurring thioether, diallyl sulfide. Cancer Res 48(23):6872–6875

Watson WH, Pohl J, Montfort WR, Stuchlik O, Reed MS, Powis G, Jones DP (2003) Redox potential of human thioredoxin 1 and identification of a second dithiol/disulfide motif. J Biol Chem 278(35):33408–33415. doi:10.1074/jbc.M211107200 M211107200 [pii]

Wenzel U, Nickel A, Daniel H (2005) alpha-Lipoic acid induces apoptosis in human colon cancer cells by increasing mitochondrial respiration with a concomitant O2-*-generation. Apoptosis 10(2):359–368. doi:10.1007/s10495-005-0810-x

Wu X, Kassie F, Mersch-Sundermann V (2005) Induction of apoptosis in tumor cells by naturally occurring sulfur-containing compounds. Mutat Res 589(2):81–102. doi:S1383-5742(04)00070-5 [pii] 10.1016/j.mrrev.2004.11.001

Xiao D (2005) Diallyltrisulfide, a constituent of processed garlic, inactivates Akt to trigger mitochondrial translocation of BAD and caspase-mediated apoptosis in human prostate cancer cells. Carcinogenesis 27(3):533–540

Xiao D, Choi S, Johnson DE, Vogel VG, Johnson CS, Trump DL, Lee YJ, Singh SV (2004) Diallyl trisulfide-induced apoptosis in human prostate cancer cells involves c-Jun N-terminal kinase and extracellular-signal regulated kinase-mediated phosphorylation of Bcl-2. Oncogene 23(33):5594–5606. doi:10.1038/sj.onc.1207747 1207747 [pii]

Xiao D, Herman-Antosiewicz A, Antosiewicz J, Xiao H, Brisson M, Lazo JS, Singh SV (2005) Diallyl trisulfide-induced G(2)-M phase cell cycle arrest in human prostate cancer cells is caused by reactive oxygen species-dependent destruction and hyperphosphorylation of Cdc 25 C. Oncogene 24(41):6256–6268. doi:1208759 [pii] 10.1038/sj.onc.1208759

Xiao D, Lew KL, Kim YA, Zeng Y, Hahm ER, Dhir R, Singh SV (2006) Diallyl trisulfide suppresses growth of PC-3 human prostate cancer xenograft in vivo in association with Bax and Bak induction. Clin Cancer Res 12(22):6836–6843. doi:12/22/6836 [pii] 10.1158/1078-0432.CCR-06-1273

Xu S, Simon Cho BH (1999) Allyl mercaptan, a major metabolite of garlic compounds, reduces cellular cholesterol synthesis and its secretion in Hep-G2 cells. J Nutr Biochem 10(11):654–659. doi:S0955-2863(99)00056-X [pii]

Xu B, Monsarrat B, Gairin JE, Girbal-Neuhauser E (2004) Effect of ajoene, a natural antitumor small molecule, on human 20 S proteasome activity in vitro and in human leukemic HL60 cells. Fundam Clin Pharmacol 18(2):171–180. doi:10.1111/j.1472-8206.2004.00219.x FCP219 [pii]

Yakovlev AG, Wang GP, Stoica BA, Boulares HA, Spoonde AY, Yoshihara K, Smulson ME (2000) A role of the Ca2+/Mg2+-dependent endonuclease in apoptosis and its inhibition by poly(ADP-ribose) polymerase. J Biol Chem 275(28):21302–21308. doi:10.1074/jbc.M001087200

Yang JY, Della-Fera MA, Nelson-Dooley C, Baile CA (2006) Molecular mechanisms of apoptosis induced by ajoene in 3 T3-L1 adipocytes. Obesity (Silver Spring) 14(3):388–397. doi:14/3/388 [pii] 10.1038/oby.2006.52

Yoshida H, Iwata N, Katsuzaki H, Naganawa R, Ishikawa K, Fukuda H, Fujino T, Suzuki A (1998) Antimicrobial activity of a compound isolated from an oil-macerated garlic extract. Biosci Biotechnol Biochem 62(5):1014–1017

Yu L, Guo N, Meng R, Liu B, Tang X, Jin J, Cui Y, Deng X (2010) Allicin-induced global gene expression profile of Saccharomyces cerevisiae. Appl Microbiol Biotechnol 88(1):219–229. doi:10.1007/s00253-010-2709-x

Zeng T, Zhang CL, Zhu ZP, Yu LH, Zhao XL, Xie KQ (2008) Diallyl trisulfide (DATS) effectively attenuated oxidative stress-mediated liver injury and hepatic mitochondrial dysfunction in acute ethanol-exposed mice. Toxicology 252(1–3):86–91. doi:S0300-483X(08)00370-3 [pii] 10.1016/j.tox.2008.07.062

Zuo Y, Xiang B, Yang J, Sun X, Wang Y, Cang H, Yi J (2009) Oxidative modification of caspase-9 facilitates its activation via disulfide-mediated interaction with Apaf-1. Cell Res 19(4):449–457. doi:cr200919 [pii] 10.1038/cr.2009.19

Chapter 13
Diallyl Sulfides and the Decision About Life and Death of a Cell

Mathias Montenarh

Abstract The medicinal benefits of garlic have been documented throughout recorded history. These known health benefits of garlic include cardiovascular protective effects, stimulation of the immune system, reduction of blood glucose, protection against microbial, viral and fungal infections as well as anticancer effects. Most of the effects of garlic are attributed to organosulfur compounds and in particular to diallyl sulfides. The molecular basis for the biological activities of diallyl sulfides remain elusive, but there is increasing experimental evidence that these compounds induce the cellular redox system, and target multiple signal transduction pathways regulating cell cycle progression and apoptosis induction. The aim of this review is to accomplish the present knowledge about cellular targets of diallyl sulfides with regard to cell cycle regulation and apoptosis induction.

13.1 Structure and Function of Diallyl Sulfides

It is clear from studies over the last 50 years that nutrition plays an essential role in preventing a variety of different diseases. Diets rich in fruits and vegetables are thought to play a protective role for the formation of different types of cancer. This protective role has long been associated with vitamins that have antioxidant properties. Intensive research and a variety of epidemiological studies have revealed that *Allium* vegetables including garlic and onions that are rich in organo sulfur compounds also play a protective role in cancer. Garlic was already a component of diets at the beginning of recorded history. Moreover, it is known from ancient medical

M. Montenarh (✉)
Medizinische Biochemie und Molekularbiologie, Universität des Saarlandes, Gebäude 44, 66424 Homburg, Germany
e-mail: Mathias.Montenarh@uks.eu

M. Diederich and K. Noworyta (eds.), *Natural Compounds as Inducers of Cell Death: Volume 1*, DOI 10.1007/978-94-007-4575-9_13,

texts that garlic was used not only to flavour food but also for medicinal applications. A nice historical overview about the medical use of garlic is presented by Rivlin (2001) and by Milner (2001).

A number of epidemiological studies suggest that protection from many different types of cancer may be related to the consumption of garlic (for review see: Fleischauer and Arab 2001). However, it was not clear from all these studies what the minimum dose of garlic necessary to elicit a protective effect might be. For instance, a population-based case–control study showed that the risk of prostate cancer was significantly lower in men consuming >10 g/day of total *Allium* vegetables than in men with total *Allium* vegetable intake of <2.2 g/day (Hsing et al. 2002). Cancer chemoprevention with garlic and its constituents has been the subjects of numerous recent reviews (Nagini 2008; Powolny and Singh 2008; Stan et al. 2008; Gullett et al. 2010; Kim and Kwon 2009).

Garlic was not only recommended for protection against cancer. In China, garlic tea has long been recommended for fever, headache, cholera and dysentery (Corzo-Martinez et al. 2007). It was thought that garlic has antiseptic, diaphoretic, diuretic and expectorant properties. Garlic has long been recommended for the treatment of tuberculosis as well. The antiparasitic effects of freshly crushed garlic were already known by ancient cultures.

From data published in the last two decades, it is evident that garlic may influence the risk for heart disease and cancer (Milner 1996; Kendler 1987). It was reported that garlic suppresses tumour incidence in breast, colon, skin, uterine, oesophagus and lung cancer (Amagase and Milner 1993; Hussain et al. 1990; Ip et al. 1992; Song and Milner 1999; Sumiyoshi and Wargovich 1990; Wargovich et al. 1988).

Dion et al. (1997) have provided evidence that several oil-soluble allylsulfur compounds are also effective antimicrobial agents. Others found evidence for a repression of redox enzymes such as NADPH/quinone oxidoreductase (Singh et al. 1998), cyclooxygenase, lipoxygenase (Schreiber et al. 1989) and glutathione-S-transferase (Hatono et al. 1996).

Alliums are all odorless until the plant cells are crushed or otherwise damaged. The anticarcinogenic effect of *Allium* vegetables is attributed to organosulfur compounds which are generated upon processing, cutting or chewing, of these vegetables (Block 1992). At this point they generate characteristic, volatile sulfur containing chemicals. These strong-smelling and -tasting compounds are classified as secondary metabolites, because they are not directly involved in normal growth, development or reproduction of the plants. Organic sulfur compounds are found everywhere in nature. A great number of sulfur compounds found in plants, fungi, bacteria and in animals and humans have chemical and biochemical properties, which are connected somehow with redox processes, metal binding and catalytic activities. Some of theses sulfur compounds function as antibiotics, anticancer or anti inflammatory agents making them interesting from pharmacological perspectives.

In the middle of the nineteenth century a French chemist first reported the isolation of garlic oil form garlic plants. It turned out that the properties described for garlic oil closely resembled the today known properties for diallyl sulfides (Hofmann and Cahours 1857). In 1892 the German chemist F.W. Semmler reported that garlic

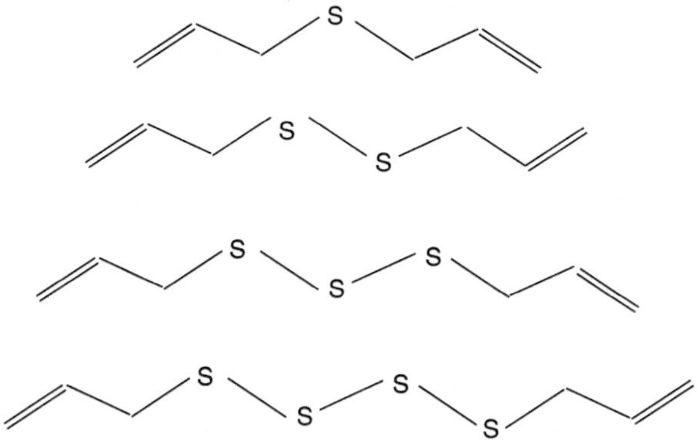

Fig. 13.1 Structure of diallyl mono- and diallyl polysulfides

oil when fractionally distilled at low pressure contained diallyl disulfide, diallyl trisulfide and diallyl tetrasulfide (Semmler 1892). Figure 13.1 shows the structure of the different diallyl sulfides.

Nowadays the highly active diallyl trisulfide is synthesized from allyl chloride, sodium thiosulfate and sodium sulfide according to the method of Milligan et al. (1961) Diallyl tetrasulfide which is analyzed recently is synthesized from allylmercaptan and disulfur dichloride as described by Derbesy and Horpp (1994).

These diallyl polysulfides are among the most studied organosulfur compounds from garlic. They are highly effective in affording protection against various cancers in animal models induced by a variety of chemical carcinogens (for review see: Stan et al. 2008). A review of the literature suggests that diallyl polysulfides may prevent cancer by multiple mechanisms including impairment of carcinogen activation, inhibition of post-translational modifications of proteins, induction of apoptosis, histone modification, inhibition of angiogenesis and metastasis (for review see: Shukla and Kalra 2007; Herman-Antosiewicz et al. 2007). It is also becoming clear that diallyl polysulfides are promiscuous because they target multiple signal transduction pathways to trigger growth arrest and eventually apoptosis. The anti-proliferative effects of the polysulfides seem to be related to their capacity to cause oxidative damage by increasing the production of reactive oxygen species. Cells lacking antioxidants are quite susceptible to polysulfides whereas cells well equipped with antioxidants such as glutathione peroxidase, copper- or zinc- superoxide dismutase are resistant to at least diallyl disulfide (Filomeni et al. 2003, 2005). Most of the experiments published up to now are performed with diallyl sulfide, diallyl disulfide and diallyl trisulfide. The corresponding tetrasulfide is almost recently used. The number of sulfur atoms in the molecule can influence the anticancer properties where diallyl trisulfide is more active than diallyl disulfide which is more active than diallyl sulfide (Sakamoto et al. 1997; Tsai et al. 1996; Sundaram and Milner 1996b). Similarly the presence of the allyl group generally enhances protection over that provided by the propyl moiety (Hu et al. 1997). Replacement of the sulfur atoms in diallyl polysulfides by carbon atoms results in inactive molecules (Busch et al. 2010) with regard to cell cycle arrest or apoptosis induction. It was long believed that the allyl sulfur compounds in garlic do not function in isolation but are influenced by several components of the diet. Moreover, there may be metabolites produced in living organisms which have another or additional activity. In rats diallyl disulfide is absorbed and transformed into allyl-mercaptan, allyl methyl sulfide, allyl methyl sulfoxide and allyl methyl sulfone. In addition the half-lives of these compounds in the cells may be different which may also contribute to the effect originally produced by diallyl disulfide (Germain et al. 2002). It was assumed that cancer protection may arise from blockage of N-nitroso compounds (NOC). However, not all allyl sulfur compounds were effective in inhibiting the formation of NOC, in particular diallyl sulfide and diallyl disulfide (Dion et al. 1997). Active cellular proliferation appears to be a factor in enhancing the growth inhibitory effect ascribed to allyl sulfides (Sigounas et al. 1997). The present chapter will address the cell cycle regulators and apoptosis pathways which are targeted by diallyl polysulfides.

13.2 Upstream Events of Cell Cycle Arrest and Apoptosis

Cell-cell communication is at least partially mediated via gap junctions. These gap junctional intercellular communications together with connexins play roles in cancer development, growth and metastasis. Gap junctions provide coupled cells with a direct pathway for sharing ions, nutrients or small metabolites. Thus, gap junctions are crucial for diverse physiological processes (Laird 2010). Diallyl disulfides improves the gap-junctional intercellular communication in rat liver epithelial cells. This effect seems to be due to an increase in the level of the connexin Cx43 protein, whereas, the phosphorylation and localization of the protein in the cell-cell contact regions of the plasma membrane is not affected (Huard et al. 2004). In the course of these studies, a rapid inhibition of protein glycosylation was observed.

The cytoskeleton is a dynamic component of the cell as it is involved in the maintenance of cell shape, intracellular trafficking, cell division, cell migration and adhesion. Oxidative stress causes both microfilament and microtubules disruption owing to oxidative modifications of specific cysteine residues of actin and tubulin. Cytoskeleton disrupting agents such as taxols or vinca alkaloids are used to perturb microtubules dynamics of proliferating cells.

Cytoskeleton and cytoskeleton-associated proteins have a fundamental role in the processes leading to apoptosis. The dramatic morphological changes typical of apoptotic cells are due to a complete reorganization of the cytoskeleton ensuring the breakdown of the cell into apoptotic bodies and the maintenance of an intact plasma membrane. Diallyl disulfide and diallyl trisulfide directly oxidize sulfhydryl groups of specific cysteine residues on the polypeptide chain of tubulin thus inhibiting the mitotic spindle (Xiao et al. 2003, 2005b; Hosono et al. 2005, 2008).

It was demonstrated that diallyl disulfide induces alterations of cell morphology, microfilament disruption and alterations in the microtubules network in neuroblastoma cells, SH-SY5Y. Furthermore, diallyl disulfide induces microtubules depolymerization in these neuroblastoma cells. Cells with a stable overexpression

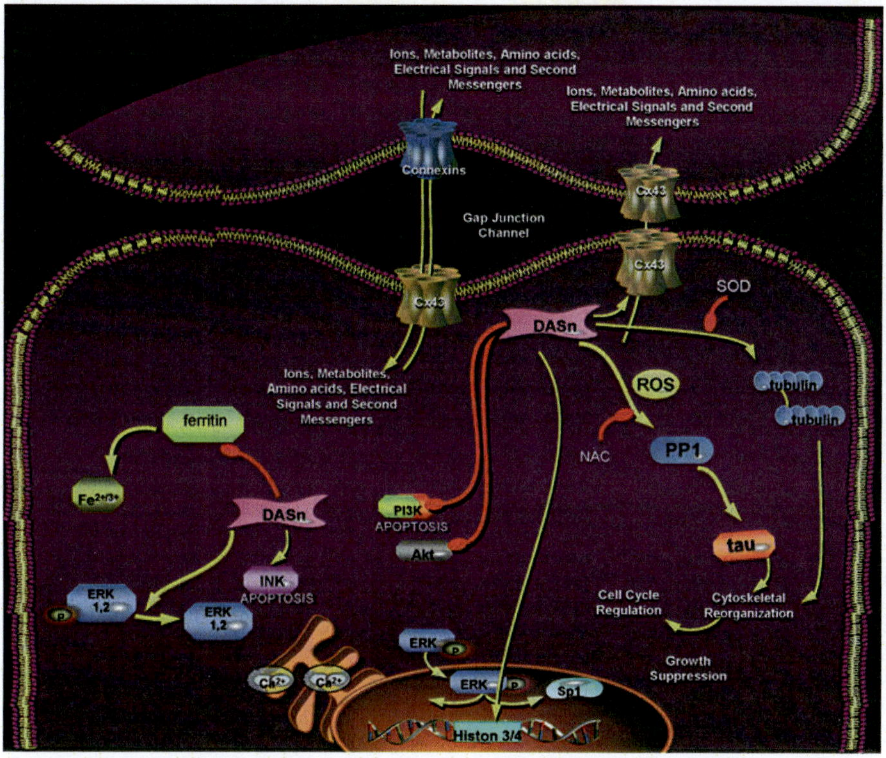

Fig. 13.2 Influence of diallyl sulfides on cell- cell communication and intra- cellular signaling. *DASn* diallyl sulfides, n = 1, n = 2, n = 3, n = 4, *ROS* reactive oxygen species

of superoxide dismutase are protected against cytoskeletal disruption, indicating a contribution of ROS to these processes. Diallyl disulfide induces a protein phosphatase −1 (PP-1) mediated dephosphorylation of tau. This dephosphorylation of tau is mediated by ROS which can be also abrogated in the presence of the ROS scavenger N-acetylcysteine (NAC) (Aquilano et al. 2010). Cells which do not express cytoskeletal tau such as HeLa cells are more resistant to diallyl disulfide induced apoptosis, which further supports the idea of an active role of tau in diallyl disulfide induced processes (Fig. 13.2).

Treatment of prostate cancer cells with diallyl trisulfide also leads to the formation of multinucleated cells (Herman-Antosiewicz and Singh 2005). Diallyl disulfide causes an increased acetylation of histones H4 and H3 in human leukemic cells and in colon cancer cells, whereas, diallyl monosulfide exhibit only a weak activity (Lea et al. 1999; Lea and Randolph 2001; Druesne et al. 2004a, b). The elevated level of acetylated histones is due to the inhibition of the nuclear histone deacetylase activity.

To gain more insight into the mechanism by which diallyl sulfides induce intracellular pathways, an increase in labile iron concentration was found. Iron is necessary for normal cell proliferation because iron containing proteins catalyze various key biochemical processes such as energy metabolism, respiration, folate metabolism

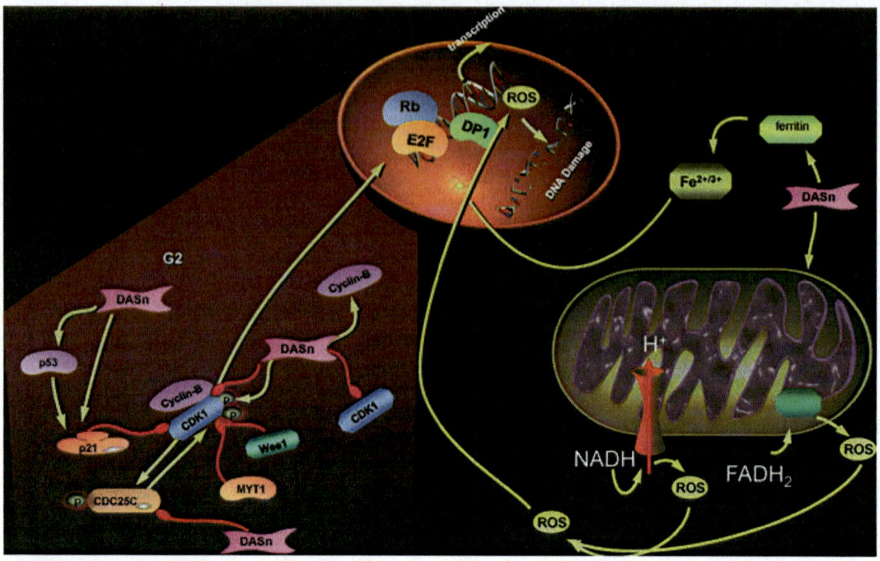

Fig. 13.3 Diallyl sulfide mediated alterations of DNA function and integrity

and DNA synthesis. The increase in labile iron concentration observed after diallyl trisulfide treatment of prostate cancer cells is caused by ferritin degradation (Antosiewicz et al. 2006) (Fig. 13.2).

Diallyl sulfides can undergo a network of different redox reactions as described by (Jacob 2006). These redox reactions differ widely and can include one- or two-electron reactions and radical reactions. Furthermore, sulfides are able to coordinate metal ions, which may play a role in metal transport and detoxification reactions.

Diallyl monosulfide and diallyl disulfide were shown to induce reactive oxygen species (ROS) in glioblastoma cells as measured with the dye 2′,7′-dichlorofluorescein diacetate (DCF-DA) (Fig. 13.3). The optimum results were obtained with 100 μM of each of the diallyl sulfide (Das et al. 2007). Interestingly ascorbic acid was shown to counteract ROS induction. A similar observation was also reported for human lung carcinoma cells where ROS production was detected as early as 0.5 h after treatment of cells with diallyl disulfide. Diallyl disulfide induced ROS formation in neuroblastoma cells is evident after 15 min of treatment (Filomeni et al. 2003). A range of 50–500 μM diallyl disulfide was used showing a dose dependent ROS production. These results demonstrate that ROS production is an early event after treatment of cells with diallyl disulfides (Wu et al. 2005). A mimetic of superoxide dismutase and catalase, namely EUK134 significantly attenuated the diallyl trisulfide induced ROS generations (Antosiewicz et al. 2006).

The level of reduced glutathione was increased in the liver and lung by diallyl sulfide and diallyl trisulfide administration, but not by the non-allylic analogue dipropyl sulfide (Hu et al. 1996). Reactive oxygen species (ROS) can either directly cause DNA damage or oxidize nucleotides, which may lead to DNA double strand breaks (Haber 1999). The phosphorylation of serine 139 of histone H2AX has emerged as a sensitive marker for the presence of DNA double strand breaks (Tanaka et al. 2006; Löbrich et al. 2010). Diallyl trisulfide was shown to cause serine 139 phosphorylation of H2AX indicating the induction of DNA double strand breaks (Herman-Antosiewicz and Singh 2005). Treatment of neuronally differentiated PC12 cells with diallyl disulfide results in higher levels of free radicals and lipid peroxidation at concentrations of 50 μM diallyl disulfide. At 100 μM, diallyl disulfide cells were killed by inhibiting PI3K/Akt and by promoting activation of GSK-3 and caspase-3, release of cytochrome c and cleavage of PARP which indicates the induction of apoptosis (Koh et al. 2005). Diallyl sulfide, diallyl disulfide and diallyl trisulfide have been shown to be inducers of rat liver cytochrome P-450 variants (Wu et al. 2002) indicating that the hepatic detoxification system was induced. Diallyl disulfide and diallyl sulfide were also found to be potent inducers of quinone reductase activity and protein level (Hu et al. 1997) where the diallyl disulfide or diallyl trisulfide are more potent than the diallyl sulfide.

$p21^{WAF1}$ is an important regulator of cell cycle progression (Gartel 2009) and the expression of $p21^{WAF1}$ has being somehow linked to histone acetylation (Yamaguchi et al. 2010). Therefore, it was not surprising that diallyl disulfide treatment of colon cancer cells led to a markedly increased $p21^{WAF1}$ mRNA and protein level (Druesne et al. 2004a). This increase seems to be p53 independent. The level of p53 increases after diallyl disulfide treatment of non small cell lung cancer cells. However, both p53 positive and p53 negative cells show apoptosis. Diallyl sulfide treatment induced a rise in the level of Bax and a decrease in the level of Bcl-2 (Hong et al. 2000).

p38 MAP kinase is a member of the mitogen-activated protein kinase signalling cascade which has been shown to regulate a variety of cellular events such as proliferation, differentiation and apoptosis (Keshet and Seger 2010). Treatment of gastric cancer cells with diallyl disulfide leads to an increase of the phosphorylation and thereby activation of the p38 MAP protein (Yuan et al. 2004).

13.3 Diallyl Polysulfide Targets of the Regulatory Network of the Cell Cycle

Cell cycle arrest can be achieved by targeting factors that control G_1/S transition or G_2/M transition of the cell cycle. There are a number of reports demonstrating that diallyl poylsulfides mostly target regulators of the G_2/M transition.

Milner and co-workers were the first to show that diallyl disulfide caused a dose-dependent and time-dependent accumulation of human colon cancer cells in the G_2/M phase of the cell cycle (Knowles and Milner 1998, 2000). Diallyl trisulfide was much more effective than either diallyl disulfide or diallyl sulfide in causing G_2/M phase cell cycle arrest (Xiao et al. 2005a) (Fig. 13.3)

The diallyl disulfide mediated G_2/M arrest is accompanied by a decrease in the kinase activity of the cyclin B1/cdk1 kinase complex, reduction in the complex formation between both proteins and a decrease in the level of the cdc25C phosphatase (Knowles and Milner 2000). This cdk1 kinase activity is necessary for the progression of the cells from G_2 into the M-phase of the cell cycle. The cdk1 kinase activity is regulated by its association with regulatory cyclin B_1 and by phosphorylation and dephosphorylation of cdk1 (Fig. 13.3). It was further shown that diallyl disulfide influenced the complex formation between cdk1 and cyclin B_1 and the phosphorylation of cdk1 (Knowles and Milner 2000). This G_2/M phase cell cycle arrest is not limited to the colon cancer cells but also found in prostate cancer cells and in promyelocytic HL-60 cells. Diallyl trisulfide treatment of prostate cancer cells caused an increase in the nuclear level of cyclin B1 as early as 1 h post-exposure (Herman-Antosiewicz et al. 2010). In hormone refractory prostate cancer and in colon cancer cells, diallyl disulfide treatment causes an increase in the level of cyclin B1 and a decrease in the level of cdk1 (Arunkumar et al. 2006; Song et al. 2009).

The diallyl trisulfide-induced G_2/M phase cell cycle arrest in prostate cancer cells was associated with an increase in tyr15 phosphorylation of cdk1, inhibition of cyclin B1/cdk1 kinase activity, an increase in the phosphorylation of cdc25C at serine 216 and a down regulation of the cdc25C level (Cerella et al. 2009). This down-regulation of the level of cdc25C was also observed in human colon carcinoma cell line (Busch et al. 2010). Some years ago, it was demonstrated that transcription of cdc25C is repressed by the growth suppressor protein p53 in a dose-dependent manner (Krause et al. 2001). After incubation of human colon carcinoma cells with diallyl di-, tri- and tetrasulfide the protein level of p53 increased considerably. However, $p53^{-/-}$ cells also show a down-regulation of cdc25C indicating that down-regulation is not necessarily connected to p53 transrepression (Busch et al. 2010) (Fig. 13.4).

Diallyl trisulfide treatment of prostate cancer cells results in an activating phosphorylation of chk1 and chk2 which is usually induced by oxidants or ionizing radiation (Herman-Antosiewicz and Singh 2005). However, by chk1/chk2 depletion experiments it was shown that chk1 but not chk2 is responsible for the phosphorylation of serine 216 of cdc25C. The diallyl polysulfide mediated hyperphosphorylation and the decrease in the cdc25C protein level were abrogated in the presence of antioxidants such as vitamin C or N-acetyl cysteine (Busch et al. 2010; Cerella et al. 2009) (Fig. 13.4).

Diallyl trisulfide treatments of prostate cancer cells cause a marked increase in the kinase activity of the c-Jun NH_2-terminal kinase (INK) which is known to play a role in the decision of cell survival and apoptosis (Bogoyevitch et al. 2010). Diallyl trisulfide induced ROS generation and cell cycle arrest were significantly reduced by ectopic expression of a catalytically inactive mutant of INK2 (Antosiewicz et al. 2006) indicating a link between the INK pathway and ROS formation. In neuroblastoma cells diallyl sulfide induces apoptosis via ROS production and activation of the INK/c-jun pathway by phosphorylation (Filomeni et al. 2003). However, ROS production was observed within minutes after treatment of cells with diallyl polysulfides. It remains to be shown whether INK activation occurs before or after ROS induction.

The effect of diallyl disulfides on cell cycle arrest and apoptosis induction seems to be cell type specific. A human adeno carcinoma gastric cell line is able to recover from a $p53/p21^{WAF1}$ mediated cell cycle arrest in the G_2/M phase upon diallyl disulfide treatment. The surviving pathways in these cells include the formation of mixed

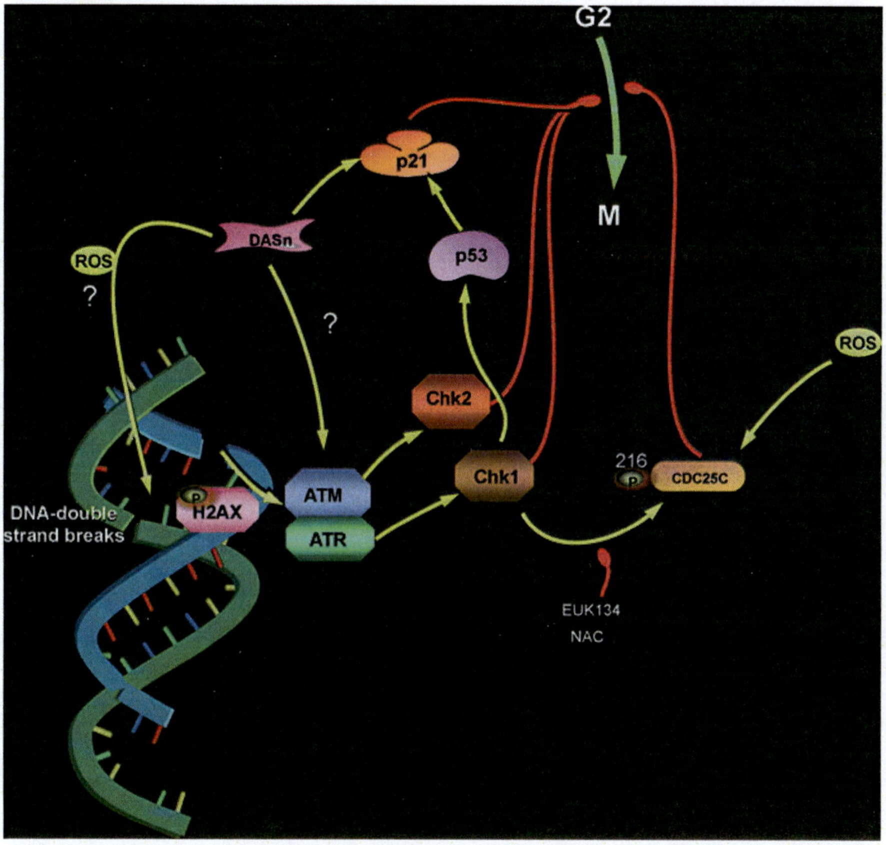

Fig. 13.4 Diallyl sulfide mediated G_2/M arrest of the cell cycle. *NAC* N-acetyl cysteine, *EUK134* a synthetic superoxide/catalase mimetic

disulfides between glutathione and protein thiol groups and a higher glutathione peroxidase activity. Furthermore, diallyl disulfide treatment induces dephosphorylation of the ERK1/2 kinase, which goes along with growth arrest (Filomeni et al. 2005).

Interestingly a normal prostate epithelial cell line was resistant to growth inhibition and cell cycle arrest by diallyl trisulfide (Xiao et al. 2005a). A similar observation was also made for peripheral blood mononuclear cells (Cerella et al. 2009). Thus, these results might indicate that diallyl polysulfide can be used for cancer treatment because normal cells are not affected, at least at low concentrations of diallyl polysulfides. This might be explained by the fact that in tumour cells the redox balance is altered, whereas, in normal cells the redox balance is hardly affected. Pertubations to the redox balance are characteristic of many pathological states of a cell. Oxidative stress is prevalent in cancer where many malignant cell types possess an abnormal redox system due to a down-regulation of antioxidant enzymes and to an impaired mitochondrial function.

13.4 Cell Death After Treatment of Cells with Diallyl Polysulfides

Apoptosis, also known as programmed cell death, is a tightly controlled and evolutionarily highly conserved process of cellular suicide. Dysregulation of apoptosis occurs under numerous pathological conditions including cancer. Targeting apoptotic pathways is therefore an interesting option in cancer treatment and probably its prevention (Fulda 2010; Blankenberg 2009). Apoptosis or programmed cell death can occur via an intrinsic or mitochondria-mediated pathway or via an extrinsic pathway. Activation of the intrinsic pathway is regulated by the anti-apoptotic Bcl-2 family of proteins and by the pro-apoptotic Bax and Bak proteins. Treatment of neuroblastoma, breast or lung cancer cells with diallyl sulfide or diallyl disulfide leads to an increase of the Bax/Bcl-2 ratio (Hong et al. 2000; Karmakar et al. 2007; Nakagawa et al. 2001). The diallyl trisulfide induced apoptosis in prostate cancer cells correlates with a decrease in the Bcl-2 level as well as with an elevated phosphorylation of Bcl-2 (Xiao et al. 2004). The hyperphosphorylation of Bcl-2 is caused by the INK kinase. An overexpression of Bcl-2 confers a protection against diallyl trisulfide induced apoptosis only in hormone refractory but not in hormone sensitive prostate cancer cells. The reason for this difference is not known. In breast cancer cells and in a myeloid leukemia cell line apoptosis induction goes along with the activation of caspase-3 (Nakagawa et al. 2001). In prostate cancer cells and in colon carcinoma cells it was shown that the diallyl trisulfide and the diallyl tetrasulfide are more potent inducers of apoptosis than diallyl sulfide and diallyl disulfide (Xiao et al. 2004; Busch et al. 2010; Cerella et al. 2009). The simultaneous activation of caspase-8 and caspase-9 in myeloid leukemia cells indicated a crosstalk between the intrinsic and extrinsic pathway of apoptosis (Cerella et al. 2009). Furthermore, diallyl tetrasulfide induces the activation of Bcl-2 and Bim which trigger the intrinsic pathway of apoptosis. Activated Bim binds to the anti-apoptotic proteins Bcl-2 and Bcl-xL preventing them from regulating Bax and Bak, which results in their translocation to the mitochondria triggering the release of cytochrome c (Cerella et al. 2009). The diallyl trisulfide induced apoptosis in hormone sensitive prostate cancer cells correlates with a collapse of the mitochondrial membrane potential, an increase in the level of the Bak protein and a down-regulation of Bcl-2 and Bcl-xL (Kim et al. 2007) whereas, the Bid level is not affected. The diallyl trisulfide induced apoptosis was significantly attenuated by knocking down Bax and Bak whereas an overexpression of Bcl-2 and Bcl-xL had no effect. These results indicated that at least in hormone sensitive prostate carcinoma cells, the diallyl trisulfide induced apoptosis is regulated by Bax and Bak but not by Bcl-2 and Bcl-xL (Fig. 13.5).

Treatment of hormone refractory prostate cancer cells with diallyl trisulfide results in a rapid decrease of the phosphorylation of serine 473 and threonine 308 of the Akt kinase, leading to a down-regulation of its kinase activity (Xiao and Singh 2006). This down-regulation results in a down-regulation of the phosphorylation of Bad, promoting a translocation of Bad to the mitochondria. These results show a contribution of the Akt signalling pathway in the diallyl polysulfide induced

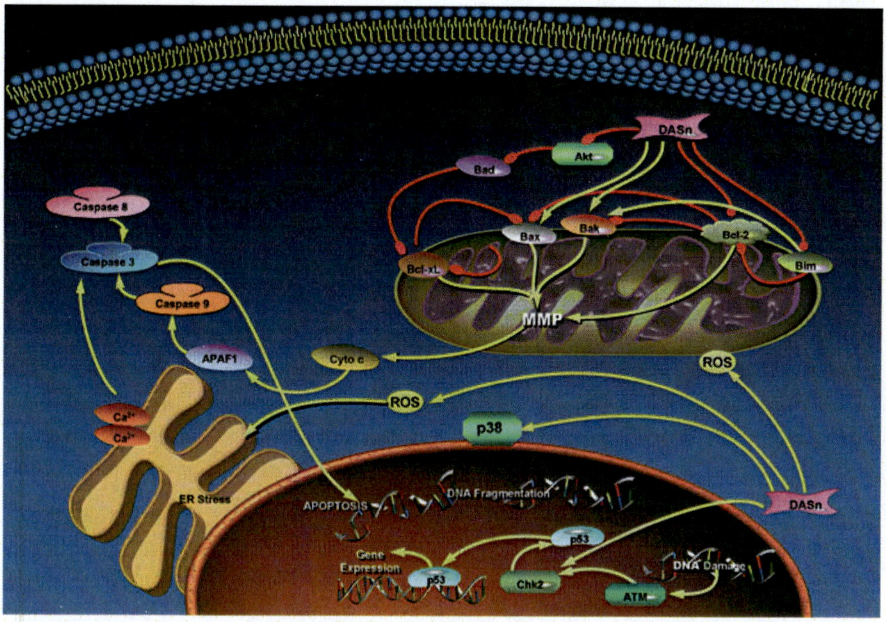

Fig. 13.5 Implication of diallyl sulfides in the regulation of apoptosis

apoptosis. Consequently, overexpression of constitutively active Akt confers a significant protection against diallyl trisulfide induced apoptosis.

A few studies described an increase in the intra-cellular free Ca^{2+} ion concentration after treatment of cells with diallyl polysulfides (Karmakar et al. 2007; Sakamoto et al. 1997; Sundaram and Milner 1996a, b). In a human colon carcinoma cell line diallyl disulfide induced a biphasic elevation of cytosolic Ca^{2+} ion concentration, a rapid induction within 3 min followed by a slow and sustained elevation until 3 h after treatment (Park et al. 2002). Apoptosis is blocked by intracellular Ca^{2+} chelators, which results also in an inhibition of the formation of ROS and blockage of the caspase dependent apoptotic pathway. These data indicate that the increase in intracellular free Ca^{2+} ion concentration is an early signalling event.

Some of the studies have compared cellular responses and in particular apoptosis responses to diallyl polysulfides in normal versus cancer cells. In general malignant cells appear more sensitive to diallyl polysulfide treatment than normal non-transformed cells. The mechanism behind the differential sensitivity of normal and cancer cells remains to be elucidated.

There are contradictory results concerning the role of p53 in diallyl disulfide induced apoptosis in human colon cancer cells. Song et al reported no change in the expression of p53 by less than 12 h post-exposure (Song et al. 2009) whereas others reported an increase in the p53 level (Busch et al. 2010). Furthermore, down-regulation of p53 by siRNA technology prevented the accumulation of cleaved PARP and sub-G_1 cells after diallyl disulfide treatment (Song et al. 2009) whereas others have shown that diallyl disulfide, diallyl trisulfide and diallyl tetrasulfide causes apoptosis in p53 negative colon carcinoma cells (Busch et al. 2010). These results indicate a role of p53 in the apoptotic signalling, on the other hand p53 seems to be dispensable for apoptosis induction

In gastric cancer cells diallyl disulfide induces the accumulation of phosphorylated chk1 but not of chk2 and a down-regulation of cdc25C and cyclin B which is in contrast to the situation in prostate and colon carcinoma cells (Arunkumar et al. 2006; Song et al. 2009). chk1 is activated by ATM kinase and indeed an increase in phosphorylated ATM kinase, which means activated kinase, was demonstrated after diallyl disulfide treatment (Ling et al. 2010).

13.5 Concluding Remarks

A large number of reports have demonstrated a growth inhibiting and apoptosis inducing effect of diallyl polysulfides mostly on cancer cells, whereas normal non-transformed cells are rather unaffected. The sulfur chain rather than the diallyl groups are responsible for the observed effects on cells. Moreover, the activity of the diallyl polysulfides increases with the length of the sulfur chains. Treatment of cells with diallyl polysulfides leads to alterations in cell-cell communication, changes in the cytoskeleton organisation as well as multi- nucleation and alterations of nuclear proteins. One of the immediate cellular events is the induction of reactive oxygen species, followed by alterations in intracellular signalling pathways. These alterations result in a G_2/M-phase arrest of the cell cycle. Subsequently intracellular and extracellular pathways of apoptosis are induced and finally cells go into apoptosis. So far it is an open question whether DNA double strand break is a direct consequence of ROS or whether it occurs in the course of apoptosis. Furthermore, it is not clear at all whether DNA repair mechanisms are turned on and whether apoptosis is the consequence of a failure in successful DNA repair. Another open question is the contribution of sulfur radicals to the activation of the apoptosis pathways. Although there are a number of open questions the present knowledge about the cellular effects of diallyl polysulfide enables us to describe the benefit of garlic uptake for molecular processes finally preventing or treating diseases such as cancer and others.

References

Amagase H, Milner JA (1993) Impact of various sources of garlic and their constituents on 7,12-dimethylbenz[a]anthracene binding to mammary cell DNA. Carcinogenesis 14:1627–1631

Antosiewicz J, Herman-Antosiewicz A, Marynowski SW, Singh SV (2006) c-Jun NH(2)-terminal kinase signaling axis regulates diallyl trisulfide-induced generation of reactive oxygen species and cell cycle arrest in human prostate cancer cells. Cancer Res 66:5379–5386

Aquilano K, Vigilanza P, Filomeni G, Rotilio G, Ciriolo MR (2010) Tau dephosphorylation and microfilaments disruption are upstream events of the anti-proliferative effects of DADS in SH-SY5Y cells. J Cell Mol Med 14:564–577

Arunkumar A, Vijayababu MR, Srinivasan N, Aruldhas MM, Arunakaran J (2006) Garlic compound, diallyl disulfide induces cell cycle arrest in prostate cancer cell line PC-3. Mol Cell Biochem 288:107–113

Blankenberg FG (2009) Apoptosis imaging: anti-cancer agents in medicinal chemistry. Anticancer Agents Med Chem 9:944–951

Block E (1992) Die Organoschwefelchemie der Gattung *Allium* und ihre Bedeutung fiir die organische Chemie des Schwefels. Angew Chem Int Ed Engl 104:1158–1203

Bogoyevitch MA, Ngoei KR, Zhao TT, Yeap YY, Ng DC (2010) c-Jun N-terminal kinase (JNK) signaling: recent advances and challenges. Biochim Biophys Acta 1804:463–475

Busch C, Jacob C, Anwar A, Burkholz T, Ba LA, Cerella C, Diederich M, Brandt W, Wessjohann L, Montenarh M (2010) Diallylpolysulfides induce growth arrest and apoptosis. Int J Oncol 36:743–749

Cerella C, Scherer C, Cristofanon S, Henry E, Anwar A, Busch C, Montenarh M, Dicato M, Jacob C, Diederich M (2009) Cell cycle arrest in early mitosis and induction of caspase-dependent apoptosis in U937 cells by diallyltetrasulfide (Al2S4). Apoptosis 14:641–646

Corzo-Martinez M, Corzo N, Villamiel M (2007) Biological properties of onions and garlic. Trends Food Sci Technol 18:609–625

Das A, Banik NL, Ray SK (2007) Garlic compounds generate reactive oxygen species leading to activation of stress kinases and cysteine proteases for apoptosis in human glioblastoma T98G and U87MG cells. Cancer 110:1083–1095

Derbesy G, Harpp DN (1994) A simple method to prepare unsymmetrical disulfide, trisulfide and tetrasulfide. Tetrahedron Lett 35:5381–5384

Dion ME, Agler M, Milner JA (1997) S-allyl cysteine inhibits nitrosomorpholine formation and bioactivation. Nutr Cancer 28:1–6

Druesne N, Pagniez A, Mayeur C, Thomas M, Cherbuy C, Duee PH, Martel P, Chaumontet C (2004a) Diallyl disulfide (DADS) increases histone acetylation and p21(waf1/cip1) expression in human colon tumor cell lines. Carcinogenesis 25:1227–1236

Druesne N, Pagniez A, Mayeur C, Thomas M, Cherbuy C, Duee PH, Martel P, Chaumontet C (2004b) Repetitive treatments of colon HT-29 cells with diallyl disulfide induce a prolonged hyperacetylation of histone H3 K14. Ann N Y Acad Sci 1030:612–621

Filomeni G, Aquilano K, Rotilio G, Ciriolo MR (2003) Reactive oxygen species-dependent c-Jun NH2-terminal kinase/c-Jun signaling cascade mediates neuroblastoma cell death induced by diallyl disulfide. Cancer Res 63:5940–5949

Filomeni G, Aquilano K, Rotilio G, Ciriolo MR (2005) Glutathione-related systems and modulation of extracellular signal-regulated kinases are involved in the resistance of AGS adenocarcinoma gastric cells to diallyl disulfide-induced apoptosis. Cancer Res 65:11735–11742

Fleischauer AT, Arab L (2001) Garlic and cancer: a critical review of the epidemiologic literature. J Nutr 131:1032S–1040S

Fulda S (2010) Modulation of apoptosis by natural products for cancer therapy. Planta Med 76:1075–1079

Gartel AL (2009) p21(WAF1/CIP1) and cancer: a shifting paradigm? Biofactors 35:161–164

Germain E, Auger J, Ginies C, Siess MH, Teyssier C (2002) In vivo metabolism of diallyl disulphide in the rat: identification of two new metabolites. Xenobiotica 32:1127–1138

Gullett NP, Ruhul Amin AR, Bayraktar S, Pezzuto JM, Shin DM, Khuri FR, Aggarwal BB, Surh YJ, Kucuk O (2010) Cancer prevention with natural compounds. Semin Oncol 37:258–281

Haber JE (1999) DNA recombination: the replication connection. Trends Biochem Sci 24:271–275

Hatono S, Jimenez A, Wargovich MJ (1996) Chemopreventive effect of S-allylcysteine and its relationship to the detoxification enzyme glutathione S-transferase. Carcinogenesis 17:1041–1044

Herman-Antosiewicz A, Singh SV (2005) Checkpoint kinase 1 regulates diallyl trisulfide-induced mitotic arrest in human prostate cancer cells. J Biol Chem 280:28519–28528

Herman-Antosiewicz A, Powolny AA, Singh SV (2007) Molecular targets of cancer chemoprevention by garlic-derived organosulfides. Acta Pharmacol Sin 28:1355–1364

Herman-Antosiewicz A, Kim YA, Kim SH, Xiao D, Singh SV (2010) Diallyl trisulfide-induced G2/M phase cell cycle arrest in DU145 cells is associated with delayed nuclear translocation of cyclin-dependent kinase 1. Pharm Res 27:1072–1079

Hofmann AW, Cahours A (1857) Researches on a new class of alcohols. Philos Trans R Soc Lond (Biol) 147:555–574

Hong YS, Ham YA, Choi JH, Kim J (2000) Effects of allyl sulfur compounds and garlic extract on the expression of Bcl-2, Bax, and p53 in non small cell lung cancer cell lines. Exp Mol Med 32:127–134

Hosono T, Fukao T, Ogihara J, Ito Y, Shiba H, Seki T, Ariga T (2005) Diallyl trisulfide suppresses the proliferation and induces apoptosis of human colon cancer cells through oxidative modification of beta-tubulin. J Biol Chem 280:41487–41493

Hosono T, Hosono-Fukao T, Inada K, Tanaka R, Yamada H, Iitsuka Y, Seki T, Hasegawa I, Ariga T (2008) Alkenyl group is responsible for the disruption of microtubule network formation in human colon cancer cell line HT-29 cells. Carcinogenesis 29:1400–1406

Hsing AW, Chokkalingam AP, Gao YT, Madigan MP, Deng J, Gridley G, Fraumeni JF Jr (2002) *Allium* vegetables and risk of prostate cancer: a population-based study. J Natl Cancer Inst 94:1648–1651

Hu X, Benson PJ, Srivastava SK, Mack LM, Xia H, Gupta V, Zaren HA, Singh SV (1996) Glutathione S-transferases of female A/J mouse liver and forestomach and their differential induction by anti-carcinogenic organosulfides from garlic. Arch Biochem Biophys 336:199–214

Hu X, Benson PJ, Srivastava SK, Xia H, Bleicher RJ, Zaren HA, Awasthi S, Awasthi YC, Singh SV (1997) Induction of glutathione S-transferase pi as a bioassay for the evaluation of potency of inhibitors of benzo(a)pyrene-induced cancer in a murine model. Int J Cancer 73:897–902

Huard C, Druesne N, Guyonnet D, Thomas M, Pagniez A, Le Bon AM, Martel P, Chaumontet C (2004) Diallyl disulfide (DADS) enhances gap-junctional intercellular communication by both direct and indirect mechanisms in rat liver cells. Carcinogenesis 25:91–98

Hussain SP, Jannu LN, Rao AR (1990) Chemopreventive action of garlic on methylcholanthrene-induced carcinogenesis in the uterine cervix of mice. Cancer Lett 49:175–180

Ip C, Lisk DJ, Stoewsand GS (1992) Mammary cancer prevention by regular garlic and selenium-enriched garlic. Nutr Cancer 17:279–286

Jacob C (2006) A scent of therapy: pharmacological implications of natural products containing redox-active sulfur atoms. Nat Prod Rep 23:851–863

Karmakar S, Banik NL, Patel SJ, Ray SK (2007) Garlic compounds induced calpain and intrinsic caspase cascade for apoptosis in human malignant neuroblastoma SH-SY5Y cells. Apoptosis 12:671–684

Kendler BS (1987) Garlic (*Allium* sativum) and onion (*Allium* cepa): a review of their relationship to cardiovascular disease. Prev Med 16:670–685

Keshet Y, Seger R (2010) The MAP kinase signaling cascades: a system of hundreds of components regulates a diverse array of physiological functions. Methods Mol Biol 661:3–38

Kim JY, Kwon O (2009) Garlic intake and cancer risk: an analysis using the Food and Drug Administration's evidence-based review system for the scientific evaluation of health claims. Am J Clin Nutr 89:257–264

Kim YA, Xiao D, Xiao H, Powolny AA, Lew KL, Reilly ML, Zeng Y, Wang Z, Singh SV (2007) Mitochondria-mediated apoptosis by diallyl trisulfide in human prostate cancer cells is associated with generation of reactive oxygen species and regulated by Bax/Bak. Mol Cancer Ther 6:1599–1609

Knowles LM, Milner JA (1998) Depressed p34cdc2 kinase activity and G2/M phase arrest induced by diallyl disulfide in HCT-15 cells. Nutr Cancer 30:169–174

Knowles LM, Milner JA (2000) Diallyl disulfide inhibits p34(cdc2) kinase activity through changes in complex formation and phosphorylation. Carcinogenesis 21:1129–1134

Koh SH, Kwon H, Park KH, Ko JK, Kim JH, Hwang MS, Yum YN, Kim OH, Kim J, Kim HT, Do BR, Kim KS, Kim H, Roh H, Yu HJ, Jung HK, Kim SH (2005) Protective effect of diallyl disulfide on oxidative stress-injured neuronally differentiated PC12 cells. Brain Res Mol Brain Res 133:176–186

Krause K, Haugwitz U, Wasner M, Wiedmann M, Mössner J, Engeland K (2001) Expression of the cell cycle phosphatase *cdc25*C is down-regulated by the tumor suppressor protein p53 but not by p73. Biochem Biophys Res Commun 284:743–750

Laird DW (2010) The gap junction proteome and its relationship to disease. Trends Cell Biol 20:92–101

Lea MA, Randolph VM (2001) Induction of histone acetylation in rat liver and hepatoma by organosulfur compounds including diallyl disulfide. Anticancer Res 21:2841–2845

Lea MA, Randolph VM, Patel M (1999) Increased acetylation of histones induced by diallyl disulfide and structurally related molecules. Int J Oncol 15:347–352

Ling H, Wen L, Ji XX, Tang YL, He J, Tan H, Xia H, Zhou JG, Su Q (2010) Growth inhibitory effect and Chk1-dependent signaling involved in G2/M arrest on human gastric cancer cells induced by diallyl disulfide. Braz J Med Biol Res 43:271–278

Löbrich M, Shibata A, Beucher A, Fisher A, Ensminger M, Goodarzi AA, Barton O, Jeggo PA (2010) gammaH2AX foci analysis for monitoring DNA double-strand break repair: strengths, limitations and optimization. Cell Cycle 9:662–669

Milligan B, Saville B, Swan JM (1961) New syntheses of trisulfides. J Chem Soc 1961:4850–4853

Milner JA (1996) Garlic: its anticarcinogenic and antitumorigenic properties. Nutr Rev 54:S82–S86

Milner JA (2001) A historical perspective on garlic and cancer. J Nutr 131:1027S–1031S

Nagini S (2008) Cancer chemoprevention by garlic and its organosulfur compounds-panacea or promise? Anticancer Agents Med Chem 8:313–321

Nakagawa H, Tsuta K, Kiuchi K, Senzaki H, Tanaka K, Hioki K, Tsubura A (2001) Growth inhibitory effects of diallyl disulfide on human breast cancer cell lines. Carcinogenesis 22:891–897

Park EK, Kwon KB, Park KI, Park BH, Jhee EC (2002) Role of Ca(2+) in diallyl disulfide-induced apoptotic cell death of HCT-15 cells. Exp Mol Med 34:250–257

Powolny AA, Singh SV (2008) Multitargeted prevention and therapy of cancer by diallyl trisulfide and related *Allium* vegetable-derived organosulfur compounds. Cancer Lett 269:305–314

Rivlin RS (2001) Historical perspective on the use of garlic. J Nutr 131:951S–954S

Sakamoto K, Lawson LD, Milner JA (1997) Allyl sulfides from garlic suppress the in vitro proliferation of human A549 lung tumor cells. Nutr Cancer 29:152–156

Schreiber J, Foureman GL, Hughes MF, Mason RP, Eling TE (1989) Detection of glutathione thiyl free radical catalyzed by prostaglandin H synthase present in keratinocytes. Study of co-oxidation in a cellular system. J Biol Chem 264:7936–7943

Semmler FW (1892) Essential oil of garlic (*Allium* sativum). Arch Pharm 230:434–448

Shukla Y, Kalra N (2007) Cancer chemoprevention with garlic and its constituents. Cancer Lett 247:167–181

Sigounas G, Hooker JL, Li W, Anagnostou A, Steiner M (1997) S-allylmercaptocysteine, a stable thioallyl compound, induces apoptosis in erythroleukemia cell lines. Nutr Cancer 28:153–159

Singh SV, Pan SS, Srivastava SK, Xia H, Hu X, Zaren HA, Orchard JL (1998) Differential induction of NAD(P)H:quinone oxidoreductase by anti-carcinogenic organosulfides from garlic. Biochem Biophys Res Commun 244:917–920

Song K, Milner JA (1999) Heating garlic inhibits its ability to suppress 7, 12-dimethylbenz(a) anthracene-induced DNA adduct formation in rat mammary tissue. J Nutr 129:657–661

Song JD, Lee SK, Kim KM, Park SE, Park SJ, Kim KH, Ahn SC, Park YC (2009) Molecular mechanism of diallyl disulfide in cell cycle arrest and apoptosis in HCT-116 colon cancer cells. J Biochem Mol Toxicol 23:71–79

Stan SD, Kar S, Stoner GD, Singh SV (2008) Bioactive food components and cancer risk reduction. J Cell Biochem 104:339–356

Sumiyoshi H, Wargovich MJ (1990) Chemoprevention of 1,2-dimethylhydrazine-induced colon cancer in mice by naturally occurring organosulfur compounds. Cancer Res 50:5084–5087

Sundaram SG, Milner JA (1996a) Diallyl disulfide induces apoptosis of human colon tumor cells. Carcinogenesis 17:669–673
Sundaram SG, Milner JA (1996b) Diallyl disulfide inhibits the proliferation of human tumor cells in culture. Biochim Biophys Acta 1315:15–20
Tanaka T, Halicka HD, Huang X, Traganos F, Darzynkiewicz Z (2006) Constitutive histone H2AX phosphorylation and ATM activation, the reporters of DNA damage by endogenous oxidants. Cell Cycle 5:1940–1945
Tsai SJ, Jenq SN, Lee H (1996) Naturally occurring diallyl disulfide inhibits the formation of carcinogenic heterocyclic aromatic amines in boiled pork juice. Mutagenesis 11:235–240
Wargovich MJ, Woods C, Eng VW, Stephens LC, Gray K (1988) Chemoprevention of N-nitrosomethylbenzylamine-induced esophageal cancer in rats by the naturally occurring thioether, diallyl sulfide. Cancer Res 48:6872–6875
Wu CC, Sheen LY, Chen HW, Kuo WW, Tsai SJ, Lii CK (2002) Differential effects of garlic oil and its three major organosulfur components on the hepatic detoxification system in rats. J Agric Food Chem 50:378–383
Wu XJ, Kassie F, Mersch-Sundermann V (2005) The role of reactive oxygen species (ROS) production on diallyl disulfide (DADS) induced apoptosis and cell cycle arrest in human A549 lung carcinoma cells. Mutat Res 579:115–124
Xiao D, Singh SV (2006) Diallyl trisulfide, a constituent of processed garlic, inactivates Akt to trigger mitochondrial translocation of BAD and caspase-mediated apoptosis in human prostate cancer cells. Carcinogenesis 27:533–540
Xiao D, Pinto JT, Soh JW, Deguchi A, Gundersen GG, Palazzo AF, Yoon JT, Shirin H, Weinstein IB (2003) Induction of apoptosis by the garlic-derived compound S-allylmercaptocysteine (SAMC) is associated with microtubule depolymerization and c-Jun NH(2)-terminal kinase 1 activation. Cancer Res 63:6825–6837
Xiao D, Choi S, Johnson DE, Vogel VG, Johnson CS, Trump DL, Lee YJ, Singh SV (2004) Diallyl trisulfide-induced apoptosis in human prostate cancer cells involves c-Jun N-terminal kinase and extracellular-signal regulated kinase-mediated phosphorylation of Bcl-2. Oncogene 23:5594–5606
Xiao D, Herman-Antosiewicz A, Antosiewicz J, Xiao H, Brisson M, Lazo JS, Singh SV (2005a) Diallyl trisulfide-induced G(2)-M phase cell cycle arrest in human prostate cancer cells is caused by reactive oxygen species-dependent destruction and hyperphosphorylation of Cdc 25 C. Oncogene 24:6256–6268
Xiao D, Pinto JT, Gundersen GG, Weinstein IB (2005b) Effects of a series of organosulfur compounds on mitotic arrest and induction of apoptosis in colon cancer cells. Mol Cancer Ther 4:1388–1398
Yamaguchi T, Cubizolles F, Zhang Y, Reichert N, Kohler H, Seiser C, Matthias P (2010) Histone deacetylases 1 and 2 act in concert to promote the G1-to-S progression. Genes Dev 24:455–469
Yuan JP, Wang GH, Ling H, Su Q, Yang YH, Song Y, Tang RJ, Liu Y, Huang C (2004) Diallyl disulfide-induced G2/M arrest of human gastric cancer MGC803 cells involves activation of p38 MAP kinase pathways. World J Gastroenterol 10:2731–2734

Part V
Effect of Natural Compounds on Cell Signaling Pathways

Chapter 14
Natural Compounds as Specific Inhibitors of Cyclin-Dependent Kinases – Past, Present and Future

***Margarita Maurer, Oxana Komina, and Józefa Węsierska-Gądek**

Abstract Deregulation of the cell cycle is one of the first events during malignant transformations that convert normal cells into tumor cells. Cyclin-dependent kinases (CDKs) are key elements of the mammalian genome surveillance machinery that controls the cell cycle. Their activity (which is normally regulated *via* cyclin binding, phosphorylation events and interactions with endogenous inhibitors of CDKs, CKIs) is frequently altered in human cancers. Therefore, strenuous efforts are being made to develop means to counter cell cycle malfunctions using pharmacological inhibitors of CDKs.

Many of the most promising CDK inhibitors originate from natural sources, e. g. flavopiridol, staurosporine, indirubin and olomoucine. More selective and less cytotoxic analogues have also been developed, based on their chemical structures, that have anti-cancer potential operating through several mechanisms, including modulation of the cell cycle, transcription and apoptosis in cancer cells. Some of the CDK inhibitors derived from natural compounds or their analogues are in clinical trials or already in use. Considering the huge numbers of compounds in plant species (~300,000), which might include powerful, as yet unidentified anti-cancer agents, it seems reasonable to assume that that even more potent and selective CDK inhibitors will be discovered and characterized in the future.

Keywords Apoptosis • Cancer • Cell cycle • Cyclin • Kinase • Cytokinin • Pharmacological CDK inhibitor • Roscovitine • Staurosporine • Transcription

---

*Margarita Maurer and Oxana Komina both of these authors equally contributed to the work

M. Maurer • O. Komina • J. Węsierska-Gądek (✉)
Cell Cycle Regulation Group, Department of Medicine I, Division: Institute of Cancer Research, Comprehensive Cancer Center, Medical University of Vienna, Borschkegasse 8a, 1090 Vienna, Austria
e-mail: Jozefa.Gadek-Wesierski@meduniwien.ac.at

M. Diederich and K. Noworyta (eds.), *Natural Compounds as Inducers of Cell Death: Volume 1*, DOI 10.1007/978-94-007-4575-9_14,

Abbreviations

Bcl-2	B-cell lymphoma 2
CAK	CDK-activating kinase
CDK	cyclin-dependent kinase
Chk1	checkpoint kinase 1
CKI	cyclin-dependent kinase inhibitor
CLL	chronic lymphocytic leukemia
c-myc	cellular homolog of avian myelocytomatosis virus oncogene
CTD	carboxy-terminal domain
DRB	5,6-dichlorobenzimidazole 1-β-D-ribofuranoside
DSIF	DRB sensitivity-inducing factor
EGF	epidermal growth factor
EGFR	epidermal growth factor receptor
EMA	European Medicines Agency
GSK3 β	glycogen synthase kinase 3 β
IAPs	inhibitors of apoptosis
MAT1	ménage-a-trois
Mcl-1	myeloid cell leukemia sequence 1
MDR	multi-drug resistance
NELF	negative elongation factor
NF-κB	nuclear factor-κB
p53AIP-1	p53 apoptosis-inducing protein 1
PARP-1	poly(ADP-ribose) polymerase-1
PKA	protein kinase A
PKC	protein kinase C
pRb	retinoblastoma
P-TEFb	positive transcription elongation factor b
XIAP	X-linked inhibitor of apoptosis

14.1 CDKs and the Cell Cycle

Accurate reproduction and transmittance of genetic information carried by cells to following generations is essential for any organism. Hence, cell division is a strictly regulated process.

The systematic regulation of this process minimizes the risk of genomic instability and aberrant chromosome segregation. Therefore, it is not surprising that deregulation of the cell cycle has fatal consequences and facilitates conversion of healthy cells into tumor cells.

The importance of regulation of the cell cycle (and the critical role of regulatory malfunctions in carcinogenesis) was highlighted when Leland Hartwell, Paul Nurse and Timothy Hunt were awarded the Nobel Prize in Physiology or Medicine in 2001

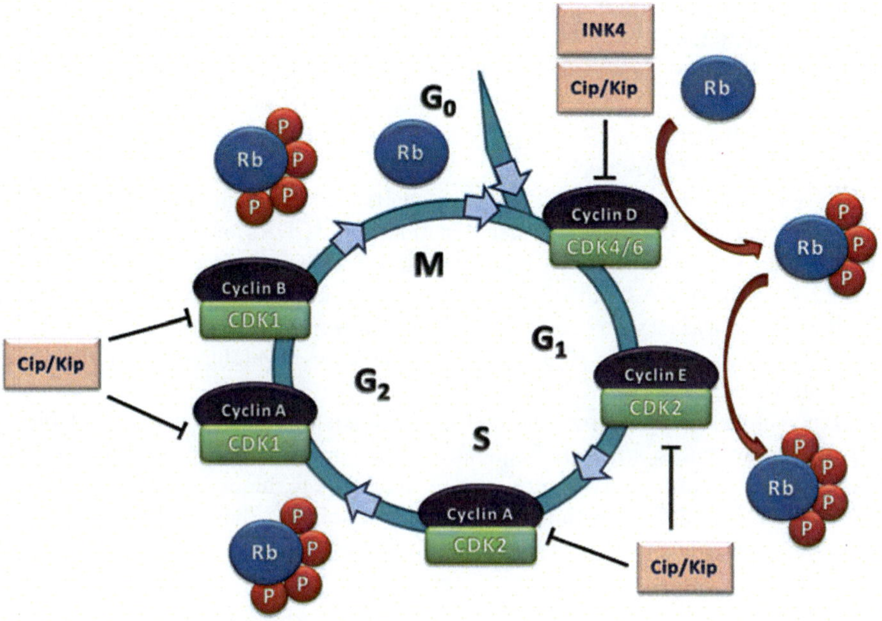

Fig. 14.1 Scheme depicting the regulation of the different phases of the cell cycle. Progression through the cell cycle is driven by CDK/cyclin complexes. INK4 and Cip/Kip family members of endogenous CKIs negatively regulate cell cycle progression

for elucidating eukaryotic cell cycling mechanisms, and identifying key molecules involved in the mechanisms (Nobelprize.org 2001).

Key elements of the surveillance machinery controlling the cell cycle are cyclin-dependent kinases (CDKs) and their regulatory partners, cyclins. Cyclins are periodically synthesized and degraded, while CDKs are constantly expressed during the cell cycle, and the sequential activation of the CDK/cyclin complexes regulates the progression of cells through the phases of the cell cycle. In addition to their association with cyclins, the activity of CDKs requires phosphorylation, catalyzed by CDK-activating kinase (CAK), of a strongly conserved threonine located within an activation loop.

CAK is a complex of CDK7, cyclin H and the RING finger protein known as ménage-a-trois (MAT1). CDKs are also negatively regulated in several ways, including: inhibitory phosphorylation of residues within the ATP-binding pocket, and through binding to endogenous CDK inhibitors (CKIs), which can reversibly inhibit their enzymatic activity (reviewed by Satyanarayana and Kaldis 2009) (Fig. 14.1).

During the early G_1 phase of the cell cycle CDK4/CDK6/cyclin D complexes, and subsequently CDK2/cyclin E complexes, inactivate Rb pocket proteins (Sherr 1994). G_1 progression is also regulated by members of the INK4 family of endogenous CKIs that specifically inhibit CDK4 and CDK6. The proteins of another group of CDK inhibitors, belonging to the Cip/Kip family, contribute to G_1 arrest by inhibiting

CDK2 and CDK4/6 (Sherr and Roberts 1999; Gartel et al. 1996). Active CDK2/cyclin A and CDK1/cyclin A complexes are essential for S-phase progression (Petersen et al. 1999; Coverley et al. 2000), S/G_2 transition is controlled by CDK1/cyclin A (Furuno et al. 1999), while G_2/M transition and mitosis are controlled by CDK1/cyclin B complexes (Riabowol et al. 1989). The Cip/Kip family also regulates these checkpoints (O'Connor 1997).

However, this classical model has been challenged in recent years. Analyses of knockout mouse models have revealed that most of the CDKs and cyclins are largely dispensable because CDK1 can replace their functions in mitotic cycles (Ortega et al. 2003). Cyclins A2 and B1 have emerged as the most non-redundant cyclins (reviewed by Satyanarayana and Kaldis 2009). However, although CDK2 seems to be easily bypassed (Martin et al. 2005), in some cases it might still be a potential target for therapy (Du et al. 2004).

Hyperactivation of the positive cell cycle regulators and inactivation of their negative counterparts, which is frequently observed in malignancies, substantially contributes to uncontrolled cell proliferation and hence to tumor development. Thus, selective CDK inhibition is thought to provide a valuable therapeutic tool, which may (for instance) be beneficial for treating certain neoplasms.

14.2 CDKs and Transcription

Besides the cell cycle regulatory CDKs, other CDKs promote initiation and elongation of nascent RNA transcripts by phosphorylating the carboxy-terminal domain (CTD) of RNA-polymerase II (RNA-Pol II) (Prelich 2002; Palancade and Bensaude 2003; Meinhart et al. 2005). CDK9/cyclin T (P-TEFb) and the previously mentioned CDK7/cyclin H complex (CAK) belong to this group (Fig. 14.2).

However, CDK7 cannot be classified so easily because it acts at a crossroads between the two cellular processes, cell cycling and transcription. It phosphorylates as CAK cell cycle-related CDKs thereby promoting cell cycle progression, and as a catalytic constituent of the general transcription factor TFIIH phosphorylates specific serine residues of the CTD of RNA-Pol II (Palancade and Bensaude 2003). These dual functions operate at different functional levels. On the one side CDK7 is an upstream cell cycle regulator, on the other side it acts as a downstream effector kinase. Interestingly, the two functions demand the capacity to recognize two types of substrates with different structures (Poon and Hunter 1995). Moreover, it does not recognize the sequence around the phosphorylation site on its own activation T-loop, which shows similarity with target CDKs (Fisher 2005). The activity and abundance of all three units of CAK are almost constant during all phases of the cell cycle (Brown et al. 1994). It has been previously suggested that MAT1 association and dissociation/degradation or binding to THIIH could regulate the activity of the complex (Adamczewski et al. 1996; Rossignol et al. 1997; Yankulov and Bentley 1997). Later studies have revealed that since kinase activity targeting CTD is selectively stimulated, it occurs without loss of CAK activity. The formation of a stable unit

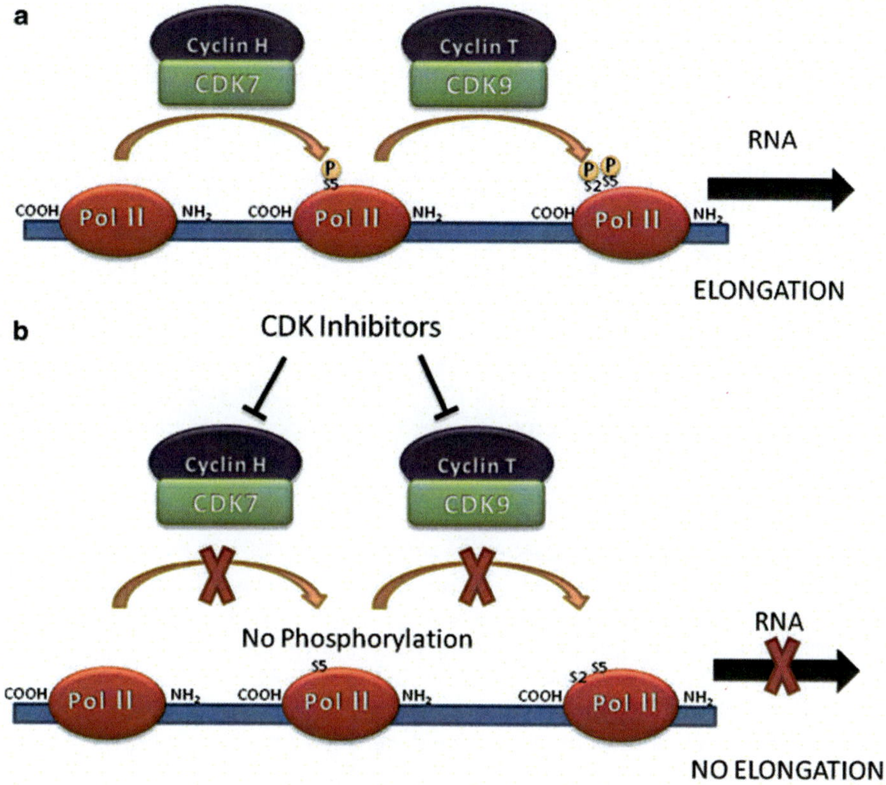

Fig. 14.2 The involvement of CDK/cyclin complexes in regulation of transcription. CDK7 and CDK9 in complex with their appropriate cyclins phosphorylate the CTD of RNA Pol II, thereby facilitating transcriptional elongation. Inhibition of these CDK/cyclin complexes results in blockage of transcription elongation. Consequently diminished levels of some anti-apoptotic proteins (e.g. Mcl-1) promote apoptosis

requires the presence of MAT1 and phosphorylation of at least one of two residues (Ser164 or Thr170) (Larochelle et al. 2001). Further studies on fruit flies substantiated the conclusion that phosphorylation at Thr170 is essential for CTD activity (Larochelle et al. 2001; Leclerc et al. 2000), and the importance of MAT1 has been demonstrated in experiments performed on *MAT1*$^{-/-}$ mice and blastocysts (Rossi et al. 2001).

Effective targeting of CDK7 for anti-cancer therapy would not only delay G_1/S transition and prevent mitosis (Larochelle et al. 2007), but would particularly affect the transcription of genes required for further steps of cell division (reviewed by Fisher 2005; Węsierska-Gądek et al. 2009; Wesierska-Gadek and Schmid 2006). Therefore, CDK7 can be considered a very promising target for anti-cancer agents.

CDK9, in complexes with cyclin T or K, forms the positive transcription elongation factor b (P-TEFb) (Wang and Fischer 2008). Since P-TEFb is a global transcription factor, its activity has to be tightly regulated. This is largely ensured by its dynamic recruitment to and release from activating and inhibitory complexes, although autophosphorylation and the involvement of small RNAs in its regulation have also been described (Marshall and Grana 2006; Wang and Fischer 2008). P-TEFb promotes transcriptional elongation by phosphorylating the CTD of the largest subunit of RNA-Pol II, as follows. First, the general transcription factor TFIIH complex containing CDK7 phosphorylates the Ser5 residues of the CTD heptad repeats, initiating transcription and promoter escape. Shortly thereafter, two negative elongation factors – DRB sensitivity-inducing factor (DSIF) and negative elongation factor (NELF) – block the elongation of pre-mRNA, thereby ensuring its capping (Wen and Shatkin 1999). This promoter-proximal pausing process seems to be a general rate-limiting step after transcription initiation (Core and Lis 2008). Subsequently, active CDK9 phosphorylates both CTD at Ser2 residues and two elongation regulators (DSIF and NELF), thereby promoting elongation. Other functions of P-TEFb, involving pre-mRNA processing, synthesis and export of mRNA, and post-translational modification of histones have also been described (Bres et al. 2008).

Given their involvement in basic cellular processes, targeting these CDKs may appear extremely toxic at first glance. However, it has been recently suggested that inhibition of CDK7 by pharmacological inhibitors mainly affects tumor cells via repression of their high CAK activity. Therefore, the limitation of mRNA synthesis may primarily affect cancer cells without shutting down transcription globally in non-dividing cells (Fisher 2005). Moreover, current knowledge strongly suggests that targeting CDK9 is a promising strategy not only for cancer therapy but also for treating AIDS, cardiac hypertrophy and inflammation-associated diseases (Wang and Fischer 2008).

14.3 CDKs and Cell Death

As yet, the ways in which CDKs may contribute to the induction of apoptosis are not clear; indeed whether their involvement is direct or indirect is uncertain. However, several lines of evidence indicate that there is a link between the activity of CDK/cyclin complexes and induction of programmed cell death.

It seems that the effector phase of cell death involves not only the caspase-3-like proteases, but also the nuclear recruitment and activation of *CDKs*, which (in turn) depends on the caspase cascade (Harvey et al. 1998). Activation of the cyclin A-dependent protein kinases CDK1 and CDK2 during apoptosis has been shown by Meinkrantz et al. (1994), while Li et al. found evidence that HIV-Tat-induced apoptosis in T-lymphocytes is associated with enhanced activation of CDKs (Li et al. 1995). Furthermore, site-specific phosphorylation of survivin mediated by activated CDK1/cyclin B complexes in late G_2 phase prevents apoptosis (O'Connor et al. 2000). Following phosphorylation at Thr34, survivin (a member of the protein family of inhibitors of apoptosis, IAPs), prevents final activation of caspase-3 (Altieri 2010) thereby protecting Wee1 kinase, which catalyzes phosphorylation of CDK1 at Thr15, from degradation (Guzman et al. 2009).

These few (of many) examples clearly show that there is a link between CDKs and apoptosis, and there is evidence that targeting of CDKs by selective inhibitors can affect cell death *via* multiple mechanisms.

14.4 CDK5: A Special Member of the CDK Family

CDK5 is not directly involved in either cell cycle regulation or transcription, and unlike other CDKs it is not activated upon binding to cyclin D or E. Discovered in 1992 by four independent groups, CDK5 was originally given several names (Dhariwala and Rajadhyaksha 2008). However, within a year of identifying the 30 kDa protein subunit of the active enzyme the nomenclature settled on CDK5 (Kobayashi et al. 1993). It has been identified as a part of a family showing >60% sequence homology to the mammalian CDK2 and yeast cdc2 (Hellmich et al. 1992; Meyerson et al. 1992; Lew et al. 1992). Though it occurs ubiquitously, the highest expression of CDK5 has been found in post-mitotic neurons and glial cells.

The association of CDK5 with its activators, p35, the p35 isoform p39 and p25, leads to formation of a functional holoenzyme (Dhavan and Tsai 2001). These activators show little similarity to the classical cyclins, but they have three-dimensional domains resembling the cyclin CDK-binding domains (Dhariwala and Rajadhyaksha 2008). p25 is a proteolytic fragment of p35 protein with a three-times longer half-life, generated by calpain, a calcium-activated protease. Binding of p25 to CDK5 activates it and facilitates translocation of the complex into the nucleus. Consequently, CDK5 persists in its hyperactive state, which is often associated with neurotoxicity (Patrick et al. 1999; Lee et al. 2000). An analogous fragment of p39, p29, contributes to the deregulation of CDK5 (Patzke and Tsai 2002).

The activity of CDK5 is modulated by its phosphorylation at specific sites similar to those of other CDKs, but with markedly different effects. The phosphorylation of CDK5 at Thr15 enhances its activity, while phosphorylation at Thr159 (which is analogous to activating phosphorylation of mitotic CDKs) is not obligatory and may even have opposing effects.

CKIs seem to have little effect on CDK5 activity (reviewed by Dhariwala and Rajadhyaksha 2008). CDK5 phosphorylates p35, its own activator, targeting it for polyubiquitination and subsequent proteasomal degradation. Therefore, under physiological conditions the activity of CDK5 is regulated by a negative feedback loop (Dhariwala and Rajadhyaksha 2008).

CDK5 is most abundant in the nervous system, where it appears to be important in almost all basic processes of neuronal development, e.g. migration, formation of cell-cell contacts and apoptosis (Paglini and Caceres 2001; Tanaka et al. 2001). CDK5 is also involved in axonal elongation and synaptogenesis (Dhariwala and Rajadhyaksha 2008). It participates in neurophysiological processes such as associative learning and memory (Fischer et al. 2002; Fischer et al. 2005) and regulation of pain reception (Wang et al. 2005). CDK5 may cause apoptosis in two distinct ways: a cytoplasmic mechanism *via* cytoskeleton disruption and a nuclear mechanism *via* interference with pro-survival genes (Dhariwala and Rajadhyaksha 2008;

Patrick et al. 1999). The pro- or anti-apoptotic capabilities of CDK5 strongly depend on the cellular context, the cellular state and (clearly) the presence of distinct activators (Dhariwala and Rajadhyaksha 2008).

Given the above observations, it is not surprising that CDK5 is involved in pathological processes associated with neurodegenerative diseases. It plays a role in the formation of intraneuronal neurofibrillary tangles and senile plaques in Alzheimer's disease (Augustinack et al. 2002; Otth et al. 2002), and it has been found in Lewy-bodies in the midbrain of Parkinson's disease patients (Brion and Couck 1995). Aberrant activation of CDK5 also seems to be involved in the pathogenesis of amyotrophic lateral sclerosis (Nguyen et al. 2001), and there is increasing evidence that CDK5 is linked to Huntington's and Niemann-Pick diseases as well as neuronal injury, especially in post-ischemic and hypoxia-related conditions (Dhariwala and Rajadhyaksha 2008; Timsit and Menn 2007).

14.5 CDK Inhibitors from Natural Origins and Their Derivatives

Proper function and activity of CDKs is essential for various cellular processes. Increases in the expression and/or activity of cell cycle regulators, and/or inactivation of endogenous CDK inhibitors, are frequent events leading to enhanced proliferation and cell growth, especially (but not only) during malignant transformation. Furthermore, as mentioned above, impaired or improper CDK activity is linked to many diseases apart from malignancies. Therefore, there are broad potential applications of pharmacological CDK inhibitors; *inter alia* they are considered to be suitable for treating human malignancies and both viral and neurodegenerative diseases (Malumbres and Barbacid 2009; Schang 2005; Monaco and Vallano 2003). Hence, there is a strong rationale for the extensive research on pharmacological CDK inhibitors and searches for new compounds that target CDKs potently and more selectively (Wesierska-Gadek and Krystof 2009; Wesierska-Gadek et al. 2011).

Most of the recently developed CDK inhibitors compete with ATP for the kinase active site (Węsierska-Gądek et al. 2009; Senderowicz 2003). However, another group of inhibitors influence CDK activity by targeting the upstream pathways, altering the expression and synthesis of cyclins, manipulating the proteolytic machinery that regulates the catabolism of CDK complexes (or their regulators), or modulating the phosphorylation status of CDKs (Senderowicz 2003).

Since the discovery of the first CDK inhibitor, dimethylaminopurine, in 1988 (Meijer and Pondaven 1988), a number of potential inhibitors have been described. Within 11 years, six classes of CDK inhibitors had been characterized and a number of new inhibitors had been identified, including flavopiridol, butyrolactone, suramin, 9-hydroxyellipticine, olomoucine and its several analogues, staurosporine, and its related compound UCN-01 (Garrett and Fattaey 1999). The number of patent applications for new CDK inhibitors has also risen, from one in 1992 to a peak in 2002

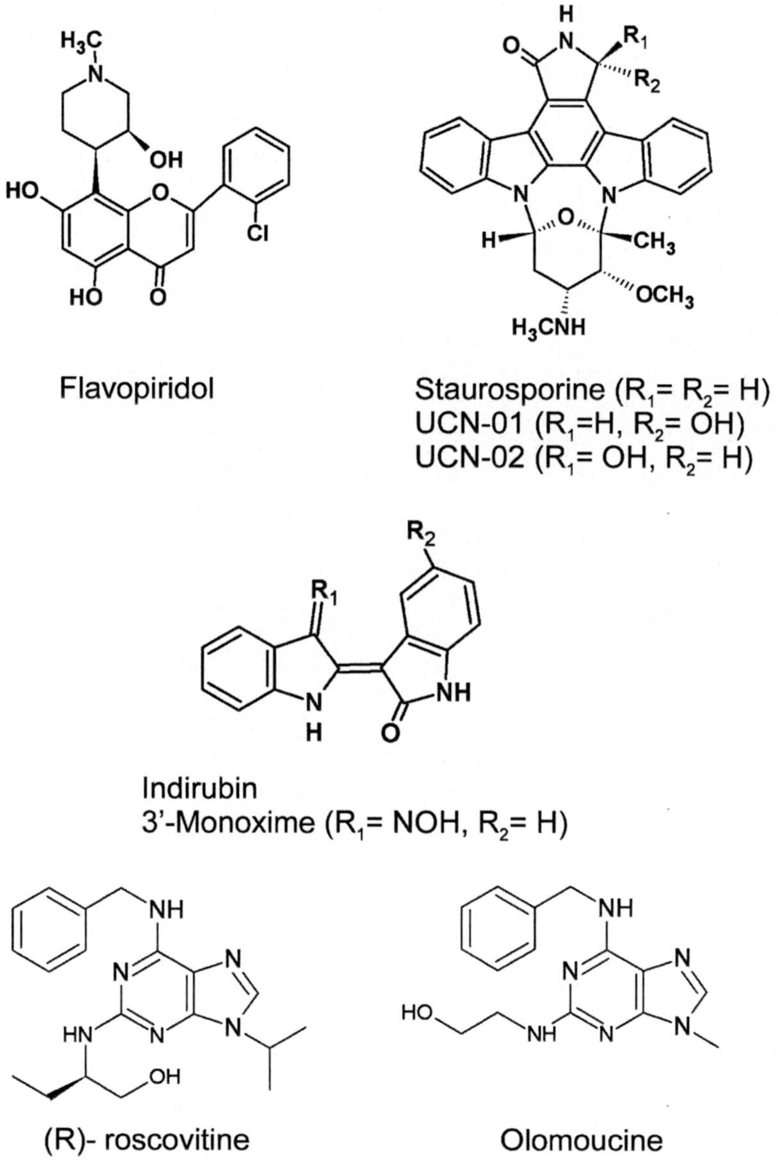

Fig. 14.3 Inhibitors of CDKs from natural origin and their derivatives

(114 applications). To date, 16 classes of CDK inhibitors have been described (Ip Overview - CDK Inhibitors 2009). Known CDK inhibitors include a wide range of natural substances and their derivatives. Of the many CDK inhibitors derived from natural origins, the focus in this article is on flavopiridol, staurosporine, indirubin, olomoucine and some of their most potent and prominent derivatives (Fig. 14.3).

14.6 Flavopiridol, the First CDK Inhibitor Administered to Patients

Flavopiridol (Alvocidib™; L86-8275; HMR 1275; NSC-649890), a semi-synthetic flavonoid derived from rohitukine, was the first compound to enter clinical trials (Senderowicz 1999). This alkaloid was first isolated from the leaves and stems of *Amoora rohituka* (0.083% dry weight), and subsequently from stem bark of *Dysoxylum binectariferum* (0.9% dry weight), both belonging to the family Meliaceae, and endogenous in India (Garrett and Fattaey 1999; Mohanakumara et al. 2010).

Flavopiridol was initially identified by screening for EGF receptor kinase (EGFR) and protein kinase A (PKA) inhibitors (IC_{50} = 21 and 122 μM, respectively) (Sedlacek et al. 1996). However, testing of 60 cell lines at the US National Cancer Institute revealed an IC_{50} for growth inhibition of 66 nM; approximately 1,000-fold lower than the concentration required to inhibit PKA and EGFR (Sedlacek et al. 1996). In further studies this anti-proliferative effect was attributed to inhibition of CDKs 1, 2, 4 and 6 (Sedlacek et al. 1996; Losiewicz et al. 1994; Worland et al. 1993). However, its inhibition of CDK9 seems to be even more potent (Chao et al. 2000; Chao and Price 2001; Shima et al. 2003). Interestingly, whereas flavopiridol competes with ATP for binding to CDKs 1, 2 and 4, the inhibition of CDK9 is non-competitive (Chao et al. 2000). Recently, the exact mechanism of this inhibition has been characterized; binding of flavopiridol to the active site of CDK9 induces a conformational change of the glycine-rich loop, which closes and folds over the active site, preventing ATP binding (Baumli et al. 2008).

This inhibition affects cellular transcription, predominantly that of transcripts with a short half-life (reviewed by Shapiro 2006). The rapid degradation of these mRNAs and simultaneous inhibition of transcriptional initiation and elongation leads to their decrease and exhaustion. This process particularly affects transcripts of several gene classes, including immediate early transcription factor-, cytokine- and apoptosis-regulating genes. The last group includes genes encoding anti-apoptotic proteins, such as Bcl-2, Mcl-1 and XIAP. Cell cycle regulators, like *c-myc*, mitotic regulatory kinases, NF-κB target genes, and genes contributing to the p53 pathway, are also involved (Lam et al. 2001).

In the first clinical trial of flavopiridol, in patients with refractory neoplasms and disease progression, the compound elicited some minor responses and stabilized the disease to some degree. Moreover, one patient with refractory metastatic gastric cancer showed a complete, sustained response with no evidence of disease even >2 years after discontinuation of flavopiridol treatment.

However, in one of the first trials with continuous infusion unexpected secretory diarrhea, reversible hypotension and a significant pro-inflammatory syndrome with fever, fatigue, local tumor pain and modulation of acute phase reactants appeared. Another approach, administering flavopiridol as bolus, led to nausea, vomiting, neutropenia, fatigue, diarrhea, local tumor pain and anorexia.

Hence, although the mechanism whereby diarrhea was induced has been ascertained, and a successful anti-diarrhea prophylaxis has been developed, these trials provided the first evidence that applying wide-spectrum CDK inhibitors can be problematic (reviewed by Senderowicz et al. 1998).

Interestingly, whereas prolonged infusion of flavopiridol was largely ineffective, bolus infusion led to cure in mice with lymphoma xenografts (Shapiro 2006). Flavopiridol has a high capacity to bind to plasma proteins. Therefore, it is difficult to achieve the required therapeutic concentrations *in vivo* (Shapiro 2006). A further optimized schedule, consisting of 30 min bolus in combination with 4 h infusion used to treat refractory high-risk CLL patients achieved a response rate of 41% in 22 assessable patients (Byrd et al. 2007). Recently, a PEGylated liposomal formulation of flavopiridol has also been developed. Such carriers have already been successfully used to deliver other anti-cancer agents, and this formulation might further optimize the administration of flavopiridol to patients. (Yang et al. 2009).

Flavopiridol is now being tested in more than 50 clinical trials as either a single agent or in combination with other chemotherapeutics (Solomon et al. 1991). Clearly, flavopiridol treatment has not proved advantageous in every trial (Carvajal et al. 2009). However, recently published findings show that flavopiridol administered as a single agent or in combination with other drugs like oxaliplatin, fluorouracil, leucovorin, fludarabine and rituximab, is effective against some solid tumors like germ cell, pancreatic, gastric and sweat gland tumors, and in hematological neoplasms, like CLL, mantle-cell lymphoma and indolent B-cell non-Hodgkin lymphoma (Rathkopf et al. 2009; Phelps et al. 2009; Lin et al. 2009, 2010; Karp et al. 2010).

In 2007 the European Medicines Agency designated flavopiridol as an orphan drug for chronic lymphocytic leukaemia (Węsierska-Gądek et al. 2009). However, although knowledge of its mechanism of action, pharmacodynamics and pharmacokinetics has improved, further studies are required to overcome its negative side effects and to optimize flavopiridol therapy.

14.7 Staurosporine and Its Derivatives

Since it became known that protein kinase C (PKC) plays a pivotal role in cell proliferation, differentiation, malignant transformation and apoptosis, PKC inhibitors have been intensively sought. An important lead, staurosporine, was discovered more than 30 years ago, by screening extracts from the bacterium *Streptomyces staurosporeus* (Omura et al. 1977).

Staurosporine, an indolo[2,3-alpha]carbazole with an IC_{50} for PKC inhibition of ~1 nM, is still one of the leading compounds used to inhibit PKC. It has strong affinity for PKC's ATP-binding site and binds to several kinases with little selectivity (Karaman et al. 2008). However, its lack of selectivity, and consequently high cytotoxicity, has precluded its clinical application and promoted the development of more specific and less cytotoxic derivatives, including 7-hydroxystaurosporine (UCN-01) (Takahashi et al. 1987) and N-benzoyl staurosporine (CGP 41251) (Meyer et al. 1989).

Although UCN-01 and CPG 41251 were initially developed as PKC inhibitors, their strong anti-proliferative effects seem to be related to CDK inhibition rather than to the repression of PKC activity (Gescher 2000). Staurosporine and UCN-01 significantly block the activity of multiple CDKs, including (for staurosporine) CDK2/cyclinA (Meijer 1996; Gadbois et al. 1992) and CDK4/cyclinD, with IC_{50} values of 7 nM and 3.10 μM, respectively, and (for UCN-01) CDK1 and CDK2 with IC_{50} values of 31 and 30 nM, respectively.

In addition to its effects on PKC and CDKs, UCN-01 also inhibits checkpoint kinase 1 (Chk1).

The mechanism of the interference of staurosporine and its analogues with CDKs is highly complex and strongly depends on the cell type. In many cell types staurosporine induces G_1 arrest (Gadbois et al. 1995; Kwon et al. 1997), depending on pRb (Schnier et al. 1996). Moreover, the endogenous CDK inhibitor $p27^{Kip1}$ is upregulated after staurosporine treatment, suggesting that the G_1 arrest strongly depends on the action of $p27^{Kip1}$ (Nishi et al. 1998).

UCN-01 affects the CDK system in many ways. For example, it inhibits the activity of CDK2, leads to accumulation of the hypophosphorylated form of pRb, decreases expression of cyclins A and D1, and enhances expression of $p21^{Cip1}$ and $p27^{Kip1}$ in human epidermoid carcinoma cells (Akiyama et al. 1997). UCN-01 also negatively affects the activity of CDK1, thus abrogating the G_2 checkpoint control in cells lacking functional p53 (Wang et al. 1996). This may explain UCN-01's ability to enhance the effects of DNA-damaging agents in cells lacking functional p53.

CDK inhibitors are known to especially affect rapidly dividing cells, which is normally a feature of cancer cells. However, slowly growing cancer cells pose especially major problems for anti-tumor therapy and often lead to a recurrence of cancer cells despite good initial responses to therapy. Kondoh et al. recently showed that UCN-01 is able to target slowly-proliferating as well as quiescent ovarian cancer cells, thus reducing the probability of latent disease (Kondoh et al. 2010). Staurosporine (and to a lesser extent UCN-01) is not only a cell cycle inhibitor, but also a very potent inducer of apoptosis, primarily *via* activation of caspase-3 (Harkin et al. 1998). Interestingly, CGP 41251 does not induce apoptosis when applied alone, but potentiates the apoptosis-inducing action of the anti-cancer drug cytosine arabinoside in leukaemia cells (Hunakova et al. 1996). Staurosporine and UCN-01, but not CGP 41251, induce apoptosis, indicating that PKC inhibition alone is not sufficient to induce programmed cell death.

Belmokhtar et al. reported that staurosporine can induce at least two apoptosis pathways, depending on the cellular context: a rapid cell death pathway involving the activation of caspases, or a slow pathway without caspase involvement (Belmokhtar et al. 2001). Since some cancer cells lack caspase activity, leading to increased resistance to conventional chemotherapy, the ability of staurosporine to induce either of these pathways could be beneficial for the treatment of cancer.

Very recently, a phase I study in which UCN-01 was administered in combination with irinotecan to patients with resistant solid tumor malignancies showed it to have acceptable toxicity, target inhibition and anti-tumor activity (Fracasso et al. 2010). Another study in which it was administered in combination with prednisone confirmed its good tolerability and ability to prolong stable disease in patients with refractory solid tumors and lymphomas (Kummar et al. 2010). However, in some trials UCN-01 has not shown convincing anti-cancer potential; notably in a phase II clinical study a combination of UCN-01 and topotecan did not show enhanced antitumor activity in patients with advanced recurrent ovarian cancer (Welch et al. 2007).

However, the cited authors suggest that the negative outcome of the study may have been due to inappropriate sequences of the drug combination.

Taken together, these observations suggest that UCN-01 and CGP 41251 can be considered as potent anticancer agents, especially in combination with other agents, like cisplatin. The findings that UCN-01 potentiates the antitumoral effects of DNA-damaging agents in cells lacking functional p53 (Wang et al. 1996) and that CGP 42151 can modulate MDR (Utz et al. 1994) may offer real advantages for anti-cancer therapy.

14.8 Indirubins

Indirubin is a 3, 2′-bisindole isomer of indigo that was initially discovered as the active compound in a traditional Chinese preparation consisting of 11 herbal constituents, named Danggui Longhui Wan (Han 1994). In 1985 a clinical study showed it to be highly effective against chronic myelocytic leukemia, with good tolerability and few side effects.

Indirubin inhibits CDKs by binding to their ATP binding site with high affinity (Hoessel et al. 1999). Early studies with indirubin and its first derivatives showed that almost all investigated cell lines were arrested in the G_2/M phase of the cell cycle. Jurkat cells were arrested at the G_1/S transition, which is consistent with CDK2 inhibition and inhibition of pRb phosphorylation (Hoessel et al. 1999). Indirubin-3′-monixime, a quite prominent derivative of indirubin, seems to affect the cell cycle at the G_1/S and G_2/M checkpoints, in accordance with its ability to inhibit both CDK2 and CDK1 (Marko et al. 2001). Following cell cycle arrest most cell lines undergo apoptosis (Marko et al. 2001), and derivatives of indirubin have recently been shown to sensitize melanoma cells to ligand-induced apoptosis (Berger et al. 2010), suggesting that indirubin derivatives also have a chemosensitizing effect.

Furthermore, indirubins are not only potent inhibitors of CDK2/cyclin A, CDK2/cyclin E, CDK5/p25 and CDK1/cyclin B complexes (Hoessel et al. 1999), but they also inhibit another kinase, glycogen synthase kinase 3 β (GSK3 β) (Leclerc et al. 2001). A very recent report also indicates that GSK3 β inhibition may have a cardioprotective role (Yadav et al. 2010).

Some unfavorable features of indirubin, like poor solubility, poor absorption and gastrointestinal toxicity led to the early development of several analogues (Hoessel et al. 1999), such as N-methyl isoindigo, 5-chloro-indirubin and indirubin-3′-monoxime (Marko et al. 2001). The design and synthesis of new derivatives of indirubin is continuing (Choi et al. 2010; Moon et al. 2006; Cheng et al. 2010; Kim et al. 2009).

The fact that indirubin derivatives can inhibit not only cell cycle regulatory kinases (CDK2 and CDK1), but also CDK5 and another kinase (GSK3 β) broadens their potential applicability to Alzheimer's disease (Ding et al. 2010), atherosclerosis (Kim et al. 2010), restenosis (Schwaiberger et al. 2010), angiogenesis (Zahler et al. 2010) and dermatophytosis (Ponnusamy et al. 2010).

14.9 Olomoucine – The First Specific CDK Inhibitor

The broad specificity of staurosporine and flavopiridol towards numerous kinases led to the search for new more specific inhibitors of CDKs. Notably, screening of the plant hormones cytokinins (N6-substituted adenine derivatives) showed that these compounds are also quite unspecific protein kinase inhibitors. Surprisingly, an aromatic cytokinin derivative, olomoucine (a 2,6,9-trisubstituted purine; 2-(2-hydroxyethylamino)-6-benzylamino-9-methylpurine) was the first discovered selective inhibitor of CDK1 and CDK2 (Vesely et al. 1994). This finding was contrary to the current dogma that no highly specific inhibitor targeting the ATP-binding pocket of kinases would ever be discovered (Meijer and Raymond 2003).

Indeed, olomoucine is a competitive inhibitor for ATP binding (Vesely et al. 1994) and has unexpectedly high selectivity. The compound was named olomoucine since one of its discoverers, Jaroslav Vesely, was based at Palacký University in Olomouc (the Czech Republic).

As expected, olomoucine strongly affects the cell cycle of various types of cancer cells and also induces apoptosis. For a few examples (of many) see references (Schutte et al. 1997; Wandl and Wesierska-Gadek 2009; Wesierska-Gadek et al. 2004, 2007a).

However, soon after the discovery of olomoucine, new more potent derivatives were synthesized, one of the most prominent being roscovitine (2-(R)-(1-ethyl-2-hydroxyethylamino)-6-benzylamino-9-isopropylpurine, CYC202, Seliciclib). This was the first 2,6,8-trisubstituted purine to enter clinical trials (Meijer and Raymond 2003), following pre-clinical trials initiated by Sir David Lane, founder of Cyclacel Ltd.

Roscovitine proved to have good oral bioavailability, which is a pre-requisite for potential clinical applications, thus offering the possibility for oral treatment over extended periods of time at active plasma levels. In studies with a panel of 19 different human cancer cell lines it showed an average cytotoxic IC_{50} of 15.3 μM. Moreover, roscovitine primarily affects rapidly diving cells rather than non-proliferating cells, thus offering selectivity for cancer cells over normal healthy cells (McClue et al. 2002).

In recent years strenuous efforts have been made to elucidate the precise mechanisms whereby roscovitine modulates biological functions, which include: accumulation of cells in G_1, S or G_2 phase of the cell cycle, induction of apoptosis, inhibition of transcription, inhibition of rRNA processing and disruption of nuclei (McClue et al. 2002; Alessi et al. 1998; Ljungman and Paulsen 2001; Lu et al. 2001; Sirri et al. 2002; David-Pfeuty et al. 2001; Whittaker et al. 2004). Apart from inhibiting the cell cycle regulatory CDKs, CDK2 and CDK1, roscovitine also inhibits CDK5 and the transcription regulating CDKs, CDK7 and CDK9 (Havlicek et al. 1997). Thus, roscovitine can repress the transcription of important anti-apoptotic proteins, leading to apoptosis. For instance, multiple myeloma cells that depend on the anti-apoptotic protein Mcl-1 are extremely sensitive to treatment with roscovitine (MacCallum et al. 2005). MacCullum et al. also showed that roscovitine inhibits RNA Polymerase II via inhibition of CDK7, leading to blockage of transcription and hence down-regulation of Mcl-1. In addition, roscovitine not only promotes accumulation of G_2 phase cells in MCF-7 breast cancer cells, which are normally quite resistant to conventional chemotherapy (Janicke et al. 1998), but concomitantly induces apoptosis in these cells (Maurer et al. 2009; Wesierska-Gadek et al. 2003, 2004, 2005, 2007b; Wojciechowski et al. 2003).

The potential applications of roscovitine are not limited to cancer therapy, but include the treatment of various other human diseases, including: viral infections (Guendel et al. 2010; Rowe et al. 2010), neurodegeneration (Camins et al. 2006; Lopes et al. 2007) and cardiovascular diseases (Yarotskyy et al. 2010). Phase I clinical studies with roscovitine have already been completed (McClue et al. 2002; Benson et al. 2007; de la Motte and Gianella-Borradori 2004; Fischer and Gianella-Borradori 2003; Le Tourneau et al. 2010). Currently, roscovitine is in phase II clinical studies in combination with gemicitabine/cisplatin, for non-small cell lung cancer and as a single agent for hematological malignancies, including multiple myeloma (Fischer and Gianella-Borradori 2003, 2005; Meijer and Raymond 2003).

To conclude, roscovitine is a pan-specific and very potent inhibitor of CDKs 1, 2, 5, 7 and 9 that can be considered for the treatment of diverse human diseases. However, this is not the end of the story; since the discovery of roscovitine the search for still more specific, more potent and less cytotoxic CDK inhibitors has continued, and a number of roscovitine derivatives have been synthesized (Popowycz et al. 2009; Bettayeb et al. 2008a, b; Sroka et al. 2010).

14.10 Future Perspectives

Since the discovery of the first, quite unspecific, natural CDK inhibitor a large number of new natural compounds and derivatives targeting CDKs have been discovered and developed. There have been considerable efforts to elucidate the mechanisms whereby pharmacological CDK inhibitors exert their numerous cellular activities. However, we still need to increase our understanding of the cell cycle to develop even more potent and specific CDK inhibitors, and to distinguish between inhibition of cell cycle regulatory and transcription regulatory CDKs. If there is an advantage of inhibiting one or the other or both depends on the nature of the disease.

Furthermore, we have to assess the full capability of the CDK inhibitors in combination with other natural compounds or standard chemotherapeutics as they also act as chemosensitizers or might synergistically potentiate their beneficial effects.

Last, but not least, we have to further investigate and screen the existing pool of natural sources for potent new CDK inhibitors.

Acknowledgments This review is based on research carried out over several years, during which the authors have been supported by grants from the Austrian Funding Agency FWF (No. P19894-B11) and the Austrian Academy of Science (OEAW) (project No. AP00401OFF).

References

Adamczewski JP, Rossignol M, Tassan JP, Nigg EA, Moncollin V, Egly JM (1996) MAT1, cdk7 and cyclin H form a kinase complex which is UV light-sensitive upon association with TFIIH. EMBO J 15(8):1877–1884

Akiyama T, Yoshida T, Tsujita T, Shimizu M, Mizukami T, Okabe M, Akinaga S (1997) G1 phase accumulation induced by UCN-01 is associated with dephosphorylation of Rb and CDK2 proteins as well as induction of CDK inhibitor p21/Cip1/WAF1/Sdi1 in p53-mutated human epidermoid carcinoma A431 cells. Cancer Res 57(8):1495–1501

Alessi F, Quarta S, Savio M, Riva F, Rossi L, Stivala LA, Scovassi AI, Meijer L, Prosperi E (1998) The cyclin-dependent kinase inhibitors olomoucine and roscovitine arrest human fibroblasts in G1 phase by specific inhibition of CDK2 kinase activity. Exp Cell Res 245(1):8–18. doi:S0014-4827(98)94216-1 [pii] 10.1006/excr.1998.4216

Altieri DC (2010) Survivin and IAP proteins in cell-death mechanisms. Biochem J 430(2):199–205. doi:BJ20100814 [pii] 10.1042/BJ20100814

Augustinack JC, Sanders JL, Tsai LH, Hyman BT (2002) Colocalization and fluorescence resonance energy transfer between cdk5 and AT8 suggests a close association in pre-neurofibrillary tangles and neurofibrillary tangles. J Neuropathol Exp Neurol 61(6):557–564

Baumli S, Lolli G, Lowe ED, Troiani S, Rusconi L, Bullock AN, Debreczeni JE, Knapp S, Johnson LN (2008) The structure of P-TEFb (CDK9/cyclin T1), its complex with flavopiridol and regulation by phosphorylation. EMBO J 27(13):1907–1918. doi:emboj2008121 [pii] 10.1038/emboj.2008.121

Belmokhtar CA, Hillion J, Segal-Bendirdjian E (2001) Staurosporine induces apoptosis through both caspase-dependent and caspase-independent mechanisms. Oncogene 20(26):3354–3362. doi:10.1038/sj.onc.1204436

Benson C, White J, De Bono J, O'Donnell A, Raynaud F, Cruickshank C, McGrath H, Walton M, Workman P, Kaye S, Cassidy J, Gianella-Borradori A, Judson I, Twelves C (2007) A phase I trial of the selective oral cyclin-dependent kinase inhibitor seliciclib (CYC202; R-Roscovitine), administered twice daily for 7 days every 21 days. Br J Cancer 96(1):29–37. doi:6603509 [pii] 10.1038/sj.bjc.6603509

Berger A, Quast SA, Plotz M, Hein M, Kunz M, Langer P, Eberle J (2010) Sensitization of melanoma cells for death ligand-induced apoptosis by an indirubin derivative – enhancement of both extrinsic and intrinsic apoptosis pathways. Biochem Pharmacol. doi:S0006-2952(10)00693-3 [pii] 10.1016/j.bcp. 2010.09.010

Bettayeb K, Oumata N, Echalier A, Ferandin Y, Endicott JA, Galons H, Meijer L (2008a) CR8, a potent and selective, roscovitine-derived inhibitor of cyclin-dependent kinases. Oncogene 27(44):5797–5807. doi:onc2008191 [pii] 10.1038/onc.2008.191

Bettayeb K, Sallam H, Ferandin Y, Popowycz F, Fournet G, Hassan M, Echalier A, Bernard P, Endicott J, Joseph B, Meijer L (2008b) N-&-N, a new class of cell death-inducing kinase inhibitors derived from the purine roscovitine. Mol Cancer Ther 7(9):2713–2724. doi:7/9/2713 [pii] 10.1158/1535-7163.MCT-08-0080

Bres V, Yoh SM, Jones KA (2008) The multi-tasking P-TEFb complex. Curr Opin Cell Biol 20(3):334–340. doi:S0955-0674(08)00080-X [pii] 10.1016/j.ceb.2008.04.008

Brion JP, Couck AM (1995) Cortical and brainstem-type Lewy bodies are immunoreactive for the cyclin-dependent kinase 5. Am J Pathol 147(5):1465–1476

Brown AJ, Jones T, Shuttleworth J (1994) Expression and activity of p40MO15, the catalytic subunit of cdk-activating kinase, during Xenopus oogenesis and embryogenesis. Mol Biol Cell 5(8):921–932

Byrd JC, Lin TS, Dalton JT, Wu D, Phelps MA, Fischer B, Moran M, Blum KA, Rovin B, Brooker-McEldowney M, Broering S, Schaaf LJ, Johnson AJ, Lucas DM, Heerema NA, Lozanski G, Young DC, Suarez JR, Colevas AD, Grever MR (2007) Flavopiridol administered using a pharmacologically derived schedule is associated with marked clinical efficacy in refractory, genetically high-risk chronic lymphocytic leukemia. Blood 109(2):399–404. doi:blood-2006-05-020735 [pii] 10.1182/blood-2006-05-020735

Camins A, Verdaguer E, Folch J, Canudas AM, Pallas M (2006) The role of CDK5/P25 formation/inhibition in neurodegeneration. Drug News Perspect 19(8):453–460. doi:1043961 [pii] 10.1358/dnp. 2006.19.8.1043961

Carvajal RD, Tse A, Shah MA, Lefkowitz RA, Gonen M, Gilman-Rosen L, Kortmansky J, Kelsen DP, Schwartz GK, O'Reilly EM (2009) A phase II study of flavopiridol (Alvocidib) in combination with docetaxel in refractory, metastatic pancreatic cancer. Pancreatology 9(4):404–409. doi:000187135 [pii] 10.1159/000187135

Chao SH, Price DH (2001) Flavopiridol inactivates P-TEFb and blocks most RNA polymerase II transcription in vivo. J Biol Chem 276(34):31793–31799. doi:10.1074/jbc.M102306200 M102306200 [pii]

Chao SH, Fujinaga K, Marion JE, Taube R, Sausville EA, Senderowicz AM, Peterlin BM, Price DH (2000) Flavopiridol inhibits P-TEFb and blocks HIV-1 replication. J Biol Chem 275(37):28345–28348. doi:10.1074/jbc.C000446200 C000446200 [pii]

Cheng X, Rasque P, Vatter S, Merz KH, Eisenbrand G (2010) Synthesis and cytotoxicity of novel indirubin-5-carboxamides. Bioorg Med Chem 18(12):4509–4515. doi:S0968-0896(10)00378-0 [pii] 10.1016/j.bmc.2010.04.066

Choi SJ, Lee JE, Jeong SY, Im I, Lee SD, Lee EJ, Lee SK, Kwon SM, Ahn SG, Yoon JH, Han SY, Kim JI, Kim YC (2010) 5,5′-Substituted indirubin-3′-oxime derivatives as potent cyclin-dependent kinase inhibitors with anticancer activity. J Med Chem 53(9):3696–3706. doi:10.1021/jm100080z

Core LJ, Lis JT (2008) Transcription regulation through promoter-proximal pausing of RNA polymerase II. Science 319(5871):1791–1792. doi:319/5871/1791 [pii] 10.1126/science.1150843

Coverley D, Pelizon C, Trewick S, Laskey RA (2000) Chromatin-bound Cdc6 persists in S and G2 phases in human cells, while soluble Cdc6 is destroyed in a cyclin A-cdk2 dependent process. J Cell Sci 113(Pt 11):1929–1938

David-Pfeuty T, Nouvian-Dooghe Y, Sirri V, Roussel P, Hernandez-Verdun D (2001) Common and reversible regulation of wild-type p53 function and of ribosomal biogenesis by protein kinases in human cells. Oncogene 20(42):5951–5963. doi:10.1038/sj.onc.1204741

de la Motte S, Gianella-Borradori A (2004) Pharmacokinetic model of R-roscovitine and its metabolite in healthy male subjects. Int J Clin Pharmacol Ther 42(4):232–239

Dhariwala FA, Rajadhyaksha MS (2008) An unusual member of the Cdk family: Cdk5. Cell Mol Neurobiol 28(3):351–369. doi:10.1007/s10571-007-9242-1

Dhavan R, Tsai LH (2001) A decade of CDK5. Nat Rev Mol Cell Biol 2(10):749–759. doi:10.1038/35096019 35096019 [pii]

Ding Y, Qiao A, Fan GH (2010) Indirubin-3′-monoxime rescues spatial memory deficits and attenuates beta-amyloid-associated neuropathology in a mouse model of Alzheimer's disease. Neurobiol Dis 39(2):156–168. doi:S0969-9961(10)00094-X [pii] 10.1016/j.nbd.2010.03.022

Du J, Widlund HR, Horstmann MA, Ramaswamy S, Ross K, Huber WE, Nishimura EK, Golub TR, Fisher DE (2004) Critical role of CDK2 for melanoma growth linked to its melanocyte-

specific transcriptional regulation by MITF. Cancer Cell 6(6):565–576. doi:S1535610804003095 [pii] 10.1016/j.ccr.2004.10.014
Fischer PM, Gianella-Borradori A (2003) CDK inhibitors in clinical development for the treatment of cancer. Expert Opin Investig Drugs 12(6):955–970. doi:10.1517/13543784.12.6.955
Fischer PM, Gianella-Borradori A (2005) Recent progress in the discovery and development of cyclin-dependent kinase inhibitors. Expert Opin Investig Drugs 14(4):457–477. doi:EID140409 [pii] 10.1517/13543784.14.4.457
Fischer A, Sananbenesi F, Schrick C, Spiess J, Radulovic J (2002) Cyclin-dependent kinase 5 is required for associative learning. J Neurosci 22(9):3700–3707. doi:20026286 22/9/3700 [pii]
Fischer A, Sananbenesi F, Pang PT, Lu B, Tsai LH (2005) Opposing roles of transient and prolonged expression of p25 in synaptic plasticity and hippocampus-dependent memory. Neuron 48(5):825–838. doi:S0896-6273(05)00951-7 [pii] 10.1016/j.neuron.2005.10.033
Fisher RP (2005) Secrets of a double agent: CDK7 in cell-cycle control and transcription. J Cell Sci 118(Pt 22):5171–5180. doi:118/22/5171 [pii] 10.1242/jcs.02718
Fracasso PM, Williams KJ, Chen RC, Picus J, Ma CX, Ellis MJ, Tan BR, Pluard TJ, Adkins DR, Naughton MJ, Rader JS, Arquette MA, Fleshman JW, Creekmore AN, Goodner SA, Wright LP, Guo Z, Ryan CE, Tao Y, Soares EM, Cai SR, Lin L, Dancey J, Rudek MA, McLeod HL, Piwnica-Worms H (2010) A Phase 1 study of UCN-01 in combination with irinotecan in patients with resistant solid tumor malignancies. Cancer Chemother Pharmacol. doi:10.1007/s00280-010-1410-1
Furuno N, den Elzen N, Pines J (1999) Human cyclin A is required for mitosis until mid prophase. J Cell Biol 147(2):295–306
Gadbois DM, Hamaguchi JR, Swank RA, Bradbury EM (1992) Staurosporine is a potent inhibitor of p34cdc2 and p34cdc2-like kinases. Biochem Biophys Res Commun 184(1):80–85. doi:0006-291X(92)91160-R [pii]
Gadbois DM, Peterson S, Bradbury EM, Lehnert BE (1995) CDK4/Cyclin D1/PCNA complexes during staurosporine-induced G1 arrest and G0 arrest of human fibroblasts. Exp Cell Res 220(1):220–225. doi:S0014-4827(85)71309-2 [pii] 10.1006/excr.1995.1309
Garrett MD, Fattaey A (1999) CDK inhibition and cancer therapy. Curr Opin Genet Dev 9(1):104–111. doi:S0959-437X(99)80015-X [pii]
Gartel AL, Serfas MS, Tyner AL (1996) p21–Negative regulator of the cell cycle. Proc Soc Exp Biol Med 213(2):138–149
Gescher A (2000) Staurosporine analogues - pharmacological toys or useful antitumour agents? Crit Rev Oncol Hematol 34(2):127–135. doi:S1040-8428(00)00058-5 [pii]
Guendel I, Agbottah ET, Kehn-Hall K, Kashanchi F (2010) Inhibition of human immunodeficiency virus type-1 by cdk inhibitors. AIDS Res Ther 7(1):7. doi:1742-6405-7-7 [pii] 10.1186/1742-6405-7-7
Guzman JR, Fukuda S, Pelus LM (2009) Inhibition of caspase-3 by Survivin prevents Wee1 Kinase degradation and promotes cell survival by maintaining phosphorylation of p34Cdc2. Gene Ther Mol Biol 13B:264–273
Han R (1994) Highlight on the studies of anticancer drugs derived from plants in China. Stem Cells 12(1):53–63. doi:10.1002/stem.5530120110
Harkin ST, Cohen GM, Gescher A (1998) Modulation of apoptosis in rat thymocytes by analogs of staurosporine: lack of direct association with inhibition of protein kinase C. Mol Pharmacol 54(4):663–670
Harvey KJ, Blomquist JF, Ucker DS (1998) Commitment and effector phases of the physiological cell death pathway elucidated with respect to Bcl-2 caspase, and cyclin-dependent kinase activities. Mol Cell Biol 18(5):2912–2922
Havlicek L, Hanus J, Vesely J, Leclerc S, Meijer L, Shaw G, Strnad M (1997) Cytokinin-derived cyclin-dependent kinase inhibitors: synthesis and cdc2 inhibitory activity of olomoucine and related compounds. J Med Chem 40(4):408–412. doi:10.1021/jm960666x jm960666x [pii]
Hellmich MR, Pant HC, Wada E, Battey JF (1992) Neuronal cdc2-like kinase: a cdc2-related protein kinase with predominantly neuronal expression. Proc Natl Acad Sci USA 89(22):10867–10871
Hoessel R, Leclerc S, Endicott JA, Nobel ME, Lawrie A, Tunnah P, Leost M, Damiens E, Marie D, Marko D, Niederberger E, Tang W, Eisenbrand G, Meijer L (1999) Indirubin, the active

constituent of a Chinese antileukaemia medicine, inhibits cyclin-dependent kinases. Nat Cell Biol 1(1):60–67. doi:10.1038/9035

Hunakova L, Sulikova M, Duraj J, Sedlak J, Chorvath B (1996) Stimulation of 1-(beta-D-arabinofuranosyl)cytosine (AraC)-induced apoptosis in the multidrug resistant human promyelocytic leukemia cell lines with protein kinase inhibitors. Neoplasma 43(5):291–295

IP Overview - CDK Inhibitors (2009) First SA, Frinnov. http://www.fist.fr/en/ip-overview/sciences-de-la-vie/cdk-inhibitors-bientot-disponible.html. Accessed 15 Sept 2010

Janicke RU, Sprengart ML, Wati MR, Porter AG (1998) Caspase-3 is required for DNA fragmentation and morphological changes associated with apoptosis. J Biol Chem 273(16):9357–9360

Karaman MW, Herrgard S, Treiber DK, Gallant P, Atteridge CE, Campbell BT, Chan KW, Ciceri P, Davis MI, Edeen PT, Faraoni R, Floyd M, Hunt JP, Lockhart DJ, Milanov ZV, Morrison MJ, Pallares G, Patel HK, Pritchard S, Wodicka LM, Zarrinkar PP (2008) A quantitative analysis of kinase inhibitor selectivity. Nat Biotechnol 26(1):127–132. doi:nbt1358 [pii] 10.1038/nbt1358

Karp JE, Blackford A, Smith BD, Alino K, Seung AH, Bolanos-Meade J, Greer JM, Carraway HE, Gore SD, Jones RJ, Levis MJ, McDevitt MA, Doyle LA, Wright JJ (2010) Clinical activity of sequential flavopiridol, cytosine arabinoside, and mitoxantrone for adults with newly diagnosed, poor-risk acute myelogenous leukemia. Leuk Res 34(7):877–882. doi:S0145-2126(09)00529-3 [pii] 10.1016/j.leukres.2009.11.007

Kim SH, Choi SJ, Kim YC, Kuh HJ (2009) Anti-tumor activity of noble indirubin derivatives in human solid tumor models in vitro. Arch Pharm Res 32(6):915–922. doi:10.1007/s12272-009-1614-2

Kim EJ, Park WH, Ahn SG, Yoon JH, Kim SW, Kim SA (2010) 5′-Nitro-indirubinoxime inhibits inflammatory response in TNF-alpha stimulated human umbilical vein endothelial cells. Atherosclerosis 211(1):77–83. doi:S0021-9150(10)00088-2 [pii] 10.1016/j.atherosclerosis.2010.01.040

Kobayashi S, Ishiguro K, Omori A, Takamatsu M, Arioka M, Imahori K, Uchida T (1993) A cdc2-related kinase PSSALRE/cdk5 is homologous with the 30 kDa subunit of tau protein kinase II, a proline-directed protein kinase associated with microtubule. FEBS Lett 335(2):171–175. doi:0014-5793(93)80723-8 [pii]

Kondoh E, Mori S, Yamaguchi K, Baba T, Matsumura N, Cory Barnett J, Whitaker RS, Konishi I, Fujii S, Berchuck A, Murphy SK (2010) Targeting slow-proliferating ovarian cancer cells. Int J Cancer 126(10):2448–2456. doi:10.1002/ijc.24919

Kummar S, Gutierrez ME, Gardner ER, Figg WD, Melillo G, Dancey J, Sausville EA, Conley BA, Murgo AJ, Doroshow JH (2010) A phase I trial of UCN-01 and prednisone in patients with refractory solid tumors and lymphomas. Cancer Chemother Pharmacol 65(2):383–389. doi:10.1007/s00280-009-1154-y

Kwon TK, Buchholz MA, Ponsalle P, Chrest FJ, Nordin AA (1997) The regulation of p27Kip1 expression following the polyclonal activation of murine G0 T cells. J Immunol 158(12):5642–5648

Lam LT, Pickeral OK, Peng AC, Rosenwald A, Hurt EM, Giltnane JM, Averett LM, Zhao H, Davis RE, Sathyamoorthy M, Wahl LM, Harris ED, Mikovits JA, Monks AP, Hollingshead MG, Sausville EA, Staudt LM (2001) Genomic-scale measurement of mRNA turnover and the mechanisms of action of the anti-cancer drug flavopiridol. Genome Biol 2(10):RESEARCH0041

Larochelle S, Chen J, Knights R, Pandur J, Morcillo P, Erdjument-Bromage H, Tempst P, Suter B, Fisher RP (2001) T-loop phosphorylation stabilizes the CDK7-cyclin H-MAT1 complex in vivo and regulates its CTD kinase activity. EMBO J 20(14):3749–3759. doi:10.1093/emboj/20.14.3749

Larochelle S, Merrick KA, Terret ME, Wohlbold L, Barboza NM, Zhang C, Shokat KM, Jallepalli PV, Fisher RP (2007) Requirements for Cdk7 in the assembly of Cdk1/cyclin B and activation of Cdk2 revealed by chemical genetics in human cells. Mol Cell 25(6):839–850. doi:S1097-2765(07)00083-4 [pii] 10.1016/j.molcel.2007.02.003

Le Tourneau C, Faivre S, Laurence V, Delbaldo C, Vera K, Girre V, Chiao J, Armour S, Frame S, Green SR, Gianella-Borradori A, Dieras V, Raymond E (2010) Phase I evaluation of seliciclib (R-roscovitine), a novel oral cyclin-dependent kinase inhibitor, in patients with advanced malignancies. Eur J Cancer. doi:S0959-8049(10)00782-3 [pii] 10.1016/j.ejca.2010.08.001

Leclerc V, Raisin S, Leopold P (2000) Dominant-negative mutants reveal a role for the Cdk7 kinase at the mid-blastula transition in Drosophila embryos. EMBO J 19(7):1567–1575. doi:10.1093/emboj/19.7.1567

Leclerc S, Garnier M, Hoessel R, Marko D, Bibb JA, Snyder GL, Greengard P, Biernat J, Wu YZ, Mandelkow EM, Eisenbrand G, Meijer L (2001) Indirubins inhibit glycogen synthase kinase-3 beta and CDK5/p25, two protein kinases involved in abnormal tau phosphorylation in Alzheimer's disease. A property common to most cyclin-dependent kinase inhibitors? J Biol Chem 276(1):251–260. doi:10.1074/jbc.M002466200 M002466200 [pii]

Lee MS, Kwon YT, Li M, Peng J, Friedlander RM, Tsai LH (2000) Neurotoxicity induces cleavage of p35 to p25 by calpain. Nature 405(6784):360–364. doi:10.1038/35012636

Lew J, Beaudette K, Litwin CM, Wang JH (1992) Purification and characterization of a novel proline-directed protein kinase from bovine brain. J Biol Chem 267(19):13383–13390

Li CJ, Friedman DJ, Wang C, Metelev V, Pardee AB (1995) Induction of apoptosis in uninfected lymphocytes by HIV-1 Tat protein. Science 268(5209):429–431

Lin TS, Ruppert AS, Johnson AJ, Fischer B, Heerema NA, Andritsos LA, Blum KA, Flynn JM, Jones JA, Hu W, Moran ME, Mitchell SM, Smith LL, Wagner AJ, Raymond CA, Schaaf LJ, Phelps MA, Villalona-Calero MA, Grever MR, Byrd JC (2009) Phase II study of flavopiridol in relapsed chronic lymphocytic leukemia demonstrating high response rates in genetically high-risk disease. J Clin Oncol 27(35):6012–6018. doi:JCO.2009.22.6944 [pii] 10.1200/JCO.2009.22.6944

Lin TS, Blum KA, Fischer DB, Mitchell SM, Ruppert AS, Porcu P, Kraut EH, Baiocchi RA, Moran ME, Johnson AJ, Schaaf LJ, Grever MR, Byrd JC (2010) Flavopiridol, fludarabine, and rituximab in mantle cell lymphoma and indolent B-cell lymphoproliferative disorders. J Clin Oncol 28(3):418–423. doi:JCO.2009.24.1570 [pii] 10.1200/JCO.2009.24.1570

Ljungman M, Paulsen MT (2001) The cyclin-dependent kinase inhibitor roscovitine inhibits RNA synthesis and triggers nuclear accumulation of p53 that is unmodified at Ser15 and Lys382. Mol Pharmacol 60(4):785–789

Lopes JP, Oliveira CR, Agostinho P (2007) Role of cyclin-dependent kinase 5 in the neurodegenerative process triggered by amyloid-Beta and prion peptides: implications for Alzheimer's disease and prion-related encephalopathies. Cell Mol Neurobiol 27(7):943–957. doi:10.1007/s10571-007-9224-3

Losiewicz MD, Carlson BA, Kaur G, Sausville EA, Worland PJ (1994) Potent inhibition of CDC2 kinase activity by the flavonoid L86-8275. Biochem Biophys Res Commun 201(2):589–595. doi:S0006-291X(84)71742-6 [pii] 10.1006/bbrc.1994.1742

Lu W, Chen L, Peng Y, Chen J (2001) Activation of p53 by roscovitine-mediated suppression of MDM2 expression. Oncogene 20(25):3206–3216. doi:10.1038/sj.onc.1204412

MacCallum DE, Melville J, Frame S, Watt K, Anderson S, Gianella-Borradori A, Lane DP, Green SR (2005) Seliciclib (CYC202, R-Roscovitine) induces cell death in multiple myeloma cells by inhibition of RNA polymerase II-dependent transcription and down-regulation of Mcl-1. Cancer Res 65(12):5399–5407. doi:65/12/5399 [pii] 10.1158/0008-5472.CAN-05-0233

Malumbres M, Barbacid M (2009) Cell cycle, CDKs and cancer: a changing paradigm. Nat Rev Cancer 9(3):153–166. doi:nrc2602 [pii] 10.1038/nrc2602

Marko D, Schatzle S, Friedel A, Genzlinger A, Zankl H, Meijer L, Eisenbrand G (2001) Inhibition of cyclin-dependent kinase 1 (CDK1) by indirubin derivatives in human tumour cells. Br J Cancer 84(2):283–289. doi:10.1054/bjoc.2000.1546 S0007092000915465 [pii]

Marshall RM, Grana X (2006) Mechanisms controlling CDK9 activity. Front Biosci 11:2598–2613. doi:1994 [pii]

Martin A, Odajima J, Hunt SL, Dubus P, Ortega S, Malumbres M, Barbacid M (2005) Cdk2 is dispensable for cell cycle inhibition and tumor suppression mediated by p27(Kip1) and p21(Cip1). Cancer Cell 7(6):591–598. doi:S1535-6108(05)00155-8 [pii] 10.1016/j.ccr.2005.05.006

Maurer M, Komina O, Wesierska-Gadek J (2009) Roscovitine differentially affects asynchronously growing and synchronized human MCF-7 breast cancer cells. Ann N Y Acad Sci 1171:250–256. doi:NYAS4717 [pii] 10.1111/j.1749-6632.2009.04717.x

McClue SJ, Blake D, Clarke R, Cowan A, Cummings L, Fischer PM, MacKenzie M, Melville J, Stewart K, Wang S, Zhelev N, Zheleva D, Lane DP (2002) In vitro and in vivo antitumor properties of the cyclin dependent kinase inhibitor CYC202 (R-roscovitine). Int J Cancer 102(5):463–468. doi:10.1002/ijc.10738

Meijer L (1996) Chemical inhibitors of cyclin-dependent kinases. Trends Cell Biol 6(10):393–397. doi:0962-8924(96)10034-9 [pii]

Meijer L, Pondaven P (1988) Cyclic activation of histone H1 kinase during sea urchin egg mitotic divisions. Exp Cell Res 174(1):116–129. doi:0014-4827(88)90147-4 [pii]

Meijer L, Raymond E (2003) Roscovitine and other purines as kinase inhibitors. From starfish oocytes to clinical trials. Acc Chem Res 36(6):417–425. doi:10.1021/ar0201198

Meikrantz W, Gisselbrecht S, Tam SW, Schlegel R (1994) Activation of cyclin A-dependent protein kinases during apoptosis. Proc Natl Acad Sci USA 91(9):3754–3758

Meinhart A, Kamenski T, Hoeppner S, Baumli S, Cramer P (2005) A structural perspective of CTD function. Genes Dev 19(12):1401–1415. doi:19/12/1401 [pii] 10.1101/gad.1318105

Meyer T, Regenass U, Fabbro D, Alteri E, Rosel J, Muller M, Caravatti G, Matter A (1989) A derivative of staurosporine (CGP 41 251) shows selectivity for protein kinase C inhibition and in vitro anti-proliferative as well as in vivo anti-tumor activity. Int J Cancer 43(5):851–856

Meyerson M, Enders GH, Wu CL, Su LK, Gorka C, Nelson C, Harlow E, Tsai LH (1992) A family of human cdc2-related protein kinases. EMBO J 11(8):2909–2917

Mohanakumara P, Sreejayan N, Priti V, Ramesha BT, Ravikanth G, Ganeshaiah KN, Vasudeva R, Mohan J, Santhoshkumar TR, Mishra PD, Ram V, Shaanker RU (2010) Dysoxylum binectariferum Hook.f (Meliaceae), a rich source of rohitukine. Fitoterapia 81(2):145–148. doi:10.1016/j.fitote.2009.08.010

Monaco EA 3rd, Vallano ML (2003) Cyclin-dependent kinase inhibitors: cancer killers to neuronal guardians. Curr Med Chem 10(5):367–379

Moon MJ, Lee SK, Lee JW, Song WK, Kim SW, Kim JI, Cho C, Choi SJ, Kim YC (2006) Synthesis and structure-activity relationships of novel indirubin derivatives as potent anti-proliferative agents with CDK2 inhibitory activities. Bioorg Med Chem 14(1):237–246. doi:S0968-0896(05)00743-1 [pii] 10.1016/j.bmc.2005.08.008

Nguyen MD, Lariviere RC, Julien JP (2001) Deregulation of Cdk5 in a mouse model of ALS: toxicity alleviated by perikaryal neurofilament inclusions. Neuron 30(1):135–147. doi:S0896-6273(01)00268-9 [pii]

Nishi K, Schnier JB, Bradbury EM (1998) The accumulation of cyclin-dependent kinase inhibitor p27kip1 is a primary response to staurosporine and independent of G1 cell cycle arrest. Exp Cell Res 243(2):222–231. doi:S0014-4827(98)94166-0 [pii] 10.1006/excr.1998.4166

Nobelprize.org (17 Sept 2001) Physiology or Medicine for 2001 – Press Release. http://nobelprize.org/nobel_prizes/medicine/laureates/2001/press.html

O'Connor PM (1997) Mammalian G1 and G2 phase checkpoints. Cancer Surv 29:151–182

O'Connor DS, Grossman D, Plescia J, Li F, Zhang H, Villa A, Tognin S, Marchisio PC, Altieri DC (2000) Regulation of apoptosis at cell division by p34cdc2 phosphorylation of survivin. Proc Natl Acad Sci USA 97(24):13103–13107. doi:10.1073/pnas.240390697 240390697 [pii]

Omura S, Iwai Y, Hirano A, Nakagawa A, Awaya J, Tsuchya H, Takahashi Y, Masuma R (1977) A new alkaloid AM-2282 OF Streptomyces origin. Taxonomy, fermentation, isolation and preliminary characterization. J Antibiot (Tokyo) 30(4):275–282

Ortega S, Prieto I, Odajima J, Martin A, Dubus P, Sotillo R, Barbero JL, Malumbres M, Barbacid M (2003) Cyclin-dependent kinase 2 is essential for meiosis but not for mitotic cell division in mice. Nat Genet 35(1):25–31. doi:10.1038/ng1232 ng1232 [pii]

Otth C, Concha II, Arendt T, Stieler J, Schliebs R, Gonzalez-Billault C, Maccioni RB (2002) AbetaPP induces cdk5-dependent tau hyperphosphorylation in transgenic mice Tg2576. J Alzheimers Dis 4(5):417–430

Paglini G, Caceres A (2001) The role of the Cdk5–p35 kinase in neuronal development. Eur J Biochem 268(6):1528–1533. doi:ejb2023 [pii]

Palancade B, Bensaude O (2003) Investigating RNA polymerase II carboxyl-terminal domain (CTD) phosphorylation. Eur J Biochem 270(19):3859–3870. doi:3794 [pii]

Patrick GN, Zukerberg L, Nikolic M, de la Monte S, Dikkes P, Tsai LH (1999) Conversion of p35 to p25 deregulates Cdk5 activity and promotes neurodegeneration. Nature 402(6762):615–622. doi:10.1038/45159

Patzke H, Tsai LH (2002) Calpain-mediated cleavage of the cyclin-dependent kinase-5 activator p39 to p29. J Biol Chem 277(10):8054–8060. doi:10.1074/jbc.M109645200 M109645200 [pii]

Petersen BO, Lukas J, Sorensen CS, Bartek J, Helin K (1999) Phosphorylation of mammalian CDC6 by cyclin A/CDK2 regulates its subcellular localization. EMBO J 18(2):396–410. doi:10.1093/emboj/18.2.396

Phelps MA, Lin TS, Johnson AJ, Hurh E, Rozewski DM, Farley KL, Wu D, Blum KA, Fischer B, Mitchell SM, Moran ME, Brooker-McEldowney M, Heerema NA, Jarjoura D, Schaaf LJ, Byrd JC, Grever MR, Dalton JT (2009) Clinical response and pharmacokinetics from a phase 1 study of an active dosing schedule of flavopiridol in relapsed chronic lymphocytic leukemia. Blood 113(12):2637–2645. doi:blood-2008-07-168583 [pii] 10.1182/blood-2008-07-168583

Ponnusamy K, Petchiammal C, Mohankumar R, Hopper W (2010) In vitro antifungal activity of indirubin isolated from a South Indian ethnomedicinal plant Wrightia tinctoria R. Br. J Ethnopharmacol. doi:S0378-8741(10)00543-X [pii] 10.1016/j.jep. 2010.07.050

Poon RY, Hunter T (1995) Cell regulation. Innocent bystanders or chosen collaborators? Curr Biol 5(11):1243–1247. doi:S0960-9822(95)00248-X [pii]

Popowycz F, Fournet G, Schneider C, Bettayeb K, Ferandin Y, Lamigeon C, Tirado OM, Mateo-Lozano S, Notario V, Colas P, Bernard P, Meijer L, Joseph B (2009) Pyrazolo[1,5-a]-1,3,5-triazine as a purine bioisostere: access to potent cyclin-dependent kinase inhibitor (R)-roscovitine analogue. J Med Chem 52(3):655–663. doi:10.1021/jm801340z 10.1021/jm801340z [pii]

Prelich G (2002) RNA polymerase II carboxy-terminal domain kinases: emerging clues to their function. Eukaryot Cell 1(2):153–162

Rathkopf D, Dickson MA, Feldman DR, Carvajal RD, Shah MA, Wu N, Lefkowitz R, Gonen M, Cane LM, Dials HJ, Winkelmann JL, Bosl GJ, Schwartz GK (2009) Phase I study of flavopiridol with oxaliplatin and fluorouracil/leucovorin in advanced solid tumors. Clin Cancer Res 15(23):7405–7411. doi:1078-0432.CCR-09-1502 [pii] 10.1158/1078-0432.CCR-09-1502

Riabowol K, Draetta G, Brizuela L, Vandre D, Beach D (1989) The cdc2 kinase is a nuclear protein that is essential for mitosis in mammalian cells. Cell 57(3):393–401. doi:0092-8674(89)90914-8 [pii]

Rossi DJ, Londesborough A, Korsisaari N, Pihlak A, Lehtonen E, Henkemeyer M, Makela TP (2001) Inability to enter S phase and defective RNA polymerase II CTD phosphorylation in mice lacking Mat1. EMBO J 20(11):2844–2856. doi:10.1093/emboj/20.11.2844

Rossignol M, Kolb-Cheynel I, Egly JM (1997) Substrate specificity of the cdk-activating kinase (CAK) is altered upon association with TFIIH. EMBO J 16(7):1628–1637. doi:10.1093/emboj/16.7.1628

Rowe J, Greenblatt RJ, Liu D, Moffat JF (2010) Compounds that target host cell proteins prevent varicella-zoster virus replication in culture, ex vivo, and in SCID-Hu mice. Antiviral Res 86(3):276–285. doi:S0166-3542(10)00544-9 [pii] 10.1016/j.antiviral.2010.03.007

Satyanarayana A, Kaldis P (2009) Mammalian cell-cycle regulation: several Cdks, numerous cyclins and diverse compensatory mechanisms. Oncogene 28(33):2925–2939. doi:onc2009170 [pii] 10.1038/onc.2009.170

Schang LM (2005) Advances on cyclin-dependent kinases (CDKs) as novel targets for antiviral drugs. Curr Drug Targets Infect Disord 5(1):29–37

Schnier JB, Nishi K, Goodrich DW, Bradbury EM (1996) G1 arrest and down-regulation of cyclin E/cyclin-dependent kinase 2 by the protein kinase inhibitor staurosporine are dependent on the retinoblastoma protein in the bladder carcinoma cell line 5637. Proc Natl Acad Sci USA 93(12):5941–5946

Schutte B, Nieland L, van Engeland M, Henfling ME, Meijer L, Ramaekers FC (1997) The effect of the cyclin-dependent kinase inhibitor olomoucine on cell cycle kinetics. Exp Cell Res 236(1):4–15. doi:S0014-4827(97)93700-9 [pii] 10.1006/excr.1997.3700

Schwaiberger AV, Heiss EH, Cabaravdic M, Oberan T, Zaujec J, Schachner D, Uhrin P, Atanasov AG, Breuss JM, Binder BR, Dirsch VM (2010) Indirubin-3′-monoxime blocks vascular smooth muscle cell proliferation by inhibition of signal transducer and activator of transcription

3 signaling and reduces neointima formation in vivo. Arterioscler Thromb Vasc Biol. doi:ATVBAHA.110.212654 [pii] 10.1161/ATVBAHA.110.212654

Sedlacek HH, Czech J, Naik R, Kaur G, Worland P, Losiewicz M, Parker B, Carlson B, Smith A, Senderowicz A, Sausville E (1996) Flavopiridol (L86 8275; NSC 649890), a new kinase inhibitor for tumor therapy. Int J Oncol 9(6):1143–1168

Senderowicz AM (1999) Flavopiridol: the first cyclin-dependent kinase inhibitor in human clinical trials. Invest New Drugs 17(3):313–320

Senderowicz AM (2003) Novel small molecule cyclin-dependent kinases modulators in human clinical trials. Cancer Biol Ther 2(4 Suppl 1):S84–S95. doi:206 [pii]

Senderowicz AM, Headlee D, Stinson SF, Lush RM, Kalil N, Villalba L, Hill K, Steinberg SM, Figg WD, Tompkins A, Arbuck SG, Sausville EA (1998) Phase I trial of continuous infusion flavopiridol, a novel cyclin-dependent kinase inhibitor, in patients with refractory neoplasms. J Clin Oncol 16(9):2986–2999

Shapiro GI (2006) Cyclin-dependent kinase pathways as targets for cancer treatment. J Clin Oncol 24(11):1770–1783. doi:24/11/1770 [pii] 10.1200/JCO.2005.03.7689

Sherr CJ (1994) G1 phase progression: cycling on cue. Cell 79(4):551–555. doi:0092-8674(94)90540-1 [pii]

Sherr CJ, Roberts JM (1999) CDK inhibitors: positive and negative regulators of G1-phase progression. Genes Dev 13(12):1501–1512

Shima D, Yugami M, Tatsuno M, Wada T, Yamaguchi Y, Handa H (2003) Mechanism of H-8 inhibition of cyclin-dependent kinase 9: study using inhibitor-immobilized matrices. Genes Cells 8(3):215–223. doi:627 [pii]

Sirri V, Hernandez-Verdun D, Roussel P (2002) Cyclin-dependent kinases govern formation and maintenance of the nucleolus. J Cell Biol 156(6):969–981. doi:10.1083/jcb.200201024 jcb.200201024 [pii]

Solomon MJ, Gautier J, Lee T, Kirschner MW (1991) Control of p34cdc2 activation. Cold Spring Harb Symp Quant Biol 56:427–435

Sroka IM, Heiss EH, Havlicek L, Totzke F, Aristei Y, Pechan P, Kubbutat MH, Strnad M, Dirsch VM (2010) A novel roscovitine derivative potently induces G1-phase arrest in platelet-derived growth factor-BB-activated vascular smooth muscle cells. Mol Pharmacol 77(2):255–261. doi:mol.109.060327 [pii] 10.1124/mol.109.060327

Takahashi I, Kobayashi E, Asano K, Yoshida M, Nakano H (1987) UCN-01, a selective inhibitor of protein kinase C from Streptomyces. J Antibiot (Tokyo) 40(12):1782–1784

Tanaka T, Veeranna OT, Rajan P, Amin ND, Cho A, Sreenath T, Pant HC, Brady RO, Kulkarni AB (2001) Neuronal cyclin-dependent kinase 5 activity is critical for survival. J Neurosci 21(2):550–558. doi:21/2/550 [pii]

Timsit S, Menn B (2007) Cerebral ischemia, cell cycle elements and Cdk5. Biotechnol J 2(8):958–966. doi:10.1002/biot.200700072

Utz I, Hofer S, Regenass U, Hilbe W, Thaler J, Grunicke H, Hofmann J (1994) The protein kinase C inhibitor CGP 41251, a staurosporine derivative with antitumor activity, reverses multidrug resistance. Int J Cancer 57(1):104–110

Vesely J, Havlicek L, Strnad M, Blow JJ, Donella-Deana A, Pinna L, Letham DS, Kato J, Detivaud L, Leclerc S et al (1994) Inhibition of cyclin-dependent kinases by purine analogues. Eur J Biochem 224(2):771–786

Wandl S, Wesierska-Gadek J (2009) Is olomoucine, a weak CDK2 inhibitor, able to induce apoptosis in cancer cells? Ann N Y Acad Sci 1171:242–249. doi:NYAS4700 [pii] 10.1111/j.1749-6632.2009.04700.x

Wang S, Fischer PM (2008) Cyclin-dependent kinase 9: a key transcriptional regulator and potential drug target in oncology, virology and cardiology. Trends Pharmacol Sci 29(6): 302–313. doi:S0165-6147(08)00078-3 [pii] 10.1016/j.tips.2008.03.003

Wang Q, Fan S, Eastman A, Worland PJ, Sausville EA, O'Connor PM (1996) UCN-01: a potent abrogator of G2 checkpoint function in cancer cells with disrupted p53. J Natl Cancer Inst 88(14):956–965

Wang CH, Chou WY, Hung KS, Jawan B, Lu CN, Liu JK, Hung YP, Lee TH (2005) Intrathecal administration of roscovitine inhibits Cdk5 activity and attenuates formalin-induced nociceptive response in rats. Acta Pharmacol Sin 26(1):46–50. doi:APHS007 [pii] 10.1111/j.1745-7254.2005.00007.x

Welch S, Hirte HW, Carey MS, Hotte SJ, Tsao MS, Brown S, Pond GR, Dancey JE, Oza AM (2007) UCN-01 in combination with topotecan in patients with advanced recurrent ovarian cancer: a study of the Princess Margaret Hospital Phase II consortium. Gynecol Oncol 106(2):305–310. doi:S0090-8258(07)00146-1 [pii] 10.1016/j.ygyno.2007.02.018

Wen Y, Shatkin AJ (1999) Transcription elongation factor hSPT5 stimulates mRNA capping. Genes Dev 13(14):1774–1779

Wesierska-Gadek J, Krystof V (2009) Selective cyclin-dependent kinase inhibitors discriminating between cell cycle and transcriptional kinases: future reality or utopia? Ann N Y Acad Sci 1171:228–241. doi:NYAS4726 [pii] 10.1111/j.1749-6632.2009.04726.x

Wesierska-Gadek J, Schmid G (2006) Dual action of the inhibitors of cyclin-dependent kinases: targeting of the cell-cycle progression and activation of wild-type p53 protein. Expert Opin Investig Drugs 15(1):23–38. doi:10.1517/13543784.15.1.23

Wesierska-Gadek J, Gueorguieva M, Horky M (2003) Dual action of cyclin-dependent kinase inhibitors: induction of cell cycle arrest and apoptosis. A comparison of the effects exerted by roscovitine and cisplatin. Pol J Pharmacol 55(5):895–902

Wesierska-Gadek J, Gueorguieva M, Wojciechowski J, Horky M (2004) Cell cycle arrest induced in human breast cancer cells by cyclin-dependent kinase inhibitors: a comparison of the effects exerted by roscovitine and olomoucine. Pol J Pharmacol 56(5):635–641

Wesierska-Gadek J, Gueorguieva M, Horky M (2005) Roscovitine-induced up-regulation of p53AIP1 protein precedes the onset of apoptosis in human MCF-7 breast cancer cells. Mol Cancer Ther 4(1):113–124. doi:4/1/113 [pii]

Wesierska-Gadek J, Gueorguieva M, Kramer MP, Ranftler C, Sarg B, Lindner H (2007a) A new, unexpected action of olomoucine, a CDK inhibitor, on normal human cells: up-regulation of CLIMP-63, a cytoskeleton-linking membrane protein. J Cell Biochem 102(6):1405–1419. doi:10.1002/jcb.21596

Wesierska-Gadek J, Schmitz ML, Ranftler C (2007b) Roscovitine-activated HIP2 kinase induces phosphorylation of wt p53 at Ser-46 in human MCF-7 breast cancer cells. J Cell Biochem 100(4):865–874. doi:10.1002/jcb.21211

Węsierska-Gądek J, Chamrád I, Kryštof V (2009) Novel potent pharmacological cyclin-dependent kinase inhibitors. Future Med Chem 1(9):1561–1581. doi:10.4155/fmc.09.110

Wesierska-Gadek J, Maurer M, Zulehner N, Komina O (2011) Whether to target single or multiple CDKs for therapy? That is the question. J Cell Physiol. doi:10.1002/jcp.22426

Whittaker SR, Walton MI, Garrett MD, Workman P (2004) The Cyclin-dependent kinase inhibitor CYC202 (R-roscovitine) inhibits retinoblastoma protein phosphorylation, causes loss of Cyclin D1, and activates the mitogen-activated protein kinase pathway. Cancer Res 64(1):262–272

Wojciechowski J, Horky M, Gueorguieva M, Wesierska-Gadek J (2003) Rapid onset of nucleolar disintegration preceding cell cycle arrest in roscovitine-induced apoptosis of human MCF-7 breast cancer cells. Int J Cancer 106(4):486–495. doi:10.1002/ijc.11290

Worland PJ, Kaur G, Stetler-Stevenson M, Sebers S, Sartor O, Sausville EA (1993) Alteration of the phosphorylation state of p34cdc2 kinase by the flavone L86-8275 in breast carcinoma cells. Correlation with decreased H1 kinase activity. Biochem Pharmacol 46(10):1831–1840. doi:0006-2952(93)90590-S [pii]

Yadav HN, Singh M, Sharma PL (2010) Involvement of GSK-3beta in attenuation of the cardio-protective effect of ischemic preconditioning in diabetic rat heart. Mol Cell Biochem 343(1–2):75–81. doi:10.1007/s11010-010-0500-z

Yang X, Zhao X, Phelps MA, Piao L, Rozewski DM, Liu Q, Lee LJ, Marcucci G, Grever MR, Byrd JC, Dalton JT, Lee RJ (2009) A novel liposomal formulation of flavopiridol. Int J Pharm 365(1–2):170–174. doi:S0378-5173(08)00552-8 [pii] 10.1016/j.ijpharm.2008.08.008

Yankulov KY, Bentley DL (1997) Regulation of CDK7 substrate specificity by MAT1 and TFIIH. EMBO J 16(7):1638–1646. doi:10.1093/emboj/16.7.1638

Yarotskyy V, Gao G, Du L, Ganapathi SB, Peterson BZ, Elmslie KS (2010) Roscovitine binds to novel L-channel (CaV1.2) sites that separately affect activation and inactivation. J Biol Chem 285(1):43–53. doi:M109.076448 [pii] 10.1074/jbc.M109.076448

Zahler S, Liebl J, Furst R, Vollmar AM (2010) Anti-angiogenic potential of small molecular inhibitors of cyclin dependent kinases in vitro. Angiogenesis 13(3):239–249. doi:10.1007/s10456-010-9181-1

Chapter 15
Plant-Derived Isoprenoids Mediate Regulation of mTOR Signaling in Tumor Cells

Dennis M. Peffley and Patricia Hentosh

Abstract It is widely recognized that metabolites derived from plants behave as preemptive nutrients that provide cytoprotection or modify disease risk through processes regulating gene expression at the levels of transcription, DNA methylation as well as formation or bioactivation of proteins. In contrast, lipid-related terpenes, commonly referred to as isoprenoids, are bioactive secondary products of plant mevalonate metabolism that modulate mammalian cell growth, survival, differentiation and autophagic cell death through their effects on gene expression at the level of mRNA translation via the mammalian target of rapamycin (mTOR) pathway. Early findings from our laboratory established that isoprenoids such as perillyl alcohol suppressed 3-hydroxy-methylglutaryl coenzyme A (HMG-CoA) reductase, the rate-limiting enzyme of mevalonate/cholesterol biosynthesis, through a mechanism regulating mRNA translational efficiency. Additionally, our studies found that perillyl alcohol suppressed 4E-BP1 phosphorylation in tumor cells via the mTOR pathway, and disrupted the m^7GpppX mRNA cap binding complex, eIF4F, by suppressing interaction of eukaryotic initiation factor 4E (eIF4E) with eIF4G. Furthermore, isoprenoids exhibit certain rapamycin-like inhibitory effects on the rapamycin-sensitive mTORC1 complex, but also have distinct effects on the rapamycin-insensitive TSC1/2-mediated regulation of mTOR signaling. Overall, these effects on mTOR signaling suppress cap-dependent protein translation and set-up conditions for cap-independent translation that in part mediate isoprenoid-induced tumor cell death through a caspase-independent mechanism similar to autophagy. Additionally, other studies have reported that polyphenols, flavonoids and triterpenes induced cell death through a similar mechanism.

D.M. Peffley, Ph.D. (✉)
Department of Biochemistry, Edward Via College of Osteopathic Medicine,
350 Howard Street, Spartonburg, SC 29303, USA
e-mail: dpeffley@corolinas.vcom.edu

P. Hentosh
Medical Laboratory and Radiation Sciences Department, College of Health Sciences,
Old Dominion University, 4608 Hampton Blvd, Norfolk, VA 23509, USA

M. Diederich and K. Noworyta (eds.), *Natural Compounds as Inducers of Cell Death: Volume 1*, DOI 10.1007/978-94-007-4575-9_15,

15.1 The Role of Isoprenoids as Dietary/Nutritional Factors in Cancer Prevention and Treatment

Epidemiological findings have shown a lower risk for a number of cancers among populations that consume large amounts of plant foods (Gullett et al. 2010) A large body of evidence indicates that anutrients (non-nutrient phytochemicals) such as anti-oxidants, dithiothriones, phenols, indoles, flavonoids, protease inhibitors and allium compounds can either block or suppress carcinogenic processes (Guilford and Pezzuto 2008; Khan et al. 2008; Gullett et al. 2010; Mehta et al. 2010). Lipid-related terpenes (commonly called isoprenoids) found in fruits and vegetables represent secondary products of plant mevalonate metabolism. The ~25,000 plant isoprenoids differ in size, complexity and function and have been widely recognized for their cancer preventive and treatment capability. Some are "pure" isoprenoids of varying structures but consisting only of multiples of the five-carbon isoprene unit (see Fig. 15.1 for examples and structures). "Mixed" isoprenoids comprise the isoflavones

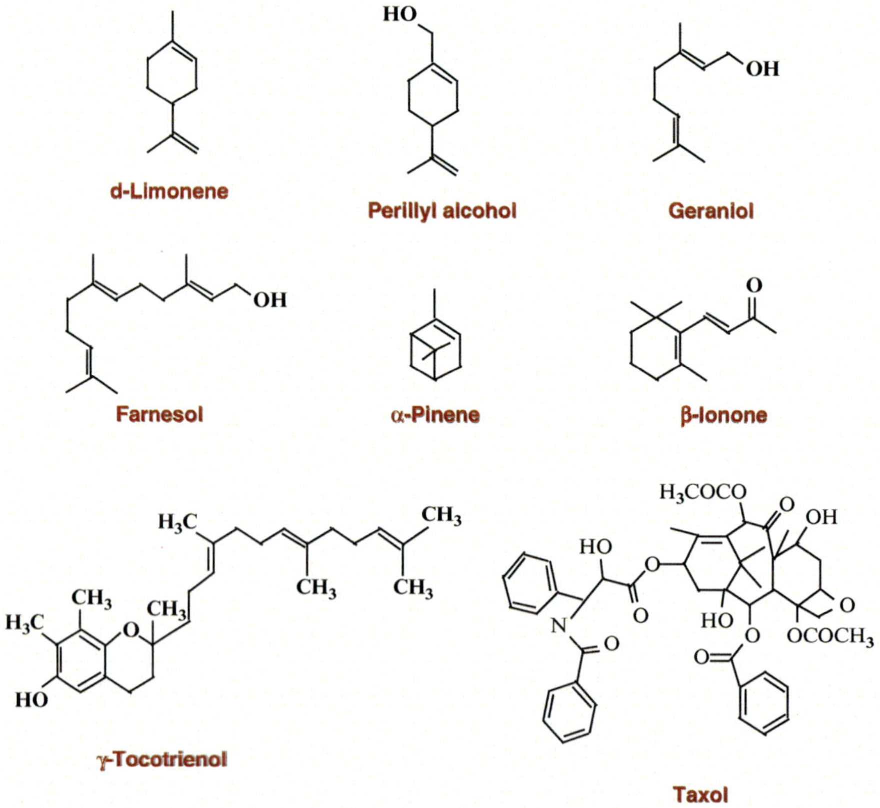

Fig. 15.1 Representative structures of pure and mixed isoprenoids

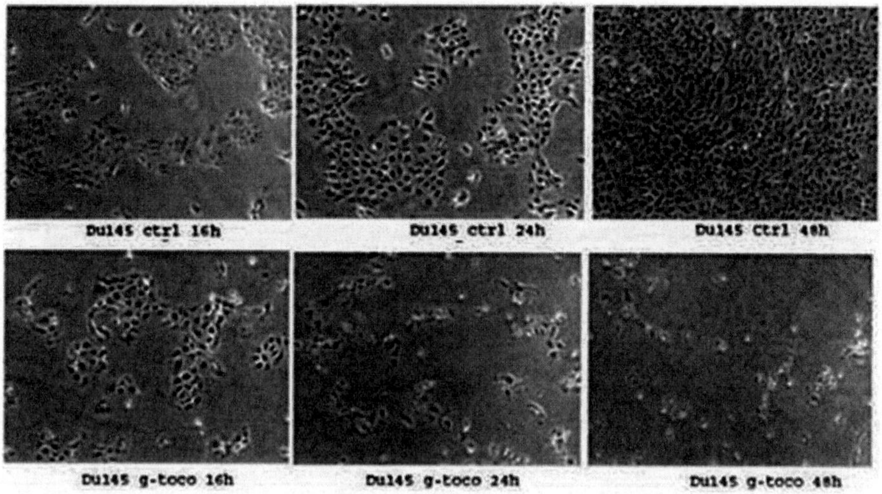

Fig. 15.2 Isoprenoid-mediated suppression of cell growth. DU145 prostate tumor cells were treated with 20 μM γ-tocotrienol for the times indicated. Note the marked suppression of cell growth at 24 and 48 h

(genistein), prenylated coumarins, flavones, flavanols, chalcones, quinones, and chromanols, each with only a part of the molecule derived via the mevalonate pathway.

Numerous studies have established the anti-tumorigenic properties of pure isoprenoids. Limonene, perillyl alcohol, γ-tocotrienol, β-ionone and farnesol all initiate apoptosis and concomitantly arrest tumor cells in the G1 phase of the cell cycle (Gould 1997; Elson et al. 1999; Mo and Elson 1999; Yu et al. 1999; McIntyre et al. 2000; Nesaretnam et al. 2000). Tocotrienols are especially effective at inhibiting growth of both murine and human breast cancer cells in culture (Aggarwal et al. 2010; Hsieh et al. 2010; Park et al. 2010) as well as human prostate tumor cells (Fig. 15.2). Numerous groups have demonstrated that pure and mixed isoprenoids suppress growth of a vast number of whole animal tumor models including implanted leukemic cells, melanomas, pancreatic tumors and hepatomas (Gould 1997; Elson et al. 1999; Rabi and Bishayee 2009; Aggarwal et al. 2010). Topical perillyl alcohol inhibited the development of squamous cell carcinomas and inhibited UVB-induced activator protein-1 activation (Barthelman et al. 1998). Additionally, topical administration of perillyl alcohol significantly reduced 7,12-dimethylbenz(a)antracene-induced melanoma formation in an in vivo murine mouse model, suggesting that perillyl alcohol has chemopreventive properties for melanoma (Lluria-Prevatt et al. 2002). In mouse tumor models, the incidence of isoprenoid-related toxic side effects is small if any (Mo et al. 1999). Moreover, perillyl alcohol has been tested in clinical studies against a number of solid tumors (Hudes et al. 2000; Ripple et al. 2000). A Phase 2a study of topically applied perillyl alcohol cream demonstrated that perillyl alcohol was effective in reversing actinic damage in patients with sun-damaged skin, further supporting the efficacy of perillyl alcohol as a chemopreventive for skin cancer (Stratton et al. 2010). The main toxicities in patients are minimal and include primarily gastrointestinal effects (Ripple et al. 1998, 2000; Hudes et al. 2000). The mechanisms of isoprenoid-mediated suppression of tumor growth are unclear. Possible sites of action include inhibition of protein isoprenylation including small G proteins such as p21ras, and other member of the ras family that modulate signal transduction (Crowell et al. 1991; Ren et al. 1997; Stayrook et al. 1998). Perillyl alcohol induces expression of transforming growth factor beta and the mannose 6-phosphate/insulin-like growth factor II receptor (Ariazi et al. 1999), an effect associated with attenuated response to growth factors.

15.2 Role of Phytochemicals as Bioactive Nutritional Factors in Modulating Gene Expression

Lipophilic isoprenoids function through a process of nutritional preemption, whereby they act as either cytoprotectors or modifiers of disease risk by regulating signal transduction processes that control gene expression (nutrigenomics). The advent of various advanced molecular techniques in genomics and proteomics has permitted identification of specific processes and genes modified by various plant metabolites. An early study by Ariazi et al. (Ariazi and Gould 1996) using subtractive display identified 42 monoterpene-induced genes and 58 monoterpene-repressed genes in perillyl alcohol-treated rat mammary carcinoma. Overall, this initial study demonstrated that monoterpene-induced/repressed genes act in concert to regulate carcinogenesis through differentiation and cell death (Ariazi and Gould 1996). A later study by Berchtold et al. (Berchtold et al. 2005) determined that perillyl alcohol decreased cellular calcium levels, rapidly decreased NF-κB DNA-binding activity and concomitantly repressed expression of NF-κB target genes in B lymphoma cells. These results indicated that perillyl alcohol suppresses the ability of NF-κB to modulate gene expression in lymphoma cells and affects cell survival (Berchtold et al. 2005). More recently, a proteomic study on perillyl alcohol-treated glioblastoma cells has provided a compelling look into effects of this terpene on a tumorigenic proteome (Fischer Jde et al. 2010). Cells were exposed for periods of time ranging from 1 min to 24 h after which a semi-quantitative proteomic analysis was employed. More than 4,000 proteins were identified and linked to Ras signaling, tissue homeostasis, induction of apoptosis, metallopeptidase activity, and ubiquitin-protein ligase activity (Fischer Jde et al. 2010).

Terpenes such as perillyl alcohol have profound cytostatic and cytotoxic effects on tumor cells and multiple reports indicate that perillyl alcohol also induces apoptosis in a variety of cell lines that include lung (Xu et al. 2004; Yeruva et al. 2007), leukocyte (Clark 2006), prostate (Chung et al. 2006), and breast (Yuri et al. 2004). However, as discussed below, we have observed that perillyl alcohol induces a caspase-independent cell death in human prostate tumor cells that closely resembles autophagy. Cytostatic effects from perillyl alcohol are linked in part to cell cycle arrest mediated via either p21Cip1 and p27Kip1 as reported by Wiseman et al. in pancreatic adenocarcinoma cells (Wiseman et al. 2007). Similarly, studies from our

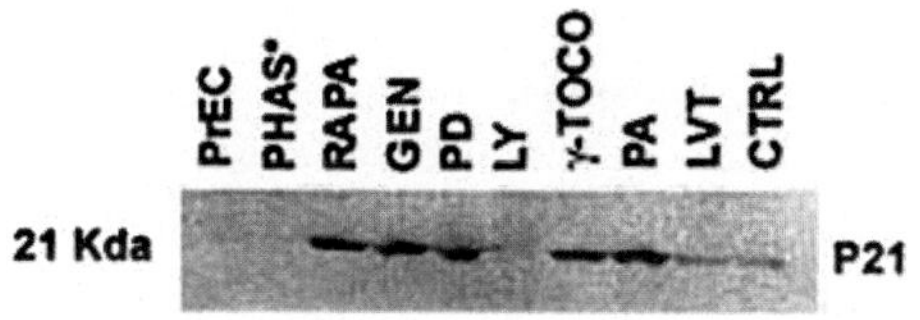

Fig. 15.3 Western blot showing effects of isoprenoids, genistein or LVT on p21 levels in DU145 prostate tumor cells. Cells were treated with perillyl alcohol (*PA*), lovastatin (*LVT*), the PI3 kinase inhibitor LY 94002 (*LY*) or genistein (*GEN*) as described. Treatment with Tocotrienol (*TOCO*, 20 μM) or the MEK1 inhibitor, PD098059 (*PD*, 50 μM) was for 16 h. Rapamycin (*RAPA*) was used at 10 nM for 4 h . Cell lysis, electrophoresis and immunodetection with a p21 specific antibody were conducted as described by Peffley et al. (2007). *PrEC* Normal human prostate epithelial cells, PHAS (4E-BP) was loaded as a control for antibody specificity

laboratory on human prostate tumor PC3 cells show robust induction of p21Cip1 in response to perillyl alcohol treatment (Fig. 15.3).

Epidemiological studies have also suggested that the structurally-related isoprenoid-related isoflavones, in particular genistein and daidzein, may provide chemopreventive effects against hormone-related cancers (Fournier et al. 1998). An antiproliferative effect of genistein has been demonstrated against a wide variety of tumor cells including breast cancer (Pagliacci et al. 1994), leukemia and lymphoma (Spinozzi et al. 1994), melanoma (Constantinou and Huberman 1995), lung cancer, and head and neck squamous carcinoma (Alhasan et al. 2001). Soy extracts rich in genistein suppress transplanted and chemically-induced prostate cancer cells in rodents (Makela et al. 1995; Pollard and Luckert 1997). The molecular effects of genistein are multifaceted and include inhibition of tyrosine protein kinases (Adlercreutz 1990), topoisomerases I and II (Okura et al. 1988), 5α-reductase (Hiipakka et al. 2002), and protein histidine kinase (Huang et al. 1992) as well as suppression of angiogenesis, growth factor-stimulated responses, oncogene activity, and prostaglandin synthesis. Genistein also induces a G2/M cell cycle arrest, which in turn suppresses cell growth (Matsukawa et al. 1993). Other effects include downregulation of cyclin B and upregulation of the growth-inhibitory protein p21WAF1 (Davis et al. 1998). Treatment of the androgen-responsive prostate tumor cell line, LNCaP, with genistein concentrations above 20 μM induces apoptosis, a response most likely associated with increased p21WAF1 expression (Shen et al. 2000). Overall, reports have shown that genistein can inhibit growth of human prostate cancer cells in culture, but generally at supraphysiological concentrations (>50 μmol) (Zhou et al. 1999). More recent studies have shown that genistein protects cells from oxidative stress by suppressing nuclear factor-kappa B activation and decreasing DNA adduct level in healthy volunteers (Davis et al. 2001). A study by Handayani et al. (Handayani et al. 2006) using DNA microarrays demonstrated that genistein and daidzein upregulated 28 genes and downregulated 47 genes. Those significantly reduced included IL-8, matrix metalloproteinase 13, inhibin beta A, follistatin and fibronectin, which are involved in modulation of cell cycle progression, metastasis and angiogenesis. Conversely, the expression of p21Cip1, a cell cycle inhibitor, was increased significantly. Genistein also has a role in modifying obesity via effects on hepatic gene expression. Mice fed a high fat diet developed abnormal lipid profiles and accumulated visceral fat compared to low fat diet fed mice. Genistein supplementation improved lipid profiles and attenuated increased visceral fat accumulation in those mice. Microarray gene expression analysis showed that 97 genes were altered in mice on the high fat diet; genistein normalized 84 of these genes. Thus, genistein modified gene expression patterns that underlie maintenance of the obesity phenotype (Kim et al. 2005).

An alternative mechanism of cytoprotection provided by nutritional factors has been postulated for isothiocyanates found in broccoli, turnips and watercress as well as phenolic compounds such as epigallocatechin-3-gallate from green tea, curcumin and resveratrol from grapes. These phytochemicals are thought to generate cellular stress and activate phase II detoxifying/antioxidant enzymes (Nair et al. 2007). Such agents modulate levels of reactive oxygen species (ROS) in cells, which act as second messengers in the activation of several signaling pathways leading to mitogenesis or apoptosis (Forman et al. 2002; Trachootham et al. 2006). The change in redox status is sensed by redox-sensitive transcription factors such as nuclear factor-E2-related factor 2 (Nrf2), AP-1, and NF-kappa B, which in turn modulate gene expression responses via sulfhydryl modification of specific cysteine residues found on proteins involved in signal transduction (Nair et al. 2007).

15.3 Impact of Isoprenoids on Mevalonate Regulation in Tumor Cells

In plants, both pure and mixed isoprenoids function in growth regulation, in host defense systems against insects and act as chemoattractants. In mammalian cells, many isoprenoid products derived from mevalonate via the cholesterol biosynthetic pathway—ubiquinone, dolichol, isopentenyl tRNA, farnesyl and geranylgeranyl for protein isoprenylation, and cholesterol—are essential for cell growth, for maintenance of cholesterol homeostasis, and for posttranslational modification and biological activity of more than 50 proteins including the Ras family of proteins, nuclear lamins A and B, and growth factor receptors (Coleman et al. 1997; Mo et al. 1999). A finely tuned metabolic feedback mechanism involving transcriptional and post-transcriptional input maintains the pool of mevalonate pathway intermediates mentioned above that are important for normal cell survival and homeostasis.

The major rate-limiting enzyme of the mevalonate/cholesterol pathway in mammalian cells is 3-hydroxy-3-methylglutaryl coenzyme A (HMG-CoA) reductase. HMG-CoA reductase is subject to negative feedback inhibition by both cholesterol and oxysterols as well as by isoprenoid or non-sterol mevalonate-derived metabolic intermediates (DeBose-Boyd 2008), and is highly regulated at transcriptional (Espenshade and Hughes 2007), translational (posttranscriptional) (Buechler and Peffley 2004) and posttranslational levels (Goldstein and Brown 1990; Peffley 1992; Correll and Edwards 1994; Correll et al. 1994; Peffley and Gayen 1997, 2003; Peffley et al. 1998).

The mevalonate pathway provides many small signaling molecules that trigger cellular events including proliferation and death (Prendergast et al. 1995; Lebowitz et al. 1997; Lebowitz and Prendergast 1998; Ghosh et al. 1999; Zerial and McBride 2001). Farnesyl-PP and geranylgeranyl-PP intermediates of the cholesterol pathway are important lipid post-translational modifications for protein activity (Liao 2002). The Ras, Rab, Rac and Rho family of small GTP-binding proteins is an important regulator of signaling, vesicle trafficking, exocytosis and cytoskeletal organization in eukaryotic cells (Martinez and Goud 1998; Haluska et al. 2002). Such proteins have a farnesylation or geranylgeranylation moiety near or at the carboxyl terminus that functions in anchoring or tethering vesicles to an acceptor membrane. Prenylation is also important in both protein:protein and protein:lipid interactions (Poon et al. 1995). For example, prenylation of RhoB is required for its cell transforming function (Huang and Prendergast 2006). Additionally, the Ser/Thr kinase Raf, a key mediator in cellular signaling, has a CAAX sequence at its carboxy terminus (Lebowitz et al. 1997); farnesylation may have a role in its association with cholesterol-rich caveolae domains in the cell membrane (Hekman et al. 2002). Further, Rubio et al. (1997) demonstrated that p21Ras farnesylation was essential for its interaction with phosphatidylinositol (PI) 3-kinase gamma.

Tumor cell growth and survival are highly reliant on attenuation of sterol-mediated reductase gene regulation, a phenomenon referred to as sterol-independent regulation of reductase. As a consequence, reductase mRNA levels are elevated in many tumor cell lines (Engstrom and Schofield 1987; Azrolan and Coleman 1989; Hentosh et al. 2001), and translational efficiency of these transcripts is increased to ensure adequate isoprenoid production in a sterol-rich environment (Fritz et al. 1998).

15.4 Isoprenoid-Mediated Effects on HMG-CoA Reductase Regulation

The Peffley laboratory was the first to identify that exogenously added dietary monoterpenes to cultured cells modulated HMG-CoA reductase gene expression by attenuating the translational efficiency of reductase transcripts (Table 15.1). Specifically, with limonene and perillyl alcohol treatment, reductase synthesis was reduced by 70% and 80%, respectively compared to control or lovastatin-treated cells, but no such corresponding decrease in reductase mRNA levels was observed. The discrepancy between changes in reductase synthesis and mRNA levels is referred to as a translational effect on mRNA efficiency mediated by these isoprenoids. Additionally, these monoterpenes did not enhance HMG-CoA reductase degradation, as was the case with mevalonate treatment (Table 15.1). Therefore, these plant-derived isoprenoids cannot mimic the effects of endogenously-derived isoprenoid intermediates from the cholesterol biosynthetic pathways required to initiate binding of reductase to endoplasmic reticulum membrane Insig-1 and –2 proteins and subsequent ubiquination of reductase (Jo and Debose-Boyd 2010). Further, the lack of mRNA suppression indicates that limonene and perillyl alcohol do not activate

Table 15.1 Summary: Effects of isoprenoids on reductase synthesis and mRNA levels

Treatment	Rate of synthesis (%)	mRNA Levels	Half-life (h)
Lovastatin	100 ± 15	100 ± 5%	10.0
Lovastatin + Mevalonate (10 mM)	35 ± 5	34 ± 3%	4.0
Lovastatin + limonene (5 mM)	30 ± 6	115 ± 7%	10.5
Lovastatin + perillyl OH (0.7 mM)	11 ± 3	112 ± 5%	16.0
Lovastatin + geraniol (0.4 mM)	1.4 ± .3	34 ± 6%	9.6

Rates of HMG-CoA reductase synthesis are based on the dpm of ^{35}S-labeled immunoprecipitable HMG-CoA reductase after a 1 h labeling period. Rates of HMG-CoA reductase synthesis in lovastatin-treated cells were set at 100% and all other values are reported as a percentage of this value

HMG-CoA reductase mRNA values were determined by ribonuclease protection assay and corrected for RNA loading effects on the basis of the amount of ribosomal (RP) S17 mRNA. Corrected HMG-CoA reductase RNA values in lovastatin-treated cells were set at 100% and all other values are reported as a percentage of this value

To assess HMG-CoA reductase degradation, cells were labeled in the presence of lovastatin and the ^{35}S-labeled HMG-CoA reductase immuniprecipitated at various time points after addition of mevalonate, limonene, perillyl alcohol, or geraniol. ^{35}S-labeled HMG-CoA reductase was immunoprecipitated and quantitated as described by Peffley and Gayen (2003)

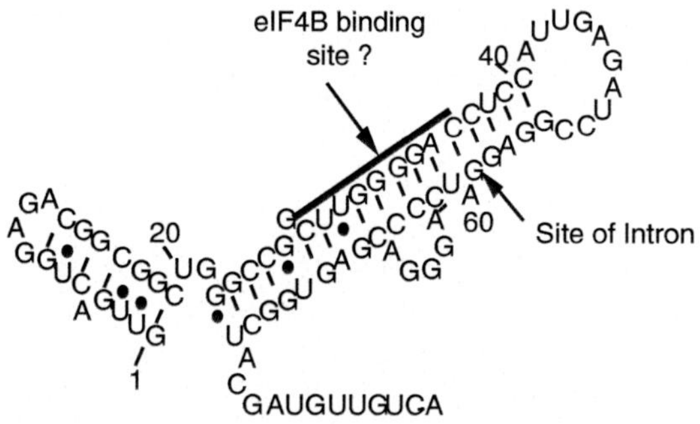

Fig. 15.4 Putative secondary structure of the HMG-CoA reductase 5′ untranslated leader (UTL): Using an M-fold software program, a computer predicted stem loop was generated from the GC-rich UTL of the reductase 5′end. The loop contains a potential binding site for eIF4B, which may alter the loop's stability

SREBP cleavage proteases required for cleavage and transposition of SREBP into the nucleus and subsequent binding to the sterol regulatory element binding protein (SREBP) (Sato 2010). An exception to the above findings was treatment with the acyclic monoterpene, geraniol, in which reductase mRNA levels were reduced by 66% suggesting that this isoprenoid exhibited transcriptional regulatory properties similar to those characteristic of side chain sterols.

15.5 Translational Control Mechanisms

Regulation of translation occurs at the level of both initiation (Kozak 2001a, b, c, 2005; von der Haar et al. 2004; Piccinelli and Samuelsson 2007), and elongation of protein synthesis (Fernandez et al. 2005; Le Sourd et al. 2006), and all reported mechanisms depend on specific sequences and structural features of RNA transcripts, especially 5′-untranslated leader (**5-UTL**) (Pelletier et al. 1991; Gayen and Peffley 1995; Fritz et al. 1998; De Gregorio et al. 2001; Fernandez et al. 2001; Wilkie et al. 2003; Buechler and Peffley 2004; Origanti and Shantz 2007) and 3′ untranslated (**3′-UT**) sequences (Choi and Peffley 1995; Izquierdo and Cuezva 2000; Cao and Richter 2002; Espel 2005; Kozak 2005; Komarova et al. 2006; van den Beucken et al. 2006; Halaby and Yang 2007). In addition, specific protein interactions with such RNA sequences have a role in translational control (van der Velden and Thomas 1999; Kozak 2005; Morley et al. 2005; Vary et al. 2005; Lee and Jeong 2006; van den Beucken et al. 2006; Halaby and Yang 2007).

The 5′-UTL for HMG-CoA reductase is heterogeneous in length, GC-rich, and exhibits the potential to form stable secondary structures (Reynolds et al. 1985; Babendure et al. 2006; Kozak 2007) (Fig. 15.4). Secondary structure associated with 5′UTLs attenuates translation initiation, and efficient translation of these mRNA sequences is regulated through cellular levels of the m7GpppX cap binding protein, eukaryotic initiation factor 4E (eIF4E) (Svitkin et al. 2005; Van Der Kelen et al. 2009). eIF4E is the rate limiting translation initiation factor and is part of the cap-binding complex, eIF4F, along with eIF4A and eIF4G (Lawrence et al. 1997; Mamane et al. 2004).

The relationship between cellular eIF4E levels and translational control of HMG-CoA reductase was demonstrated in a study by Buechler and Peffley in which eIF4E over-expression in Chinese Hamster Ovary cells attenuated mevalonate-mediated suppression of HMG-CoA reductase synthesis (Buechler and Peffley 2004). Specifically, over-expression of eIF4E increased HMG-CoA reductase protein levels fivefold compared to control cells, with no concomitant elevation in reductase mRNA levels. This effect was specific for HMG-CoA reductase because general cellular protein synthesis was only increased by 15% in eIF4E over-expressing cells. Additionally, rapamycin, an inhibitor of the mammalian target of rapamycin (mTOR), suppressed HMG-CoA reductase significantly in lovastatin-treated cells (Buechler and Peffley 2004). These results linked regulation of HMG-CoA reductase mRNA translation to the PI3K/Akt/mTOR/4E-BP1 signaling pathway and as discussed below, this discovery was crucial in determining the mechanism of action for terpene-mediated suppression of HMG-CoA reductase synthesis (Sonenberg and Hinnebusch 2009; Van Der Kelen et al. 2009).

15.6 Isoprenoid-Mediated Effects on mTOR Signaling

In quiescent cells, most eIF4E is associated with its inhibitor, 4E-BP1 (Abraham and Gibbons 2007). In response to mitogenic stimulation, 4E-BP1 becomes heavily phosphorylated via the phosphatidylinositol 3-kinase related kinase family of kinases (PIKK), mTOR, and releases eIF4E (Averous and Proud 2006). The upstream sequence of effector proteins for mTOR includes PTEN, PI3 kinase, PDK1, and Akt/PKB (Corradetti and Guan 2006). Release of eIF4E results in a small increase for basal protein synthesis, but a markedly greater stimulation of translation from specific mRNAs, especially those coding for growth promoting factors such as ornithine decarboxylase (Shantz 2004; Origanti and Shantz 2007), cyclin D1 (Graff and Zimmer 2003; Mamane et al. 2004), vascular endothelial growth factor (Goldson et al. 2007), ribonucleotide reductase (Abid et al. 1999) as well as HMG-CoA reductase (Buechler and Peffley 2004). The above mRNAs have as a common feature 5′-UTL sequences that are GC-rich with extensive 2° structure (Kozak 2005).

Specific translational regulation also occurs via mTOR-mediated phosphorylation of p70 ribosomal S6 kinase (p70S6 kinase) (Corradetti and Guan 2006). Phosphorylated p70S6 kinase dissociates from eIF3 and phosphorylates ribosomal protein S6 as well as eIF4B, which assists the eIF4F complex in translation initiation and increases translation of mRNAs with 5′ terminal oligopyrimidine tract sequences (5′TOP) (Holz et al. 2005). Examples of proteins coded by TOP mRNAs include components of the translational apparatus – ribosomal proteins, elongation factors eEF1A and eEF2, and poly (A)-binding protein (Stolovich et al. 2002). It was previously

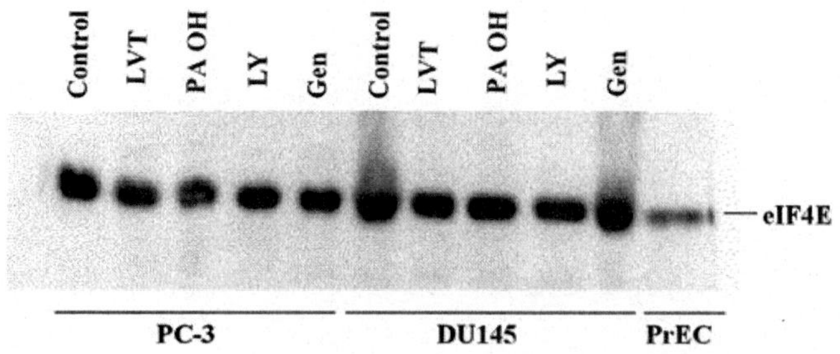

Fig. 15.5 Western blot analysis of eIF4E levels in PC-3, DU145, and normal PrEC cells treated with lovastatin (*Lvt*, 1 μM for 16 h), perillyl alcohol (*PA OH*; 400 μM for 16 h), genistein (*Gen*; 40 μM for 4 h), or LY 294002 (*LY* [PI3 kinase inhibitor]; 10 μM for 4 h). Cells were lysed and protein extracts quantitated. Aliquots (100 μg) were electrophoresed and transferred to PVDF membranes; eIF4E levels were detected with a eIF4E-specific antibody by chemoluminescence using a Kodak Image Station

thought that p70S6 kinase increased translation of mRNAs with 5′TOP sequences (Lawrence and Abraham 1997), but Stolovich et al. (2002) reported that mTOR regulates translation of these mRNAs through a mechanism independent of p70S6 kinase and S6 ribosomal protein.

Mitogenic activation of cell proliferation can also phosphorylate eIF4E, the significance of which is under debate although it has been associated with modulation of ornithine decarboxylase mRNA IRES-mediated translation (Shantz 2004; Origanti and Shantz 2007). eIF4E phosphorylation is mediated in vivo through the protein kinase mitogen- and stress-activated kinase, Mnk1 (Waskiewicz et al. 1999). Tumorigenic cell lines characteristically express high eIF4E levels (Fig. 15.5) compared to normal counterparts where it behaves as a proto-oncogene (DeFatta et al. 1999, 2000, 2002; Berkel et al. 2001; Li et al. 2002; Defatta and De Benedetti 2003; Thornton et al. 2003; Chen et al. 2004; De Benedetti and Graff 2004; Byrnes et al. 2006; Salehi and Mashayekhi 2006; Trachootham et al. 2006).

mTOR is a protein of ~289 kDA also belongs to the PIKK family (Corradetti and Guan 2006); but when purified by gel filtration, it exists as a large multi-protein complex 1.5–2 MDa (Hekman et al. 2002). The mTOR sequence has domains—HEAT repeats, focal adhesion targeting domain, FRB domain, kinase domain and a focal adhesion targeting C-terminal domain—that can form complexes with other proteins, although the nature and extent of these binding partners remain unclear (Levy et al. 1991; Chiu et al. 1994; Corradetti and Guan 2006).

In mammals, there is one TOR protein that exists in two functional complexes–mTORC1 and mTORC2 (Corradetti and Guan 2006). mTORC1 is inhibited by rapamycin, a process that is mediated by binding of a rapamycin-FKBP12 complex (Chiu et al. 1994; Corradetti and Guan 2006). Conversely, mTORC2 excludes binding of the rapamycin-FKBP12 complex and is resistant to rapamycin-mediated inhibition (Inoki and Guan 2006). mTORC1 complexes with the proteins mLST8 (or GβL) and Raptor (regulatory-associated protein of mTOR); this complex primarily regulates translation and cell proliferation in response to mitogenic stimuli (Sarbassov et al. 2005;

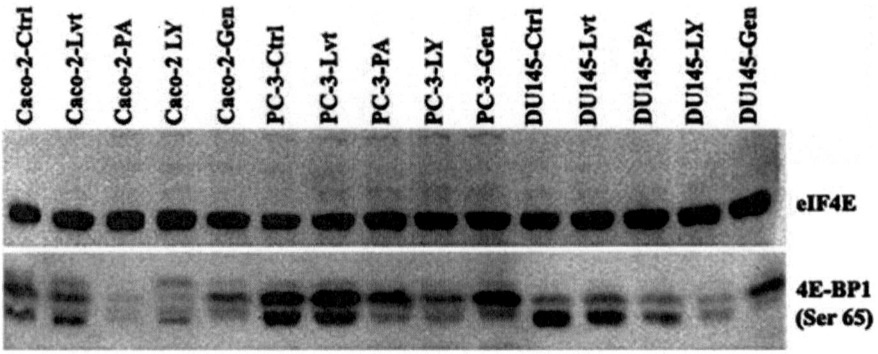

Fig. 15.6 Effects of perillyl alcohol and genistein on 4E-BP phosphorylation. PC-3, DU145 and CaCo2 cells were plated in RPMI plus 10% FBS and cells allowed to grow for 24 h. Medium was supplemented with lovastatin (*Lvt*, 1 μM for 16 h), perillyl alcohol (*PA*; 400 μM for 16 h), genistein (*Gen*; 40 μM for 4 h), or the PI3 kinase inhibitor LY 294002 (*LY*; 10 μM for 4 h). Cells were lysed in RIPA buffer and protein extracts quantitated. Aliquots (100 μg) were electrophoresed and transferred to PVDF membranes. Phospho-4E-BP1 (Ser65) was detected using an antibody specific for phospho-Ser65 (Cell Signaling). Specific proteins were detected by ECL using a Kodak Image Station. *Ctrl* Untreated control cells. Reprinted with permission from Elsevier (Peffley et al. 2007)

Corradetti and Guan 2006). The mTORC2 complex is also associated with mLST8 but differs from mTORC2 by binding Rictor (rapamycin-insensitive companion of mTOR) (Sarbassov et al. 2005; Inoki and Guan 2006). The function of mTORC2 is to control actin cytoskeleton dynamics, cell morphology and cell adhesion (Kim et al. 2003; Sarbassov et al. 2005). The mTORC1 component Raptor binds to 4E-BP1 and p70S6 kinase 1 and facilitates their phosphorylation (Sumitani et al. 2002). Conversely, Rictor in the rapamycin-insensitive mTORC2 complex functions to direct activity away from 4E-BP1 and p70S6 kinase 1 and facilitates activation of Akt/PKB (Sarbassov et al. 2004, 2005, 2006). The protein component mLST8 is common to both complexes and enhances mTORC1 kinase activity towards 4E-BP1 and S6 kinase 1 as well as facilitating the role of mTORC2 in actin polymerization and cell spreading (Kim et al. 2003; Jacinto et al. 2004).

The Peffley laboratory recently established that perillyl alcohol, γ-tocotrienol and genistein differentially impact m^7GpppX cap-dependent translation in human prostate tumor cell lines via effects on the PI3 kinase/Akt/PKB/mTOR cascade (Peffley et al. 2007). Specifically, our experiments found that perillyl alcohol and genistein suppressed 4E-BP1(Ser65) phosphorylation in prostate tumor cell lines, DU145 and PC-3, and in Caco2 adenocarcinoma cells (Fig. 15.6). Suppressive effects were similar to or greater than that observed with a PI3 kinase inhibitor or rapamycin, an mTOR inhibitor (Fig. 15.7). Phosphorylation of 4E-BP1(Thr37) was also reduced by perillyl alcohol and genistein in DU145 cells (Fig. 15.8). Our results are significant because they provide a mechanism of action for terpenes on the mTOR-4E-BP1 pathway and cap-dependent translation. Because terpenes reduce 4E-BP1 phosphorylation leading to eIF4E sequestering on 4E-BP1, cap-dependent translation is suppressed. Support for a link between terpenes and HMG-CoA reductase translation is further provided by the observation that perillyl alcohol

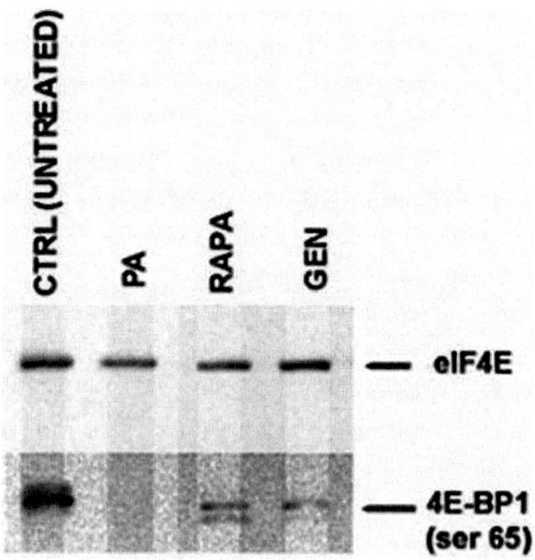

Fig. 15.7 Western blot comparing the effects of perillyl alcohol (*PA*) and rapamycin (*RAPA*) on 4E-BP1 (Ser65) phosphorylation in DU145 prostate cells. Perillyl alcohol treatment was done as described in Fig. 15.3. Cells were incubated in rapamycin for 4 h. PVDF membranes were incubated with an antibody specific for phospho-4E-BP1 (Ser65). Reprinted with permission from Elsevier (Peffley et al. 2007)

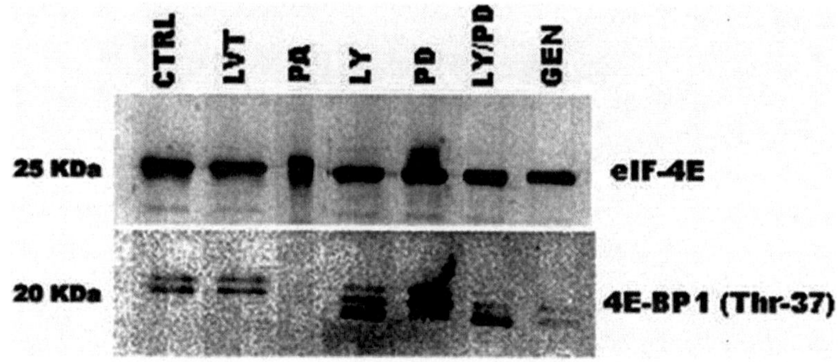

Fig. 15.8 Western blot comparing the effects of genistein and perillyl alcohol on 4E-BP1 (Thr37) in human prostate tumor cells. DU145 cells were treated with either perillyl alcohol, genistein, or lovastatin as described in Fig. 15.3. Cells were also treated with the PI3 kinase inhibitor LY294002 or the MEK1 inhibitor PD098059. Cell lysates were prepared and equal amounts of protein were electrophoresed and transferred to PVDF membranes. Membranes were incubated with a phospho-4E-BP1 (Thr37) specific antibody. Reprinted with permission from Elsevier (Peffley et al. 2007)

blocks initiation of translation on HMG-CoA reductase mRNA when added to CHO fibroblasts. In Fig. 15.9, polysome-associated reductase mRNA was reduced in perillyl alcohol-treated cells while the amount of reductase mRNA in translationally inactive messenger ribonucleoprotein particles increased. The results are interpreted to mean that perillyl alcohol specifically disrupted formation of the cap-binding complex.

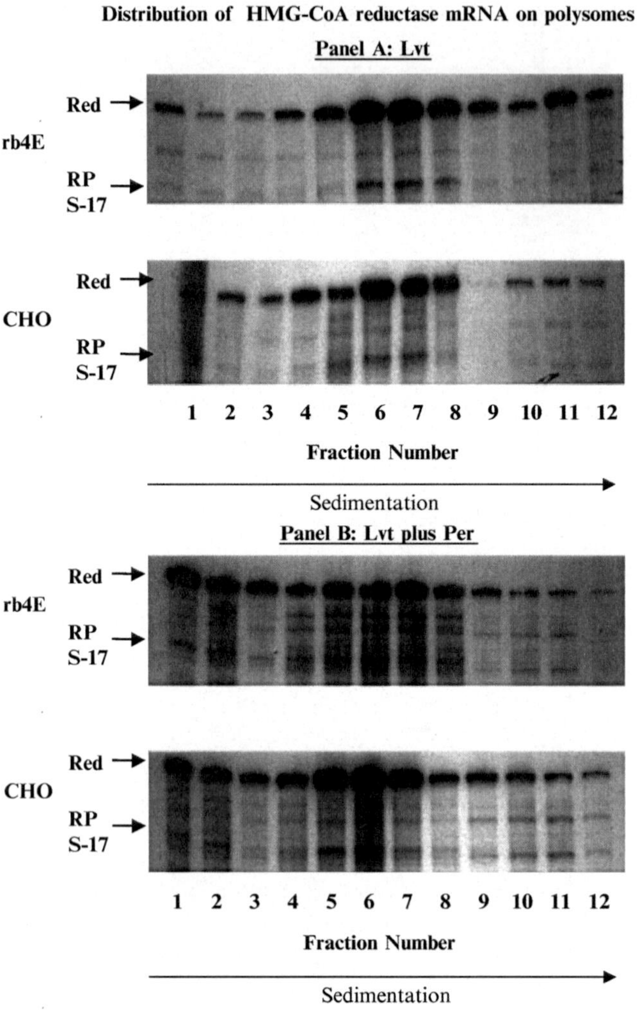

Fig. 15.9 Autoradiogram of polysome-associated HMG-CoA reductase (*Red*) and RP S-17 mRNA in CHO and the CHO cell line overexpressing eIF4E, or rb4E cells. Cells were incubated with or without perillyl alcohol as described in Fig. 15.3. Postmitochondrial supernatants were prepared and fractionated on linear 15–45% sucrose gradients. RNA (4 μg) from each of 12 gradient fractions was electrophoresed on a 7 M urea polyacrylamide gel, and HMG-CoA reductase and RP S-17 mRNA measured by RNase protection. Fractions 1–5 represent initiation and preinitiation complexes, and translationally inactive messenger ribonucleotide particles (mRNPs). Fractions 6–12 are polysome associate messenger RNAs that are translationally active

Additional studies likewise reported effects of phytochemicals on signaling pathways that mediate regulation of protein synthesis. Beevers et al. (2006) found that curcumin blocked mTOR-mediated signaling in tumor cells and inhibited both phosphorylation of p70 S6 kinase I and 4E-BP1. Another study has reported that phenethyl isothiocyanate–a component of cruciferous vegetables–inhibited cap-dependent translation by regulating levels and phosphorylation of 4E-BP1 (Hu et al. 2007). A more recent study found that curcumin-mediated inhibition of mTORC1 signaling occurred independently of protein phosphatase 2A or AMP-activating protein kinase AMPK-tuberous sclerosis complex (Beevers et al. 2009).

Furthermore, curcumin dissociated raptor from mTOR, resulting in inhibition of mTORC1 activity (Beevers et al. 2009). Overall, these results as well as our findings for perillyl alcohol support the role of phytochemicals in mediating the mTOR pathway and downstream translation of proteins.

15.7 Relationship of Terpenes to Cap-Independent Translation Through Internal Ribosomal Entry Sites

As discussed above, lipid-related terpenes such as isoprenoids, flavonoids and others exert their anti-proliferative effects in part by targeting cap-dependent protein translation. An expected effect would be changes in protein expression and protein posttranslational modifications that would ultimately change key signal transduction pathways that mediate cell survival and cell stasis or death.

Elevated translational control of protein synthesis is mediated through increased eIF4E levels associated with cell proliferation, suppression of apoptosis and tumorigenicity (Gingras et al. 2001a, b). Conversely, inhibition of eIF4E-mediated translational control via suppression of 4E-BP1 phosphorylation in transformed cells suppresses cell cycle progression, increases the pro-apoptotic potential, and decreases tumorigenicity (Gingras et al. 2001a, b). Cellular treatments that suppress tumor cell growth and induce apoptosis suppress eIF4E-mediated cap-dependent protein synthesis through mechanisms that in part involve cleavage of translation initiation factors (Clemens and Bommer 1999; Herbert et al. 2000; Marissen et al. 2000; Polunovsky et al. 2000; Subkhankulova et al. 2001; Wittke et al. 2001; Jeffrey et al. 2002). However, translation of certain mRNAs is not suppressed under eIF4F rate-limiting conditions. These mRNAs contain an internal ribosomal entry sequence (IRES) element in their respective 5′-UTLs (Nevins et al. 2003). Translation of such mRNAs is associated with cell cycle progression, apoptosis, amino acid availability and endoplasmic stress (Pyronnet et al. 2000; Gingras et al. 2001a, b; Nevins et al. 2003; Sonenberg and Dever 2003). Examples of such proteins include XIAP (Holcik et al. 2003), IGF-IR (Giraud et al. 2001), FGF2 (Kevil et al. 1995; Humar et al. 2002), PDGF (Bernstein et al. 1997), IFGII (Teerink et al. 1995; van der Velden and Thomas 1999), c-Myc (Schmidt 1999; Tan Tan et al. 2000; Subkhankulova et al. 2001), c-JUN (Sehgal et al. 2000), and DAP5 (Henis-Korenblit et al. 2000; Nevins et al. 2003). mRNAs for these proteins contain long, GC-rich 5′-UTLs with secondary structure. Under normal cellular conditions, their translation occurs via a scanning mechanism that involves eIF4F binding (cap-dependent). However, under conditions of cellular stress where eIF4F levels are depleted, translation is initiated through a mechanism independent of the cap structure. It is generally considered that translation via IRES elements in the 5′-UTL of these mRNAs has a critical role in determining cell fate (Nevins et al. 2003). More importantly, up-regulation of IRES-mediated translation of pro-survival proteins such as XIAP results in resistance to cell death when tumor cells are treated with chemotherapeutic agents (Holcik et al. 2003).

In addition, cellular stress-related responses result in the caspase-mediated cleavage of eIF4G family members (eIF4G, eIF4GII, and p97/DAP5) (Henis-Korenblit et al. 2000; Nevins et al. 2003). The middle fragment of eIF4G (M-FAG/p76) can bind eIF3 and eIF4A and thus support translation initiation via IRES elements (De Gregorio et al. 2001). The p86/DAP5 fragment has been shown to increase IRES-mediated translation of pro-apoptotic Apaf-1 and DAP5 but not other IRES elements. Therefore, physiological stress can differentially regulate IRES elements of various proteins and modify protein expression ("protein quality") to either support cell survival or promote cell death. It is believed that transient stress of tumor cells favors translation of pro-survival proteins such as XIAP (X-chromosome-linked inhibitor of apoptosis) (Perkins et al. 2000; Holcik et al. 2003). Conversely, severe apoptotic conditions support translation of pro-death proteins such as DAP5 or Apaf-1 (Henis-Korenblit et al. 2000; Nevins et al. 2003).

Findings from the Peffley lab (unpublished results) support the role of both terpenes and genistein in mediating a switch from cap-dependent to cap-independent translation. The most compelling evidence supporting this function was the finding that isoprenoids and genistein mediate cleavage of Death-associated protein 5 (DAP5/p97/NAT1) to DAP5/p86. DAP5—also known as p97 or NAT1—is a 97-kDa protein that has homology to eIF4G1 (Henis-Korenblit et al. 2000, 2002; Nevins et al. 2003). Unlike eIF4G1, DAP5 lacks an eIF4E-binding site and is unable to support cap-dependent translation (Henis-Korenblit et al. 2000, 2002; Nevins et al. 2003). However, like eIF4G, DAP5 interacts with both eIF4A and eIF3 and supports cap-independent translation through its own IRES (Henis-Korenblit et al. 2000, 2002; Nevins et al. 2003). During programmed cell death, DAP5 is cleaved by caspases to yield DAP5/p86 (Henis-Korenblit et al. 2002). The p86 fragment of DAP5 is capable of supporting translation through the death IRESs of DAP5, c-Myc, and Apaf-1 (Henis-Korenblit et al. 2000, 2002; Nevins et al. 2003). Consequently, DAP5 cleavage is an important regulatory step in programmed cell death that facilitates death IRES-mediated translation. As shown in Fig. 15.10, in DU145 and Caco2 cells, perillyl alcohol, genistein and tocotrienol enhanced cleavage of DAP5 to its p86 form. These results indicate that isoprenoids and genistein induce cleavage of DAP5/p97 to p86, which promotes cap-independent translation of death-associated proteins. We also noted a persistence of the DAP5/p86 fragment in control (untreated) cells. Although the presence of DAP5/p86 would suggest a pro-death condition, the effects of this translation factor in control cells could be negated by the relatively high levels of pro-survival proteins XIAP and Bcl-X_L measured in DU145 and PC3 cells (Li et al. 2001; Yang et al. 2003).

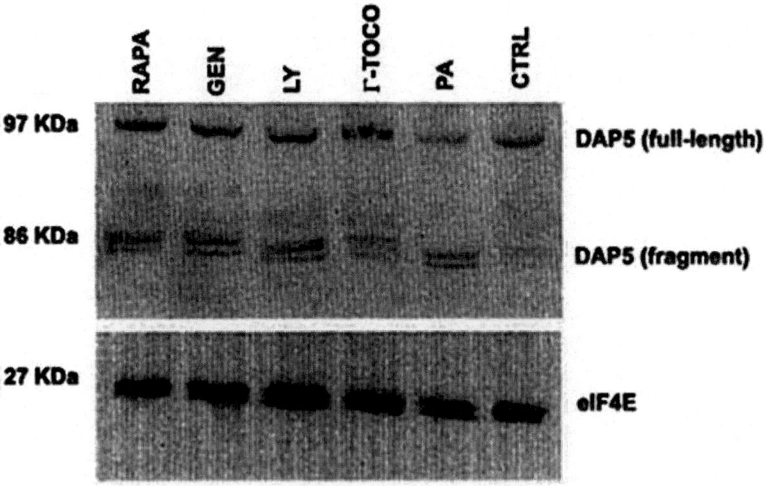

Fig. 15.10 Western blots demonstrating effects of isoprenoids and genistein on cleavage of DAP5/p97 to DAP5/p86. DU145 cells were treated as described in Fig. 15.3. Cell lysis, electrophoresis, and transfer to membranes were done as described in Fig. 15.3. Membranes were incubated with a DAP5 antibody that recognizes both the p97 and p86 forms

15.8 Isoprenoid-Induced Cell Death via a Caspase-Independent Mechanism Resembling Autophagy

Lipid-related terpenes affect gene expression at the level of mRNA translational efficiency and modulate several key protein factors involved in cell stasis and autophagic (non caspase-mediated) cell death (Peffley and Gayen 2003; Buechler and Peffley 2004; Peffley et al. 2007). mTOR is a key regulator of autophagy and growth and coordinately controls the balance between growth and autophagy as mediated through cellular stress (Jung et al. 2010). Suppression of mTOR either through rapamycin treatment or nutrient starvation is a critical step in autophagy induction in mammalian cells (Codogno and Meijer 2005; Jung et al. 2010). Availability of either cellular amino acids or glucose regulates mTOR activity(Jung et al. 2010). Loss of amino acid transport function inhibits cell growth and initiates autophagy in response to leucine deprivation and mTOR suppression (Nicklin et al. 2009). Glucose is also an important signaling molecule in mediating cell homeostasis because it regulates the cellular energy state and subsequently mTORC1 (Corradetti et al. 2004; Shaw et al. 2004). Glucose deprivation decreases the ratio of ATP and AMP and consequently activates AMPK (Corradetti et al. 2004; Shaw et al. 2004). This results in phosphorylation and activation of TSC2, which is a negative regulator of mTORC1(Jung et al. 2010). The suppression of mTORC1 and activation of AMPK results in activation of autophagy (Meigs and Simoni 1997; Meley et al. 2006; Jung et al. 2010).

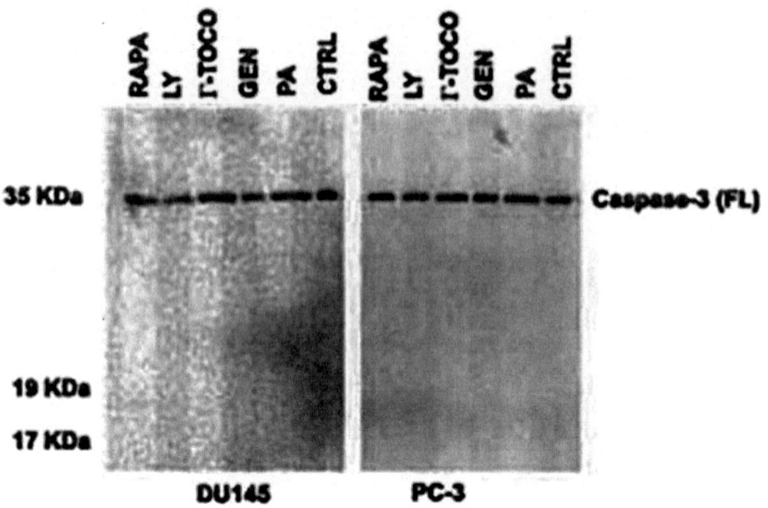

Fig. 15.11 Western blots illustrating the effects of isoprenoids and genistein on caspase 3 cleavage (activation) in human prostate tumor cells. Cells were treated with perillyl alcohol (*PA*), γ-tocotrienol (*γ-TOCO*), LY294002 (*LY*) or rapamycin (*RAPA*) as described in Fig. 15.3. Antibodies used recognize both procaspase (inactive) and cleaved (active) fragments

Nutrient-mediated signaling upstream of mTORC1 is also regulated through human ortholog of yeast vacuolar protein sorting 34 (hVps34) or phosphoinositide 3-kinase class III (PI3KIII), a lipid kinase conserved in eukaryotes (Petiot et al. 2000; Galluzzi et al. 2008). PI3KIII catalyzes the phosphorylation of phosphatidylinositol (PtdIns) into phosphatidylinositol-3-phosphate (PtdIns(3)P), a molecular signal that promotes formation of phagophores by facilitating recruitment of autophagy (Atg) proteins (Nobukuni et al. 2007; Yan and Backer 2007). In contrast, class I PI3K acts an inhibitor of autophagy, an effect presumably mediated by phosphoinositides which activate mTOR by its upstream regulator Akt1/PKB (Yorimitsu and Klionsky 2005). Phagophore formation and induction of autophagy under these conditions also involves association of Atg proteins with the multiprotein complex that includes Beclin 1 (Bcn-1–the mammalian ortholog of Atg6), UV irradiation resistance-associated tumor suppressor gene (UVRAG) and the myristylated kinase p150 (ortholog of Vps15) (Galluzzi et al. 2008).

Compelling evidence that supports the role of isoprenoids and genistein in mediating autophagic cell death is that neither of these phytonutrients initiates cleavage of caspase 3 or 7 in prostate tumor cells (Fig. 15.11). We estimated caspase 3 and 7 cleavage by western blot analyses using antibodies that recognize procaspase 3 and 7 as well as cleaved caspase. Procaspase 3 was readily detectible in both prostate cell lines but no apparent cleavage was detected in treated and untreated cells (caspase 7 data not shown). Detection of cleaved caspases may be confounded by the relatively high XIAP levels (Yang et al. 2003) in prostate tumor cells. Not only does XIAP interact with and block caspase 3 activity but it also enhances degradation of cleaved caspase via the proteosome complex (Suzuki et al. 2001). However, the absence of proteins corresponding to cleaved and activated caspases does not preclude low level caspase-mediated eIF4G cleavage. It is also important to point out that activation of other non-caspase proteases such as calpains, cathepsin B, D and L, and granzymes A and B also cooperate with caspases in programmed cell death (Kitanaka and Kuchino 1999; Blagosklonny 2000). Consequently, eIF4G cleavage may be due to these proteases as well. Overall, these results suggest that isoprenoid and genistein-mediated programmed cell death in human prostate tumor cells is caspase-independent. This is also in agreement with other studies that now recognize that programmed cell death can occur in the absence of caspase activity (Blagosklonny 2000). This type of cell death is referred to as programmed cell death II or autophagic cell death (Lefranc et al. 2007).

Nutrient-mediated induction of autophagy has been reported in several other cell systems, and in all cases it is associated with mTOR suppression. In malignant glioma cells, curcumin induced G2/M arrest, inhibited the Akt/mTOR/p70S6k pathway and activated the ERK1/2 pathway, and induced autophagic cell death (Aoki et al. 2007). Phenethyl isothiocyanate is a cancer chemopreventive that was shown to induce Atg5-dependent autophagic cell death in human prostate cancer cells (Bommareddy et al. 2009) . This effect was due in part to suppressed activating phosphorylations of Akt and mTOR. However, ectopic expression of active Akt or overexpression of the mTOR-positive regulator Rheb only partially reversed phenethyl isothiocyanate-induced autophagy indicating that other pathways were involved (Bommareddy et al. 2009). A related isothiocyanate from cruciferous vegetables, sulforaphane, induced autophagy in human prostate tumor cells (Herman-Antosiewicz et al. 2006). Sulforaphane-induced autophagy was unique because it inhibited the cytosolic release of cytochrome c and apoptotic cell death in prostate cancer cells. These results suggest that autophagy may be a defense mechanism against isothiocyantate-induced apoptotic cell death (Herman-Antosiewicz et al. 2006). The plant phytoalexin resveratrol was shown to trigger autophagy in imatinib-sensitive and imatinib-resistant chronic myelogenous leukemia cells, an effect associated with inhibition of the mTOR pathway (Puissant et al. 2010). Likewise, prostate tumor cells exposed to the dietary flavonoid, fisetin, underwent autophagic cell death, a process linked to suppression of the mTOR pathway (Suh et al. 2010). Overall, these studies support the hypothesis that autophagy is a principle mechanism through which nutrients act as cancer chemopreventives.

15.9 Conclusion

Nutritional patterns are intimately associated with major disease development and mortality arising from those diseases including cancer, obesity, diabetes, and cardiovascular disorders (Walker and Blackburn 2004). The fields of nutrigenomics (understanding how genes and bioactive food components interact) and nutriproteomics (understanding how food components affect protein synthesis and protein:protein interactions) have resulted to unravel the complexities of responses to dietary factors at a molecular level. This overview has provided insight into novel molecular targets for nutritional preemption, i.e., for optimizing health, reducing one's risk for disease and/or limiting disease progression. Studies from the Peffley group have defined how simple lipophilic compounds like perillyl alcohol regulate gene expression through modulation of a key nutrient sensing pathway, mTOR. Specifically this group has defined the unique effects of dietary isoprenoids on translational processes that are aberrantly up-regulated in tumor cells (Graff et al. 2008; Sonenberg 2008). The mTOR pathway is important not only in cell proliferation but also in physiologic and pathologic tissue hypertrophy (Lee et al. 2007) of both skeletal and cardiac muscle, vascular restenosis and compensatory nephritic hypertrophy. The health relatedness of the mTOR signaling pathway is supported by its demonstrated role in the etiology of cancer, Huntington's and cardiovascular disease, as well as metabolic syndromes such as diabetes and obesity (Lee et al. 2007). Clearly, other studies on nutritional preemption of cancer and other diseases will uncover more details linking the mTOR pathway to autophagic cell death.

References

Abid MR, Li Y et al (1999) Translational regulation of ribonucleotide reductase by eukaryotic initiation factor 4E links protein synthesis to the control of DNA replication. J Biol Chem 274(50):35991–35998

Abraham RT, Gibbons JJ (2007) The mammalian target of rapamycin signaling pathway: twists and turns in the road to cancer therapy. Clin Cancer Res 13(11):3109–3114

Adlercreutz H (1990) Western diet and Western diseases: some hormonal and biochemical mechanisms and associations. Scand J Clin Lab Invest Suppl 201:3–23

Aggarwal BB, Sundaram C et al (2010) Tocotrienols, the vitamin E of the 21st century: its potential against cancer and other chronic diseases. Biochem Pharmacol 80(11):1613–1631

Alhasan SA, Aranha O et al (2001) Genistein elicits pleiotropic molecular effects on head and neck cancer cells. Clin Cancer Res 7(12):4174–4181

Aoki H, Takada Y et al (2007) Evidence that curcumin suppresses the growth of malignant gliomas in vitro and in vivo through induction of autophagy: role of Akt and extracellular signal-regulated kinase signaling pathways. Mol Pharmacol 72(1):29–39

Ariazi EA, Gould MN (1996) Identifying differential gene expression in monoterpene-treated mammary carcinomas using subtractive display. J Biol Chem 271(46):29286–29294

Ariazi EA, Satomi Y et al (1999) Activation of the transforming growth factor beta signaling pathway and induction of cytostasis and apoptosis in mammary carcinomas treated with the anticancer agent perillyl alcohol. Cancer Res 59(8):1917–1928

Averous J, Proud CG (2006) When translation meets transformation: the mTOR story. Oncogene 25(48):6423–6435

Azrolan NI, Coleman PS (1989) A discoordinate increase in the cellular amount of 3-hydroxy-3-methylglutaryl-CoA reductase results in the loss of rate-limiting control over cholesterogenesis in a tumour cell-free system. Biochem J 258(2):421–425

Babendure JR, Babendure JL et al (2006) Control of mammalian translation by mRNA structure near caps. RNA 12(5):851–861

Barthelman M, Chen W et al (1998) Inhibitory effects of perillyl alcohol on UVB-induced murine skin cancer and AP-1 transactivation. Cancer Res 58(4):711–716

Beevers CS, Li F et al (2006) Curcumin inhibits the mammalian target of rapamycin-mediated signaling pathways in cancer cells. Int J Cancer 119(4):757–764

Beevers CS, Chen L et al (2009) Curcumin disrupts the Mammalian target of rapamycin-raptor complex. Cancer Res 69(3):1000–1008
Berchtold CM, Chen KS et al (2005) Perillyl alcohol inhibits a calcium-dependent constitutive nuclear factor-kappaB pathway. Cancer Res 65(18):8558–8566
Berkel HJ, Turbat-Herrera EA et al (2001) Expression of the translation initiation factor eIF4E in the polyp-cancer sequence in the colon. Cancer Epidemiol Biomarkers Prev 10(6):663–666
Bernstein J, Sella O et al (1997) PDGF2/c-sis mRNA leader contains a differentiation-linked internal ribosomal entry site (D-IRES). J Biol Chem 272(14):9356–9362
Blagosklonny MV (2000) Cell death beyond apoptosis. Leukemia 14(8):1502–1508
Bommareddy A, Hahm ER et al (2009) Atg5 regulates phenethyl isothiocyanate-induced autophagic and apoptotic cell death in human prostate cancer cells. Cancer Res 69(8):3704–3712
Buechler RD, Peffley DM (2004) Proto oncogene/eukaryotic translation initiation factor (eIF) 4E attenuates mevalonate-mediated regulation of 3-hydroxy-3-methylglutaryl coenzyme A (HMG-CoA) reductase synthesis. Mol Carcinog 41(1):39–53
Byrnes K, White S et al (2006) High eIF4E, VEGF, and microvessel density in stage I to III breast cancer. Ann Surg 243(5):684–690, discussion 691–682
Cao Q, Richter JD (2002) Dissolution of the maskin-eIF4E complex by cytoplasmic polyadenylation and poly(A)-binding protein controls cyclin B1 mRNA translation and oocyte maturation. EMBO J 21(14):3852–3862
Chen CN, Hsieh FJ et al (2004) Expression of eukaryotic initiation factor 4E in gastric adenocarcinoma and its association with clinical outcome. J Surg Oncol 86(1):22–27
Chiu MI, Katz H et al (1994) RAPT1, a mammalian homolog of yeast Tor, interacts with the FKBP12/rapamycin complex. Proc Natl Acad Sci USA 91(26):12574–12578
Choi JW, Peffley DM (1995) 3′-untranslated sequences mediate post-transcriptional regulation of 3-hydroxy-3-methylglutaryl-CoA reductase mRNA by 25-hydroxycholesterol. Biochem J 307(Pt 1):233–238
Chung BH, Lee HY et al (2006) Perillyl alcohol inhibits the expression and function of the androgen receptor in human prostate cancer cells. Cancer Lett 236(2):222–228
Clark SS (2006) Perillyl alcohol induces c-Myc-dependent apoptosis in Bcr/Abl-transformed leukemia cells. Oncology 70(1):13–18
Clemens MJ, Bommer UA (1999) Translational control: the cancer connection. Int J Biochem Cell Biol 31(1):1–23
Codogno P, Meijer AJ (2005) Autophagy and signaling: their role in cell survival and cell death. Cell Death Differ 12(Suppl 2):1509–1518
Coleman PS, Chen LC et al (1997) Cholesterol metabolism and tumor cell proliferation. Subcell Biochem 28:363–435
Constantinou A, Huberman E (1995) Genistein as an inducer of tumor cell differentiation: possible mechanisms of action. Proc Soc Exp Biol Med 208(1):109–115
Corradetti MN, Guan KL (2006) Upstream of the mammalian target of rapamycin: do all roads pass through mTOR? Oncogene 25(48):6347–6360
Corradetti MN, Inoki K et al (2004) Regulation of the TSC pathway by LKB1: evidence of a molecular link between tuberous sclerosis complex and Peutz-Jeghers syndrome. Genes Dev 18(13):1533–1538
Correll CC, Edwards PA (1994) Mevalonic acid-dependent degradation of 3-hydroxy-3-methylglutaryl-coenzyme A reductase in vivo and in vitro. J Biol Chem 269(1):633–638
Correll CC, Ng L et al (1994) Identification of farnesol as the non-sterol derivative of mevalonic acid required for the accelerated degradation of 3-hydroxy-3-methylglutaryl-coenzyme A reductase. J Biol Chem 269(26):17390–17393
Crowell PL, Chang RR et al (1991) Selective inhibition of isoprenylation of 21-26-kDa proteins by the anticarcinogen d-limonene and its metabolites. J Biol Chem 266(26):17679–17685
Davis JN, Singh B et al (1998) Genistein-induced upregulation of p21WAF1, downregulation of cyclin B, and induction of apoptosis in prostate cancer cells. Nutr Cancer 32(3):123–131
Davis JN, Kucuk O et al (2001) Soy isoflavone supplementation in healthy men prevents NF-kappa B activation by TNF-alpha in blood lymphocytes. Free Radic Biol Med 30(11):1293–1302

De Benedetti A, Graff JR (2004) eIF-4E expression and its role in malignancies and metastases. Oncogene 23(18):3189–3199
De Gregorio E, Baron J et al (2001) Tethered-function analysis reveals that elF4E can recruit ribosomes independent of its binding to the cap structure. RNA 7(1):106–113
DeBose-Boyd RA (2008) Feedback regulation of cholesterol synthesis: sterol-accelerated ubiquitination and degradation of HMG CoA reductase. Cell Res 18(6):609–621
Defatta RJ, De Benedetti A (2003) Translational upregulation of yes accompanies eIF4E-mediated oncogenic transformation. Int J Oncol 23(6):1709–1713
DeFatta RJ, Turbat-Herrera EA et al (1999) Elevated expression of eIF4E in confined early breast cancer lesions: possible role of hypoxia. Int J Cancer 80(4):516–522
DeFatta RJ, Nathan CA et al (2000) Antisense RNA to eIF4E suppresses oncogenic properties of a head and neck squamous cell carcinoma cell line. Laryngoscope 110(6):928–933
DeFatta RJ, Li Y et al (2002) Selective killing of cancer cells based on translational control of a suicide gene. Cancer Gene Ther 9(7):573–578
Elson CE, Peffley DM et al (1999) Isoprenoid-mediated inhibition of mevalonate synthesis: potential application to cancer. Proc Soc Exp Biol Med 221(4):294–311
Engstrom W, Schofield PN (1987) Expression of the 3-hydroxy-3-methylglutaryl coenzyme A-reductase and LDL-receptor genes in human embryonic tumours and in normal foetal tissues. Anticancer Res 7(3 Pt B):337–342
Espel E (2005) The role of the AU-rich elements of mRNAs in controlling translation. Semin Cell Dev Biol 16(1):59–67
Espenshade PJ, Hughes AL (2007) Regulation of sterol synthesis in eukaryotes. Annu Rev Genet 41:401–427
Fernandez J, Yaman I et al (2001) Internal ribosome entry site-mediated translation of a mammalian mRNA is regulated by amino acid availability. J Biol Chem 276(15):12285–12291
Fernandez J, Yaman I et al (2005) Ribosome stalling regulates IRES-mediated translation in eukaryotes, a parallel to prokaryotic attenuation. Mol Cell 17(3):405–416
Fischer Jde S, Liao L et al (2010) Dynamic proteomic overview of glioblastoma cells (A172) exposed to perillyl alcohol. J Proteomics 73(5):1018–1027
Forman HJ, Torres M et al (2002) Redox signaling. Mol Cell Biochem 234–235(1–2):49–62
Fournier DB, Erdman JW Jr et al (1998) Soy, its components, and cancer prevention: a review of the in vitro, animal, and human data. Cancer Epidemiol Biomarkers Prev 7(11):1055–1065
Fritz T, Buechler R, Peffley DM (1998) Translational efficiency of 3-hydroxy-3-methylglutaryl coenzyme A (HMG-CoA) reductase is regulated by 5′-untranslated (UTR) mRNA secondary structure. Circ Res 98:379
Galluzzi L, Vicencio JM et al (2008) To die or not to die: that is the autophagic question. Curr Mol Med 8(2):78–91
Gayen AK, Peffley DM (1995) The length of 5′-untranslated leader sequences influences distribution of 3-hydroxy-3-methylglutaryl-coenzyme A reductase mRNA in polysomes: effects of lovastatin, oxysterols, and mevalonate. Arch Biochem Biophys 322(2):475–485
Ghosh PM, Ghosh-Choudhury N et al (1999) Role of RhoA activation in the growth and morphology of a murine prostate tumor cell line. Oncogene 18(28):4120–4130
Gingras AC, Raught B et al (2001a) Control of translation by the target of rapamycin proteins. Prog Mol Subcell Biol 27:143–174
Gingras AC, Raught B et al (2001b) Regulation of translation initiation by FRAP/mTOR. Genes Dev 15(7):807–826
Giraud S, Greco A et al (2001) Translation initiation of the insulin-like growth factor I receptor mRNA is mediated by an internal ribosome entry site. J Biol Chem 276(8):5668–5675
Goldson TM, Vielhauer G et al (2007) Eukaryotic initiation factor 4E variants alter the morphology, proliferation, and colony-formation properties of MDA-MB-435 cancer cells. Mol Carcinog 46(1):71–84
Goldstein JL, Brown MS (1990) Regulation of the mevalonate pathway. Nature 343(6257):425–430
Gould MN (1997) Cancer chemoprevention and therapy by monoterpenes. Environ Health Perspect 105(Suppl 4):977–979

Graff JR, Zimmer SG (2003) Translational control and metastatic progression: enhanced activity of the mRNA cap-binding protein eIF-4E selectively enhances translation of metastasis-related mRNAs. Clin Exp Metastasis 20(3):265–273
Graff JR, Konicek BW et al (2008) Targeting the eukaryotic translation initiation factor 4E for cancer therapy. Cancer Res 68(3):631–634
Guilford JM, Pezzuto JM (2008) Natural products as inhibitors of carcinogenesis. Expert Opin Investig Drugs 17(9):1341–1352
Gullett NP, Ruhul Amin AR et al (2010) Cancer prevention with natural compounds. Semin Oncol 37(3):258–281
Halaby MJ, Yang DQ (2007) p53 translational control: a new facet of p53 regulation and its implication for tumorigenesis and cancer therapeutics. Gene 395(1–2):1–7
Haluska P, Dy GK et al (2002) Farnesyl transferase inhibitors as anticancer agents. Eur J Cancer 38(13):1685–1700
Handayani R, Rice L et al (2006) Soy isoflavones alter expression of genes associated with cancer progression, including interleukin-8, in androgen-independent PC-3 human prostate cancer cells. J Nutr 136(1):75–82
Hekman M, Hamm H et al (2002) Associations of B- and C-Raf with cholesterol, phosphatidylserine, and lipid second messengers: preferential binding of Raf to artificial lipid rafts. J Biol Chem 277(27):24090–24102
Henis-Korenblit S, Strumpf NL et al (2000) A novel form of DAP5 protein accumulates in apoptotic cells as a result of caspase cleavage and internal ribosome entry site-mediated translation. Mol Cell Biol 20(2):496–506
Henis-Korenblit S, Shani G et al (2002) The caspase-cleaved DAP5 protein supports internal ribosome entry site-mediated translation of death proteins. Proc Natl Acad Sci USA 99(8):5400–5405
Hentosh P, Yuh SH et al (2001) Sterol-independent regulation of 3-hydroxy-3-methylglutaryl coenzyme A reductase in tumor cells. Mol Carcinog 32(3):154–166
Herbert TP, Fahraeus R et al (2000) Rapid induction of apoptosis mediated by peptides that bind initiation factor eIF4E. Curr Biol 10(13):793–796
Herman-Antosiewicz A, Johnson DE et al (2006) Sulforaphane causes autophagy to inhibit release of cytochrome C and apoptosis in human prostate cancer cells. Cancer Res 66(11):5828–5835
Hiipakka RA, Zhang HZ et al (2002) Structure-activity relationships for inhibition of human 5alpha-reductases by polyphenols. Biochem Pharmacol 63(6):1165–1176
Holcik M, Gordon BW et al (2003) The internal ribosome entry site-mediated translation of antiapoptotic protein XIAP is modulated by the heterogeneous nuclear ribonucleoproteins C1 and C2. Mol Cell Biol 23(1):280–288
Holz MK, Ballif BA et al (2005) mTOR and S6K1 mediate assembly of the translation preinitiation complex through dynamic protein interchange and ordered phosphorylation events. Cell 123(4):569–580
Hsieh TC, Elangovan S et al (2010) Gamma-Tocotrienol controls proliferation, modulates expression of cell cycle regulatory proteins and up-regulates quinone reductase NQO2 in MCF-7 breast cancer cells. Anticancer Res 30(7):2869–2874
Hu J, Straub J et al (2007) Phenethyl isothiocyanate, a cancer chemopreventive constituent of cruciferous vegetables, inhibits cap-dependent translation by regulating the level and phosphorylation of 4E-BP1. Cancer Res 67(8):3569–3573
Huang M, Prendergast GC (2006) RhoB in cancer suppression. Histol Histopathol 21(2):213–218
Huang J, Nasr M et al (1992) Genistein inhibits protein histidine kinase. J Biol Chem 267(22): 15511–15515
Hudes GR, Szarka CE et al (2000) Phase I pharmacokinetic trial of perillyl alcohol (NSC 641066) in patients with refractory solid malignancies. Clin Cancer Res 6(8):3071–3080
Humar R, Kiefer FN et al (2002) Hypoxia enhances vascular cell proliferation and angiogenesis in vitro via rapamycin (mTOR)-dependent signaling. FASEB J 16(8):771–780
Inoki K, Guan KL (2006) Complexity of the TOR signaling network. Trends Cell Biol 16(4):206–212

Izquierdo JM, Cuezva JM (2000) Internal-ribosome-entry-site functional activity of the 3′-untranslated region of the mRNA for the beta subunit of mitochondrial H+–ATP synthase. Biochem J 346 (Pt 3):849–855

Jacinto E, Loewith R et al (2004) Mammalian TOR complex 2 controls the actin cytoskeleton and is rapamycin insensitive. Nat Cell Biol 6(11):1122–1128

Jeffrey IW, Bushell M et al (2002) Inhibition of protein synthesis in apoptosis: differential requirements by the tumor necrosis factor alpha family and a DNA-damaging agent for caspases and the double-stranded RNA-dependent protein kinase. Cancer Res 62(8):2272–2280

Jo Y, Debose-Boyd RA (2010) Control of cholesterol synthesis through regulated ER-associated degradation of HMG CoA reductase. Crit Rev Biochem Mol Biol 45(3):185–198

Jung CH, Ro SH et al (2010) mTOR regulation of autophagy. FEBS Lett 584(7):1287–1295

Kevil C, Carter P et al (1995) Translational enhancement of FGF-2 by eIF-4 factors, and alternate utilization of CUG and AUG codons for translation initiation. Oncogene 11(11):2339–2348

Khan N, Afaq F et al (2008) Cancer chemoprevention through dietary antioxidants: progress and promise. Antioxid Redox Signal 10(3):475–510

Kim DH, Sarbassov DD et al (2003) GbetaL, a positive regulator of the rapamycin-sensitive pathway required for the nutrient-sensitive interaction between raptor and mTOR. Mol Cell 11(4):895–904

Kim S, Sohn I et al (2005) Hepatic gene expression profiles are altered by genistein supplementation in mice with diet-induced obesity. J Nutr 135(1):33–41

Kitanaka C, Kuchino Y (1999) Caspase-independent programmed cell death with necrotic morphology. Cell Death Differ 6(6):508–515

Komarova AV, Brocard M et al (2006) The case for mRNA 5′ and 3′ end cross talk during translation in a eukaryotic cell. Prog Nucleic Acid Res Mol Biol 81:331–367

Kozak M (2001a) Constraints on reinitiation of translation in mammals. Nucleic Acids Res 29(24):5226–5232

Kozak M (2001b) New ways of initiating translation in eukaryotes? Mol Cell Biol 21(6):1899–1907

Kozak M (2001c) A progress report on translational control in eukaryotes. Sci STKE 2001(71):PE1

Kozak M (2005) Regulation of translation via mRNA structure in prokaryotes and eukaryotes. Gene 361:13–37

Kozak M (2007) Lessons (not) learned from mistakes about translation. Gene 403(1–2):194–203

Lawrence JC Jr, Abraham RT (1997) PHAS/4E-BPs as regulators of mRNA translation and cell proliferation. Trends Biochem Sci 22(9):345–349

Lawrence JC Jr, Fadden P et al (1997) PHAS proteins as mediators of the actions of insulin, growth factors and cAMP on protein synthesis and cell proliferation. Adv Enzyme Regul 37:239–267

Le Sourd F, Boulben S et al (2006) eEF1B: At the dawn of the 21st century. Biochim Biophys Acta 1759(1–2):13–31

Lebowitz PF, Prendergast GC (1998) Functional interaction between RhoB and the transcription factor DB1. Cell Adhes Commun 6(4):277–287

Lebowitz PF, Du W et al (1997) Prenylation of RhoB is required for its cell transforming function but not its ability to activate serum response element-dependent transcription. J Biol Chem 272(26):16093–16095

Lee HK, Jeong S (2006) Beta-Catenin stabilizes cyclooxygenase-2 mRNA by interacting with AU-rich elements of 3′-UTR. Nucleic Acids Res 34(19):5705–5714

Lee CH, Inoki K et al (2007) mTOR pathway as a target in tissue hypertrophy. Annu Rev Pharmacol Toxicol 47:443–467

Lefranc F, Facchini V et al (2007) Proautophagic drugs: a novel means to combat apoptosis-resistant cancers, with a special emphasis on glioblastomas. Oncologist 12(12):1395–1403

Levy S, Avni D et al (1991) Oligopyrimidine tract at the 5′ end of mammalian ribosomal protein mRNAs is required for their translational control. Proc Natl Acad Sci USA 88(8):3319–3323

Li X, Marani M et al (2001) Overexpression of BCL-X(L) underlies the molecular basis for resistance to staurosporine-induced apoptosis in PC-3 cells. Cancer Res 61(4):1699–1706

Li B, Gruner JS et al (2002) Prospective study of eukaryotic initiation factor 4E protein elevation and breast cancer outcome. Ann Surg 235(5):732–738; discussion 738–739

Liao JK (2002) Isoprenoids as mediators of the biological effects of statins. J Clin Invest 110(3):285–288
Lluria-Prevatt M, Morreale J et al (2002) Effects of perillyl alcohol on melanoma in the TPras mouse model. Cancer Epidemiol Biomarkers Prev 11(6):573–579
Makela SI, Pylkkanen LH et al (1995) Dietary soybean may be antiestrogenic in male mice. J Nutr 125(3):437–445
Mamane Y, Petroulakis E et al (2004) eIF4E–from translation to transformation. Oncogene 23(18):3172–3179
Marissen WE, Gradi A et al (2000) Cleavage of eukaryotic translation initiation factor 4GII correlates with translation inhibition during apoptosis. Cell Death Differ 7(12):1234–1243
Martinez O, Goud B (1998) Rab proteins. Biochim Biophys Acta 1404(1–2):101–112
Matsukawa Y, Marui N et al (1993) Genistein arrests cell cycle progression at G2-M. Cancer Res 53(6):1328–1331
McIntyre BS, Briski KP et al (2000) Antiproliferative and apoptotic effects of tocopherols and tocotrienols on normal mouse mammary epithelial cells. Lipids 35(2):171–180
Mehta RG, Murillo G et al (2010) Cancer chemoprevention by natural products: how far have we come? Pharm Res 27(6):950–961
Meigs TE, Simoni RD (1997) Farnesol as a regulator of HMG-CoA reductase degradation: characterization and role of farnesyl pyrophosphatase. Arch Biochem Biophys 345(1):1–9
Meley D, Bauvy C et al (2006) AMP-activated protein kinase and the regulation of autophagic proteolysis. J Biol Chem 281(46):34870–34879
Mo H, Elson CE (1999) Apoptosis and cell-cycle arrest in human and murine tumor cells are initiated by isoprenoids. J Nutr 129(4):804–813
Mo H, Peffley DM, Elson CE (1999) Targeting the action of isoprenoids and related phytochemicals to tumors. In: Heber D, Blackburn GL, Go VLW (eds) Nutritional oncology. Academic, San Diego, pp 379–391
Morley SJ, Coldwell MJ et al (2005) Initiation factor modifications in the preapoptotic phase. Cell Death Differ 12(6):571–584
Nair S, Li W et al (2007) Natural dietary anti-cancer chemopreventive compounds: redox-mediated differential signaling mechanisms in cytoprotection of normal cells versus cytotoxicity in tumor cells. Acta Pharmacol Sin 28(4):459–472
Nesaretnam K, Dorasamy S et al (2000) Tocotrienols inhibit growth of ZR-75-1 breast cancer cells. Int J Food Sci Nutr 51(Suppl):S95–S103
Nevins TA, Harder ZM et al (2003) Distinct regulation of internal ribosome entry site-mediated translation following cellular stress is mediated by apoptotic fragments of eIF4G translation initiation factor family members eIF4GI and p97/DAP5/NAT1. J Biol Chem 278(6):3572–3579
Nicklin P, Bergman P et al (2009) Bidirectional transport of amino acids regulates mTOR and autophagy. Cell 136(3):521–534
Nobukuni T, Kozma SC et al (2007) hvps34, an ancient player, enters a growing game: mTOR Complex1/S6K1 signaling. Curr Opin Cell Biol 19(2):135–141
Okura A, Arakawa H et al (1988) Effect of genistein on topoisomerase activity and on the growth of [Val 12] Ha-ras-transformed NIH 3T3 cells. Biochem Biophys Res Commun 157(1):183–189
Origanti S, Shantz LM (2007) Ras transformation of RIE-1 cells activates cap-independent translation of ornithine decarboxylase: regulation by the Raf/MEK/ERK and phosphatidylinositol 3-kinase pathways. Cancer Res 67(10):4834–4842
Pagliacci MC, Smacchia M et al (1994) Growth-inhibitory effects of the natural phyto-oestrogen genistein in MCF-7 human breast cancer cells. Eur J Cancer 30A(11):1675–1682
Park SK, Sanders BG et al (2010) Tocotrienols induce apoptosis in breast cancer cell lines via an endoplasmic reticulum stress-dependent increase in extrinsic death receptor signaling. Breast Cancer Res Treat 124(2):361–375
Peffley DM (1992) Regulation of 3-hydroxy-3-methylglutaryl coenzyme A reductase synthesis in Syrian hamster C100 cells by mevinolin, 25-hydroxycholesterol, and mevalonate: the role of posttranscriptional control. Somat Cell Mol Genet 18(1):19–32

Peffley DM, Gayen AK (1997) Inhibition of squalene synthase but not squalene cyclase prevents mevalonate-mediated suppression of 3-hydroxy-3-methylglutaryl coenzyme A reductase synthesis at a posttranscriptional level. Arch Biochem Biophys 337(2):251–260

Peffley DM, Gayen AK (2003) Plant-derived monoterpenes suppress hamster kidney cell 3-hydroxy-3-methylglutaryl coenzyme a reductase synthesis at the post-transcriptional level. J Nutr 133(1):38–44

Peffley DM, Gayen AK et al (1998) Down-regulation of 3-hydroxy-3-methylglutaryl coenzyme A reductase mRNA levels and synthesis in syrian hamster C100 cells by the oxidosqualene cyclase inhibitor [4′-(6-allyl-ethyl-amino-hexyloxy)-2′-fluoro-phenyl]-(4-bromophenyl)-me thanone (Ro 48–8071): comparison to simvastatin. Biochem Pharmacol 56(4):439–449

Peffley DM, Sharma C et al (2007) Perillyl alcohol and genistein differentially regulate PKB/Akt and 4E-BP1 phosphorylation as well as eIF4E/eIF4G interactions in human tumor cells. Arch Biochem Biophys 465(1):266–273

Pelletier J, Brook JD et al (1991) Assignment of two of the translation initiation factor-4E (EIF4EL1 and EIF4EL2) genes to human chromosomes 4 and 20. Genomics 10(4):1079–1082

Perkins CL, Fang G et al (2000) The role of Apaf-1, caspase-9, and bid proteins in etoposide- or paclitaxel-induced mitochondrial events during apoptosis. Cancer Res 60(6):1645–1653

Petiot A, Ogier-Denis E et al (2000) Distinct classes of phosphatidylinositol 3′-kinases are involved in signaling pathways that control macroautophagy in HT-29 cells. J Biol Chem 275(2):992–998

Piccinelli P, Samuelsson T (2007) Evolution of the iron-responsive element. RNA 13(7):952–966

Pollard M, Luckert PH (1997) Influence of isoflavones in soy protein isolates on development of induced prostate-related cancers in L-W rats. Nutr Cancer 28(1):41–45

Polunovsky VA, Gingras AC et al (2000) Translational control of the antiapoptotic function of Ras. J Biol Chem 275(32):24776–24780

Poon RY, Toyoshima H et al (1995) Redistribution of the CDK inhibitor p27 between different cyclin.CDK complexes in the mouse fibroblast cell cycle and in cells arrested with lovastatin or ultraviolet irradiation. Mol Biol Cell 6(9):1197–1213

Prendergast GC, Khosravi-Far R et al (1995) Critical role of Rho in cell transformation by oncogenic Ras. Oncogene 10(12):2289–2296

Puissant A, Robert G et al (2010) Resveratrol promotes autophagic cell death in chronic myelogenous leukemia cells via JNK-mediated p62/SQSTM1 expression and AMPK activation. Cancer Res 70(3):1042–1052

Pyronnet S, Pradayrol L et al (2000) A cell cycle-dependent internal ribosome entry site. Mol Cell 5(4):607–616

Rabi T, Bishayee A (2009) Terpenoids and breast cancer chemoprevention. Breast Cancer Res Treat 115(2):223–239

Ren Z, Elson CE et al (1997) Inhibition of type I and type II geranylgeranyl-protein transferases by the monoterpene perillyl alcohol in NIH3T3 cells. Biochem Pharmacol 54(1):113–120

Reynolds GA, Goldstein JL et al (1985) Multiple mRNAs for 3-hydroxy-3-methylglutaryl coenzyme A reductase determined by multiple transcription initiation sites and intron splicing sites in the 5′-untranslated region. J Biol Chem 260(18):10369–10377

Ripple GH, Gould MN et al (1998) Phase I clinical trial of perillyl alcohol administered daily. Clin Cancer Res 4(5):1159–1164

Ripple GH, Gould MN et al (2000) Phase I clinical and pharmacokinetic study of perillyl alcohol administered four times a day. Clin Cancer Res 6(2):390–396

Rubio I, Rodriguez-Viciana P et al (1997) Interaction of Ras with phosphoinositide 3-kinase gamma. Biochem J 326(Pt 3):891–895

Salehi Z, Mashayekhi F (2006) Expression of the eukaryotic translation initiation factor 4E (eIF4E) and 4E-BP1 in esophageal cancer. Clin Biochem 39(4):404–409

Sarbassov DD, Ali SM et al (2004) Rictor, a novel binding partner of mTOR, defines a rapamycin-insensitive and raptor-independent pathway that regulates the cytoskeleton. Curr Biol 14(14): 1296–1302

Sarbassov DD, Ali SM et al (2005) Growing roles for the mTOR pathway. Curr Opin Cell Biol 17(6):596–603
Sarbassov DD, Ali SM et al (2006) Prolonged rapamycin treatment inhibits mTORC2 assembly and Akt/PKB. Mol Cell 22(2):159–168
Sato R (2010) Sterol metabolism and SREBP activation. Arch Biochem Biophys 501(2):177–181
Schmidt EV (1999) The role of c-myc in cellular growth control. Oncogene 18(19):2988–2996
Sehgal A, Briggs J et al (2000) The chicken c-Jun 5′ untranslated region directs translation by internal initiation. Oncogene 19(24):2836–2845
Shantz LM (2004) Transcriptional and translational control of ornithine decarboxylase during Ras transformation. Biochem J 377(Pt 1):257–264
Shaw RJ, Bardeesy N et al (2004) The LKB1 tumor suppressor negatively regulates mTOR signaling. Cancer Cell 6(1):91–99
Shen JC, Klein RD et al (2000) Low-dose genistein induces cyclin-dependent kinase inhibitors and G(1) cell-cycle arrest in human prostate cancer cells. Mol Carcinog 29(2):92–102
Sonenberg N (2008) eIF4E, the mRNA cap-binding protein: from basic discovery to translational research. Biochem Cell Biol 86(2):178–183
Sonenberg N, Dever TE (2003) Eukaryotic translation initiation factors and regulators. Curr Opin Struct Biol 13(1):56–63
Sonenberg N, Hinnebusch AG (2009) Regulation of translation initiation in eukaryotes: mechanisms and biological targets. Cell 136(4):731–745
Spinozzi F, Pagliacci MC et al (1994) The natural tyrosine kinase inhibitor genistein produces cell cycle arrest and apoptosis in Jurkat T-leukemia cells. Leuk Res 18(6):431–439
Stayrook KR, McKinzie JH et al (1998) Effects of the antitumor agent perillyl alcohol on H-Ras vs. K-Ras farnesylation and signal transduction in pancreatic cells. Anticancer Res 18(2A):823–828
Stolovich M, Tang H et al (2002) Transduction of growth or mitogenic signals into translational activation of TOP mRNAs is fully reliant on the phosphatidylinositol 3-kinase-mediated pathway but requires neither S6K1 nor rpS6 phosphorylation. Mol Cell Biol 22(23):8101–8113
Stratton SP, Alberts DS et al (2010) A phase 2a study of topical perillyl alcohol cream for chemoprevention of skin cancer. Cancer Prev Res (Phila) 3(2):160–169
Subkhankulova T, Mitchell SA et al (2001) Internal ribosome entry segment-mediated initiation of c-Myc protein synthesis following genotoxic stress. Biochem J 359(Pt 1):183–192
Suh Y, Afaq F et al (2010) Fisetin induces autophagic cell death through suppression of mTOR signaling pathway in prostate cancer cells. Carcinogenesis 31(8):1424–1433
Sumitani S, Goya K et al (2002) Akt1 and Akt2 differently regulate muscle creatine kinase and myogenin gene transcription in insulin-induced differentiation of C2C12 myoblasts. Endocrinology 143(3):820–828
Suzuki Y, Nakabayashi Y et al (2001) Ubiquitin-protein ligase activity of X-linked inhibitor of apoptosis protein promotes proteasomal degradation of caspase-3 and enhances its anti-apoptotic effect in Fas-induced cell death. Proc Natl Acad Sci USA 98(15):8662–8667
Svitkin YV, Herdy B et al (2005) Eukaryotic translation initiation factor 4E availability controls the switch between cap-dependent and internal ribosomal entry site-mediated translation. Mol Cell Biol 25(23):10556–10565
Tan A, Bitterman P et al (2000) Inhibition of Myc-dependent apoptosis by eukaryotic translation initiation factor 4E requires cyclin D1. Oncogene 19(11):1437–1447
Teerink H, Voorma HO et al (1995) The human insulin-like growth factor II leader 1 contains an internal ribosomal entry site. Biochim Biophys Acta 1264(3):403–408
Thornton S, Anand N et al (2003) Not just for housekeeping: protein initiation and elongation factors in cell growth and tumorigenesis. J Mol Med 81(9):536–548
Trachootham D, Zhou Y et al (2006) Selective killing of oncogenically transformed cells through a ROS-mediated mechanism by beta-phenylethyl isothiocyanate. Cancer Cell 10(3):241–252
van den Beucken T, Koritzinsky M et al (2006) Translational control of gene expression during hypoxia. Cancer Biol Ther 5(7):749–755
Van Der Kelen K, Beyaert R et al (2009) Translational control of eukaryotic gene expression. Crit Rev Biochem Mol Biol 44(4):143–168

van der Velden AW, Thomas AA (1999) The role of the 5′ untranslated region of an mRNA in translation regulation during development. Int J Biochem Cell Biol 31(1):87–106

Vary TC, Goodman S et al (2005) Nutrient Regulation of PKC{epsilon} is Mediated by Leucine, not Insulin in Skeletal Muscle. Am J Physiol Endocrinol Metab 289(4):E684–E694

von der Haar T, Gross JD et al (2004) The mRNA cap-binding protein eIF4E in post-transcriptional gene expression. Nat Struct Mol Biol 11(6):503–511

Walker WA, Blackburn G (2004) Symposium introduction: nutrition and gene regulation. J Nutr 134(9):2434S–2436S

Waskiewicz AJ, Johnson JC et al (1999) Phosphorylation of the cap-binding protein eukaryotic translation initiation factor 4E by protein kinase Mnk1 in vivo. Mol Cell Biol 19(3):1871–1880

Wilkie GS, Dickson KS et al (2003) Regulation of mRNA translation by 5′- and 3′-UTR-binding factors. Trends Biochem Sci 28(4):182–188

Wiseman DA, Werner SR et al (2007) Cell cycle arrest by the isoprenoids perillyl alcohol, geraniol, and farnesol is mediated by p21(Cip1) and p27(Kip1) in human pancreatic adenocarcinoma cells. J Pharmacol Exp Ther 320(3):1163–1170

Wittke I, Madge B et al (2001) DAP-5 is involved in MycN/IFNgamma-induced apoptosis in human neuroblastoma cells. Cancer Lett 162(2):237–243

Xu M, Floyd HS et al (2004) Perillyl alcohol-mediated inhibition of lung cancer cell line proliferation: potential mechanisms for its chemotherapeutic effects. Toxicol Appl Pharmacol 195(2):232–246

Yan Y, Backer JM (2007) Regulation of class III (Vps34) PI3Ks. Biochem Soc Trans 35(Pt 2): 239–241

Yang L, Cao Z et al (2003) Coexistence of high levels of apoptotic signaling and inhibitor of apoptosis proteins in human tumor cells: implication for cancer specific therapy. Cancer Res 63(20): 6815–6824

Yeruva L, Pierre KJ et al (2007) Perillyl alcohol and perillic acid induced cell cycle arrest and apoptosis in non small cell lung cancer cells. Cancer Lett 257(2):216–226

Yorimitsu T, Klionsky DJ (2005) Autophagy: molecular machinery for self-eating. Cell Death Differ 12(Suppl 2):1542–1552

Yu W, Simmons-Menchaca M et al (1999) Induction of apoptosis in human breast cancer cells by tocopherols and tocotrienols. Nutr Cancer 33(1):26–32

Yuri T, Danbara N et al (2004) Perillyl alcohol inhibits human breast cancer cell growth in vitro and in vivo. Breast Cancer Res Treat 84(3):251–260

Zerial M, McBride H (2001) Rab proteins as membrane organizers. Nat Rev Mol Cell Biol 2(2):107–117

Zhou JR, Gugger ET et al (1999) Soybean phytochemicals inhibit the growth of transplantable human prostate carcinoma and tumor angiogenesis in mice. J Nutr 129(9):1628–1635

Chapter 16
Regulation of MicroRNAs by Natural Compounds: Implications for Cancer Therapy

Devarajan Karunagaran, Maitreyi Subramanian, and Rao Srinivasa Rao

MicroRNAs (miRNAs) are evolutionarily conserved short (19–22 nucleotides) noncoding RNA sequences that bind to target mRNAs, leading to their degradation or inhibition of translation. They have received a lot of attention in recent years as fine regulators of gene expression thus influencing many biological processes including the development and progression of cancers. Many miRNAs with a role in cancer including invasion and metastasis as well as those having tumor suppressor activities have been characterized. Expression profiling of miRNAs classifies cancers and even serves to predict prognosis. Aberrations in miRNA expression affect that of their target proteins eventually altering the chemosensitivity of tumor cells. Targeting miRNAs for cancer therapy is thus an emerging field for treatment optimization aiming to inhibit proliferation of cancer cells and/or to increase their sensitivity to conventional chemotherapy by inducing apoptosis. Natural compounds and dietary constituents such as curcumin, epigallocatechin-3-gallate, ellagitannin, folates, retinoids and some isoflavones are known to have antiproliferative and/or apoptotic effects in cancer cells and have been shown to modulate the miRNA expression profiles. However, detailed mechanisms as to how curcumin or other natural compounds regulate miRNAs are not known. The natural compounds are relatively non-toxic and their combination with conventional chemotherapy could be a novel and safer approach to eliminate the resistant cancer stem cells or those undergoing epithelial to mesenchymal transition (EMT) and realize the ultimate goal of improving the drug sensitivity (Kawasaki et al. 2008; Kakarala et al. 2010; Tang et al. 2010a). Deep understanding on the mechanisms of miRNA regulation by natural compounds would offer promising hopes to overcome anticancer drug resistance.

D. Karunagaran (✉) • M. Subramanian • R.S. Rao
Department of Biotechnology, Indian Institute of Technology Madras, Chennai 600 036, India

M. Diederich and K. Noworyta (eds.), *Natural Compounds as Inducers of Cell Death: Volume 1*, DOI 10.1007/978-94-007-4575-9_16,

16.1 MicroRNAs

In recent years, there has been a great deal of interest in studying the role of microRNAs (miRNAs) as tiny regulators of gene expression that influence various cellular processes including development, proliferation, differentiation, apoptosis and survival. miRNAs are 19–22 nucleotide-long evolutionarily conserved RNA molecules which act by binding to complementary sequences on the 3′-untranslated regions (3′-UTRs) of target mRNAs leading to their degradation or translational inhibition (Bartel 2009). Approximately 3% of human genes encode for miRNAs, and up to one-third of human protein-coding genes may be regulated by miRNAs (Lewis et al. 2005). The miRNA genes are present in the intergenic regions or are hosted within the introns and exons of other protein coding genes. The intragenic miRNAs are usually transcribed along with the host genes whereas the intergenic miRNA genes have their own promoters and regulatory elements (Lagos-Quintana et al. 2001; Rodriguez et al. 2004; Kim and Kim 2007). The expression of miRNAs may also be affected by epigenetic changes, such as DNA methylation, histone acetylation and chromatin remodeling (Saito and Jones 2006). miRNA genes are transcribed by RNA polymerase II and sometimes by RNA polymerase III to give pri-miRNAs which can be 200 bases to several kilobases in length with 5′ 7-methylguanosine cap and 3′ poly(A) tail. This pri-miRNA may have multiple stem loops when it is transcribed from a miRNA cluster (Lee et al. 2004; Altuvia et al. 2005; Cai et al. 2004; Faller and Guo 2008). The pri-miRNA is then cleaved by the nuclear RNase III (Drosha) – DGCR8 complexes at regions flanking the stem-loop structure to form ~70 nucleotides long precursor called 'pre-miRNA' having a hairpin structure with a monophosphate at the 5′ end and a 2-nucleotide overhang at the 3′ end (Gregory et al. 2006). The miRNAs transcribed from introns may bypass the Drosha machinery and the pre-miRNAs are formed after splicing (Berezikov et al. 2007). This precursor is exported out into the cytoplasm by the exportin-Ran GTP complex where it is processed by Dicer (endonuclease III) forming ~21 bp miRNA duplex. The miRNA strand which has an energetically less stable 5′ end is considered to be the 'guide strand' which is loaded onto the RISC (RNA-induced-silencing complex) for processing while the other strand is considered as inactive or carrier strand called miRNA* (miRNA star) or passenger strand that is usually degraded (Murchison and Hannon 2004; Lund and Dahlberg 2006; Ji 2008; Pratt and MacRae 2009). The main components of the RISC complex are the argonaute proteins having two conserved RNA binding domains: the PAZ and PIWI domains which bind to the 3′- and 5′-end of the guide strand, respectively, and orient the miRNA to bind to the complementary sites on the mRNA. The double stranded RNA is then cleaved by the argonaute proteins or accessory proteins are recruited to the RISC complex to enable translational repression (Pratt and MacRae 2009). However, recently, some miRNA* sequences have been shown to function as mature miRNAs and their expression varies dramatically during developmental stages (Okamura et al. 2008; Ro et al. 2007). In animals, miRNAs are partially complementary to their mRNA targets at the seed sequence, a heptameric sequence beginning at the first or second position from the 5′ end of the miRNA

(Ambros 2004; Doench and Sharp 2004). This partial complementarity prevents translation of the mRNA but in some cases, can also cause acceleration of deadenylation and mRNA degradation (Eulalio et al. 2009). Some miRNAs have binding sites in the 5′-UTRs or the coding or promoter regions (causing histone modification and/or DNA methylation) ultimately affecting the expression of the target genes (Hawkins and Morris 2008). Each miRNA has multiple targets and each mRNA is targeted by multiple miRNAs and various bioinformatics programs score the predictions based primarily on the extent of sequence complementarity between the target mRNA and miRNA and the stability of the hybrid. Other considerations include conservation of target sites across species, correlation of available expression profiles, proximity to stop codon and AU rich regions on the 3′-UTRs and the proximity to sites targeted by co-regulated miRNAs (Stark et al. 2003; Robins et al. 2005; Krek et al. 2005; Lewis et al. 2005; Long et al. 2007; Grimson et al. 2007). Many recent reviews on miRNA biogenesis, mode of action and their therapeutic potential in cancer are available (Fabian et al. 2010; Sotiropoulou et al. 2009; Esquela-Kerscher and Slack 2006; Voorhoeve 2010; Cho 2010) and further discussion here is focused on the involvement of miRNAs in apoptosis and cancer.

16.2 Role of MicroRNAs in Cancer and Apoptosis

Aberrant miRNA expression in cancer can be the result of several different mechanisms, including chromosomal abnormalities, genomic mutations and polymorphism, epigenetic changes, and alterations in miRNA biogenesis. Many miRNA genes in humans are located at fragile sites or chromosomal break points, regions of loss of heterozygosity or viral integration sites which are associated with cancer. Cancer cells from every type of tumor analyzed have significantly different miRNA expression profiles as compared to normal cells from the same tissue underlining the biological significance of miRNA function in cancer progression. Tumor samples of epithelial origin differed in miRNA expression profiles from those of hematopoietic origin (Lu et al. 2005; Yanaihara et al. 2006; Volinia et al. 2006). Microarray technologies for analysis of miRNAs enabled rapid identification of miRNAs that are up or downregulated in various cancers. Cancer subtypes can be identified by using such expression profiling of miRNAs more accurately than using the expression profiles of protein-coding genes and hence miRNA profiling also has the potential to become a powerful tool for diagnosis and treatment of cancer (Esquela-Kerscher and Slack 2006; Calin et al. 2004). miRNAs promoting cell proliferation or tumour formation are called oncomirs and their expression is often upregulated in cancers. miRNAs that act as tumor suppressors by downregulating the expression of oncogenes and/or antagonizing tumor formation are called antioncomirs and are usually underexpressed in cancers (Goga and Benz 2007). miR-15 and miR-16 are antioncomirs encoded in the 13q14 chromosomal region that is often deleted in Chronic Lymphocytic Leukemia (Calin and Croce 2006a) and the miR-99a/let-7c/miR-125b2 cluster and the homologous cluster, miR-100/let-7a/miR-125b, are found in regions whose deletion is associated with lung cancers and breast carcinoma, respectively (Calin et al. 2004). Malignant lymphomas are often characterized by amplification/overexpression of miR-17-92 gene cluster (Ota et al. 2004; He et al. 2005) and miR-155 (Metzler et al. 2004; Eis et al. 2005), both of which are typical oncomirs. Oncomirs generally target proapoptotic genes and antioncomirs target the antiapoptotic genes stabilizing the apoptotic pathways contributing to the regulation of cancer progression (Voorhoeve and Agami 2007). miR-15 and miR-16 that target the antiapoptotic factor BCL2 (Cimmino et al. 2005), miR-34 that targets genes like CDK6, CCND1, SIRT1, E2F3, MYCN (Sun et al. 2008a; Yamakuchi et al. 2008; Welch et al. 2007; Wei et al. 2008) involved in cell proliferation, miR-29a/b/c that target antiapoptotic factors like MCL1 and TCL1 (Mott et al. 2007; Pekarsky et al. 2006) and let-7 that targets Bcl-xL (Shimizu et al. 2010) are typical antioncomirs and are thus proapoptotic when ectopically expressed in cancer cells. In contrast, miR-21, a typical oncomir, exerts an antiapoptotic effect by downregulating the proapoptotic factors like PDCD4, TPM1, and MARCKS (Frankel et al. 2008; Zhu et al. 2007; Li et al. 2009a) and miR-17-92 cluster downregulates the proapoptotic factor BIM and confers resistance to apoptosis (Xiao et al. 2008). However, contradictory roles for some miRNAs have also been observed. For instance, let-7 (antioncomir) downregulated caspase-3 expression by directly binding to the 3′UTR of its mRNA and increased the resistance of A431 (human squamous carcinoma) and HepG2 (hepatocellular carcinoma) cells to apoptosis induced by therapeutic drugs (Tsang and Kwok 2008) whereas the miR-17-92 microRNA cluster, contrary to its demonstrated role as an oncomir in lymphomas, targets the oncogene AIB1 in breast cancer cell lines (Hossain et al. 2006). Hence, the characterization of miRNAs as oncomirs/antiapoptotic or antioncomirs/proapoptotic is highly context-dependent (Croce 2009). Some well known miRNAs involved in the regulation of apoptosis and their respective validated targets are listed in Table 16.1.

In recent years, a number of miRNA microarray profiling studies have been carried out to study the alteration of the miRNA signatures of the cells upon treatment with anticancer drugs as well as some natural compounds that are inducers of cell death to try and correlate their pharmacological activities to the miRNA profiles. As one of the mechanisms, many natural compounds such as genistein, curcumin, resveratrol and epigallocatechin-3-gallate can also cause epigenetic changes (Meeran et al. 2010) that can then influence the miRNA expression. For example mir-127 upregulation was observed upon treatment with chromatin-modifying drugs in human cancer cells (Saito et al. 2006). The chemical structures of some of the natural compounds known to induce alterations in miRNA profiles are shown in Fig. 16.1. The present review summarizes the recent available information on the alterations in miRNA expression profiles induced by natural compounds known to regulate apoptosis (Table 16.2) and discusses the implications of such alterations for cancer therapy.

Table 16.1 List of miRNAs regulating apoptosis and their validated targets

miRNA	Validated targets	Function of miRNA	References
Let-7a/b/c/d/e/f/i	RAS, MYCN, HMGA2, CCND2, CDK6, CDC25A, BCL2L1 (Bcl-xL), CASP3	Proapoptotic	Johnson et al. (2005), Sampson et al. (2007), Lee and Dutta (2007), Johnson et al. (2007), Shimizu et al. (2010), and Tsang and Kwok (2008)
miR-15, miR-16	BCL2, CCND1	Proapoptotic	Cimmino et al. (2005) and Deshpande et al. (2009)
miR-17-92 (miR-17, miR-18a, miR-19a, miR-20a, miR-19b, and miR-92a)	E2F1, BCL2L11 (BIM), PTEN, CDKN1A (p21), RBL2, CTGF, NCOA3 (AIB1)	Antiapoptotic	Xiao et al. (2008), O'Donnell et al. (2005), Olive et al. (2009), Inomata et al. (2009), Lu et al. (2007), Ernst et al. (2010), and Hossain et al. (2006)
miR-21	PTEN, PDCD4,TPM1, TIMP3	Antiapoptotic	Meng et al. (2007), Frankel et al. (2008), Zhu et al. (2007), and Zhang et al. (2008)
miR-22	ESR1, SP1, CMYB, PTEN	Proapoptotic	Sun et al. (2008b), Pandey and Picard (2009), Xiong et al. (2010), and Bar and Dikstein (2010)
miR-24	FAF1, DHFR, E2F2, MYC, AURKB, CCNA2, CDC2, CDK4, FEN1, BRCA1	Proapoptotic	Qin et al. (2010), Mishra et al. (2009), and Lal et al. (2009)
miR--25(miR-106b, miR-93, miR-25)	CDKN1A, BCL2L11	Antiapoptotic	Kan et al. (2009) and Li et al. (2009c)
miR-27a	ST14, PPARG, APC, PAX3	Antiapoptotic	Wang et al. (2009b), Karbiener et al. (2009), Wang and Xu (2010), and Crist et al. (2009)
miR-29a/b/c	MCl1, TCL1A, DNMTs, PIK3R1, CDC42, DKK1, KREMEN2, SFRP2	Proapoptotic	Mott et al. (2007), Pekarsky et al. (2006), Park et al. (2009), Fabbri et al. (2007), and Kapinas et al. (2010)
miR-34a/b/c	CCNE2, CDK6, CCND1, SIRT1, E2F3, MET, MYCN, CREB1	Proapoptotic	Sun et al. (2008a), Yamakuchi et al. (2008), Welch et al. (2007), Wei et al. (2008), Li et al. (2009d), and Pigazzi et al. (2009)
miR-106a	RB1	Antiapoptotic	Jiang et al. (2010)

(continued)

Table 16.1 (continued)

miRNA	Validated targets	Function of miRNA	References
miR-122	BCL2L2, CCNG1	Proapoptotic	Lin et al. (2008) and Gramantieri et al. (2007)
miR-125	BCL3, E2F3	Proapoptotic	Guan et al. (2010) and Huang et al. (2010b)
miR-127	BCL6	Proapoptotic	Saito et al. (2006)
miR-143	MAPK7, KRAS	Proapoptotic	Clape et al. (2009) and Chen et al. (2009)
miR-145	PPP3CA, CBFB, CLINT1, YES1, STAT1, RTKN, MYC	Proapoptotic	Ostenfeld et al. (2010), Gregersen et al. (2010), Wang et al. (2009c), and Sachdeva et al. (2009)
miR-146	CCL8, ERBB4, FAS	Antiapoptotic	Rom et al. (2010), Horie et al. (2010), and Suzuki et al. (2010)
miR-155	FOXO3, PKIA, SHIP1, TP53INP1	Antiapoptotic	Kong et al. (2010), Fassi Fehri et al. (2010), Pedersen et al. (2009), and Gironella et al. (2007)
miR-181	BCL2, TCL1A	Proapoptotic	Pekarsky et al. (2006) and Zhu et al. (2010)
miR-200	PTPN13 (FAP-1), ZEB1, ZEB2	Proapoptotic	Schickel et al. (2010) and Park et al. (2008)
miR-214	LTF, PTEN	Antiapoptotic	Liao et al. (2010) and Yang et al. (2008)
miR-221, miR-222	KIT, PSMD9 (p27), CDKN1C (p57), BBC3 (PUMA), BMF	Antiapoptotic	Felli et al. (2005), le Sage et al. (2007), Fornari et al. (2008), Zhang et al. (2010c), and Gramantieri et al. (2009)
miR-372, miR-373	LATS2	Antiapoptotic	Cho et al. (2009) and Lee et al. (2009)

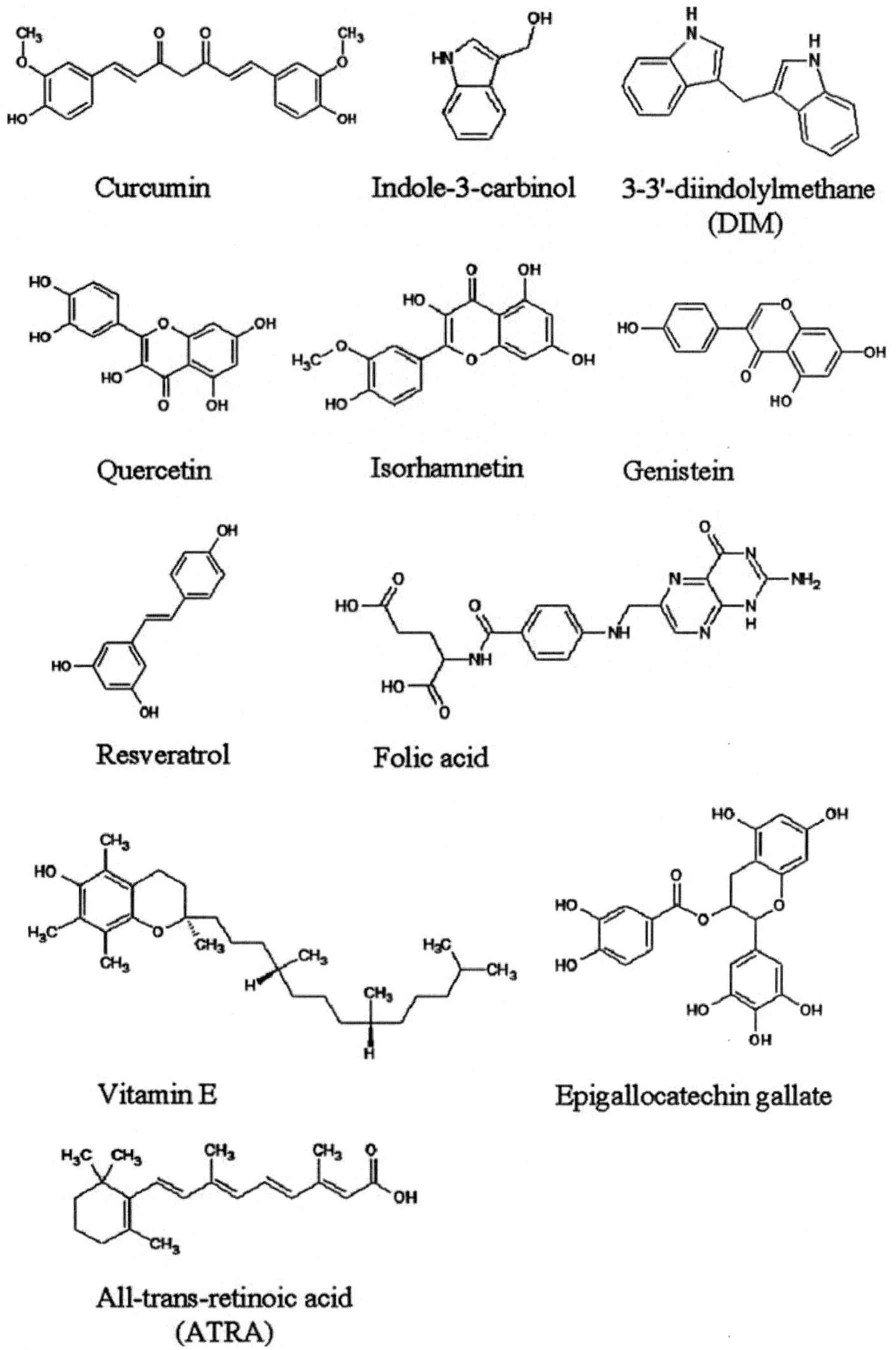

Fig. 16.1 Chemical structures of natural compounds known to alter miRNA expression profiles

Table 16.2 Alterations in miRNA expression profile induced by natural compounds

Chemical	Downregulated miRNA	Upregulated miRNA	References
Curcumin	miR-21, miR-140, miR-146b, miR-148a, miR-15b, miR-195, miR-196 s, miR-199a*, miR-204, miR-25, miR-26a, miR-374, miR-510, miR-7, mR-92, miR-93, miR-98	miR-103, miR-181a, miR-181b, miR-181d, miR-21, miR-22, miR-23a, miR-23b, miR-24, miR-27a, miR-34a, miR-200	Sun et al. (2008b), Mudduluru et al. (2010), and Ali et al. (2010)
EGCG	miR-10a, miR-18a, miR-19a, miR-26b, miR-29b, miR-34b, miR-98, miR-99b, miR-129, miR-138, miR-181d, miR-182, miR-186, miR-193b, miR-196a, miR-196b, miR-199a, miR-200a, miR-205, miR-210, miR-217, miR-222, miR-302b/c, miR-335, miR-342, miR-361, miR-373, miR-376, miR-409, miR-422, miR-423, miR-425, miR-450, miR-484, miR-491, miR-494, miR-497, miR-505, miR-507, miR-516, miR-517c, miR-518a/c, miR-519, miR-522, miR-524, miR-526, miR-125b, miR-27a, miR-27b, miR-100, miR-224, miR-23a, miR-24, miR-31, miR-93, miR-99b, miR-20a, miR-15b, miR-767-5p	miR-182*, miR-498, let-7a/b/c/d, miR-16, miR-18b, miR-20a, miR-25, miR-92, miR-93, miR-221, miR-320, miR-377	Tsang and Kwok (2010) and Ahn et al. (2010)
Genistein	miR-27a	Let-7a/b/c/d/e/f, miR-200b/c	Sun et al. (2009) and Li et al. (2009b)

Resveratrol	miR-181a-2, miR-21, miR-424, miR-196a-1, miR-657, miR-92a-2, miR-23a, miR-16-1, miR-25, miR-146a, miR-100-1/2, miR-26a, miR-594, miR-30a-3p, miR-17, miR-565, miR-103-1, miR-631, miR-30d, miR-23b, miR-102, miR-205, miR-629, miR-30e-5p, miR-155	miR-206, miR-560, miR-194-2, miR-639, miR-1, miR-801, miR-659, miR-323, miR-572, miR-560, miR-497, miR-30c-1, miR-615, miR-663, miR-565, miR-340, miR-363*-5p, miR-638, miR-494, miR-622, miR-574, miR-146b-5p, miR-663	Lukiw et al. (2008) and Tili et al. (2010b, c)
Quercetin	miR-155		Boesch-Saadatmandi et al. (2010)
I3C, DIM	miR-21	Let-7a/b/c/d/e/f, miR-200b/c	Li et al. (2009b) and Melkamu et al. (2010)
Ellagitannin	miR-542-3p, let-7d, miR-299-3p, let-7c, -miR-200a*, let-7f, let-7i, let-7a	miR-443, miR-526b, miR-370, miR-452, miR-194, miR-373*, miR-518f*-526a, miR-302a*, miR-424, let-7e, miR-525, miR-519e*, miR-510, miR-513, miR-518c*, miR-512-5p, miR-346	Wen et al. (2009)
Ethanol	miR-200a, miR-496, miR-296, miR-30e-5p, miR-362, miR-339, miR-29c, miR-154	miR-10a, miR-10b, miR-9, miR-145, miR-30a-3p, miR-152	Wang et al. (2009a)
Folate, Retinoids	miR-10a, miR-9/9*, miR-124a, and miR-125b, miR-181b,	let-7a-3, let-7c, let-7d, miR-16-1, miR-223, miR-15a, miR-15b, miR-342, miR-107d, miR-147d, miR-10a	Wang et al. (2009a), Zhao et al. (2008), Garzon et al. (2007), and Huang et al. (2010a)

16.3 Regulation of miRNA Expression by Curcumin

Curcumin (Diferuloyl methane) is an active polyphenolic ingredient present in the rhizomes of *Curcuma longa*, used over several centuries in culinary and medical practices in Asia. Curcumin is a potent antioxidant, antiinflammatory, chemopreventive and chemotherapeutic agent (Hatcher et al. 2008). Anticancer activity of curcumin has been demonstrated in cancer cell lines of different tissue origin, including breast, cervical, colon, brain, gastric, hepatic, leukemia, oral epithelial, ovarian, pancreatic, melanoma, and prostate (Karunagaran et al. 2007). Anticancer effects of curcumin are mainly attributed to its ability to induce apoptosis in cancer cells by influencing multiple signaling pathways including those mediated by STAT, p53, NF-κB, MAPK, jun and cyclooxygenase (Karunagaran et al. 2005). Curcumin also potentiates the effects of chemotherapy in animal models and is safe as it is tolerated in doses as high as 8,000 mg/day in human patients (Cheng et al. 2001; Sharma et al. 2001). As fine regulators of cellular functions including apoptosis, miRNAs are expected to be involved in curcumin-induced apoptosis in cancer cells. Curcumin indeed upregulated the expression of miR-22 and consequently downregulated its target genes (ESR1 and SP1) in BxPC-3 (human pancreatic cancer) cells (Sun et al. 2008b). miR-22 is a proapoptotic miRNA that targets and downregulates ESR1 (estrogen receptor 1) (Pandey and Picard 2009) and cMYB (Xiong et al. 2010) leading to a decrease in proliferation of MCF7-SH and MCF7 breast cancer cells, respectively. Curcumin also upregulated miR-34a in BxPC-3 cells having a mutant p53 (Sun et al. 2008b). miR-34a is a p53-inducible miRNA that promotes apoptosis (Chang et al. 2007) and restoration of its expression in p53 mutant pancreatic cancer cells (BxPC-3 and MiaPaCa2) induced apoptosis and sensitized them to chemotherapy and radiation (Ji et al. 2009). Interestingly, B-RAF induced miR-34a in immortalized fibroblasts independent of p53 (Christoffersen et al. 2010) but curcumin decreased B-RAF protein in canine kidney cells (MDCK) exposed to forskolin (Gao et al. 2011). Differences in cell types and experimental conditions used by different workers make it difficult to provide a mechanistic basis for curcumin-mediated upregulation of miR-34a. Nevertheless, the ability of curcumin to induce this miRNA highlights its potency as an inducer of apoptosis independent of p53. Curcumin also upregulates miR-15 and miR-16 in MCF7 cells thereby downregulating Bcl-2 (Yang et al. 2009a). Bcl-2 was shown to be a direct target of miR-15 and miR-16 and overexpression of these miRNAs induced apoptosis in a leukemia cell line model (Cimmino et al. 2005). Curcumin also downregulates miR-21 by repressing AP-1 transcription factor in colon cancer cells (Mudduluru et al. 2010). miR-21 is most often upregulated in human tumors and inactivation of miR-21 leads to total tumor regression in animal models (Medina et al. 2010). Although curcumin downregulates the expression of miR-199a* in BxPC-3 pancreatic cancer cells (Sun et al. 2008b), transfection of miR-199a and/or -199a* mimetics into several cancer cell lines caused prominent apoptosis with miR-199a* being more proapoptotic (Kim et al. 2008) suggesting the complex nature of curcumin-mediated regulation of miRNAs. However, the greatest hurdle for use of curcumin as a drug is its very low bioavailability and a great deal of work has been done to develop more effective strategies of delivery and new analogues of curcumin with higher bioavailability. CDF, a diflouro analog of curcumin with greater bioavailability (Padhye et al. 2009) upregulated miR-200b and miR-200c and downregulated the expression of miR-21 in gemcitabine-resistant pancreatic cancer cell lines and sensitized the cells to gemcitabine (Ali et al. 2010). The antimetastatic and proapoptotic nature of the miR-200 family of miRNAs has been demonstrated in many studies. miR-200 prevents TGF-β-induced EMT of NMuMG mouse mammary epithelial cells (Korpal et al. 2008) and miR-200c increases the susceptibility of HCT116 (human colorectal carcinoma) and CAKI-1 (human renal cell line) cells to apoptosis mediated by CD95 (Schickel et al. 2010). In A549/DDP multidrug-resistant human lung adenocarcinoma cells, curcumin downregulated miR-186* and induced apoptosis. The same effect was observed with a specific inhibitor of this miRNA whereas ectopic expression of the miRNA blocked curcumin-induced apoptosis (Zhang et al. 2010a). This demonstrates that curumin-induced downregulation of miR-186* is required for its apoptotic effects. miR-186* acts as an antiapoptotic factor by targeting caspase-10 (Zhang et al. 2010b). Human lung cancer cells (A549/DDP) treated with curcumin showed upregulation of miR-29a and downregulation of miR-34a (Tang et al. 2010b) both of which are proapoptotic in cancer cell lines of epithelial origin. It is apparent that regulation of miRNA expression is an important and novel mechanism by which curcumin induces apoptosis. It is hoped that a deeper understanding on curcumin-mediated regulation of miRNAs would offer novel and safer approaches to eliminate the resistant cancer cells and realize the ultimate goal of improving the drug sensitivity.

16.4 Role of Epigallocatechin Gallate in the Regulation of miRNAs

Epigallocatechin gallate (EGCG), a flavanoid found in green tea leaves, is well known for its antioxidant and anticancer properties. EGCG induced apoptosis in breast, cervical and pancreatic cancer cells, and human osteogenic sarcoma cells (Thangapazham et al. 2007; Qanungo et al. 2005; Siddiqui et al. 2010; Ji et al. 2006). It has been suggested that EGCG may increase the potency of other chemotherapeutic drugs when used in combination though it is contraindicated for patients undergoing treatment with Bortezomib (Velcade) (Golden et al. 2009). A microarray analysis of HepG2 (human hepatocarcinoma) cells showed that EGCG deregulated the expression of 61 miRNAs. miR-16, one of the miRNAs upregulated by EGCG, is known to target the antiapoptotic factor Bcl-2. EGCG-induced apoptosis was reduced when miR-16 was inhibited suggesting that the apoptotic effect of EGCG, at least in part, is carried out through the induction of miR-16 (Tsang and Kwok 2010). Other miRNAs upregulated by EGCG in HepG2 cells include the let-7 family of miRNAs (Tsang and Kwok 2010) that targets the RAS family of oncogenes (Johnson et al. 2005). In contrast, some miRNAs upregulated by EGCG (miR-20a and miR-25) are known to have antiapoptotic effects (Tsang and Kwok 2010). Inhibition of miR-20a of the mir-17-92 cluster impedes cell cycle progression by a G_1 checkpoint involving p21, p53 and 53BP1 (Pickering et al. 2009). miR-25 from the miR-106b-25 cluster, overexpressed in gastric cancers, downregulated the expression of Bcl-2-interacting mediator of cell death (BIM), which is essential for TGF-β-dependent apoptosis (Kan et al. 2009). In addition, miRNAs downregulated by EGCG include miR-29b, miR-34b, miR-200a and miR-199a which have been shown to be proapoptotic. miR-29b downregulates Mcl-1 (Mott et al. 2007) and upregulates p53 (Park et al. 2009) promoting apoptosis and miR-34b is a p53-inducible proapoptotic miRNA (Corney et al. 2007). Transfection of miR-199a mimetics into PC3 (prostate cancer cell line), KB (oral epidermoid carcinoma) and MCF7 (breast carcinoma) cells caused prominent apoptosis (Kim et al. 2008). These results suggest that the apoptotic effect of EGCG in HepG2 cells cannot be clearly explained by looking at the changes in the miRNA profile alone as there is no discernible pattern to the induction or repression of miRNAs by it. Furthermore the results may vary in a time or concentration dependent manner and are complicated by the variations in miRNA-mRNA target pairs induced by EGCG. Two miRNA-mRNA target pairs (miR-125b, miR-27a) changed in a time-dependent manner and nine pairs (miR-100, miR-182*, miR-224, miR-23a, miR-24, miR-31, miR-498, miR-miR-93, miR-99b) changed in a concentration-dependent manner and four pairs changed in a time and concentration dependent manner (miR-15b, miR-27b, miR-20a, miR-767-5p) upon treatment with EGCG in HepG2 cells (Ahn et al. 2010). In spite of these conflicting results by EGCG in HepG2 cells, the overall effect of this compound in many cell types including HepG2 appears to be proapoptotic (Thangapazham et al. 2007; Qanungo et al. 2005; Siddiqui et al. 2010; Ji et al. 2006). This shows that the regulation of cellular processes by miRNAs is more complicated and a better understanding of such regulatory circuits is required to elucidate the mechanism of action of EGCG.

16.5 Effects of Genistein on the Expression of miRNAs

Genistein, an isoflavone isolated from soybean, inhibited the growth of uveal melanoma cells and their tumor xenografts in nude mice and its antiproliferative activity, at least in part, is due to the downregulation of miR-27a expression and increase in its target (ZBTB10) expression with genistein treatment in a concentration-dependent manner (Sun et al. 2009). miR-27a had oncogenic activity in ER-α negative MDA-MB-231 cells and this effect was partly attributed to the suppression of its direct targets, ZBTB10 and MYT1 (Mertens-Talcott et al. 2007). miR-27a induced the expression of P-glycoprotein (encoded by the MDR1 gene), known to be associated with the resistance of cancer cells to chemotherapeutic drugs (Zhu et al. 2008). Drug resistance is also associated with EMT (Fuchs et al. 2008; Cheng et al. 2007;

Sabbah et al. 2008). miR-200 and let-7 families of miRNAs are negative regulators of EMT (Park et al. 2008; Peter 2009) and were downregulated in gemcitabine-resistant pancreatic cancer cells (Li et al. 2009b). G2535, an isoflavone mixture (70.54% genistein, 26.34% diadzin, and 0.31% glycitein), upregulated miR-200 and let-7 miRNAs in gemcitabine-resistant pancreatic cancer cells thereby reversing the EMT and sensitizing the cells to gemcitabine, an effect that was also observed upon ectopic expression of these miRNAs (Li et al. 2009b). Genistein, nutlin and miR-16 synergistically induced apoptosis in malignant B-1 cells from New Zealand Black mice with chronic lymphoblastic leukemia (Salerno et al. 2009). It will be of interest to know whether the genistein-mediated regulation of miRNAs would be useful to sensitize cancer cells to many other chemotherapeutic agents.

16.6 Modulation of miRNA Expression by Resveratrol

Resveratrol (3,4′,5-trihydroxy-trans-stilbene) is a polyphenol that is found mainly in red grapes, berries, plums, peanuts, pines and other plant sources. It has been shown to induce apoptosis in human prostate carcinoma cells, human breast cancer xenografts, transformed follicular lymphoma cells, human retinoblastoma cells and other cancer cell lines (Aziz et al. 2006; Benitez et al. 2007; Garvin et al. 2006; Faber and Chiles 2006; Sareen et al. 2006). Preclinical *in vivo* studies highlighted the potential of resveratrol to be used as an anticancer agent for breast cancer (Levi et al. 2005). Treatment of SW480 (human colon adenocarcinoma) cells with 50 μM resveratrol significantly increased the expression levels of 22 miRNAs and decreased that of 26 other miRNAs many of which are oncomirs (miR-17, miR-21, miR-25, or miR-92a-2) (Tili et al. 2007, 2010a; Calin and Croce 2006b) known to be overexpressed in colorectal carcinomas (Rossi et al. 2010; Yang et al. 2009b). Resveratrol also downregulated miRNAs that target Dicer1 (miR-103-1 and miR-103-2) (Tili et al. 2010a). The lower levels of miR-103 in SW480 cells correlated with the lower metastatic potential of these cells as compared to SW620 cells, derived from the metastatic sites of the same patient from whom SW480 cells were derived (primary tumor cells) (Martello et al. 2010). Targeting Dicer1 by miR-103 may result in a global downregulation of miRNAs, a trend seen in cancer cells (Lu et al. 2005). Resveratrol also downregulated two proapoptotic miRNAs (miR-16-1 and miR-29c) (Tili et al. 2010a). CAY10512, an analog of resveratrol decreased NF-κB-dependent activation of miR-146a promoter though the effect of this compound on the levels of mature miRNA was not studied (Lukiw et al. 2008). Resveratrol upregulated miR-663, in human THP-1 monocytic cells and blood monocytes and decreased endogenous AP-1 activity and impaired the upregulation of miR-155 by lipopolysaccharide in a miR-663-dependent manner. Considering the role of miR-155 in the innate immune response and its upregulation in many cancers, these results suggest that one can optimize the use of resveratrol as anti-inflammatory and/or anticancer agent against tumors with high levels of miR-155 by manipulating miR-663 levels (Tili et al. 2010b).

16.7 Effects of Indole-3-Carbinol (I3C) and Its Derivative on miRNAs

Indole-3-carbinol (I3C), a naturally occurring component of *Brassica* vegetables (cabbage, broccoli and brussels sprouts), and its di-indole derivative 3-3′-diindolylmethane (DIM), are known to have antiproliferative effects on cancer cells (Rahman et al. 2000; Srivastava and Shukla 1998; Hong et al. 2002; Leong et al. 2001). DIM induced the expression of miR-200 and let-7 family of miRNAs (miR-200b, miR-200c, let-7b, let-7c, let-7d, and let-7e) in pancreatic cancer cells making them more susceptible to gemcitabine-induced cell death and reversed the EMT observed in the gemcitabine-resistant cells (Li et al. 2009b). Dietary administration of Indole-3-carbinol reversed the carcinogenic effects of vinyl carbamate-induced lung tumors in A/J mice partially by downregulating miR-21, miR-31 and miR-146a which were upregulated by vinyl carbamate. Levels of these miRNAs were higher in A549 lung adenocarcinoma cells and hTERT immortalized normal human bronchial epithelial (NHBE) cells as compared with the non-immortalized NHBE cells. Indole-3-carbinol significantly downregulated miR-21 and upregulated its targets (PTEN, PDCD4 and RECK) in A549 cells (Melkamu et al. 2010). These results suggest that I3C and DIM have the ability to alter miRNA expression and, if carefully exploited, this could serve to sensitize the cancer cells resistant to chemotherapy.

16.8 miRNAs Regulated by All-Trans-Retinoic Acid (ATRA)

All-trans-retinoic acid (ATRA)-treated pregnant rats showed downregulation of Bcl-2, miR-9/9*, miR-124a/125b and P53 expression in their fetuses showing spina bifida and further studies may reveal the mechanisms by which ATRA induces cell death (Zhao et al. 2008). ATRA induced granulocytic differentiation of acute promyelocytic leukemia cells and downregulated miR-181b but upregulated let-7a-3, let-7c, let-7d, miR-16-1, miR-223, miR-15a, miR-15b, miR-342, miR-107d, and miR-147d. Similar changes except for the downregulation of miR-181b were seen after ATRA treatment of primary blast cells isolated from acute promyelocytic leukemia patients (Fazi et al. 2005). miR-181 family had a tumor suppressor role in human glioma cells (Shi et al. 2008) but acted as an oncomir in acute myeloid leukemia cells (Chen et al. 2010). Interestingly, ATRA-induced miR-107 targeted NF1-A transcription factor (negative regulator of miR-223) thereby upregulating miR-223 (Fazi et al. 2005). miR-107 acted as a tumor suppressor in human non small cell lung cancer cell lines (Takahashi et al. 2009) and also inhibited tumor angiogenesis (Yamakuchi et al. 2010). miR-223 is a myeloid specific miRNA that inhibited hematopoietic cell proliferation and fine tuned granulocytic differentiation and erythropoiesis (Sun et al. 2010; Johnnidis et al. 2008; Felli et al. 2009). NF-κB-induced transcription of the let-7a-3/let7b cluster was upregulated by ATRA in human acute promyelocytic leukemia. ATRA-mediated downregulation of antiapoptotic proteins, RAS and Bcl-2, correlated with the activation of known miRNA regulators of those proteins, let-7a and miR-15a/miR-16-1, respectively (Garzon et al. 2007). Retinoic acid induced the binding of NF-κB to the promoter of miR-10a and the resultant increase in miR-10a enhanced smooth muscle cell differentiation from embryonic stem cells via repression of HDAC4, a negative regulator of differentiation (Huang et al. 2010a). A recent report has shown that upon treatment with ATRA, 402 gene promoters became demethylated whereas, 88 were hypermethylated (Das et al. 2010). mRNA expression microarrays revealed that 82 of the demethylated genes were overexpressed by >twofold, whereas 13 of the hypermethylated genes were underexpressed in neuroblastoma cells. miRNA-mediated DNA demethylation changes contributed to the process of ATRA-induced differentiation resulting in the activation of NOS1, a critical determinant of neural cell differentiation (Das et al. 2010). These results clearly suggest that ATRA-mediated miRNA modulation influences several cellular processes such as differentiation, apoptosis and epigenetic changes relevant in cancer.

16.9 Influence of Dietary Factors and Other Natural Compounds on miRNAs

Quercetin is a phytochemical found in the skins of apples and red onions and is sold as a dietary supplement. Quercetin and its metabolite, isorhamnetin, counteracted lipopolysaccharide-induced increase in proinflammatory microRNA-155 in murine RAW264.7 macrophages whereas quercetin-3-glucuronide, another metabolite of quercetin, did not change the miR-155 levels (Boesch-Saadatmandi et al. 2010). Ellagitannin (1,3-Di-O-galloyl-4,6-(s)-HHDP-β-D-glucopyranose), a polyphenolic compound isolated from *Balanophora japonica* upregulated 17 miRNAs and down-regulated 8 miRNAs in HepG2 cells. Most of the proapoptotic let-7 family members were downregulated upon treatment with ellagitannin (Wen et al. 2009). A diet deficient in Vitamin E, reduced the levels of miR-125b and miR-122a in the liver. miR-122a is known to be associated with lipid metabolism (Esau et al. 2006) and hepatocellular carcinoma (Kutay et al. 2006) and miR-125b with cancer progression and inflammation (Ozen et al. 2008; Porkka et al. 2007). Prenatal ethanol exposure is known to cause teratogenesis and out of the total 509 miRNAs screened, miR-10a, miR-10b, miR-9, miR-145, miR-30a-3p and miR-152 were upregulated, whereas miR-200a, miR-496, miR-296, miR-30e-5p, miR-362, miR-339, miR-29c and miR-154 were downregulated in fetal mouse brains that developed teratogenesis due to prenatal ethanol exposure as compared to the controls. Increased miR-10a levels caused by ethanol exposure were accompanied by a decrease in the protein levels of its target, HOXA1, and folic acid supplementation in the diet partially counteracted the upregulation of miR-10a and downregulation of HOXA1 (Wang et al. 2009a). miR-10a also plays a role in apoptosis by inducing caspase-3 activity in a tumor necrosis factor-related apoptosis-inducing ligand-dependent manner (Ovcharenko et al. 2007) and the deficiency of folate resulted in the accumulation of TK-6 (human

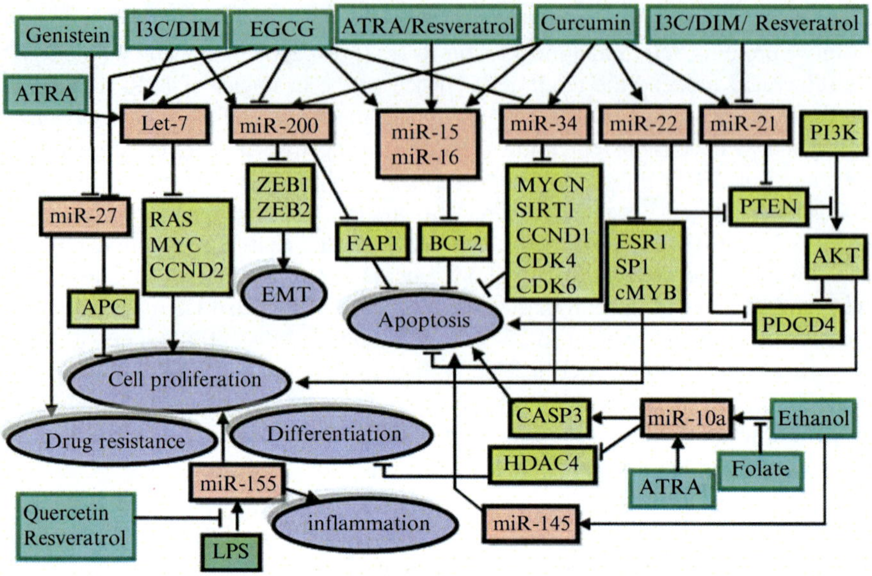

Fig. 16.2 Natural compounds alter the cellular processes by modulating the expression of miRNAs and their targets

immortalized lymphoblast) cells in S phase followed by apoptosis with the upregulation of other proapoptotic miRNAs like miR-145, miR-34a and miR-22 (Pandey and Picard 2009; Chang et al. 2007; Marsit et al. 2006; Ostenfeld et al. 2010).

It is clear from the above examples that many natural compounds that are known to induce apoptosis do so partly by modulating the expression of several miRNAs and their targets (Fig. 16.2). The natural compounds are relatively non-toxic and their combination with conventional chemotherapy could be a novel and safer approach to eliminate the resistant cancer stem cells or those undergoing EMT through the induction of apoptosis in cancer cells. As miRNAs are a novel class of regulators of signaling network and apoptosis, an understanding on the mechanisms of miRNA regulation by natural compounds would offer promising hopes to overcome anticancer drug resistance.

References

Ahn J-I, Jeong K, Ko M-J, Shin H, Kim H, Chung H, Jeong H-S (2010) Changes of miRNA and mRNA expression in HepG2 cells treated by epigallocatechin gallate. Mol Cell Toxicol 6(2):169–177. doi:10.1007/s13273-010-0024-3

Ali S, Ahmad A, Banerjee S, Padhye S, Dominiak K, Schaffert JM, Wang Z, Philip PA, Sarkar FH (2010) Gemcitabine sensitivity can be induced in pancreatic cancer cells through modulation of miR-200 and miR-21 expression by curcumin or its analogue CDF. Cancer Res 70(9):3606–3617. doi:0008-5472.CAN-09-4598 [pii] 10.1158/0008-5472.CAN-09-4598

Altuvia Y, Landgraf P, Lithwick G, Elefant N, Pfeffer S, Aravin A, Brownstein MJ, Tuschl T, Margalit H (2005) Clustering and conservation patterns of human microRNAs. Nucleic Acids Res 33(8):2697–2706. doi:33/8/2697 [pii] 10.1093/nar/gki567

Ambros V (2004) The functions of animal microRNAs. Nature 431(7006):350–355. doi:10.1038/nature02871 nature02871 [pii]

Aziz MH, Nihal M, Fu VX, Jarrard DF, Ahmad N (2006) Resveratrol-caused apoptosis of human prostate carcinoma LNCaP cells is mediated via modulation of phosphatidylinositol 3′-kinase/Akt pathway and Bcl-2 family proteins. Mol Cancer Ther 5(5):1335–1341. doi:5/5/1335 [pii] 10.1158/1535-7163.MCT-05-0526

Bar N, Dikstein R (2010) miR-22 forms a regulatory loop in PTEN/AKT pathway and modulates signaling kinetics. PLoS One 5(5):e10859. doi:10.1371/journal.pone.0010859

Bartel DP (2009) MicroRNAs: target recognition and regulatory functions. Cell 136(2):215–233. doi:S0092-8674(09)00008-7 [pii] 10.1016/j.cell.2009.01.002

Benitez DA, Pozo-Guisado E, Alvarez-Barrientos A, Fernandez-Salguero PM, Castellon EA (2007) Mechanisms involved in resveratrol-induced apoptosis and cell cycle arrest in prostate cancer-derived cell lines. J Androl 28(2):282–293. doi:jandrol.106.000968 [pii] 10.2164/jandrol.106.000968

Berezikov E, Chung WJ, Willis J, Cuppen E, Lai EC (2007) Mammalian mirtron genes. Mol Cell 28(2):328–336. doi:S1097-2765(07)00669-7 [pii] 10.1016/j.molcel.2007.09.028

Boesch-Saadatmandi C, Loboda A, Wagner AE, Stachurska A, Jozkowicz A, Dulak J, Doring F, Wolffram S, Rimbach G (2010) Effect of quercetin and its metabolites isorhamnetin and quercetin-3-glucuronide on inflammatory gene expression: role of miR-155. J Nutr Biochem. doi:S0955-2863(10)00066-5 [pii] 10.1016/j.jnutbio.2010.02.008

Cai X, Hagedorn CH, Cullen BR (2004) Human microRNAs are processed from capped, polyadenylated transcripts that can also function as mRNAs. RNA 10(12):1957–1966. doi:rna.7135204 [pii] 10.1261/rna.7135204

Calin GA, Croce CM (2006a) Genomics of chronic lymphocytic leukemia microRNAs as new players with clinical significance. Semin Oncol 33(2):167–173. doi:S0093-7754(06)00019-4 [pii] 10.1053/j.seminoncol.2006.01.010

Calin GA, Croce CM (2006b) MicroRNA signatures in human cancers. Nat Rev Cancer 6(11):857–866. doi:nrc1997 [pii] 10.1038/nrc1997

Calin GA, Sevignani C, Dumitru CD, Hyslop T, Noch E, Yendamuri S, Shimizu M, Rattan S, Bullrich F, Negrini M, Croce CM (2004) Human microRNA genes are frequently located at fragile sites and genomic regions involved in cancers. Proc Natl Acad Sci USA 101(9):2999–3004. doi:10.1073/pnas.0307323101 0307323101 [pii]

Chang TC, Wentzel EA, Kent OA, Ramachandran K, Mullendore M, Lee KH, Feldmann G, Yamakuchi M, Ferlito M, Lowenstein CJ, Arking DE, Beer MA, Maitra A, Mendell JT (2007) Transactivation of miR-34a by p53 broadly influences gene expression and promotes apoptosis. Mol Cell 26(5):745–752. doi:S1097-2765(07)00310-3 [pii] 10.1016/j.molcel.2007.05.010

Chen X, Guo X, Zhang H, Xiang Y, Chen J, Yin Y, Cai X, Wang K, Wang G, Ba Y, Zhu L, Wang J, Yang R, Zhang Y, Ren Z, Zen K, Zhang J, Zhang CY (2009) Role of miR-143 targeting KRAS in colorectal tumorigenesis. Oncogene 28(10):1385–1392. doi:onc2008474 [pii] 10.1038/onc.2008.474

Chen H, Chen Q, Fang M, Mi Y (2010) microRNA-181b targets MLK2 in HL-60 cells. Sci China Life Sci 53(1):101–106. doi:10.1007/s11427-010-0002-y

Cheng AL, Hsu CH, Lin JK, Hsu MM, Ho YF, Shen TS, Ko JY, Lin JT, Lin BR, Ming-Shiang W, Yu HS, Jee SH, Chen GS, Chen TM, Chen CA, Lai MK, Pu YS, Pan MH, Wang YJ, Tsai CC, Hsieh CY (2001) Phase I clinical trial of curcumin, a chemopreventive agent, in patients with high-risk or pre-malignant lesions. Anticancer Res 21(4B):2895–2900

Cheng GZ, Chan J, Wang Q, Zhang W, Sun CD, Wang LH (2007) Twist transcriptionally up-regulates AKT2 in breast cancer cells leading to increased migration, invasion, and resistance to paclitaxel. Cancer Res 67(5):1979–1987. doi:67/5/1979 [pii] 10.1158/0008-5472.CAN-06-1479

Cho WC (2010) MicroRNAs in cancer – from research to therapy. Biochim Biophys Acta 1805(2):209–217. doi:S0304-419X(09)00075-4 [pii] 10.1016/j.bbcan.2009.11.003

Cho WJ, Shin JM, Kim JS, Lee MR, Hong KS, Lee JH, Koo KH, Park JW, Kim KS (2009) miR-372 regulates cell cycle and apoptosis of ags human gastric cancer cell line through direct regulation of LATS2. Mol Cells 28(6):521–527. doi:10.1007/s10059-009-0158-0

Christoffersen NR, Shalgi R, Frankel LB, Leucci E, Lees M, Klausen M, Pilpel Y, Nielsen FC, Oren M, Lund AH (2010) p53-independent upregulation of miR-34a during oncogene-induced senescence represses MYC. Cell Death Differ 17(2):236–245. doi:cdd2009109 [pii] 10.1038/cdd.2009.109

Cimmino A, Calin GA, Fabbri M, Iorio MV, Ferracin M, Shimizu M, Wojcik SE, Aqeilan RI, Zupo S, Dono M, Rassenti L, Alder H, Volinia S, Liu CG, Kipps TJ, Negrini M, Croce CM (2005) miR-15 and miR-16 induce apoptosis by targeting BCL2. Proc Natl Acad Sci USA 102(39):13944–13949. doi:0506654102 [pii] 10.1073/pnas.0506654102

Clape C, Fritz V, Henriquet C, Apparailly F, Fernandez PL, Iborra F, Avances C, Villalba M, Culine S, Fajas L (2009) miR-143 interferes with ERK5 signaling, and abrogates prostate cancer progression in mice. PLoS One 4(10):e7542. doi:10.1371/journal.pone.0007542

Corney DC, Flesken-Nikitin A, Godwin AK, Wang W, Nikitin AY (2007) MicroRNA-34b and MicroRNA-34c are targets of p53 and cooperate in control of cell proliferation and adhesion-independent growth. Cancer Res 67(18):8433–8438. doi:0008-5472.CAN-07-1585 [pii] 10.1158/0008-5472.CAN-07-1585

Crist CG, Montarras D, Pallafacchina G, Rocancourt D, Cumano A, Conway SJ, Buckingham M (2009) Muscle stem cell behavior is modified by microRNA-27 regulation of Pax3 expression. Proc Natl Acad Sci USA 106(32):13383–13387. doi:0900210106 [pii] 10.1073/pnas.0900210106

Croce CM (2009) Causes and consequences of microRNA dysregulation in cancer. Nat Rev Genet 10(10):704–714. doi:nrg2634 [pii] 10.1038/nrg2634

Das S, Foley N, Bryan K, Watters KM, Bray I, Murphy DM, Buckley PG, Stallings RL (2010) MicroRNA mediates DNA demethylation events triggered by retinoic acid during neuroblastoma cell differentiation. Cancer Res. doi:0008-5472.CAN-10-1534 [pii] 10.1158/0008-5472.CAN-10-1534

Deshpande A, Pastore A, Deshpande AJ, Zimmermann Y, Hutter G, Weinkauf M, Buske C, Hiddemann W, Dreyling M (2009) 3′UTR mediated regulation of the cyclin D1 proto-oncogene. Cell Cycle 8(21):3584–3592. doi:9993 [pii]

Doench JG, Sharp PA (2004) Specificity of microRNA target selection in translational repression. Genes Dev 18(5):504–511. doi:10.1101/gad.1184404 1184404 [pii]

Eis PS, Tam W, Sun L, Chadburn A, Li Z, Gomez MF, Lund E, Dahlberg JE (2005) Accumulation of miR-155 and BIC RNA in human B cell lymphomas. Proc Natl Acad Sci USA 102(10):3627–3632. doi:0500613102 [pii] 10.1073/pnas.0500613102

Ernst A, Campos B, Meier J, Devens F, Liesenberg F, Wolter M, Reifenberger G, Herold-Mende C, Lichter P, Radlwimmer B (2010) De-repression of CTGF via the miR-17-92 cluster upon differentiation of human glioblastoma spheroid cultures. Oncogene 29(23):3411–3422. doi:onc201083 [pii] 10.1038/onc.2010.83

Esau C, Davis S, Murray SF, Yu XX, Pandey SK, Pear M, Watts L, Booten SL, Graham M, McKay R, Subramaniam A, Propp S, Lollo BA, Freier S, Bennett CF, Bhanot S, Monia BP (2006) miR-122 regulation of lipid metabolism revealed by in vivo antisense targeting. Cell Metab 3(2):87–98. doi:S1550-4131(06)00029-5 [pii] 10.1016/j.cmet.2006.01.005

Esquela-Kerscher A, Slack FJ (2006) Oncomirs – microRNAs with a role in cancer. Nat Rev Cancer 6(4):259–269. doi:nrc1840 [pii] 10.1038/nrc1840

Eulalio A, Huntzinger E, Nishihara T, Rehwinkel J, Fauser M, Izaurralde E (2009) Deadenylation is a widespread effect of miRNA regulation. RNA 15(1):21–32. doi:rna.1399509 [pii] 10.1261/rna.1399509

Fabbri M, Garzon R, Cimmino A, Liu Z, Zanesi N, Callegari E, Liu S, Alder H, Costinean S, Fernandez-Cymering C, Volinia S, Guler G, Morrison CD, Chan KK, Marcucci G, Calin GA, Huebner K, Croce CM (2007) MicroRNA-29 family reverts aberrant methylation in lung cancer by targeting DNA methyltransferases 3A and 3B. Proc Natl Acad Sci USA 104(40):15805–15810. doi:0707628104 [pii] 10.1073/pnas.0707628104

Faber AC, Chiles TC (2006) Resveratrol induces apoptosis in transformed follicular lymphoma OCI-LY8 cells: evidence for a novel mechanism involving inhibition of BCL6 signaling. Int J Oncol 29(6):1561–1566

Fabian MR, Sonenberg N, Filipowicz W (2010) Regulation of mRNA translation and stability by microRNAs. Annu Rev Biochem 79:351–379. doi:10.1146/annurev-biochem-060308-103103

Faller M, Guo F (2008) MicroRNA biogenesis: there's more than one way to skin a cat. Biochim Biophys Acta 1779(11):663–667. doi:S1874-9399(08)00177-6 [pii] 10.1016/j.bbagrm.2008.08.005

Fassi Fehri L, Koch M, Belogolova E, Khalil H, Bolz C, Kalali B, Mollenkopf HJ, Beigier-Bompadre M, Karlas A, Schneider T, Churin Y, Gerhard M, Meyer TF (2010) Helicobacter pylori induces miR-155 in T cells in a cAMP-Foxp3-dependent manner. PLoS One 5(3):e9500. doi:10.1371/journal.pone.0009500

Fazi F, Rosa A, Fatica A, Gelmetti V, De Marchis ML, Nervi C, Bozzoni I (2005) A minicircuitry comprised of microRNA-223 and transcription factors NFI-A and C/EBPalpha regulates human granulopoiesis. Cell 123(5):819–831. doi:S0092-8674(05)00977-3 [pii] 10.1016/j.cell.2005.09.023

Felli N, Fontana L, Pelosi E, Botta R, Bonci D, Facchiano F, Liuzzi F, Lulli V, Morsilli O, Santoro S, Valtieri M, Calin GA, Liu CG, Sorrentino A, Croce CM, Peschle C (2005) MicroRNAs 221 and 222 inhibit normal erythropoiesis and erythroleukemic cell growth via kit receptor down-modulation. Proc Natl Acad Sci USA 102(50):18081–18086. doi:0506216102 [pii] 10.1073/pnas.0506216102

Felli N, Pedini F, Romania P, Biffoni M, Morsilli O, Castelli G, Santoro S, Chicarella S, Sorrentino A, Peschle C, Marziali G (2009) MicroRNA 223-dependent expression of LMO2 regulates normal erythropoiesis. Haematologica 94(4):479–486. doi:haematol.2008.002345 [pii] 10.3324/haematol.2008.002345

Fornari F, Gramantieri L, Ferracin M, Veronese A, Sabbioni S, Calin GA, Grazi GL, Giovannini C, Croce CM, Bolondi L, Negrini M (2008) MiR-221 controls CDKN1C/p57 and CDKN1B/p27 expression in human hepatocellular carcinoma. Oncogene 27(43):5651–5661. doi:onc2008178 [pii] 10.1038/onc.2008.178

Frankel LB, Christoffersen NR, Jacobsen A, Lindow M, Krogh A, Lund AH (2008) Programmed cell death 4 (PDCD4) is an important functional target of the microRNA miR-21 in breast cancer cells. J Biol Chem 283(2):1026–1033. doi:M707224200 [pii] 10.1074/jbc.M707224200

Fuchs BC, Fujii T, Dorfman JD, Goodwin JM, Zhu AX, Lanuti M, Tanabe KK (2008) Epithelial-to-mesenchymal transition and integrin-linked kinase mediate sensitivity to epidermal growth factor receptor inhibition in human hepatoma cells. Cancer Res 68(7):2391–2399. doi:68/7/2391 [pii] 10.1158/0008-5472.CAN-07-2460

Gao J, Zhou H, Lei T, Zhou L, Li W, Li X, Yang B (2011) Curcumin inhibits renal cyst formation and enlargement in vitro by regulating intracellular signaling pathways. Eur J Pharmacol 654(1):92–99. doi:S0014-2999(10)01235-5 [pii] 10.1016/j.ejphar.2010.12.008

Garvin S, Ollinger K, Dabrosin C (2006) Resveratrol induces apoptosis and inhibits angiogenesis in human breast cancer xenografts in vivo. Cancer Lett 231(1):113–122. doi:S0304-3835(05)00106-0 [pii] 10.1016/j.canlet.2005.01.031

Garzon R, Pichiorri F, Palumbo T, Visentini M, Aqeilan R, Cimmino A, Wang H, Sun H, Volinia S, Alder H, Calin GA, Liu CG, Andreeff M, Croce CM (2007) MicroRNA gene expression during retinoic acid-induced differentiation of human acute promyelocytic leukemia. Oncogene 26(28):4148–4157. doi:1210186 [pii] 10.1038/sj.onc.1210186

Gironella M, Seux M, Xie MJ, Cano C, Tomasini R, Gommeaux J, Garcia S, Nowak J, Yeung ML, Jeang KT, Chaix A, Fazli L, Motoo Y, Wang Q, Rocchi P, Russo A, Gleave M, Dagorn JC, Iovanna JL, Carrier A, Pebusque MJ, Dusetti NJ (2007) Tumor protein 53-induced nuclear protein 1 expression is repressed by miR-155, and its restoration inhibits pancreatic tumor development. Proc Natl Acad Sci USA 104(41):16170–16175. doi:0703942104 [pii] 10.1073/pnas.0703942104

Goga A, Benz C (2007) Anti-oncomir suppression of tumor phenotypes. Mol Interv 7(4):199–202. doi:, 180

Golden EB, Lam PY, Kardosh A, Gaffney KJ, Cadenas E, Louie SG, Petasis NA, Chen TC, Schonthal AH (2009) Green tea polyphenols block the anticancer effects of bortezomib and other boronic acid-based proteasome inhibitors. Blood 113(23):5927–5937. doi:blood-2008-07-171389 [pii] 10.1182/blood-2008-07-171389

Gramantieri L, Ferracin M, Fornari F, Veronese A, Sabbioni S, Liu CG, Calin GA, Giovannini C, Ferrazzi E, Grazi GL, Croce CM, Bolondi L, Negrini M (2007) Cyclin G1 is a target of miR-122a, a microRNA frequently down-regulated in human hepatocellular carcinoma. Cancer Res 67(13):6092–6099. doi:67/13/6092 [pii] 10.1158/0008-5472.CAN-06-4607

Gramantieri L, Fornari F, Ferracin M, Veronese A, Sabbioni S, Calin GA, Grazi GL, Croce CM, Bolondi L, Negrini M (2009) MicroRNA-221 targets Bmf in hepatocellular carcinoma and correlates with tumor multifocality. Clin Cancer Res 15(16):5073–5081. doi:1078-0432.CCR-09-0092 [pii] 10.1158/1078-0432.CCR-09-0092

Gregersen LH, Jacobsen AB, Frankel LB, Wen J, Krogh A, Lund AH (2010) MicroRNA-145 targets YES and STAT1 in colon cancer cells. PLoS One 5(1):e8836. doi:10.1371/journal.pone.0008836

Gregory RI, Chendrimada TP, Shiekhattar R (2006) MicroRNA biogenesis: isolation and characterization of the microprocessor complex. Methods Mol Biol 342:33–47. doi:1-59745-123-1:33 [pii] 10.1385/1-59745-123-1:33

Grimson A, Farh KK, Johnston WK, Garrett-Engele P, Lim LP, Bartel DP (2007) MicroRNA targeting specificity in mammals: determinants beyond seed pairing. Mol Cell 27(1):91–105. doi:S1097-2765(07)00407-8 [pii] 10.1016/j.molcel.2007.06.017

Guan Y, Yao H, Zheng Z, Qiu G, Sun K (2010) MiR-125b targets BCL3 and suppresses ovarian cancer proliferation. Int J Cancer. doi:10.1002/ijc.25575

Hatcher H, Planalp R, Cho J, Torti F, Torti S (2008) Curcumin: from ancient medicine to current clinical trials. Cell Mol Life Sci 65(11):1631–1652. doi:10.1007/s00018-008-7452-4

Hawkins PG, Morris KV (2008) RNA and transcriptional modulation of gene expression. Cell Cycle 7(5):602–607. doi:5522 [pii]

He L, Thomson JM, Hemann MT, Hernando-Monge E, Mu D, Goodson S, Powers S, Cordon-Cardo C, Lowe SW, Hannon GJ, Hammond SM (2005) A microRNA polycistron as a potential human oncogene. Nature 435(7043):828–833. doi:nature03552 [pii] 10.1038/nature03552

Hong C, Firestone GL, Bjeldanes LF (2002) Bcl-2 family-mediated apoptotic effects of 3,3′-diindolylmethane (DIM) in human breast cancer cells. Biochem Pharmacol 63(6):1085–1097. doi:S0006295202008560 [pii]

Horie T, Ono K, Nishi H, Nagao K, Kinoshita M, Watanabe S, Kuwabara Y, Nakashima Y, Takanabe-Mori R, Nishi E, Hasegawa K, Kita T, Kimura T (2010) Acute doxorubicin cardiotoxicity is associated with miR-146a-induced inhibition of the neuregulin-ErbB pathway. Cardiovasc Res 87(4):656–664. doi:cvq148 [pii] 10.1093/cvr/cvq148 [doi]

Hossain A, Kuo MT, Saunders GF (2006) Mir-17-5p regulates breast cancer cell proliferation by inhibiting translation of AIB1 mRNA. Mol Cell Biol 26(21):8191–8201. doi:MCB.00242-06 [pii] 10.1128/MCB.00242-06

Huang H, Xie C, Sun X, Ritchie RP, Zhang J, Chen YE (2010a) miR-10a contributes to retinoid acid-induced smooth muscle cell differentiation. J Biol Chem 285(13):9383–9389. doi:M109.095612 [pii] 10.1074/jbc.M109.095612

Huang L, Luo J, Cai Q, Pan Q, Zeng H, Guo Z, Dong W, Huang J, Lin T (2010b) MicroRNA-125b suppresses the development of bladder cancer by targeting E2F3. Int J Cancer. doi:10.1002/ijc.25509

Inomata M, Tagawa H, Guo YM, Kameoka Y, Takahashi N, Sawada K (2009) MicroRNA-17-92 down-regulates expression of distinct targets in different B-cell lymphoma subtypes. Blood 113(2):396–402. doi:blood-2008-07-163907 [pii] 10.1182/blood-2008-07-163907

Ji X (2008) The mechanism of RNase III action: how dicer dices. Curr Top Microbiol Immunol 320:99–116

Ji SJ, Han DH, Kim JH (2006) Inhibition of proliferation and induction of apoptosis by EGCG in human osteogenic sarcoma (HOS) cells. Arch Pharm Res 29(5):363–368

Ji Q, Hao X, Zhang M, Tang W, Yang M, Li L, Xiang D, Desano JT, Bommer GT, Fan D, Fearon ER, Lawrence TS, Xu L (2009) MicroRNA miR-34 inhibits human pancreatic cancer tumor-initiating cells. PLoS One 4(8):e6816. doi:10.1371/journal.pone.0006816

Jiang Y, Wu Y, Greenlee AR, Wu J, Han Z, Li X, Zhao Y (2010) miR-106a-mediated malignant transformation of cells induced by anti-benzo[a]pyrene-trans-7,8-diol-9,10-epoxide. Toxicol Sci. doi:kfq306 [pii] 10.1093/toxsci/kfq306

Johnnidis JB, Harris MH, Wheeler RT, Stehling-Sun S, Lam MH, Kirak O, Brummelkamp TR, Fleming MD, Camargo FD (2008) Regulation of progenitor cell proliferation and granulocyte function by microRNA-223. Nature 451(7182):1125–1129. doi:nature06607 [pii] 10.1038/nature06607

Johnson SM, Grosshans H, Shingara J, Byrom M, Jarvis R, Cheng A, Labourier E, Reinert KL, Brown D, Slack FJ (2005) RAS is regulated by the let-7 microRNA family. Cell 120(5):635–647. doi:S0092-8674(05)00088-7 [pii] 10.1016/j.cell.2005.01.014

Johnson CD, Esquela-Kerscher A, Stefani G, Byrom M, Kelnar K, Ovcharenko D, Wilson M, Wang X, Shelton J, Shingara J, Chin L, Brown D, Slack FJ (2007) The let-7 microRNA represses cell proliferation pathways in human cells. Cancer Res 67(16):7713–7722. doi:67/16/7713 [pii] 10.1158/0008-5472.CAN-07-1083

Kakarala M, Brenner DE, Korkaya H, Cheng C, Tazi K, Ginestier C, Liu S, Dontu G, Wicha MS (2010) Targeting breast stem cells with the cancer preventive compounds curcumin and piperine. Breast Cancer Res Treat 122(3):777–785. doi:10.1007/s10549-009-0612-x

Kan T, Sato F, Ito T, Matsumura N, David S, Cheng Y, Agarwal R, Paun BC, Jin Z, Olaru AV, Selaru FM, Hamilton JP, Yang J, Abraham JM, Mori Y, Meltzer SJ (2009) The miR-106b-25 polycistron, activated by genomic amplification, functions as an oncogene by suppressing p21 and Bim. Gastroenterology 136(5):1689–1700

Kapinas K, Kessler C, Ricks T, Gronowicz G, Delany AM (2010) miR-29 modulates Wnt signaling in human osteoblasts through a positive feedback loop. J Biol Chem 285(33):25221–25231. doi:M110.116137 [pii] 10.1074/jbc.M110.116137

Karbiener M, Fischer C, Nowitsch S, Opriessnig P, Papak C, Ailhaud G, Dani C, Amri EZ, Scheideler M (2009) microRNA miR-27b impairs human adipocyte differentiation and targets PPARgamma. Biochem Biophys Res Commun 390(2):247–251. doi:S0006-291X(09)01915-9 [pii] 10.1016/j.bbrc.2009.09.098

Karunagaran D, Rashmi R, Kumar TR (2005) Induction of apoptosis by curcumin and its implications for cancer therapy. Curr Cancer Drug Targets 5(2):117–129

Karunagaran D, Joseph J, Kumar TR (2007) Cell growth regulation. Adv Exp Med Biol 595:245–268

Kawasaki BT, Hurt EM, Mistree T, Farrar WL (2008) Targeting cancer stem cells with phytochemicals. Mol Interv 8(4):174–184. doi:8/4/174 [pii] 10.1124/mi.8.4.9

Kim YK, Kim VN (2007) Processing of intronic microRNAs. EMBO J 26(3):775–783. doi:7601512 [pii] 10.1038/sj.emboj.7601512

Kim S, Lee UJ, Kim MN, Lee EJ, Kim JY, Lee MY, Choung S, Kim YJ, Choi YC (2008) MicroRNA miR-199a* regulates the MET proto-oncogene and the downstream extracellular signal-regulated kinase 2 (ERK2). J Biol Chem 283(26):18158–18166. doi:M800186200 [pii] 10.1074/jbc.M800186200

Kong W, He L, Coppola M, Guo J, Esposito NN, Coppola D, Cheng JQ (2010) MicroRNA-155 regulates cell survival, growth, and chemosensitivity by targeting FOXO3a in breast cancer. J Biol Chem 285(23):17869–17879. doi:M110.101055 [pii] 10.1074/jbc.M110.101055

Korpal M, Lee ES, Hu G, Kang Y (2008) The miR-200 family inhibits epithelial-mesenchymal transition and cancer cell migration by direct targeting of E-cadherin transcriptional repressors ZEB1 and ZEB2. J Biol Chem 283(22):14910–14914. doi:C800074200 [pii] 10.1074/jbc.C800074200

Krek A, Grun D, Poy MN, Wolf R, Rosenberg L, Epstein EJ, MacMenamin P, da Piedade I, Gunsalus KC, Stoffel M, Rajewsky N (2005) Combinatorial microRNA target predictions. Nat Genet 37(5):495–500. doi:ng1536 [pii] 10.1038/ng1536

Kutay H, Bai S, Datta J, Motiwala T, Pogribny I, Frankel W, Jacob ST, Ghoshal K (2006) Downregulation of miR-122 in the rodent and human hepatocellular carcinomas. J Cell Biochem 99(3):671–678. doi:10.1002/jcb.20982

Lagos-Quintana M, Rauhut R, Lendeckel W, Tuschl T (2001) Identification of novel genes coding for small expressed RNAs. Science 294(5543):853–858. doi:10.1126/science.1064921 294/5543/853 [pii]

Lal A, Navarro F, Maher CA, Maliszewski LE, Yan N, O'Day E, Chowdhury D, Dykxhoorn DM, Tsai P, Hofmann O, Becker KG, Gorospe M, Hide W, Lieberman J (2009) miR-24 Inhibits cell proliferation by targeting E2F2, MYC, and other cell-cycle genes via binding to "seedless" 3′UTR microRNA recognition elements. Mol Cell 35(5):610–625. doi:S1097-2765(09)00600-5 [pii] 10.1016/j.molcel.2009.08.020

le Sage C, Nagel R, Egan DA, Schrier M, Mesman E, Mangiola A, Anile C, Maira G, Mercatelli N, Ciafre SA, Farace MG, Agami R (2007) Regulation of the p27(Kip1) tumor suppressor by miR-221 and miR-222 promotes cancer cell proliferation. EMBO J 26(15):3699–3708. doi:7601790 [pii] 10.1038/sj.emboj.7601790

Lee YS, Dutta A (2007) The tumor suppressor microRNA let-7 represses the HMGA2 oncogene. Genes Dev 21(9):1025–1030. doi:gad.1540407 [pii] 10.1101/gad.1540407

Lee Y, Kim M, Han J, Yeom KH, Lee S, Baek SH, Kim VN (2004) MicroRNA genes are transcribed by RNA polymerase II. EMBO J 23(20):4051–4060. doi:10.1038/sj.emboj.7600385 7600385 [pii]

Lee KH, Goan YG, Hsiao M, Lee CH, Jian SH, Lin JT, Chen YL, Lu PJ (2009) MicroRNA-373 (miR-373) post-transcriptionally regulates large tumor suppressor, homolog 2 (LATS2) and stimulates proliferation in human esophageal cancer. Exp Cell Res 315(15):2529–2538. doi:S0014-4827(09)00261-4 [pii] 10.1016/j.yexcr.2009.06.001

Leong H, Firestone GL, Bjeldanes LF (2001) Cytostatic effects of 3,3′-diindolylmethane in human endometrial cancer cells result from an estrogen receptor-mediated increase in transforming growth factor-alpha expression. Carcinogenesis 22(11):1809–1817

Levi F, Pasche C, Lucchini F, Ghidoni R, Ferraroni M, La Vecchia C (2005) Resveratrol and breast cancer risk. Eur J Cancer Prev 14(2):139–142. doi:00008469-200504000-00009 [pii]

Lewis BP, Burge CB, Bartel DP (2005) Conserved seed pairing, often flanked by adenosines, indicates that thousands of human genes are microRNA targets. Cell 120(1):15–20. doi:S0092867404012607 [pii] 10.1016/j.cell.2004.12.035

Li T, Li D, Sha J, Sun P, Huang Y (2009a) MicroRNA-21 directly targets MARCKS and promotes apoptosis resistance and invasion in prostate cancer cells. Biochem Biophys Res Commun 383(3):280–285. doi:S0006-291X(09)00543-9 [pii] 10.1016/j.bbrc.2009.03.077

Li Y, VandenBoom TG 2nd, Kong D, Wang Z, Ali S, Philip PA, Sarkar FH (2009b) Up-regulation of miR-200 and let-7 by natural agents leads to the reversal of epithelial-to-mesenchymal transition in gemcitabine-resistant pancreatic cancer cells. Cancer Res 69(16):6704–6712. doi:0008-5472. CAN-09-1298 [pii] 10.1158/0008-5472.CAN-09-1298

Li Y, Tan W, Neo TW, Aung MO, Wasser S, Lim SG, Tan TM (2009c) Role of the miR-106b-25 microRNA cluster in hepatocellular carcinoma. Cancer Sci 100(7):1234–1242. doi:CAS1164 [pii] 10.1111/j.1349-7006.2009.01164.x

Li Y, Guessous F, Zhang Y, Dipierro C, Kefas B, Johnson E, Marcinkiewicz L, Jiang J, Yang Y, Schmittgen TD, Lopes B, Schiff D, Purow B, Abounader R (2009d) MicroRNA-34a inhibits glioblastoma growth by targeting multiple oncogenes. Cancer Res 69(19):7569–7576. doi:0008-5472.CAN-09-0529 [pii] 10.1158/0008-5472.CAN-09-0529

Liao Y, Du X, Lonnerdal B (2010) miR-214 regulates lactoferrin expression and pro-apoptotic function in mammary epithelial cells. J Nutr 140(9):1552–1556. doi:jn.110.124289 [pii] 10.3945/jn.110.124289

Lin CJ, Gong HY, Tseng HC, Wang WL, Wu JL (2008) miR-122 targets an anti-apoptotic gene, Bcl-w, in human hepatocellular carcinoma cell lines. Biochem Biophys Res Commun 375(3):315–320. doi:S0006-291X(08)01485-X [pii] 10.1016/j.bbrc.2008.07.154

Long D, Lee R, Williams P, Chan CY, Ambros V, Ding Y (2007) Potent effect of target structure on microRNA function. Nat Struct Mol Biol 14(4):287–294. doi:nsmb1226 [pii] 10.1038/nsmb1226

Lu J, Getz G, Miska EA, Alvarez-Saavedra E, Lamb J, Peck D, Sweet-Cordero A, Ebert BL, Mak RH, Ferrando AA, Downing JR, Jacks T, Horvitz HR, Golub TR (2005) MicroRNA expression profiles classify human cancers. Nature 435(7043):834–838. doi:nature03702 [pii] 10.1038/nature03702

Lu Y, Thomson JM, Wong HY, Hammond SM, Hogan BL (2007) Transgenic over-expression of the microRNA miR-17-92 cluster promotes proliferation and inhibits differentiation of lung epithelial progenitor cells. Dev Biol 310(2):442–453. doi:S0012-1606(07)01252-3 [pii] 10.1016/j.ydbio.2007.08.007

Lukiw WJ, Zhao Y, Cui JG (2008) An NF-kappaB-sensitive micro RNA-146a-mediated inflammatory circuit in Alzheimer disease and in stressed human brain cells. J Biol Chem 283(46):31315–31322. doi:M805371200 [pii] 10.1074/jbc.M805371200

Lund E, Dahlberg JE (2006) Substrate selectivity of exportin 5 and Dicer in the biogenesis of microRNAs. Cold Spring Harb Symp Quant Biol 71:59–66. doi:10.1101/sqb.2006.71.050

Marsit CJ, Eddy K, Kelsey KT (2006) MicroRNA responses to cellular stress. Cancer Res 66(22):10843–10848. doi:66/22/10843 [pii] 10.1158/0008-5472.CAN-06-1894

Martello G, Rosato A, Ferrari F, Manfrin A, Cordenonsi M, Dupont S, Enzo E, Guzzardo V, Rondina M, Spruce T, Parenti AR, Daidone MG, Bicciato S, Piccolo S (2010) A MicroRNA targeting dicer for metastasis control. Cell 141(7):1195–1207. doi:S0092-8674(10)00553-2 [pii] 10.1016/j.cell.2010.05.017

Medina PP, Nolde M, Slack FJ (2010) OncomiR addiction in an in vivo model of microRNA-21-induced pre-B-cell lymphoma. Nature 467(7311):86–90. doi:nature09284 [pii] 10.1038/nature09284

Meeran SM, Ahmed A, Tollefsbol TO (2010) Epigenetic targets of bioactive dietary components for cancer prevention and therapy. Clin Epigenetics 1(3–4):101–116. doi:10.1007/s13148-010-0011-5

Melkamu T, Zhang X, Tan J, Zeng Y, Kassie F (2010) Alteration of microRNA expression in vinyl carbamate-induced mouse lung tumors and modulation by the chemopreventive agent indole-3-carbinol. Carcinogenesis 31(2):252–258. doi:bgp208 [pii] 10.1093/carcin/bgp208

Meng F, Henson R, Wehbe-Janek H, Ghoshal K, Jacob ST, Patel T (2007) MicroRNA-21 regulates expression of the PTEN tumor suppressor gene in human hepatocellular cancer. Gastroenterology 133(2):647–658. doi:S0016-5085(07)01002-5 [pii] 10.1053/j.gastro.2007.05.022

Mertens-Talcott SU, Chintharlapalli S, Li X, Safe S (2007) The oncogenic microRNA-27a targets genes that regulate specificity protein transcription factors and the G2-M checkpoint in MDA-MB-231 breast cancer cells. Cancer Res 67(22):11001–11011. doi:67/22/11001 [pii] 10.1158/0008-5472.CAN-07-2416

Metzler M, Wilda M, Busch K, Viehmann S, Borkhardt A (2004) High expression of precursor microRNA-155/BIC RNA in children with Burkitt lymphoma. Genes Chromosomes Cancer 39(2):167–169. doi:10.1002/gcc.10316

Mishra PJ, Song B, Wang Y, Humeniuk R, Banerjee D, Merlino G, Ju J, Bertino JR (2009) MiR-24 tumor suppressor activity is regulated independent of p53 and through a target site polymorphism. PLoS One 4(12):e8445. doi:10.1371/journal.pone.0008445

Mott JL, Kobayashi S, Bronk SF, Gores GJ (2007) mir-29 regulates Mcl-1 protein expression and apoptosis. Oncogene 26(42):6133–6140. doi:1210436 [pii] 10.1038/sj.onc.1210436

Mudduluru G, George-William JN, Muppala S, Asangani IA, Regalla K, Nelson LD, Allgayer H (2010) Curcumin regulates miR-21 expression and inhibits invasion and metastasis in colorectal cancer. Biosci Rep. doi:BSR20100065 [pii] 10.1042/BSR20100065

Murchison EP, Hannon GJ (2004) miRNAs on the move: miRNA biogenesis and the RNAi machinery. Curr Opin Cell Biol 16(3):223–229. doi:10.1016/j.ceb.2004.04.003 S0955067404000547 [pii]

O'Donnell KA, Wentzel EA, Zeller KI, Dang CV, Mendell JT (2005) c-Myc-regulated microRNAs modulate E2F1 expression. Nature 435(7043):839–843. doi:nature03677 [pii] 10.1038/nature03677

Okamura K, Phillips MD, Tyler DM, Duan H, Chou YT, Lai EC (2008) The regulatory activity of microRNA* species has substantial influence on microRNA and 3′ UTR evolution. Nat Struct Mol Biol 15(4):354–363. doi:nsmb.1409 [pii] 10.1038/nsmb.1409

Olive V, Bennett MJ, Walker JC, Ma C, Jiang I, Cordon-Cardo C, Li QJ, Lowe SW, Hannon GJ, He L (2009) miR-19 is a key oncogenic component of mir-17-92. Genes Dev 23(24):2839–2849. doi:23/24/2839 [pii] 10.1101/gad.1861409

Ostenfeld MS, Bramsen JB, Lamy P, Villadsen SB, Fristrup N, Sorensen KD, Ulhoi B, Borre M, Kjems J, Dyrskjot L, Orntoft TF (2010) miR-145 induces caspase-dependent and -independent cell death in urothelial cancer cell lines with targeting of an expression signature present in Ta bladder tumors. Oncogene 29(7):1073–1084. doi:onc2009395 [pii] 10.1038/onc.2009.395

Ota A, Tagawa H, Karnan S, Tsuzuki S, Karpas A, Kira S, Yoshida Y, Seto M (2004) Identification and characterization of a novel gene, C13orf25, as a target for 13q31-q32 amplification in malignant lymphoma. Cancer Res 64(9):3087–3095

Ovcharenko D, Kelnar K, Johnson C, Leng N, Brown D (2007) Genome-scale microRNA and small interfering RNA screens identify small RNA modulators of TRAIL-induced apoptosis pathway. Cancer Res 67(22):10782–10788. doi:67/22/10782 [pii] 10.1158/0008-5472.CAN-07-1484

Ozen M, Creighton CJ, Ozdemir M, Ittmann M (2008) Widespread deregulation of microRNA expression in human prostate cancer. Oncogene 27(12):1788–1793. doi:1210809 [pii] 10.1038/sj.onc.1210809

Padhye S, Yang H, Jamadar A, Cui QC, Chavan D, Dominiak K, McKinney J, Banerjee S, Dou QP, Sarkar FH (2009) New difluoro Knoevenagel condensates of curcumin, their schiff bases and copper complexes as proteasome inhibitors and apoptosis inducers in cancer cells. Pharm Res 26(8):1874–1880. doi:10.1007/s11095-009-9900-8

Pandey DP, Picard D (2009) miR-22 inhibits estrogen signaling by directly targeting the estrogen receptor alpha mRNA. Mol Cell Biol 29(13):3783–3790. doi:MCB.01875-08 [pii] 10.1128/MCB.01875-08

Park SM, Gaur AB, Lengyel E, Peter ME (2008) The miR-200 family determines the epithelial phenotype of cancer cells by targeting the E-cadherin repressors ZEB1 and ZEB2. Genes Dev 22(7):894–907. doi:22/7/894 [pii] 10.1101/gad.1640608

Park SY, Lee JH, Ha M, Nam JW, Kim VN (2009) miR-29 miRNAs activate p53 by targeting p85 alpha and CDC42. Nat Struct Mol Biol 16(1):23–29. doi:nsmb.1533 [pii] 10.1038/nsmb.1533

Pedersen IM, Otero D, Kao E, Miletic AV, Hother C, Ralfkiaer E, Rickert RC, Gronbaek K, David M (2009) Onco-miR-155 targets SHIP1 to promote TNFalpha-dependent growth of B cell lymphomas. EMBO Mol Med 1(5):288–295. doi:10.1002/emmm.200900028

Pekarsky Y, Santanam U, Cimmino A, Palamarchuk A, Efanov A, Maximov V, Volinia S, Alder H, Liu CG, Rassenti L, Calin GA, Hagan JP, Kipps T, Croce CM (2006) Tcl1 expression in chronic lymphocytic leukemia is regulated by miR-29 and miR-181. Cancer Res 66(24):11590–11593. doi:66/24/11590 [pii] 10.1158/0008-5472.CAN-06-3613

Peter ME (2009) Let-7 and miR-200 microRNAs: guardians against pluripotency and cancer progression. Cell Cycle 8(6):843–852. doi:7907 [pii]

Pickering MT, Stadler BM, Kowalik TF (2009) miR-17 and miR-20a temper an E2F1-induced G1 checkpoint to regulate cell cycle progression. Oncogene 28(1):140–145. doi:onc2008372 [pii] 10.1038/onc.2008.372

Pigazzi M, Manara E, Baron E, Basso G (2009) miR-34b targets cyclic AMP-responsive element binding protein in acute myeloid leukemia. Cancer Res 69(6):2471–2478. doi:0008-5472.CAN-08-3404 [pii] 10.1158/0008-5472.CAN-08-3404

Porkka KP, Pfeiffer MJ, Waltering KK, Vessella RL, Tammela TL, Visakorpi T (2007) MicroRNA expression profiling in prostate cancer. Cancer Res 67(13):6130–6135. doi:67/13/6130 [pii] 10.1158/0008-5472.CAN-07-0533

Pratt AJ, MacRae IJ (2009) The RNA-induced silencing complex: a versatile gene-silencing machine. J Biol Chem 284(27):17897–17901. doi:R900012200 [pii] 10.1074/jbc.R900012200

Qanungo S, Das M, Haldar S, Basu A (2005) Epigallocatechin-3-gallate induces mitochondrial membrane depolarization and caspase-dependent apoptosis in pancreatic cancer cells. Carcinogenesis 26(5):958–967. doi:bgi040 [pii] 10.1093/carcin/bgi040

Qin W, Shi Y, Zhao B, Yao C, Jin L, Ma J, Jin Y (2010) miR-24 regulates apoptosis by targeting the open reading frame (ORF) region of FAF1 in cancer cells. PLoS One 5(2):e9429. doi:10.1371/journal.pone.0009429

Rahman KM, Aranha O, Glazyrin A, Chinni SR, Sarkar FH (2000) Translocation of Bax to mitochondria induces apoptotic cell death in indole-3-carbinol (I3C) treated breast cancer cells. Oncogene 19(50):5764–5771. doi:10.1038/sj.onc.1203959

Ro S, Park C, Young D, Sanders KM, Yan W (2007) Tissue-dependent paired expression of miRNAs. Nucleic Acids Res 35(17):5944–5953. doi:gkm641 [pii] 10.1093/nar/gkm641

Robins H, Li Y, Padgett RW (2005) Incorporating structure to predict microRNA targets. Proc Natl Acad Sci USA 102(11):4006–4009. doi:0500775102 [pii] 10.1073/pnas.0500775102
Rodriguez A, Griffiths-Jones S, Ashurst JL, Bradley A (2004) Identification of mammalian microRNA host genes and transcription units. Genome Res 14(10A):1902–1910. doi:10.1101/gr.2722704 gr.2722704 [pii]
Rom S, Rom I, Passiatore G, Pacifici M, Radhakrishnan S, Del Valle L, Pina-Oviedo S, Khalili K, Eletto D, Peruzzi F (2010) CCL8/MCP-2 is a target for mir-146a in HIV-1-infected human microglial cells. FASEB J 24(7):2292–2300. doi:fj.09-143503 [pii] 10.1096/fj.09-143503
Rossi S, Kopetz S, Davuluri R, Hamilton SR, Calin GA (2010) MicroRNAs, ultraconserved genes and colorectal cancers. Int J Biochem Cell Biol 42(8):1291–1297. doi:S1357-2725(09)00172-1 [pii] 10.1016/j.biocel.2009.05.018
Sabbah M, Emami S, Redeuilh G, Julien S, Prevost G, Zimber A, Ouelaa R, Bracke M, De Wever O, Gespach C (2008) Molecular signature and therapeutic perspective of the epithelial-to-mesenchymal transitions in epithelial cancers. Drug Resist Updat 11(4–5):123–151. doi:S1368-7646(08)00045-9 [pii] 10.1016/j.drup. 2008.07.001
Sachdeva M, Zhu S, Wu F, Wu H, Walia V, Kumar S, Elble R, Watabe K, Mo YY (2009) p53 represses c-Myc through induction of the tumor suppressor miR-145. Proc Natl Acad Sci USA 106(9):3207–3212. doi:0808042106 [pii] 10.1073/pnas.0808042106
Saito Y, Jones PA (2006) Epigenetic activation of tumor suppressor microRNAs in human cancer cells. Cell Cycle 5(19):2220–2222. doi:3340 [pii]
Saito Y, Liang G, Egger G, Friedman JM, Chuang JC, Coetzee GA, Jones PA (2006) Specific activation of microRNA-127 with downregulation of the proto-oncogene BCL6 by chromatin-modifying drugs in human cancer cells. Cancer Cell 9(6):435–443. doi:S1535-6108(06)00143-7 [pii]10.1016/j.ccr.2006.04.020
Salerno E, Scaglione BJ, Coffman FD, Brown BD, Baccarini A, Fernandes H, Marti G, Raveche ES (2009) Correcting miR-15a/16 genetic defect in New Zealand Black mouse model of CLL enhances drug sensitivity. Mol Cancer Ther 8(9):2684–2692. doi:1535-7163.MCT-09-0127 [pii] 10.1158/1535-7163.MCT-09-0127
Sampson VB, Rong NH, Han J, Yang Q, Aris V, Soteropoulos P, Petrelli NJ, Dunn SP, Krueger LJ (2007) MicroRNA let-7a down-regulates MYC and reverts MYC-induced growth in Burkitt lymphoma cells. Cancer Res 67(20):9762–9770. doi:67/20/9762 [pii] 10.1158/0008-5472.CAN-07-2462
Sareen D, van Ginkel PR, Takach JC, Mohiuddin A, Darjatmoko SR, Albert DM, Polans AS (2006) Mitochondria as the primary target of resveratrol-induced apoptosis in human retinoblastoma cells. Invest Ophthalmol Vis Sci 47(9):3708–3716. doi:47/9/3708 [pii] 10.1167/iovs.06-0119
Schickel R, Park SM, Murmann AE, Peter ME (2010) miR-200c regulates induction of apoptosis through CD95 by targeting FAP-1. Mol Cell 38(6):908–915. doi:S1097-2765(10)00380-1 [pii] 10.1016/j.molcel.2010.05.018
Sharma RA, McLelland HR, Hill KA, Ireson CR, Euden SA, Manson MM, Pirmohamed M, Marnett LJ, Gescher AJ, Steward WP (2001) Pharmacodynamic and pharmacokinetic study of oral curcuma extract in patients with colorectal cancer. Clin Cancer Res 7(7):1894–1900
Shi L, Cheng Z, Zhang J, Li R, Zhao P, Fu Z, You Y (2008) hsa-mir-181a and hsa-mir-181b function as tumor suppressors in human glioma cells. Brain Res 1236:185–193. doi:S0006-8993(08)01836-2 [pii] 10.1016/j.brainres.2008.07.085
Shimizu S, Takehara T, Hikita H, Kodama T, Miyagi T, Hosui A, Tatsumi T, Ishida H, Noda T, Nagano H, Doki Y, Mori M, Hayashi N (2010) The let-7 family of microRNAs inhibits Bcl-xL expression and potentiates sorafenib-induced apoptosis in human hepatocellular carcinoma. J Hepatol 52(5):698–704. doi:S0168-8278(10)00082-6 [pii] 10.1016/j.jhep. 2009.12.024
Siddiqui FA, Naim M, Islam N (2010) Apoptotic effect of green tea polyphenol (EGCG) on cervical carcinoma cells. Diagn Cytopathol. doi:10.1002/dc.21434
Sotiropoulou G, Pampalakis G, Lianidou E, Mourelatos Z (2009) Emerging roles of microRNAs as molecular switches in the integrated circuit of the cancer cell. RNA 15(8):1443–1461. doi:rna.1534709 [pii] 10.1261/rna.1534709

Srivastava B, Shukla Y (1998) Antitumour promoting activity of indole-3-carbinol in mouse skin carcinogenesis. Cancer Lett 134(1):91–95. doi:S0304-3835(98)00247-X [pii]

Stark A, Brennecke J, Russell RB, Cohen SM (2003) Identification of drosophila microRNA targets. PLoS Biol 1(3):E60. doi:10.1371/journal.pbio.0000060

Sun F, Fu H, Liu Q, Tie Y, Zhu J, Xing R, Sun Z, Zheng X (2008a) Downregulation of CCND1 and CDK6 by miR-34a induces cell cycle arrest. FEBS Lett 582(10):1564–1568. doi:S0014-5793(08)00306-2 [pii] 10.1016/j.febslet.2008.03.057

Sun M, Estrov Z, Ji Y, Coombes KR, Harris DH, Kurzrock R (2008b) Curcumin (diferuloylmethane) alters the expression profiles of microRNAs in human pancreatic cancer cells. Mol Cancer Ther 7(3):464–473. doi:7/3/464 [pii] 10.1158/1535-7163.MCT-07-2272

Sun Q, Cong R, Yan H, Gu H, Zeng Y, Liu N, Chen J, Wang B (2009) Genistein inhibits growth of human uveal melanoma cells and affects microRNA-27a and target gene expression. Oncol Rep 22(3):563–567

Sun W, Shen W, Yang S, Hu F, Li H, Zhu TH (2010) miR-223 and miR-142 attenuate hematopoietic cell proliferation, and miR-223 positively regulates miR-142 through LMO2 isoforms and CEBP-beta. Cell Res 20(10):1158–1169. doi:cr2010134 [pii] 10.1038/cr.2010.134

Suzuki Y, Kim HW, Ashraf M, Haider H (2010) Diazoxide potentiates mesenchymal stem cell survival via NF-kappaB-dependent miR-146a expression by targeting Fas. Am J Physiol Heart Circ Physiol 299(4):H1077–H1082. doi:ajpheart.00212.2010 [pii] 10.1152/ajpheart.00212.2010 [doi]

Takahashi Y, Forrest AR, Maeno E, Hashimoto T, Daub CO, Yasuda J (2009) MiR-107 and MiR-185 can induce cell cycle arrest in human non small cell lung cancer cell lines. PLoS One 4(8):e6677. doi:10.1371/journal.pone.0006677

Tang SN, Singh C, Nall D, Meeker D, Shankar S, Srivastava RK (2010a) The dietary bioflavonoid quercetin synergizes with epigallocathechin gallate (EGCG) to inhibit prostate cancer stem cell characteristics, invasion, migration and epithelial-mesenchymal transition. J Mol Signal 5:14. doi:1750-2187-5-14 [pii] 10.1186/1750-2187-5-14

Tang N, Zhang J, Du Y (2010b) Curcumin promoted the apoptosis of cisplain-resistant human lung carcinoma cells A549/DDP through down-regulating miR-186*. Zhongguo Fei Ai Za Zhi 13(4):301–306. doi:10.3779/j.issn.1009-3419.2010.04.06

Thangapazham RL, Singh AK, Sharma A, Warren J, Gaddipati JP, Maheshwari RK (2007) Green tea polyphenols and its constituent epigallocatechin gallate inhibits proliferation of human breast cancer cells in vitro and in vivo. Cancer Lett 245(1–2):232–241. doi:S0304-3835(06)00059-0 [pii] 10.1016/j.canlet.2006.01.027

Tili E, Michaille JJ, Gandhi V, Plunkett W, Sampath D, Calin GA (2007) miRNAs and their potential for use against cancer and other diseases. Future Oncol 3(5):521–537. doi:10.2217/14796694.3.5.521

Tili E, Michaille JJ, Alder H, Volinia S, Delmas D, Latruffe N, Croce CM (2010a) Resveratrol modulates the levels of microRNAs targeting genes encoding tumor-suppressors and effectors of TGFbeta signaling pathway in SW480 cells. Biochem Pharmacol 80(12):2057–2065. doi:S0006-2952(10)00514-9 [pii] 10.1016/j.bcp. 2010.07.003

Tili E, Michaille JJ, Adair B, Alder H, Limagne E, Taccioli C, Ferracin M, Delmas D, Latruffe N, Croce CM (2010b) Resveratrol decreases the levels of miR-155 by upregulating miR-663, a microRNA targeting JunB and JunD. Carcinogenesis 31(9):1561–1566. doi:bgq143 [pii] 10.1093/carcin/bgq143

Tili E, Michaille JJ, Alder H, Volinia S, Delmas D, Latruffe N, Croce CM (2010c) Resveratrol modulates the levels of microRNAs targeting genes encoding tumor-suppressors and effectors of TGFbeta signaling pathway in SW480 cells. Biochem Pharmacol. doi:S0006-2952(10)00514-9 [pii] 10.1016/j.bcp. 2010.07.003

Tsang WP, Kwok TT (2008) Let-7a microRNA suppresses therapeutics-induced cancer cell death by targeting caspase-3. Apoptosis 13(10):1215–1222. doi:10.1007/s10495-008-0256-z

Tsang WP, Kwok TT (2010) Epigallocatechin gallate up-regulation of miR-16 and induction of apoptosis in human cancer cells. J Nutr Biochem 21(2):140–146. doi:S0955-2863(08)00256-8 [pii] 10.1016/j.jnutbio.2008.12.003

Volinia S, Calin GA, Liu CG, Ambs S, Cimmino A, Petrocca F, Visone R, Iorio M, Roldo C, Ferracin M, Prueitt RL, Yanaihara N, Lanza G, Scarpa A, Vecchione A, Negrini M, Harris CC, Croce CM (2006) A microRNA expression signature of human solid tumors defines cancer gene targets. Proc Natl Acad Sci USA 103(7):2257–2261. doi:0510565103 [pii] 10.1073/pnas.0510565103

Voorhoeve PM (2010) MicroRNAs: oncogenes, tumor suppressors or master regulators of cancer heterogeneity? Biochim Biophys Acta 1805(1):72–86. doi:S0304-419X(09)00061-4 [pii] 10.1016/j.bbcan.2009.09.003

Voorhoeve PM, Agami R (2007) Classifying microRNAs in cancer: the good, the bad and the ugly. Biochim Biophys Acta 1775(2):274–282. doi:S0304-419X(06)00064-3 [pii] 10.1016/j.bbcan.2006.11.003

Wang T, Xu Z (2010) miR-27 promotes osteoblast differentiation by modulating Wnt signaling. Biochem Biophys Res Commun. doi:S0006-291X(10)01517-2 [pii] 10.1016/j.bbrc.2010.08.031

Wang LL, Zhang Z, Li Q, Yang R, Pei X, Xu Y, Wang J, Zhou SF, Li Y (2009a) Ethanol exposure induces differential microRNA and target gene expression and teratogenic effects which can be suppressed by folic acid supplementation. Hum Reprod 24(3):562–579. doi:den439 [pii] 10.1093/humrep/den439

Wang Y, Rathinam R, Walch A, Alahari SK (2009b) ST14 (suppression of tumorigenicity 14) gene is a target for miR-27b, and the inhibitory effect of ST14 on cell growth is independent of miR-27b regulation. J Biol Chem 284(34):23094–23106. doi:M109.012617 [pii] 10.1074/jbc.M109.012617

Wang S, Bian C, Yang Z, Bo Y, Li J, Zeng L, Zhou H, Zhao RC (2009c) miR-145 inhibits breast cancer cell growth through RTKN. Int J Oncol 34(5):1461–1466

Wei JS, Song YK, Durinck S, Chen QR, Cheuk AT, Tsang P, Zhang Q, Thiele CJ, Slack A, Shohet J, Khan J (2008) The MYCN oncogene is a direct target of miR-34a. Oncogene 27(39):5204–5213. doi:onc2008154 [pii] 10.1038/onc.2008.154

Welch C, Chen Y, Stallings RL (2007) MicroRNA-34a functions as a potential tumor suppressor by inducing apoptosis in neuroblastoma cells. Oncogene 26(34):5017–5022. doi:1210293 [pii] 10.1038/sj.onc.1210293

Wen XY, Wu SY, Li ZQ, Liu ZQ, Zhang JJ, Wang GF, Jiang ZH, Wu SG (2009) Ellagitannin (BJA3121), an anti-proliferative natural polyphenol compound, can regulate the expression of MiRNAs in HepG2 cancer cells. Phytother Res 23(6):778–784. doi:10.1002/ptr.2616

Xiao C, Srinivasan L, Calado DP, Patterson HC, Zhang B, Wang J, Henderson JM, Kutok JL, Rajewsky K (2008) Lymphoproliferative disease and autoimmunity in mice with increased miR-17-92 expression in lymphocytes. Nat Immunol 9(4):405–414. doi:ni1575 [pii] 10.1038/ni1575

Xiong J, Yu D, Wei N, Fu H, Cai T, Huang Y, Wu C, Zheng X, Du Q, Lin D, Liang Z (2010) An estrogen receptor alpha suppressor, microRNA-22, is downregulated in estrogen receptor alpha-positive human breast cancer cell lines and clinical samples. FEBS J 277(7):1684–1694. doi:EJB7594 [pii] 10.1111/j.1742-4658.2010.07594.x

Yamakuchi M, Ferlito M, Lowenstein CJ (2008) miR-34a repression of SIRT1 regulates apoptosis. Proc Natl Acad Sci USA 105(36):13421–13426. doi:0801613105 [pii] 10.1073/pnas.0801613105

Yamakuchi M, Lotterman CD, Bao C, Hruban RH, Karim B, Mendell JT, Huso D, Lowenstein CJ (2010) P53-induced microRNA-107 inhibits HIF-1 and tumor angiogenesis. Proc Natl Acad Sci USA 107(14):6334–6339. doi:0911082107 [pii] 10.1073/pnas.0911082107

Yanaihara N, Caplen N, Bowman E, Seike M, Kumamoto K, Yi M, Stephens RM, Okamoto A, Yokota J, Tanaka T, Calin GA, Liu CG, Croce CM, Harris CC (2006) Unique microRNA molecular profiles in lung cancer diagnosis and prognosis. Cancer Cell 9(3):189–198. doi:S1535-6108(06)00033-X [pii] 10.1016/j.ccr.2006.01.025

Yang H, Kong W, He L, Zhao JJ, O'Donnell JD, Wang J, Wenham RM, Coppola D, Kruk PA, Nicosia SV, Cheng JQ (2008) MicroRNA expression profiling in human ovarian cancer: miR-214 induces cell survival and cisplatin resistance by targeting PTEN. Cancer Res 68(2):425–433. doi:68/2/425 [pii]10.1158/0008-5472.CAN-07-2488

Yang J, Cao Y, Sun J, Zhang Y (2009a) Curcumin reduces the expression of Bcl-2 by upregulating miR-15a and miR-16 in MCF-7 cells. Med Oncol. doi:10.1007/s12032-009-9344-3

Yang L, Belaguli N, Berger DH (2009b) MicroRNA and colorectal cancer. World J Surg 33(4): 638–646. doi:10.1007/s00268-008-9865-5

Zhang Z, Li Z, Gao C, Chen P, Chen J, Liu W, Xiao S, Lu H (2008) miR-21 plays a pivotal role in gastric cancer pathogenesis and progression. Lab Invest 88(12):1358–1366. doi:labinvest200894 [pii] 10.1038/labinvest.2008.94

Zhang J, Zhang T, Ti X, Shi J, Wu C, Ren X, Yin H (2010a) Curcumin promotes apoptosis in A549/DDP multidrug-resistant human lung adenocarcinoma cells through an miRNA signaling pathway. Biochem Biophys Res Commun 399(1):1–6. doi:S0006-291X(10)01315-X [pii] 10.1016/j.bbrc.2010.07.013

Zhang J, Du Y, Wu C, Ren X, Ti X, Shi J, Zhao F, Yin H (2010b) Curcumin promotes apoptosis in human lung adenocarcinoma cells through miR-186* signaling pathway. Oncol Rep 24(5):1217–1223

Zhang CZ, Zhang JX, Zhang AL, Shi ZD, Han L, Jia ZF, Yang WD, Wang GX, Jiang T, You YP, Pu PY, Cheng JQ, Kang CS (2010c) MiR-221 and miR-222 target PUMA to induce cell survival in glioblastoma. Mol Cancer 9:229. doi:1476-4598-9-229 [pii] 10.1186/1476-4598-9-229

Zhao JJ, Sun DG, Wang J, Liu SR, Zhang CY, Zhu MX, Ma X (2008) Retinoic acid downregulates microRNAs to induce abnormal development of spinal cord in spina bifida rat model. Childs Nerv Syst 24(4):485–492. doi:10.1007/s00381-007-0520-5

Zhu S, Si ML, Wu H, Mo YY (2007) MicroRNA-21 targets the tumor suppressor gene tropomyosin 1 (TPM1). J Biol Chem 282(19):14328–14336. doi:M611393200 [pii] 10.1074/jbc.M611393200

Zhu H, Wu H, Liu X, Evans BR, Medina DJ, Liu CG, Yang JM (2008) Role of MicroRNA miR-27a and miR-451 in the regulation of MDR1/P-glycoprotein expression in human cancer cells. Biochem Pharmacol 76(5):582–588. doi:S0006-2952(08)00387-0 [pii] 10.1016/j.bcp. 2008.06.007

Zhu W, Shan X, Wang T, Shu Y, Liu P (2010) miR-181b modulates multidrug resistance by targeting BCL2 in human cancer cell lines. Int J Cancer 127(11):2520–2529. doi:10.1002/ijc.25260

Part VI
Phytochemicals in Inflammation and Cancer

Chapter 17
Interference with Estrogen Receptor-α by Dietary Components: Impact on the Balance Between Cell Proliferation and Cell Death

Józefa Węsierska-Gądek, Margarita Maurer, and Oxana Komina

Abstract ER-α, a major estrogen receptor, is a ligand-regulated factor that is involved in the transcriptional control of various physiological processes, including cell proliferation (by inducing progression through the G_1 phase of the cell cycle in estrogen-responsive tissues) and other effects that appear to occur too rapidly to be mediated by transcriptional activation of genes. Furthermore, increased levels of cyclin D_1 in breast cancer cells correlate with overexpression of ER-α. Epidemiological data have suggested that the consumption of some dietary components offers beneficial health effects due to their estrogenic activity, and several classes of natural products that can modulate ER-α activity and promote apoptosis have been identified. Interference with ER-α activity affects a fine balance between cell proliferation and cell death, and might have significant chemopreventive effects. Thus, the activities of natural compounds that influence ER-α activity, especially dietary components, warrant thorough characterization and evaluation.

Keywords Breast cancer • Contraceptives • Estrogens • Estrogen receptors • Genistein • Hormone replacement therapy • Multi-drug resistance • Phytoestrogens • Sex hormones

Abbreviations

AF	activating function
BCRP	breast cancer resistance protein
CDK7	cyclin-dependent kinase 7

J. Węsierska-Gądek (✉) • M. Maurer • O. Komina
Cell Cycle Regulation Group, Department of Medicine I, Division: Institute of Cancer Research, Comprehensive Cancer Center, Medical University of Vienna, Borschkegasse 8a, A-1090 Vienna, Austria
e-mail: Jozefa.Gadek-Wesierski@meduniwien.ac.at

M. Diederich and K. Noworyta (eds.), *Natural Compounds as Inducers of Cell Death: Volume 1*, DOI 10.1007/978-94-007-4575-9_17,

DBD	DNA binding domain
ER	estrogen receptor
LBD	ligand-binding domain
MAPK	mitogen-activated protein kinase
MDR	multi-drug resistance
PTEN	phosphatase and tensin homologue deleted on chromosome ten

17.1 A Causal Link Between Exposure to Sex Hormones and Development of Breast Cancer

Breast cancer is the most frequently-observed malignancy in women and is the second most common cause of death among women worldwide (Glass et al. 2007). According to recent statistics for the United States, more than 200,000 new cases of breast cancer are diagnosed each year, and more than 40,000 women die of the disease (Jemal et al. 2010). It is widely accepted that breast cancer is a very complex disease, arising from the presence of specific alleles and the interactions between them and various environmental factors that seem to affect the accumulation of mutations in essential genes (Ford et al. 1994; Hulka and Stark 1995; Nathanson et al. 2001; Peto et al. 1999).

It has been well established in numerous epidemiological studies that inherited mutations in certain genes represent risks for developing cancer. Mutations of two genes, *BRCA1* and *BRCA2* (on the long arms of chromosomes 17 and 13, respectively), induce genomic instability and confer susceptibility to cancer development (Mavaddat et al. 2010; Coate et al. 2010; O'Donovan and Livingston 2010; Kwei et al. 2010; Peto et al. 1999). Together, they give rise to approximately 90% of inherited breast cancers. However, mutations in these two genes account for only 5–10% of all breast cancer cases, clearly indicating that other factors play important roles in breast carcinogenesis. Indeed, in recent years, numerous risk factors for the development of breast cancer have been identified, many of which are linked to hormones (Hilakivi-Clarke 2000; Russo et al. 2006; Russo and Russo 2006, 2008). Notably, various studies have found indications that contraceptives and hormone replacement therapies involving administration of estrogens and/or other steroids (e.g. synthetic progesterone derivatives) significantly increase the risk of developing breast cancer (Key and Verkasalo 1999; Magnusson et al. 1999; Ross et al. 2000; Collaborative Group on Hormonal Factors in Breast Cancer 1996) . In addition, very recent experiments in which medroxyprogesterone acetate (a synthetic progesterone derivative applied in hormone therapy) (el Mahgoub et al. 1972; Hofseth et al. 1999) was administered *in vivo* to an animal model have confirmed that steroid hormones can induce breast cancer, and provided indications of the underlying mechanisms (Gonzalez-Suarez et al. 2010). The treatment strongly induced the osteoclast differentiation factor RANKL (a receptor activator of the NF-κB ligand) in mammary gland epithelial cells, while inactivation of the RANKL receptor in these cells abolished their hormone-induced proliferation (Schramek et al. 2010).

17.2 Expression and Regulation of Estrogen Receptors

It is not surprising that administration of estrogens (and other steroid hormones) can have potent, sometimes undesirable, effects since they regulate diverse cellular processes during growth, development, differentiation and subsequent events, acting *via* signalling pathways induced by their binding to specific receptors (for reviews, see Enmark and Gustafsson 1999; Matthews and Gustafsson 2003). Estrogens are required for the proliferation and differentiation of healthy breast epithelium, and control of metabolic processes, thus they have beneficial effects on the brain, heart and bones (Sherwin 2009; ESHRE Capri Workshop Group 2006). Two main estrogen receptors (ERs) are known: ER-α (Green et al. 1986a, b; Greene and Press 1986) and ER-β (Kuiper et al. 1996; Mosselman et al. 1996).

The ERs are hormone-stimulated transcription factors that belong to a large family of receptors, including (*inter alia*) receptors for thyroid and steroid hormones (Evans 1988). These proteins bind to specific estrogen response elements (EREs) in the promoter region of responsive genes (Beato et al. 1989; Ham and Parker 1989), which include tumor suppressor genes (Gudas et al. 1995; Hurd et al. 1997; Spillman and Bowcock 1996), oncogenes (Dubik et al. 1987), TGF-α and IGF-1 (El-Ashry et al. 1996). They also strongly affect the expression of several downstream genes that are components of the cell cycle machinery (e.g. *CCND1*), thereby promoting the proliferation of cells expressing ER (Clarke et al. 1997; Herman and Katzenellenbogen 1994; Prall et al. 1998; Petre et al. 2002) and/or other cellular targets involved in the regulation of cell death (Arnold and Papanikolaou 2005; Nass and Dickson 1997; Wakeling et al. 1991; Sabbah et al. 1999; Hartman et al. 2009).

Close functional links between hormone signalling and the cell division cycle have been demonstrated by experiments performed on transgenic mice (Lubahn et al. 1993). ER-α knock-out female mice are infertile and display marginal development of mammary glands as well as atrophy of the uterus (Lubahn et al. 1993). An animal experimental model established by Sicinski et al. (Sicinski et al. 1995) has also provided evidence of a close functional link between the major G_1 cyclin and sex steroid hormone-regulated processes. Cyclin D_1 knock-out mice display defects in hormone-responsive proliferation of the epithelium during pregnancy (Sicinski et al. 1995). This action of female sex hormones explains their roles in both the physiological regulation of normal mammary gland development and reproductive tracts, and the development of breast cancer.

ER-α, the first member of the steroid hormone receptor protein family to be identified, is the major estrogen receptor (Mangelsdorf et al. 1995) and functions as a ligand-dependent transcription factor (Katzenellenbogen and Katzenellenbogen 1996). ER-α has a number of splice variants, some of which affect the activity and function of the regularly-spliced ER-α form (Hopp and Fuqua 1998; Jazaeri et al. 1999). Estrogen receptors are present in discrete subcellular locations in the cell, including the nucleus and several extra-nuclear compartments (Hammes and Levin 2007). The major extra-nuclear pool of ERs is in the plasma membrane (Szego and Davis 1967; Pietras and Szego 1977).

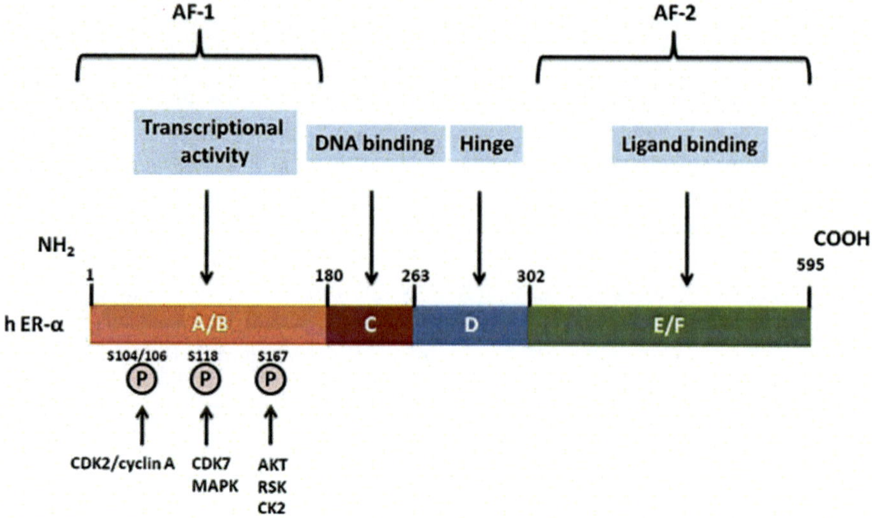

Fig. 17.1 Structural organization of ER-α. Scheme illustrating structure of ER-α and the serine residues (S) whose phosphorylations are catalyzed in response to estrogen signalling or activation of second messenger signaling pathways. The kinases known to catalyze these modifications are indicated. Structural domains correlate with the functions. *AF* activating function, *DBD* DNA binding domain, *LBD* ligand binding domain

However, ERs have also been found in other cellular organelles, including the endoplasmic reticulum and mitochondria (Hammes and Levin 2007), which may explain the rapidity of some biological effects that are induced by estrogen too quickly (within seconds or minutes) to be mediated by "classic" genomic pathways involving the transcriptional activation of genes (Revelli et al. 1998; Hammes and Levin 2007). These rapid, extra-nuclear ("non-genomic") mechanisms of ERs, more accurately termed "membrane-initiated steroid signalling" are still subject to intense debate (Hammes and Levin 2007; Moriarty et al. 2006). The ability to stimulate endothelial nitric oxide synthase (eNOS) is one of the best characterized rapid effects of estrogen. However, estrogens have also been proposed to promote energy production in mitochondria (oxidative phosphorylation) while decreasing mitochondrial production of free radicals (reactive oxygen species).

Thus, the differential subcellular localization of the estrogen receptors and the tight regulation of their intracellular trafficking seem to contribute to the fine-tuned regulation of estrogen action and broaden the biological effects of estrogens.

Like other members of the receptors superfamily, ERs have a modular structure that includes functional domains for ligand- and DNA-binding as well as two regions that modulate their transcriptional activity (Katzenellenbogen et al. 1996) (Fig. 17.1). One of these regions, designated transcription activating function-1 (AF-1), is located in the NH_2-terminal part of the protein and functions in a ligand-independent manner. The other (AF-2) is located in the COOH-domain and is ligand-dependent. The ligand-dependent activation of ERs requires recruitment of various coactivators to the promoters (Lonard and O'Malley 2006; Brzozowski et al. 1997) (Fig. 17.2).

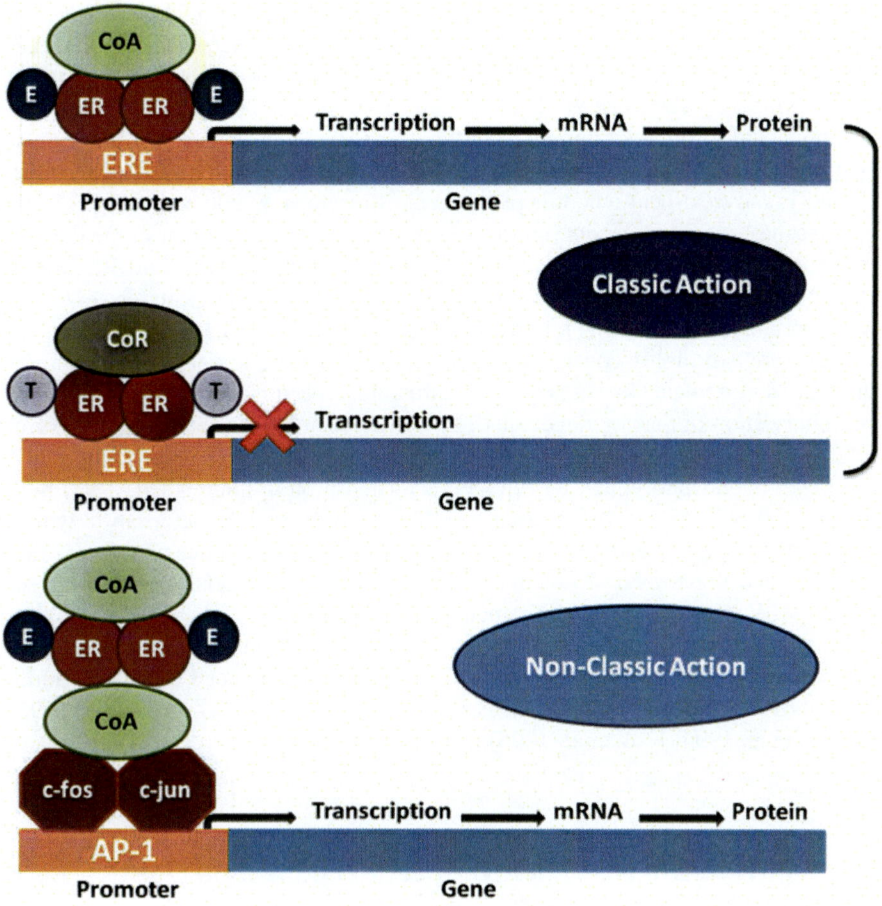

Fig. 17.2 Mechanism of transcriptional regulation of estrogen-dependent genes. Two types of action are shown: classic and non-classic. In the first type, ER directly binds to estrogen response elements (*EREs*) in the promoter region of target genes. The change of the activity of the complex depends on recruitment of additional co-regulators. Estrogen-bound ER forms complexes with co-activators what leads to activation of gene expression. ER bound to antagonist T (e.g. tamoxifen) recruits co-repressor proteins resulting in the block of transcription. In a non-classical mode of action, direct protein-protein interaction occurs at DNA sites occupied by other transcription factors e. g. AP-1

In addition, ERs are regulated by interaction with estrogen-responsive promoters and the recruitment of various cofactors to these promoters (Brzozowski et al. 1997). The presence of two separate AFs facilitates fine-tuning of the receptor's activity (Brzozowski et al. 1997). ER-α undergoes distinct posttranslational modifications, such as acetylation, methylation, palmitoylation, phosphorylation and sumoylation that have been found to regulate ER translocation, interactions with distinct proteins (e.g. caveolin-1), rapid signalling and transcriptional activity (Razandi et al. 2003).

ER-α is a phosphoprotein, and its phosphorylation is strongly enhanced in responses to ligand- and growth factor signalling pathways (Aronica and Katzenellenbogen 1993; Kato et al. 1995). It is phosphorylated at several residues by various protein kinases (Washburn et al. 1991; Ali et al. 1993; Lannigan 2003), and its phosphorylation status in human breast cancer biopsies was recently determined (Murphy et al. 2009). Phosphorylated ER-α variants appear to be associated with prognosis and treatment outcome parameters (Murphy et al. 2004a, b) (Fig. 17.1).

ER-α has several phosphorylation sites that seem to be important in the therapy and prognosis of breast cancer, including serines 104/106, 118, 167, and 305, which are reportedly modified *inter alia* by mitogen-activated protein kinases (MAPK), AKT, protein kinase A (PKA), ribosomal kinases and p21Pak1 kinase.

There are two highly conserved serine residues (Ser^{106} and Ser^{118}) in the amino-terminal AF-1 domain (Joel et al. 1995). Estradiol has been found to trigger extensive phosphorylation of Ser^{118} (Joel et al. 1995), which seems to be catalyzed by several cellular kinases (for a review, see Lannigan 2003). Kato and colleagues reported that Ser^{118} is phosphorylated by mitogen-activated protein kinases (MAPKs) both *in vitro* and in COS-1 cells exposed to EGF and IGF growth factors in a ligand-independent manner (Kato et al. 1995). However, Joel and colleagues found that ligand-dependent phosphorylation of ER-α at the same serine residue (Joel et al. 1998) seems to be catalyzed by cyclin-dependent kinase 7 (CDK7) (Chen et al. 2000). Although Ser^{118} is located in the amino-terminal ligand-independent AF-1, it has been shown to be involved in the modulation of estrogen-induced ER-α activation, since its mutation markedly reduces transactivation by ER-α (Ali et al. 1993; Le Goff et al. 1994; Kato et al. 1995).

17.3 Phytoestrogens, Their Properties and Action on Mammary Glands

Phytoestrogens comprise a diverse group of naturally occurring compounds, found in more than 300 plant species, that have structural similarities to 17-β-estradiol, and hence estrogenic and/or anti-estrogenic effects. Scientific interest in phytoestrogens, especially soya bean isoflavones, has strongly increased in the last decade, partly due to epidemiological observations that the incidence of hormone-related disorders, especially some cancers, is much lower in China and Japan (where soya beans are common constituents of the diet; (Setchell 1998)) than in USA and Europe. This has led to the hypothesis that the high soya intake among Asian women might explain their low breast cancer risks (Trock et al. 2006; Wu et al. 2008).

There is accumulating evidence that phytoestrogens may have beneficial, metabolic effects, including tendencies to reduce cholesterol levels, facilitate the maintenance of normal bone density and provide protection against diverse disorders (via equally diverse and in some cases controversial mechanisms) such as cancers, cardiovascular and brain diseases, and osteoporosis.

There are three main classes of phytoestrogens: non-steroidal isoflavones (Reinli and Block 1996), lignans (Thompson et al. 1991) and coumestans (Thompson et al. 2006) (Fig. 17.3). Genistein and daidzein (the two major isoflavones found in red clover, soya beans and other legumes) are the best characterized and most extensively studied of these compounds (Albertazzi and Purdie 2002). Soya beans and soya foods are by far the most significant dietary sources of isoflavones (Coward et al. 1993; Wang and Murphy 1994; Murphy and Hendrich 2002).

Genistein and daidzein are present in plants as the glycosides genistin and daidzin, respectively (Walter 1941; Murphy et al. 1997). These glucose conjugates are not estrogenically active (Miksicek 1995), but upon consumption they are hydrolyzed to the corresponding aglycones by β-glucosidases in the human small intestine and liver and by the gut microflora (Coldham and Sauer 2001). Since the biological properties of the precursor compounds and their hydrolyzed metabolites differ, and the gut enzymes and microflora play crucial roles in phytoestrogen metabolism, inter-individual differences in the metabolism of phytoestrogens may occur, with accompanying variations in cancer risks.

Phytoestrogens with unique diphenolic structures conferring increased stability (Adlercreutz and Mazur 1997) bind to ERs and induce estrogen signaling pathways, including kinase activation and transcriptional gene modulation. Notably, genistein has been shown to affect the cell cycle, proliferation, apoptosis, invasion and metastasis in numerous *in vitro* and *in vivo* studies. It has been shown to exert biphasic effects on the proliferation of ER(+) breast cancer cell lines; stimulating proliferation at concentrations up to 10 μM (Wang and Kurzer 1997; Zava and Duwe 1997) and blocking cell divisions at higher concentrations (Peterson and Barnes 1991; Monti and Sinha 1994). In contrast, phytoestrogens do not appear to promote the proliferation of ER(-) breast cancer cell lines. Genistein also induces cell cycle arrest in ER(+) MCF-7 cells in a concentration-dependent manner. At low dosage (10 μM) it causes reversible G_2/M arrest, while at higher concentrations (≥50 μM) it decreases the frequency of S-phase cells associated with a prolonged G_2/M block. In addition, prolonged treatment with genistein (>48 h) has been found to induce apoptosis (Pagliacci et al. 1994; Choi et al. 1998; Constantinou et al. 1998), and to affect (in a similar manner) the cell cycle progression of ER(−) breast cancer cell lines (MDA-MB-231, MDA-MB-468) and human non-malignant mammary epithelial MCF-10F cells (Frey et al. 2001).

The genistein-mediated blockage of breast cancer cells in the G_2/M transition is probably due to induction of the $p21^{waf1}$ protein and deregulation of the activity of the CDK1/cyclin B complex (Cappelletti et al. 2000). Interestingly, genistein also strongly affects some tumor suppressor proteins. Notably, expression of the phosphatase and tensin homologue deleted on chromosome ten (PTEN) in mammary gland epithelial cells can be induced by dietary exposure to the isoflavone *in vivo* and by supplying it to MCF-7 cells *in vitro* (Dave et al. 2005). PTEN encodes a dual-specificity phosphatase that negatively regulates phosphatidylinositol 3-kinase (PI3K), thereby preventing activation of the pro-survival protein kinase B/AKT pathway (Stambolic et al. 1998). Exposure of the nonmalignant human mammary epithelial cell line MCF-10A to genistein at physiologically relevant concentrations reportedly induces nuclear accumulation of PTEN and p53 tumor suppressor proteins (Rahal and Simmen 2010),

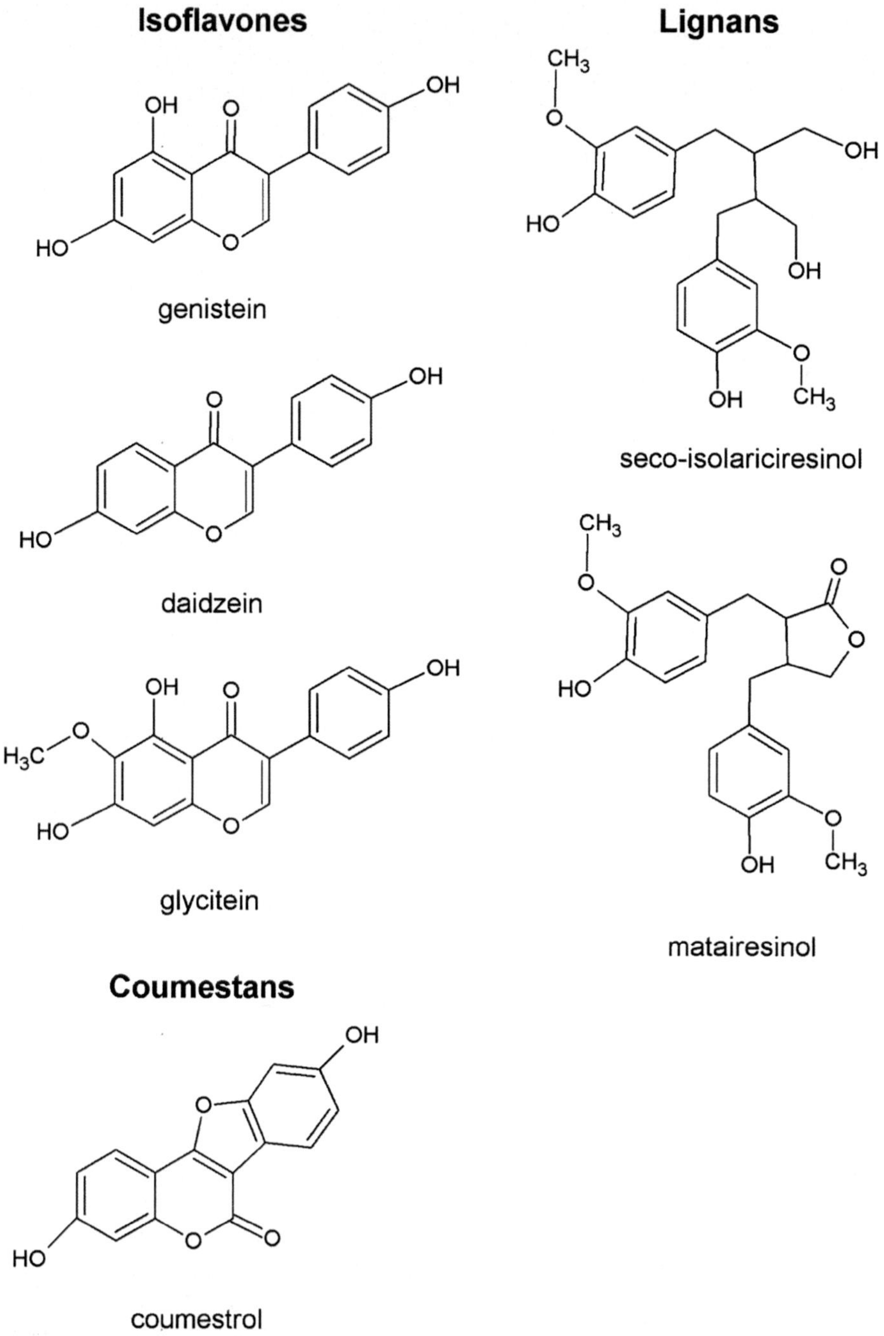

Fig. 17.3 Structure of the major groups of phytoestrogens. Isoflavonoids (genistein, daidzein and glycitein), lignans and coumestans are shown

probably through an autoregulatory loop whereby PTEN's increased interaction with nuclear wt p53 enhances PTEN promoter activity (Rahal and Simmen 2010). Genistein-induced PTEN-p53 cross-talk seems to decrease cyclin D_1 and pleiotrophin gene expression, thus markedly enhancing cell cycle arrest, and the early formation of mammary acini, which is indicative of lobuloalveolar differentiation (Rahal and Simmen 2010). Moreover, genistein inhibits the activity of topoisomerase II, and in turn decatenation of DNA, thereby inducing DNA strand breaks (Markovits et al. 1989). It can also contribute to induction of apoptosis. For instance, in Brca1 mutant mammary tumor cells, which are more sensitive to genistein than other cancer cells, it can reduce proliferation, induce cell cycle arrest and activate DNA damage checkpoints, resulting in mitotic catastrophe and apoptosis (Tominaga et al. 2007). Finally, several *in vivo* studies have shown that isoflavones can protect animals from chemically induced cancer (Barnes et al. 1990; Serraino and Thompson 1991). However, the protective effects of isoflavones strongly depend on the dose and time of exposure; notably the latent period preceding the appearance of chemically generated tumors in animals is reportedly longer if the treatment is neonatal or prepubertal rather than postpubertal (Barnes 1997; Murrill et al. 1996).

17.4 Mechanisms of Action of Genistein on Mammary Gland Epithelial Cells

As previously mentioned, genistein stimulates cell divisions of ER(+) but not ER(−) breast cancer cells, suggesting that genistein operates *via* the ERs, and it has biphasic effects on the former (Zava and Duwe 1997).

Accordingly, genistein binds to ER-α and ER-β *in vitro* with several-fold lower binding affinities than 17-β estradiol (Muthyala et al. 2004). Moreover, at natural dietary levels genistein induces the transcriptional activation of both ERs in transient transfection assays (Mavaddat et al. 2010; Jemal et al. 2010; Gonzalez-Suarez et al. 2010; Eshre Capri Workshop Group 2006). At low concentrations genistein has been shown to be a full agonist for both ER-α and ER-β (Maggiolini et al. 2001), in accordance with the observation that isoflavones can induce pS2 expression. However, since genistein appears to have anti-proliferative effects on breast cancer cells irrespective of their ER status, its growth inhibitory effects do not appear to be mediated by an ER-dependent pathway, but rather *via* activation of tumor suppressors and induction of cell cycle arrest.

17.5 Reversal of Drug Resistance in Breast Cancer by Phytoestrogens

Multidrug-resistance (MDR), i.e. cross-resistance to structurally unrelated drugs, frequently arises during chemotherapy and causes severe complications since patients developing it become nonresponsive to treatment (Gottesman et al. 1995). Breast cancer resistance protein (BCRP) is an ATP-binding cassette half-transporter (Doyle et al. 1998) that mediates concomitant resistance to chemotherapeutics such as SN-38 (an active metabolite of CPT-11), topotecan and mitoxantrone, probably by pumping the drugs out of the cells and thus reducing their anti-cancer action.

Interestingly, isoflavones including genistein have been found to strongly reverse BCRP-mediated drug resistance and, thus, increase the toxicity of drugs. It has been suggested that genistein is one of various natural substrates of BCRP, which competitively inhibits BCRP-generated drug efflux (Sugimoto et al. 2003; Imai et al. 2004).

17.6 Exposure to Phytoestrogens and Breast Cancer Risk

The evidence collected to date implies that the intake of soy phytoestrogens in the amounts traditionally consumed in Asian populations may have protective effects against the development of breast cancer (Warri et al. 2008). However, results of some animal studies do not support this hypothesis (Hilakivi-Clarke et al. 1999; Pei et al. 2003). Furthermore, in human intervention studies the administration of 100 mg isoflavone per day to premenopausal women for a year did not reduce mammographic density, which is linked to four- to six-fold variations in risks of breast cancer (Maskarinec et al. 2003), and exposure to 50 mg isoflavone daily for 2 years had no apparent effect on circulating steroid hormones or sex hormone-binding proteins (Maskarinec et al. 2004).

In summary, reports on the positive and negative effects of phytoestrogens seem to be, at least partially conflicting, reflecting the complexity of the relationships between phytoestrogens and breast cancer. The timing of exposure to phytoestrogens (exposure early in life appears to be beneficial), their digestion and the ways in which individual phytoestrogens are metabolized all appear to influence their impact on breast cancer risks. Further elucidation of the mechanisms involved may be valuable for both explaining the variations in responses to them and for identifying possible therapies (Tempfer et al. 2009).

References

Adlercreutz H, Mazur W (1997) Phyto-oestrogens and western diseases. Ann Med 29(2):95–120

Albertazzi P, Purdie D (2002) The nature and utility of the phytoestrogens: a review of the evidence. Maturitas 42(3):173–185. doi:S0378512202000245 [pii]

Ali S, Metzger D, Bornert JM, Chambon P (1993) Modulation of transcriptional activation by ligand-dependent phosphorylation of the human oestrogen receptor a/b region. EMBO J 12(3):1153–1160

Arnold A, Papanikolaou A (2005) Cyclin d1 in breast cancer pathogenesis. J Clin Oncol 23(18):4215–4224. doi:23/18/4215 [pii] 10.1200/JCO.2005.05.064

Aronica SM, Katzenellenbogen BS (1993) Stimulation of estrogen receptor-mediated transcription and alteration in the phosphorylation state of the rat uterine estrogen receptor by estrogen, cyclic adenosine monophosphate, and insulin-like growth factor-i. Mol Endocrinol 7(6):743–752

Barnes S (1997) The chemopreventive properties of soy isoflavonoids in animal models of breast cancer. Breast Cancer Res Treat 46(2–3):169–179

Barnes S, Grubbs C, Setchell KD, Carlson J (1990) Soybeans inhibit mammary tumors in models of breast cancer. Prog Clin Biol Res 347:239–253

Beato M, Chalepakis G, Schauer M, Slater EP (1989) DNA regulatory elements for steroid hormones. J Steroid Biochem 32(5):737–747

Brzozowski AM, Pike AC, Dauter Z, Hubbard RE, Bonn T, Engstrom O, Ohman L, Greene GL, Gustafsson JA, Carlquist M (1997) Molecular basis of agonism and antagonism in the oestrogen receptor. Nature 389(6652):753–758. doi:10.1038/39645

Cappelletti V, Fioravanti L, Miodini P, Di Fronzo G (2000) Genistein blocks breast cancer cells in the g(2)m phase of the cell cycle. J Cell Biochem 79(4):594–600. doi:10.1002/1097-4644(20001215)79:4<594::AID-JCB80>3.0.CO;2-4 [pii]

Chen D, Riedl T, Washbrook E, Pace PE, Coombes RC, Egly JM, Ali S (2000) Activation of estrogen receptor alpha by s118 phosphorylation involves a ligand-dependent interaction with tfiih and participation of cdk7. Mol Cell 6(1):127–137. doi:S1097-2765(05)00004-3 [pii]

Choi YH, Zhang L, Lee WH, Park KY (1998) Genistein-induced g2/m arrest is associated with the inhibition of cyclin b1 and the induction of p21 in human breast carcinoma cells. Int J Oncol 13(2):391–396

Clarke RB, Howell A, Anderson E (1997) Estrogen sensitivity of normal human breast tissue in vivo and implanted into athymic nude mice: analysis of the relationship between estrogen-induced proliferation and progesterone receptor expression. Breast Cancer Res Treat 45(2):121–133

Coate L, Cuffe S, Horgan A, Hung RJ, Christiani D, Liu G (2010) Germline genetic variation, cancer outcome, and pharmacogenetics. J Clin Oncol 28(26):4029–4037. doi:JCO.2009.27.2336 [pii] 10.1200/JCO.2009.27.2336

Coldham NG, Sauer MJ (2001) Identification, quantitation and biological activity of phytoestrogens in a dietary supplement for breast enhancement. Food Chem Toxicol 39(12):1211–1224. doi:S0278-6915(01)00081-3 [pii]

Collaborative Group on Hormonal Factors in Breast Cancer (1996) Breast cancer and hormonal contraceptives: collaborative reanalysis of individual data on 53 297 women with breast cancer and 100 239 women without breast cancer from 54 epidemiological studies. Lancet 347(9017): 1713–1727

Constantinou AI, Kamath N, Murley JS (1998) Genistein inactivates bcl-2, delays the g2/m phase of the cell cycle, and induces apoptosis of human breast adenocarcinoma mcf-7 cells. Eur J Cancer 34(12):1927–1934. doi:Doi: 10.1016/s0959-8049(98)00198-1

Coward L, Barnes NC, Setchell KDR, Barnes S (1993) Genistein, daidzein, and their Beta.-glycoside conjugates: antitumor isoflavones in soybean foods from american and asian diets. J Agric Food Chem 41(11):1961–1967. doi:10.1021/jf00035a027

Dave B, Eason RR, Till SR, Geng Y, Velarde MC, Badger TM, Simmen RC (2005) The soy isoflavone genistein promotes apoptosis in mammary epithelial cells by inducing the tumor suppressor pten. Carcinogenesis 26(10):1793–1803. doi:bgi131 [pii] 10.1093/carcin/bgi131

Doyle LA, Yang W, Abruzzo LV, Krogmann T, Gao Y, Rishi AK, Ross DD (1998) A multidrug resistance transporter from human mcf-7 breast cancer cells. Proc Natl Acad Sci USA 95(26):15665–15670

Dubik D, Dembinski TC, Shiu RP (1987) Stimulation of c-myc oncogene expression associated with estrogen-induced proliferation of human breast cancer cells. Cancer Res 47(24 Pt 1):6517–6521

El-Ashry D, Chrysogelos SA, Lippman ME, Kern FG (1996) Estrogen induction of tgf-alpha is mediated by an estrogen response element composed of two imperfect palindromes. J Steroid Biochem Mol Biol 59(3–4):261–269. doi:S0960-0760(96)00118-5 [pii]

Enmark E, Gustafsson JA (1999) Oestrogen receptors - an overview. J Intern Med 246(2):133–138. doi:jim545 [pii]

ESHRE Capri Workshop Group (2006) Hormones and cardiovascular health in women. Hum Reprod Update 12(5):483–497

Evans RM (1988) The steroid and thyroid hormone receptor superfamily. Science 240(4854): 889–895

Ford D, Easton DF, Bishop DT, Narod SA, Goldgar DE (1994) Risks of cancer in brca1-mutation carriers Breast cancer linkage consortium. Lancet 343(8899):692–695
Frey RS, Li J, Singletary KW (2001) Effects of genistein on cell proliferation and cell cycle arrest in nonneoplastic human mammary epithelial cells: involvement of cdc2, p21(waf/cip1), p27(kip1), and cdc25c expression. Biochem Pharmacol 61(8):979–989. doi:S0006-2952(01)00572-X [pii]
Glass AG, Lacey JV Jr, Carreon JD, Hoover RN (2007) Breast cancer incidence, 1980–2006: combined roles of menopausal hormone therapy, screening mammography, and estrogen receptor status. J Natl Cancer Inst 99(15):1152–1161. doi:djm059 [pii] 10.1093/jnci/djm059
Gonzalez-Suarez E, Jacob AP, Jones J, Miller R, Roudier-Meyer MP, Erwert R, Pinkas J, Branstetter D, Dougall WC (2010) Rank ligand mediates progestin-induced mammary epithelial proliferation and carcinogenesis. Nature. doi:nature09495 [pii] 10.1038/nature09495
Gottesman MM, Hrycyna CA, Schoenlein PV, Germann UA, Pastan I (1995) Genetic analysis of the multidrug transporter. Annu Rev Genet 29:607–649. doi:10.1146/annurev.ge.29.120195.003135
Green S, Kumar V, Krust A, Walter P, Chambon P (1986a) Structural and functional domains of the estrogen receptor. Cold Spring Harb Symp Quant Biol 51(Pt 2):751–758
Green S, Walter P, Greene G, Krust A, Goffin C, Jensen E, Scrace G, Waterfield M, Chambon P (1986b) Cloning of the human oestrogen receptor cdna. J Steroid Biochem 24(1):77–83
Greene GL, Press MF (1986) Structure and dynamics of the estrogen receptor. J Steroid Biochem 24(1):1–7
Gudas JM, Nguyen H, Li T, Cowan KH (1995) Hormone-dependent regulation of brca1 in human breast cancer cells. Cancer Res 55(20):4561–4565
Ham J, Parker MG (1989) Regulation of gene expression by nuclear hormone receptors. Curr Opin Cell Biol 1(3):503–511
Hammes SR, Levin ER (2007) Extranuclear steroid receptors: nature and actions. Endocr Rev 28(7):726–741. doi:er.2007-0022 [pii] 10.1210/er.2007-0022
Hartman J, Lam EW, Gustafsson JA, Strom A (2009) Hes-6, an inhibitor of hes-1, is regulated by 17beta-estradiol and promotes breast cancer cell proliferation. Breast Cancer Res 11(6):R79. doi:bcr2446 [pii] 10.1186/bcr2446
Herman ME, Katzenellenbogen BS (1994) Alterations in transforming growth factor-alpha and -beta production and cell responsiveness during the progression of mcf-7 human breast cancer cells to estrogen-autonomous growth. Cancer Res 54(22):5867–5874
Hilakivi-Clarke L (2000) Estrogens, brca1, and breast cancer. Cancer Res 60(18):4993–5001
Hilakivi-Clarke L, Cho E, Onojafe I, Raygada M, Clarke R (1999) Maternal exposure to genistein during pregnancy increases carcinogen-induced mammary tumorigenesis in female rat offspring. Oncol Rep 6(5):1089–1095
Hofseth LJ, Raafat AM, Osuch JR, Pathak DR, Slomski CA, Haslam SZ (1999) Hormone replacement therapy with estrogen or estrogen plus medroxyprogesterone acetate is associated with increased epithelial proliferation in the normal postmenopausal breast. J Clin Endocrinol Metab 84(12):4559–4565
Hopp TA, Fuqua SA (1998) Estrogen receptor variants. J Mammary Gland Biol Neoplasia 3(1):73–83
Hulka BS, Stark AT (1995) Breast cancer: cause and prevention. Lancet 346(8979):883–887. doi:S0140-6736(95)92713-1 [pii]
Hurd C, Khattree N, Dinda S, Alban P, Moudgil VK (1997) Regulation of tumor suppressor proteins, p53 and retinoblastoma, by estrogen and antiestrogens in breast cancer cells. Oncogene 15(8):991–995. doi:10.1038/sj.onc.1201233
Imai Y, Tsukahara S, Asada S, Sugimoto Y (2004) Phytoestrogens/flavonoids reverse breast cancer resistance protein/abcg2-mediated multidrug resistance. Cancer Res 64(12):4346–4352. doi:10.1158/0008-5472.CAN-04-0078 64/12/4346 [pii]
Jazaeri O, Shupnik MA, Jazaeri AA, Rice LW (1999) Expression of estrogen receptor alpha mrna and protein variants in human endometrial carcinoma. Gynecol Oncol 74(1):38–47. doi:10.1006/gyno.1999.5404 S0090-8258(99)95404-5 [pii]
Jemal A, Siegel R, Xu J, Ward E (2010) Cancer statistics, 2010. CA Cancer J Clin 60(5):277–300. doi:caac.20073 [pii] 10.3322/caac.20073

Joel PB, Traish AM, Lannigan DA (1995) Estradiol and phorbol ester cause phosphorylation of serine 118 in the human estrogen receptor. Mol Endocrinol 9(8):1041–1052

Joel PB, Traish AM, Lannigan DA (1998) Estradiol-induced phosphorylation of serine 118 in the estrogen receptor is independent of p42/p44 mitogen-activated protein kinase. J Biol Chem 273(21):13317–13323

Kato S, Endoh H, Masuhiro Y, Kitamoto T, Uchiyama S, Sasaki H, Masushige S, Gotoh Y, Nishida E, Kawashima H, Metzger D, Chambon P (1995) Activation of the estrogen receptor through phosphorylation by mitogen-activated protein kinase. Science 270(5241):1491–1494

Katzenellenbogen JA, Katzenellenbogen BS (1996) Nuclear hormone receptors: ligand-activated regulators of transcription and diverse cell responses. Chem Biol 3(7):529–536

Katzenellenbogen JA, O'Malley BW, Katzenellenbogen BS (1996) Tripartite steroid hormone receptor pharmacology: interaction with multiple effector sites as a basis for the cell- and promoter-specific action of these hormones. Mol Endocrinol 10(2):119–131

Key TJ, Verkasalo PK (1999) Endogenous hormones and the aetiology of breast cancer. Breast Cancer Res 1(1):18–21

Kuiper GG, Enmark E, Pelto-Huikko M, Nilsson S, Gustafsson JA (1996) Cloning of a novel receptor expressed in rat prostate and ovary. Proc Natl Acad Sci USA 93(12):5925–5930

Kwei KA, Kung Y, Salari K, Holcomb IN, Pollack JR (2010) Genomic instability in breast cancer: pathogenesis and clinical implications. Mol Oncol 4(3):255–266. doi:S1574-7891(10)00023-2 [pii] 10.1016/j.molonc.2010.04.001

Lannigan DA (2003) Estrogen receptor phosphorylation. Steroids 68(1):1–9. doi:S0039128X-02001101 [pii]

Le Goff P, Montano MM, Schodin DJ, Katzenellenbogen BS (1994) Phosphorylation of the human estrogen receptor identification of hormone-regulated sites and examination of their influence on transcriptional activity. J Biol Chem 269(6):4458–4466

Lonard DM, O'Malley BW (2006) The expanding cosmos of nuclear receptor coactivators. Cell 125(3):411–414. doi:S0092-8674(06)00510-1 [pii] 10.1016/j.cell.2006.04.021

Lubahn DB, Moyer JS, Golding TS, Couse JF, Korach KS, Smithies O (1993) Alteration of reproductive function but not prenatal sexual development after insertional disruption of the mouse estrogen receptor gene. Proc Natl Acad Sci USA 90(23):11162–11166

Maggiolini M, Bonofiglio D, Marsico S, Panno ML, Cenni B, Picard D, Ando S (2001) Estrogen receptor alpha mediates the proliferative but not the cytotoxic dose-dependent effects of two major phytoestrogens on human breast cancer cells. Mol Pharmacol 60(3):595–602

Magnusson CM, Persson IR, Baron JA, Ekbom A, Bergstrom R, Adami HO (1999) The role of reproductive factors and use of oral contraceptives in the aetiology of breast cancer in women aged 50 to 74 years. Int J Cancer 80(2):231–236. doi:10.1002/(SICI)1097-0215(19990118)80:2<231::AID-IJC11>3.0.CO;2-R [pii]

el Mahgoub S, Karim M, Ammar R (1972) Long-term use of depot medroxy progesterone acetate as a contraceptive. Acta Obstet Gynecol Scand 51(3):251–255

Mangelsdorf DJ, Thummel C, Beato M, Herrlich P, Schutz G, Umesono K, Blumberg B, Kastner P, Mark M, Chambon P, Evans RM (1995) The nuclear receptor superfamily: the second decade. Cell 83(6):835–839. doi:0092-8674(95)90199-X [pii]

Markovits J, Linassier C, Fosse P, Couprie J, Pierre J, Jacquemin-Sablon A, Saucier JM, Le Pecq JB, Larsen AK (1989) Inhibitory effects of the tyrosine kinase inhibitor genistein on mammalian DNA topoisomerase ii. Cancer Res 49(18):5111–5117

Maskarinec G, Williams AE, Carlin L (2003) Mammographic densities in a one-year isoflavone intervention. Eur J Cancer Prev 12(2):165–169. doi:10.1097/01.cej.0000062792.86004.69

Maskarinec G, Franke AA, Williams AE, Hebshi S, Oshiro C, Murphy S, Stanczyk FZ (2004) Effects of a 2-year randomized soy intervention on sex hormone levels in premenopausal women. Cancer Epidemiol Biomarkers Prev 13(11 Pt 1):1736–1744. doi:13/11/1736 [pii]

Matthews J, Gustafsson JA (2003) Estrogen signaling: a subtle balance between er alpha and er beta. Mol Interv 3(5):281–292. doi:10.1124/mi.3.5.281 3/5/281 [pii]

Mavaddat N, Antoniou AC, Easton DF, Garcia-Closas M (2010) Genetic susceptibility to breast cancer. Mol Oncol 4(3):174–191. doi:S1574-7891(10)00033-5 [pii] 10.1016/j.molonc.2010.04.011

Miksicek RJ (1995) Estrogenic flavonoids: structural requirements for biological activity. Proc Soc Exp Biol Med 208(1):44–50
Monti E, Sinha BK (1994) Antiproliferative effect of genistein and adriamycin against estrogen-dependent and -independent human breast carcinoma cell lines. Anticancer Res 14:1221–1226, 3A
Moriarty K, Kim KH, Bender JR (2006) Minireview: estrogen receptor-mediated rapid signaling. Endocrinology 147(12):5557–5563. doi:en.2006-0729 [pii] 10.1210/en.2006-0729
Mosselman S, Polman J, Dijkema R (1996) Er beta: identification and characterization of a novel human estrogen receptor. FEBS Lett 392(1):49–53. doi:0014-5793(96)00782-X [pii]
Murphy PA, Hendrich S (2002) Phytoestrogens in foods. Adv Food Nutr Res 44:195–246
Murphy PA, Song T, Buseman G, Barua K (1997) Isoflavones in soy-based infant formulas. J Agric Food Chem 45(12):4635–4638. doi:10.1021/jf970590t
Murphy LC, Niu Y, Snell L, Watson P (2004a) Phospho-serine-118 estrogen receptor-alpha expression is associated with better disease outcome in women treated with tamoxifen. Clin Cancer Res 10(17):5902–5906. doi:10.1158/1078-0432.CCR-04-0191 10/17/5902 [pii]
Murphy L, Cherlet T, Adeyinka A, Niu Y, Snell L, Watson P (2004b) Phospho-serine-118 estrogen receptor-alpha detection in human breast tumors in vivo. Clin Cancer Res 10(4):1354–1359
Murphy LC, Skliris GP, Rowan BG, Al-Dhaheri M, Williams C, Penner C, Troup S, Begic S, Parisien M, Watson PH (2009) The relevance of phosphorylated forms of estrogen receptor in human breast cancer in vivo. J Steroid Biochem Mol Biol 114(1–2):90–95. doi:S0960-0760(09) 00045-4 [pii] 10.1016/j.jsbmb.2009.01.017
Murrill WB, Brown NM, Zhang JX, Manzolillo PA, Barnes S, Lamartiniere CA (1996) Prepubertal genistein exposure suppresses mammary cancer and enhances gland differentiation in rats. Carcinogenesis 17(7):1451–1457
Muthyala RS, Ju YH, Sheng S, Williams LD, Doerge DR, Katzenellenbogen BS, Helferich WG, Katzenellenbogen JA (2004) Equol, a natural estrogenic metabolite from soy isoflavones: convenient preparation and resolution of r- and s-equols and their differing binding and biological activity through estrogen receptors alpha and beta. Bioorg Med Chem 12(6):1559–1567. doi:10.1016/j.bmc.2003.11.035 S0968089604000239 [pii]
Nass SJ, Dickson RB (1997) Defining a role for c-myc in breast tumorigenesis. Breast Cancer Res Treat 44(1):1–22
Nathanson KL, Wooster R, Weber BL (2001) Breast cancer genetics: what we know and what we need. Nat Med 7(5):552–556. doi:10.1038/87876 87876 [pii]
O'Donovan PJ, Livingston DM (2010) Brca1 And brca2: breast/ovarian cancer susceptibility gene products and participants in DNA double-strand break repair. Carcinogenesis 31(6):961–967. doi:bgq069 [pii] 10.1093/carcin/bgq069
Pagliacci MC, Smacchia M, Migliorati G, Grignani F, Riccardi C, Nicoletti I (1994) Growth-inhibitory effects of the natural phyto-oestrogen genistein in mcf-7 human breast cancer cells. Eur J Cancer 30A(11):1675–1682
Pei RJ, Sato M, Yuri T, Danbara N, Nikaido Y, Tsubura A (2003) Effect of prenatal and prepubertal genistein exposure on n-methyl-n-nitrosourea-induced mammary tumorigenesis in female Sprague–Dawley rats. In Vivo 17(4):349–357
Peterson G, Barnes S (1991) Genistein inhibition of the growth of human breast cancer cells: independence from estrogen receptors and the multi-drug resistance gene. Biochem Biophys Res Commun 179(1):661–667. doi:0006-291X(91)91423-A [pii]
Peto J, Collins N, Barfoot R, Seal S, Warren W, Rahman N, Easton DF, Evans C, Deacon J, Stratton MR (1999) Prevalence of brca1 and brca2 gene mutations in patients with early-onset breast cancer. J Natl Cancer Inst 91(11):943–949
Petre CE, Wetherill YB, Danielsen M, Knudsen KE (2002) Cyclin d1: mechanism and consequence of androgen receptor co-repressor activity. J Biol Chem 277(3):2207–2215. doi:10.1074/jbc.M106399200 M106399200 [pii]
Pietras RJ, Szego CM (1977) Specific binding sites for oestrogen at the outer surfaces of isolated endometrial cells. Nature 265(5589):69–72
Prall OW, Rogan EM, Sutherland RL (1998) Estrogen regulation of cell cycle progression in breast cancer cells. J Steroid Biochem Mol Biol 65(1–6):169–174

Rahal OM, Simmen RC (2010) Pten and p53 cross-regulation induced by soy isoflavone genistein promotes mammary epithelial cell cycle arrest and lobuloalveolar differentiation. Carcinogenesis 31(8):1491–1500. doi:bgq123 [pii] 10.1093/carcin/bgq123

Razandi M, Pedram A, Park ST, Levin ER (2003) Proximal events in signaling by plasma membrane estrogen receptors. J Biol Chem 278(4):2701–2712. doi:10.1074/jbc.M205692200 M205692200 [pii]

Reinli K, Block G (1996) Phytoestrogen content of foods–a compendium of literature values. Nutr Cancer 26(2):123–148

Revelli A, Massobrio M, Tesarik J (1998) Nongenomic actions of steroid hormones in reproductive tissues. Endocr Rev 19(1):3–17

Ross RK, Paganini-Hill A, Wan PC, Pike MC (2000) Effect of hormone replacement therapy on breast cancer risk: estrogen versus estrogen plus progestin. J Natl Cancer Inst 92(4):328–332

Russo J, Russo IH (2006) The role of estrogen in the initiation of breast cancer. J Steroid Biochem Mol Biol 102(1–5):89–96. doi:S0960-0760(06)00245-7 [pii] 10.1016/j.jsbmb.2006.09.004

Russo J, Russo IH (2008) Breast development, hormones and cancer. Adv Exp Med Biol 630:52–56

Russo J, Fernandez SV, Russo PA, Fernbaugh R, Sheriff FS, Lareef HM, Garber J, Russo IH (2006) 17-Beta-estradiol induces transformation and tumorigenesis in human breast epithelial cells. FASEB J 20(10):1622–1634. doi:20/10/1622 [pii] 10.1096/fj.05-5399com

Sabbah M, Courilleau D, Mester J, Redeuilh G (1999) Estrogen induction of the cyclin d1 promoter: involvement of a camp response-like element. Proc Natl Acad Sci USA 96(20):11217–11222

Schramek D, Leibbrandt A, Sigl V, Kenner L, Pospisilik JA, Lee HJ, Hanada R, Joshi PA, Aliprantis A, Glimcher L, Pasparakis M, Khokha R, Ormandy CJ, Widschwendter M, Schett G, Penninger JM (2010) Osteoclast differentiation factor rankl controls development of progestin-driven mammary cancer. Nature. doi:nature09387 [pii] 10.1038/nature09387

Serraino M, Thompson LU (1991) The effect of flaxseed supplementation on early risk markers for mammary carcinogenesis. Cancer Lett 60(2):135–142. doi:0304-3835(91)90220-C [pii]

Setchell KD (1998) Phytoestrogens: the biochemistry, physiology, and implications for human health of soy isoflavones. Am J Clin Nutr 68(6 Suppl):1333S–1346S

Sherwin BB (2009) Estrogen therapy: is time of initiation critical for neuroprotection? Nat Rev Endocrinol 5(11):620–627. doi:nrendo.2009.193 [pii] 10.1038/nrendo.2009.193

Sicinski P, Donaher JL, Parker SB, Li T, Fazeli A, Gardner H, Haslam SZ, Bronson RT, Elledge SJ, Weinberg RA (1995) Cyclin d1 provides a link between development and oncogenesis in the retina and breast. Cell 82(4):621–630. doi:0092-8674(95)90034-9 [pii]

Spillman MA, Bowcock AM (1996) Brca1 and brca2 mrna levels are coordinately elevated in human breast cancer cells in response to estrogen. Oncogene 13(8):1639–1645

Stambolic V, Suzuki A, de la Pompa JL, Brothers GM, Mirtsos C, Sasaki T, Ruland J, Penninger JM, Siderovski DP, Mak TW (1998) Negative regulation of pkb/akt-dependent cell survival by the tumor suppressor pten. Cell 95(1):29–39. doi:S0092-8674(00)81780-8 [pii]

Sugimoto Y, Tsukahara S, Imai Y, Ueda K, Tsuruo T (2003) Reversal of breast cancer resistance protein-mediated drug resistance by estrogen antagonists and agonists. Mol Cancer Ther 2(1):105–112

Szego CM, Davis JS (1967) Adenosine 3′,5′-monophosphate in rat uterus: acute elevation by estrogen. Proc Natl Acad Sci USA 58(4):1711–1718

Tempfer CB, Froese G, Heinze G, Bentz EK, Hefler LA, Huber JC (2009) Side effects of phytoestrogens: A meta-analysis of randomized trials. Am J Med 122(10):939–946. doi:S0002-9343(09)00542-7 [pii] 10.1016/j.amjmed.2009.04.018, e939

Thompson LU, Robb P, Serraino M, Cheung F (1991) Mammalian lignan production from various foods. Nutr Cancer 16(1):43–52

Thompson LU, Boucher BA, Liu Z, Cotterchio M, Kreiger N (2006) Phytoestrogen content of foods consumed in canada, including isoflavones, lignans, and coumestan. Nutr Cancer 54(2):184–201. doi:10.1207/s15327914nc5402_5

Tominaga Y, Wang A, Wang RH, Wang X, Cao L, Deng CX (2007) Genistein inhibits brca1 mutant tumor growth through activation of DNA damage checkpoints, cell cycle arrest, and mitotic catastrophe. Cell Death Differ 14(3):472–479. doi:4402037 [pii] 10.1038/sj.cdd.4402037

Trock BJ, Hilakivi-Clarke L, Clarke R (2006) Meta-analysis of soy intake and breast cancer risk. J Natl Cancer Inst 98(7):459–471. doi:98/7/459 [pii] 10.1093/jnci/djj102

Wakeling AE, Dukes M, Bowler J (1991) A potent specific pure antiestrogen with clinical potential. Cancer Res 51(15):3867–3873

Walter ED (1941) Genistin (an isoflavone glucoside) and its aglucone, genistein, from soybeans. J Am Chem Soc 63(12):3273–3276. doi:10.1021/ja01857a013

Wang C, Kurzer MS (1997) Phytoestrogen concentration determines effects on DNA synthesis in human breast cancer cells. Nutr Cancer 28(3):236–247

Wang H, Murphy PA (1994) Isoflavone content in commercial soybean foods. J Agric Food Chem 42(8):1666–1673. doi:10.1021/jf00044a016

Warri A, Saarinen NM, Makela S, Hilakivi-Clarke L (2008) The role of early life genistein exposures in modifying breast cancer risk. Br J Cancer 98(9):1485–1493. doi:6604321 [pii] 10.1038/sj.bjc.6604321

Washburn T, Hocutt A, Brautigan DL, Korach KS (1991) Uterine estrogen receptor in vivo: phosphorylation of nuclear specific forms on serine residues. Mol Endocrinol 5(2):235–242

Wu TY, Hsieh HF, West BT (2008) Demographics and perceptions of barriers toward breast cancer screening among asian-american women. Women Health 48(3):261–281

Zava DT, Duwe G (1997) Estrogenic and antiproliferative properties of genistein and other flavonoids in human breast cancer cells *in vitro*. Nutr Cancer 27(1):31–40

Chapter 18
Natural Triterpenoids from Olive Oil: Potential Activities Against Cancer

Rosalia Rodriguez-Rodriguez and Ulf Simonsen

Abstract Triterpenoids are compounds extensively distributed in numerous plants used in traditional medicine. Olive oil and specially pomace olive oil are important sources of pentacyclic triterpenoids such as oleanolic acid and maslinic acid. Because of their ability to interfere at different signalling pathways, triterpenoids from olives seem to be promising therapeutic strategies in terms of cancer and cell proliferation, cardiovascular complications, inflammation, and hepatotoxicity. Recently, an intensive research has been focused on the anti-cancer properties exhibited by olive oil triterpenoids, particularly effective against experimental colon and brain cancer. Although the exact mechanisms by which these triterpenoids induce the anti-tumor effects are not fully understood, recent investigations have provided evidence about their effect at different stages of carcinogenesis including: pro-apoptotic activity via the mitochondrial pathway (e.g.: Bax activation, caspase-3 activation), cell cycle arrest, modulation of mitochondrial ROS production, anti-angiogenesis and protective effects on inflammation related to cancer. Different approaches are in progress in order to improve bioavailability of these triterpenic compounds, thus making them more suitable for animal studies and clinical trials. Therefore, pentacyclic triterpenoids from olives and olive oil show a promising pharmacological profile that may provide future pharmaceutical development and clinical investigations against chronic diseases such as cancer.

R. Rodriguez-Rodriguez (✉)
Department of Pharmacology, School of Pharmacy, University of Seville,
C/Profesor Garcia Gonzalez 2, 41012 Seville, Spain
e-mail: rodriguezr@us.es

U. Simonsen
Department of Biomedicine - Pharmacology, Aarhus University,
Wilhelm Meyers Allé 4, DK-8000, Aarhus C, Denmark

M. Diederich and K. Noworyta (eds.), *Natural Compounds as Inducers of Cell Death: Volume 1*, DOI 10.1007/978-94-007-4575-9_18,

18.1 Diet and Chronic Diseases

Experimental and clinical studies have provided strong evidence suggesting that nutrition, dietary factors and physical activity compromise the prevalence of chronic diseases including cancer and cardiovascular pathologies, which are major causes of death worldwide. In this context, the conventional Mediterranean dietary pattern has been rediscovered as the one that best represents the need for nutrition and health promotion. Epidemiological studies have revealed that countries where populations consume the traditional Mediterranean diet have a lower incidence of major illnesses such as cancer and cardiovascular diseases than countries from Northern Europe, North America, and Australia (La Vecchia et al. 1995; Trichopoulou et al. 2000; La Vecchia 2004, 2009).

Despite conflicting results, most of the epidemiological data suggest that there is an association between dietary fat intake and risk of cancer (Kushi and Giovannucci 2002). There is also evidence suggesting that it is not only the amount but also the type of dietary fat that is important in the aetiology of some cancers (Owen et al. 2004). The traditional Mediterranean diet is characterized by a high consumption of plant-derived foods, relatively low intake of red meat, and consumption of olive oil as the main source of fat. Several studies have reported that intake of olive oil is more beneficial against cancer than other forms of lipids (Trichopoulou et al. 2000). The beneficial properties of olive oil have often been attributed to its high levels of monounsaturated fatty acids (MUFA), namely in the form of oleic acid (18:1, n–9).

18.2 Olive Oil and Cancer

Although clinical investigations have provided contradictory results, most of experimental and cohort studies have supported that consumption of diets enriched in olive oil and oleic acid are related to a decreased risk of cancer compared to dietary prototypes containing saturated fatty acids or linoleic acid as the main source of fat, which possess tumor-enhancing properties (Bosetti et al. 2009; Rodriguez-Rodriguez and Ruiz-Gutierrez 2009; López-Miranda et al. 2010). The protective effects attributed to olive oil intake and its fatty acid content have been suggested in different types of cancer, specially breast tumor in experimental animals (Costa et al. 2004; Escrich et al. 2006) and in epidemiological studies (Willett 2001; Flynn and Reinert 2010). Nevertheless, the role of oleic acid and olive oil on cancer is still under discussion due to inconsistent results derived from several studies including non-promoting, weak promoting or even promoting actions on tumor growth (Stark and Madar 2002; Escrich et al. 2007). Nowadays, investigations on the mechanisms by which dietary fat and high olive oil diets modulate cancer are in progress. Such protecting action has been proposed to involve several pathways including an influence on different stages of carcinogenesis, modulation of the immune system and hormonal balance, alterations on composition and structure of tumor cell membranes, changes in eicosanoid biosynthesis, gene expression modifications, reduced oxidative stress and DNA injuries (Colomer and Menéndez 2006; Escrich et al. 2007).

Olive oil is, however, more than a monounsaturated fat. In contrast to other vegetable oils, olive oil contains other biologically active minor components besides MUFA. Moreover, the content of oleic acid alone cannot fully explain the healthful properties of olive oil. These minor components constitute only 1–2% of the total composition of virgin olive oil and are classified in two subgroups: (a) the unsaponifiable fraction, described as the fraction extracted with solvents after saponification of the oil (including terpenoids and sterols), and (b) the soluble fraction, which includes phenolic compounds (Rodriguez-Rodriguez and Ruiz-Gutierrez 2009). The amount of these minor components on olive oil and olives vary depending on numerous factors such as growing and climatic conditions, oil extraction process and storage (Pérez-Camino and Cert 1999). Although they are in limited proportion compared to fatty acids, the presence of these minor components in olive oil is crucial not only in terms of olive oil stability and protection from auto-oxidation but also to confer important biological activities to olive oil. The beneficial effects of olive oil in cancer is considered to be mediated by a synergy of all its major and minor components generating a variety of cell responses involved in cancer prevention or treatment of cancer development at different stages (López-Miranda et al. 2010).

Particularly, several minor components from olive oil and olives have shown significant anti-cancer activities by themselves. For instance, *in vivo* and *in vitro* studies on the activity of phenolic derivatives from olive oil such as hydroxytyrosol and oleuropein have demonstrated, in addition to their antioxidant properties, antiangiogenic actions and the capacity of regulating the cell cycle inducing apoptosis (Fabiani et al. 2002; Hamdi and Castellon 2005). Besides, squalene has been considered to be responsible for the lower incidence of skin cancer exhibited in populations consuming olive oil (Newmark 1997). Among minor components from olive oil, interest on its triterpenic fraction on cancer has gained evidence in the last few years, as it will be described in the following sections.

18.3 The Triterpenic Fraction from Olive Oil

The triterpenic fraction in olive oil and olive skin is mainly constituted by pentacyclic triterpenic acids (oleanolic and maslinic acid) and diols (erythrodiol and uvaol) (Fig. 18.1), which have shown numerous biological activities (Herrera et al. 2006). The concentration range of these triterpenoids reaches values up to 400 mg kg^{-1} in the skin of the olive fruit whereas concentrations in olive oil are 25–50 mg kg^{-1} or even up to 200 mg kg^{-1} in virgin olive oil for triterpenic acids, and 6–18 mg kg^{-1} for erythrodiol and uvaol, depending on acidity and olive variety (Pérez-Camino and Cert 1999). The process applied for olive oil extraction is also determining the content of triterpenoids and other minor constituents. Thus, pomace olive oil (called "orujo" olive oil in Spain) is obtained from the residue that remains after virgin olive oil mechanical extraction. Despite of the lack of polyphenols, pomace olive oil,

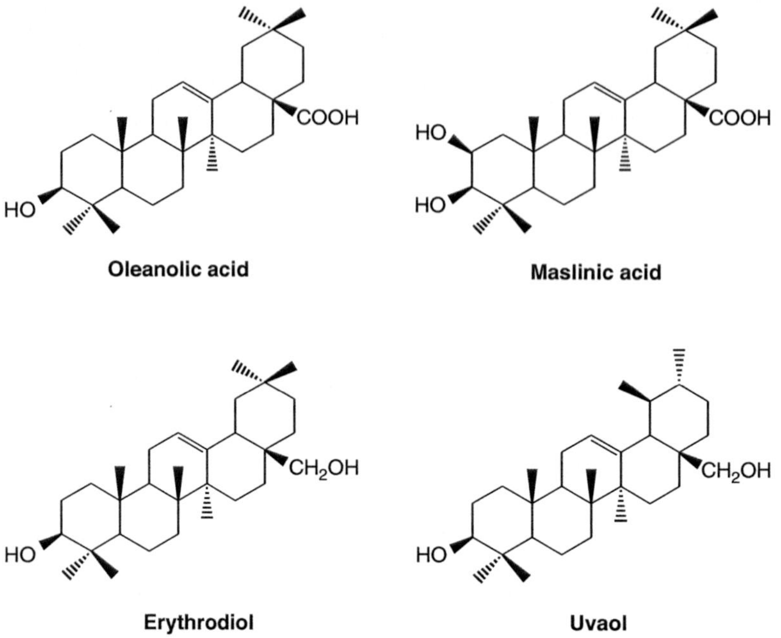

Fig. 18.1 Chemical structures of the major pentacyclic triterpenoids from olive and pomace olive oil: two acids (oleanolic and maslinic acid) and two alcohols (erythrodiol and uvaol)

extracted using a new process (patent number 200400755) contains higher concentrations of triterpenic acids and alcohols than virgin olive oil exceeding values of 200 mg kg^{-1} (Pérez-Camino and Cert 1999; Rodriguez-Rodriguez et al. 2007, 2009). Therefore, pomace olive oil and virgin olive oil are both rich sources of these bioactive triterpenic compounds.

A growing interest is focused on the pharmacological potential of these pentacyclic triterpenoids and related derivates, mainly in terms of inflammation, cancer and cardiovascular pathologies (Laszczyk 2009; Rodriguez-Rodriguez and Ruiz-Gutierrez 2010; Mullauer et al. 2010). In addition, many studies are currently investigating the mechanisms underlying their pharmacological activities. Figure 18.2 is summarizing the most important pharmacological properties exhibited by olive and pomace olive oil triterpenoids.

In vitro studies have revealed that triterpenic acids and diols from olive oil induce vasodilatation in isolated arteries from both normotensive (Rodriguez-Rodriguez et al. 2004, 2008) and hypertensive rats (Rodriguez-Rodriguez et al. 2006). In this context, endothelial NO was the main relaxing factor contributing to this response, especially in the vasodilatation induced by oleanolic acid. This NO-mediated dilatation evoked by oleanolic acid occurs by calcium-independent mechanisms via phosphoinositide-3-kinase-dependent phosphorylation of Akt-Ser^{473} followed by activation of endothelial NO synthase (eNOS)-Ser^{1177} (Rodriguez-Rodriguez et al. 2008). Furthermore, the vasoactive effects of oleanolic acid and related olive oil triterpenoids

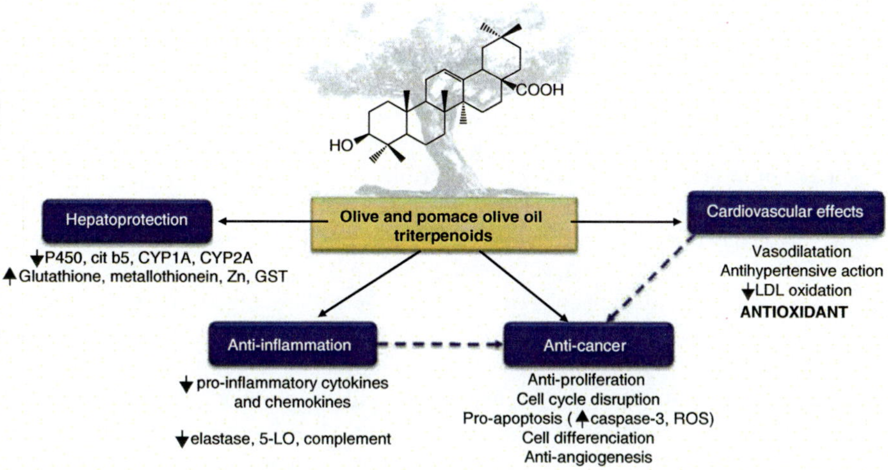

Fig. 18.2 Main functional activities induced by olive oil triterpenoids: anti-cancer, cardiovascular and antioxidant, anti-inflammatory and hepatoprotective effects. Abbreviations used: *CYP* cytochrome P450, *GST* glutathione-S-transferase, *LDL* Low-density lipoprotein, *5-LO* 5-lipoxygenase, *NO* nitric oxide, *ROS*, reactive oxygen species

such as erythrodiol are also associated to an in vitro upregulation of cyclooygenase-2 (COX-2) and prostacyclin release in human coronary smooth muscle cells, without any effect on the synthesis of the vasoconstrictor eicosanoid thromboxane A2 (Martínez-González et al. 2008). Following the line of investigations elucidating the mechanisms mediating cellular effects of olive oil triterpenoids, the main objective of our review will be directed to the potential effects of these triterpenoids on cancer and cell proliferation.

18.3.1 Anti-cancer

The process of carcinogenesis involves the sequence of the following events: tumor initiation, promotion and progression. Although chemoprevention is crucial to avoid cancer promotion, agents acting on the promotion and progression phases are also relevant. In general, natural products and food-derived chemicals can act as both chemopreventive and chemotherapeutic agents (Milner 2008; Mehta et al. 2010). In the early 1960s, two relevant types of natural compounds, vinca alkaloids and taxanes were discovered and successfully applied for treatment of cancer, with some accepted toxicity derived from their use (Johnson et al. 1963; Schiff et al. 1979). In line with subsequent investigations, chemopreventive agents can be effectively supplied within the foods or as dietary supplements with low values of toxicity (Khan et al. 2007; Mehta et al. 2010).

Particularly, plant-derived pentacyclic triterpenoids gained attention as promising anti-cancer drugs because of their cytotoxicity against cell cancer lines and their promising results at experimental and preclinical level (Ovesná et al. 2004). In addition, the wide range of pharmacological activities induced by triterpenoids including antioxidant and anti-inflammatory actions, vasoprotection and anti-angiogenesis are importantly contributing to their potential therapeutic role in chronic diseases such as cancer (Rodriguez-Rodriguez and Ruiz-Gutierrez 2010).

According to the anti-tumor effects attributed to olive oil triterpenoids, most of the research has focused on brain and colon cancer cell lines as well as other cancer types as leukaemia. The broad anticancer effects of these natural compounds involve numerous targets and molecular pathways as it will be reported below. Results derived from these investigations reveal that triterpenoids from olive oil may act at three different stages of carcinogenesis including tumor initiation (e.g. scavenging ROS), promotion (e.g. action on apoptosis) and progression (e.g. inhibition of angiogenesis), thus modifying cancer risk and tumor behaviour by several pathways. Considering the development of cancer, the most efficient therapeutic intervention would be at the promotion stage, thus eliminating premalignant cells before they become malignant or altering this transformation. Nowadays, the main therapies aim to eradicate cancer cells by inducing apoptosis or cell cycle modifications.

18.3.1.1 Apoptosis and Cell Cycle

Throughout the carcinogenesis, as a consequence of specific mutations in genes regulating cell cycle, the tumor promotion involves a deregulation of the signalling pathways that normally control cell proliferation and apoptosis. Apoptosis is defined as a well organized intrinsic mechanism of protection by which undesirable or damaged cells (pre-malignant or malignant cells) are eliminated from the system. The apoptotic process provides a normal development, turnover and replacement of healthy cells and also protects the organism against tumor development (Hengartner 2000). Therefore, induction of apoptosis by pro-apoptotic agents plays a key role in cancer therapy.

Two major pathways promote apoptosis: the extrinsic (death-receptor mediated) and the intrinsic (mitochondrial mediated) (Fig. 18.3). The death-receptor pathway is activated when a "death ligand" binds to its specific cell-surface death receptor that belongs to the tumor necrosis factor (TNF) receptor superfamily, followed by the caspase-8 activation through the adaptor molecule Fas-associated death domain (FADD) and finally activating caspase-3, which is the key executioner of programmed cell death (Hengartner 2000; Mita et al. 2008). Conversely, the mitochondrial or intrinsic pathway is mobilized in response to an external or internal stimulus (e.g. DNA damage) and is regulated by the Bcl-2 family members including proapoptotic (Bax/Bak; BH3-only proteins) and prosurvival proteins (e.g. Bcl-2) (Hengartner 2000; Cory and Adams 2002; Mita et al. 2008). An increased induction of the proapoptotic members promotes mitochondrial membrane permeabilization and release of cytochrome c that along with Apaf-1 and caspase-9, subsequently cleave the effector caspase-3 thus inducing apoptosis (Hengartner 2000; Mita et al. 2008).

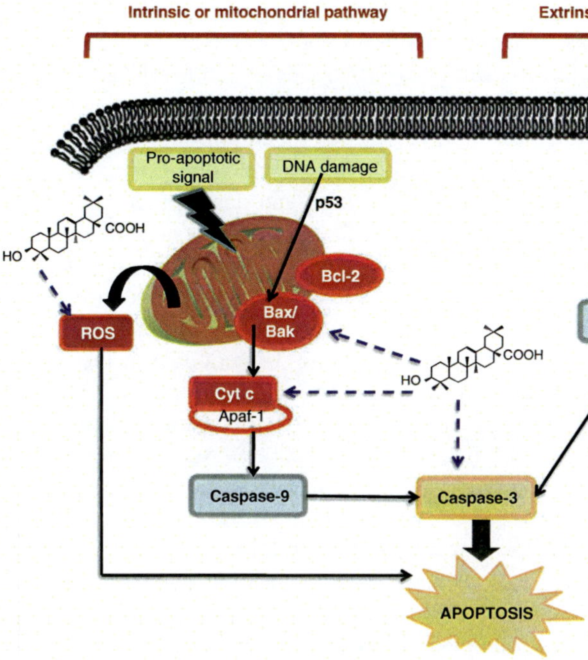

Fig. 18.3 The main actions of olive oil triterpenoids on the two apoptotic pathways in mammalian cells

Triterpenoids contained in olive and pomace olive oil have been demonstrated to trigger apoptosis with subsequent cell death by different mechanisms of action in several types of cancer. Accordingly, in the last few years an emerging interest has been directed towards the in vitro effects of maslinic acid on cell cycle and proliferation, being considered even more effective than oleanolic acid against some type of cancer cells (Juan et al. 2008a).

Triterpenic Acids and Apoptosis

Promising results have been provided from recent investigations with these olive oil triterpenic acids on colon cancer cell lines (Reyes et al. 2006; Juan et al. 2006, 2008a; Reyes-Zurita et al. 2009). In these studies, the isolated oleanolic and maslinic acids and an olive oil extract containing both triterpenoids, inhibited cell growth and proliferation in different colon cancer cell lines. The authors reported that the anti-proliferative activity evoked by these pentacyclic triterpenoids was not a consequence of their cytotoxicity but appeared to result from either inhibition of cell cycle progression or the induction of the apoptotic machinery, or both. It has recently been shown that maslinic acid inhibits selectively colon adenocarcinoma cells by cell cycle arrest in the G0 phase and direct activation of the mitochondrial apoptotic pathway (Reyes et al. 2006; Juan et al. 2008a; Reyes-Zurita et al. 2009).

They also found morphological changes in maslinic acid-treated cells that are typical in apoptosis: cell shrinkage, chromatin condensation, loss of normal nuclear structure and disruption of cell membrane integrity (Reyes et al. 2006). The intrinsic pro-apoptotic effect by maslinic acid in HT29 colon cancer cells involves the inhibition of the prosurvival protein Bcl-2 and a simultaneous induction of Bax expression with the subsequent mitochondrial permeabilization and release of cytochrome c, finally leading to caspase-9 and caspase-3 activation and death of the malignant cells (Reyes-Zurita et al. 2009). Moreover, Juan et al. (2008a) suggested that maslinic acid is able to increase mitochondrial ROS production as a previous step for the disruption of the function of the mitochondria in the pro-apoptotic action in colon cancer cells. Although oleanolic acid was also able to inhibit colon cancer cell proliferation, this effect was not mediated by caspase-3 in contrast to the results observed with maslinic acid (Juan et al. 2008a). The inability of oleanolic acid to either induce mitochondrial ROS or to activate caspase-3 explains the lack of effects of oleanolic acid on colon cancer cell lines (Juan et al. 2008a). According to several investigations on colon carcinoma, the growth-inhibition of oleanolic acid on this cancer type may be partly related to cell cycle arrest (Li et al. 2002; Juan et al. 2008a) and to its anti-inflammatory effects, as it will be discussed below.

The pro-apoptotic effects induced by oleanolic and maslinic acid from olive oil were also demonstrated in malignant astrocytic tumors, a common primary brain tumor (Martín et al. 2007). They found that oleanolic acid and maslinic acid inhibit DNA synthesis and promote the intrinsic apoptotic pathway in human astrocytoma cell lines showing similar effectiveness. The brain cell apoptosis induced by these triterpenic acids involved morphologic and cytoskeletal alterations, accumulation of intracellular ROS with loss of mitochondrial membrane integrity and final activation of caspase-3 (Martín et al. 2007). The described anti-proliferative and pro-apoptotic actions of these active triterpenes on brain cancer are in concordance with other investigations in different types of cancer including human colon adenocarcinoma (see above) (Li et al. 2002; Juan et al. 2006, 2008a; Reyes et al. 2006; Reyes-Zurita et al. 2009) and leukaemia cells (Ovesná et al. 2006; Zhang et al. 2007). According to the latter, oleanolic acid elicited apoptosis in human leukaemia HL60 cells via activation of caspase-9 and caspase-3 accompained by the cleavage of the caspase-3 substrate poly(ADP-ribose) polymerase (PARP) (Zhang et al. 2007) or by scavenging ROS (Ovesná et al. 2006).

Triterpenic Diols and Apoptosis

Regarding to the pentacyclic triterpenic diols, erythrodiol and uvaol (Fig. 18.1), they have shown promising activities in terms of arterial dilatation (Rodriguez-Rodriguez et al. 2004, 2006), anti-inflammation (De la Puerta et al. 2000) and antioxidation (Marquez-Martin et al. 2006a). It has been recently reported that erythrodiol from olives induces anti-proliferative and pro-apoptotic activity in HT-29 human colon adenocarcinoma cells. This pro-apoptotic action was associated to a reduced number of adherent cells and an increased caspase-3 activity (Juan et al. 2008b).

An anti-proliferative effect induced by both erythrodiol and uvaol was also found in human astrocytoma cells. In this brain cancer cell line, the terpenic diols effectively inhibited cell cycle and proliferation with apoptosis promotion through ROS-mediated mitochondrial depolarization and activation of c-Jun N-terminal kinases (JNK) (Martín et al. 2009), where the action of erythrodiol and uvaol on ROS production plays a crucial role. Thus, the investigation of anticancer effects of erythrodiol and uvaol are limited.

18.3.1.2 Effects on ROS

ROS are involved in different physiological processes acting as mediators in signal transductions pathways or activating proteins such as mitogen-activated protein kinases (MAPK). An overproduction of ROS mainly in the mitochondria causes oxidative stress with cell and mitochondrial damage, disruption of membrane integrity by lipid peroxidation, which is commonly associated to cardiovascular pathologies, autoimmune diseases, or inflammation (Valko et al. 2007). Therefore, regulation of ROS levels may be a crucial preventive biomarker and may be an important target for anti-cancer therapies by ameliorating oxidative stress and thus DNA damages.

Levels of ROS are tightly regulated antioxidant mechanisms that are classified in enzymatic (e.g. superoxide dismutase and catalase) and non-enzymatic (e.g. glutathione) systems in living cells. In general, pentacyclic triterpenoids are known for their antioxidant activities. Particularly, olive oil triterpenoids have been shown as potential antioxidants acting as ROS scavenger as well as increasing the activity of antioxidant enzymes (Allouche et al. 2010). In addition, the protective effect against oxidative stress provided by these triterpenoids in vivo and in vitro has been related to their beneficial action on cardiovascular pathologies (Somova et al. 2003; Rodriguez-Rodriguez et al. 2004; Herrera et al. 2006) and inflammation (Marquez-Martin et al. 2006a).

Substances able to produce cell damage especially DNA injuries and inflammatory responses, are considered as potential carcinogens, which cause oxidative stress, glutathione depletion and decrease the activity of antioxidant enzymes. The so called chemopreventive agents act against the deleterious effects derived from the carcinogens or against the substance per se. Olive oil triterpenoids have been identified as chemopreventive molecules showing protection at different levels. For instance, oleanolic acid decreased cell damage derived from oxidative stress in rat colon carcinoma induced by 1,2-dimethylhydrazine (Furtado et al. 2008). The hepatoprotective effect elicited by pentacyclic triterpenoids against toxic substances have been related to increased levels of antioxidant substances such as glutathione and metallothionein as well as simultaneous protective actions on liver mitochondria (Herrera et al. 2006). In terms of cancer, the antioxidant action of olive triterpenoids have been revealed as a crucial mechanisms for inhibition of tumor proliferation.

It has been reported that mitochondrial ROS are involved in cell death acting as mediators of apoptosis at different levels, and this participation could be even caspase- and Bax-independent (Fleury et al. 2002). Thus, an increased production of ROS at the mitochondria is activating the apoptotic machinery. As it has been reported in the preceding section, pentacyclic triterpenoids from olive oil cause ROS accumulation as a previous step for the pro-apoptotic response in cancer cell lines (Martín et al. 2009; Juan et al. 2008a).

18.3.1.3 Inflammation

It is accepted that there is a strong link between inflammation and cancer. In fact, epidemiological data have suggested that chronic inflammation predisposes individuals to several types of cancer (Mantovani et al. 2008). Therefore, the targeting of key inflammatory mediators (chemokines and cytokines, such as TNF-α and IL-1β), transcription factors involved in inflammation (e.g. NF-kβ) or inflammatory cells may attenuate incidence and promotion of cancer (Mantovani et al. 2008).

The anti-inflammatory effect is a common property of many triterpenoids. Accordingly, numerous studies have reported that olive oil pentacyclic triterpenes have beneficial effects in the inflammatory response. Different mechanisms are involved such as phospholipase A_2 inhibition (De la Puerta et al. 2000), 5-lipooxygenase inhibition (Safayhi and Sailer 1997) and attenuation of the complement system (Lee et al. 2004). In addition, a promising effect of the olive oil triterpenoids on inflammation mediated by macrophages has been reported. In these studies, maslinic acid induced a significant reduction in the generation of interleukine (IL)-6 and TNF-α in lipopolysaccharide (LPS)-stimulated murine peritoneal macrophages (Marquez-Martín et al. 2006b). The modulation of inflammatory cytokine and chemokine secretion by olive oil triterpenoids in human mononuclear cells was also found: oleanolic acid, erythrodiol and uvaol inhibited IL-1β and IL-6 production, both oleanolic acid and uvaol exhibited a biphasic response in terms of TNF-α, whereas maslinic acid only attenuated IL-6 production at high concentrations (Marquez-Martin et al. 2006a).

The expression of these inflammatory cytokines is regulated by the transcription factor NF-kβ. Carcinogen- and inflammation-induced activation of NF-kβ is an important step for cellular promotion, transformation and progression of cancer cells that often involves apoptosis inhibition (Van Waes 2007).

Although inhibition of NF-kβ has been found to be an important mechanism of action of several anti-cancer drugs, newer agents have also revealed anti-cancer activity by inducing NF-kβ activation (Van Waes 2007). The role of olive oil triterpenoids in the regulation of NF-kβ involves either activation or suppression of the action of this transcription factor. On the one hand, maslinic acid can potentiate the anti-tumor activity exhibited by TNF-α in pancreatic cancer cells through promoting apoptosis and suppressing NF-kβ activation (Li et al. 2010). In contrast to this, oleanolic acid activated NF-kβ expression in resting macrophages leading to increased levels of TNF-α and IL-1 (Choi et al. 2001). However, these triterpene-induced effects are critically affected by experimental conditions. For instance, different observations may depend on concentration-dependent effects, as described for oleanolic acid on production of TNF-α in human mononuclear cells (Marquez-Martin et al. 2006a).

18.3.1.4 Bioavailability Limitations

In general, the main limitation of natural triterpenoids is that they are lipophilic substances and consequently they have a poor solubility in aqueous solutions thus determining a limited bioavailability in vivo (Mullauer et al. 2010). In terms of olive oil triterpenoids, only pharmacokinetic and delivery studies on oleanolic acid have been reported. In this regard, it has been recently evidenced some of the pharmacokinetic parameters by which oleanolic acid is metabolized in vivo (Song et al. 2006; Jeong et al. 2007; Ji et al. 2009). Although these predictions have been considered useful for designing a dosage schedule of oleanolic acid in clinical trials in the future (Ji et al. 2009), additional approaches have been developed for enhancing the triterpenoid solubility. On the one hand, Xi et al. (2009) have suggested the potential use of a self-nanoemulsified drug delivery system to improve dissolution and oral bioavailability of oleanolic acid. Alternatively, more promising results have derived from investigations developing new synthetic oleanolic acid derivatives showing higher solubility, lower toxicity and better bioavailability and effectiveness. Among these new derivatives, it is worthy to mention the 2-cyano-3,12-dioxooleana-1,9(11)-dien-28-oic acid (CDDO) as a methyl ester or ethyl amide form. Forms of CDDO have successfully demonstrated an enhanced bioavailability and a better bioactive profile compared to oleanolic acid against inflammation and cancer (Sogno et al. 2009; Honda et al. 2010). Finally, administration of triterpenoids as part of combination treatments has been proved as another strategy to ensure higher effectiveness of the therapy in cancer (Mullauer et al. 2010). For instance, a beneficial and synergistic effect of combining triterpenoids such as oleanolic acid and betulinic acid with 5-fluorouracil was reported against esophageal squameous cell carcinoma cell lines in vitro (Yamai et al. 2009).

18.4 Conclusion

Triterpenoids are compounds extensively distributed in numerous plants used in traditional medicine. Olive oil and specially pomace olive oil are important sources of pentacyclic triterpenoids such as oleanolic acid and maslinic acid. Because of their ability to interfere at different signalling pathways, triterpenoids from olives seem to be promising therapeutic strategies in terms of cancer and cell proliferation, cardiovascular complications, inflammation, and hepatotoxicity. Particularly, these triterpenes have gained attention as potential anti-cancer drugs in relation to their efficiency against different types of cancer such as colon, brain or prostatic tumor at experimental or even preclinical level. Although the exact mechanisms by which olive oil triterpenoids induce the anti-tumor effects are not fully understood, recent investigations have evidenced their actions at different stages of the carcinogenesis process including: pro-apoptotic activity via the mitochondrial pathway (e.g.: Bax activation, cytochrome c release and finally caspase-3 activation), cell cycle arrest, modulation of mitochondrial ROS production, anti-angiogenesis and protective effects on inflammation related to cancer. The poor water solubility of these pentacyclic triterpenoids is probably the main limitation for finding a formulation suitable for their application in humans. Nevertheless, finding novel approaches for the administration of these triterpenes in humans and the discovery of new derivatives have been proved as successful strategies to ensure higher effectiveness of these olive triterpenoids in the therapy of cancer even in clinical trials. In addition, investigations in animal models and humans are required to further confirm the potential anti-cancer effects of olive oil and its triterpenic fraction. We can conclude that olives and olive oil are a rich natural pool of promising anti-cancer pentacyclic triterpenoids that, together with their pharmacological profile, may provide future pharmaceutical development and clinical investigations against chronic diseases such as cancer.

References

Allouche Y, Beltrán G, Gaforio JJ, Uceda M, Mesa MD (2010) Antioxidant and antiatherogenic activities of pentacyclic triterpenic diols and acids. Food Chem Toxicol 48:2885–2890

Bosetti C, Pelucchi C, La Vecchia C (2009) Diet and cancer in Mediterranean countries: carbohydrates and fats. Public Health Nutr 12:1595–1600

Choi CY, You HJ, Jeong HG (2001) Nitric oxide and tumor necrosis factor-alpha production by oleanolic acid via nuclear factor-kappaB activation in macrophages. Biochem Biophys Res Commun 288:49–55

Colomer R, Menéndez JA (2006) Mediterranean diet, olive oil and cancer. Clin Transl Oncol 8:15–21

Cory S, Adams JM (2002) The Bcl2 family: regulators of the cellular life-or-death switch. Nat Rev Cancer 2:647–656

Costa I, Moral R, Solanas M, Escrich E (2004) High-fat corn oil diet promotes the development of high histologic grade rat DMBA-induced mammary adenocarcinomas, while high olive oil diet does not. Breast Cancer Res Treat 86:225–235

De la Puerta R, Martinez-Dominguez E, Ruiz-Gutierrez V (2000) Effect of minor components of virgin olive oil on topical anti-inflammatory assays. Z Naturforsch C 55:814–819

Escrich E, Solanas M, Moral R, Costa I, Grau L (2006) Are the olive oil and other dietary lipids related to cancer? Experimental evidence. Clin Transl Oncol 8:868–883

Escrich E, Moral R, Grau L, Costa I, Solanas M (2007) Molecular mechanisms of the effects of olive oil and other dietary lipids on cancer. Mol Nutr Food Res 51:1279–1292

Fabiani R, De Bartolomeo A, Rosignoli P, Servili M, Montedoro GF, Morozzi G (2002) Cancer chemoprevention by hydroxytyrosol isolated from virgin olive oil through G1 cell cycle arrest and apoptosis. Eur J Cancer Prev 11:351–358

Fleury C, Mignotte B, Vayssière JL (2002) Mitochondrial reactive oxygen species in cell death signaling. Biochimie 84:131–141

Flynn MM, Reinert SE (2010) Comparing an olive oil-enriched diet to a standard lower-fat diet for weight loss in breast cancer survivors: a pilot study. J Womens Health (Larchmt) 19:1155–1161

Furtado RA, Rodrigues EP, Araújo FR, Oliveira WL, Furtado MA, Castro MB, Cunha WR, Tavares DC (2008) Ursolic acid and oleanolic acid suppress preneoplastic lesions induced by 1,2-dimethylhydrazine in rat colon. Toxicol Pathol 36:576–580

Hamdi HK, Castellon R (2005) Oleuropein, a non-toxic olive iridoid, is an anti-tumor agent and cytoskeleton disruptor. Biochem Biophys Res Commun 334:769–778

Hengartner MO (2000) The biochemistry of apoptosis. Nature 407:770–776

Herrera MD, Rodríguez-Rodríguez R, Ruiz-Gutiérrez V (2006) Functional properties of pentacyclic triterpenes contained in "orujo" olive oil. Curr Nutr Food Sci 2:45–50

Honda T, Padegimas EM, David E, Sundararajan C, Liby KT, Williams C, Sporn MB, Visnick M (2010) 2-Cyano-3,10-dioxooleana-1,9(11)-dien-28-oic acid anhydride A novel and highly potent anti-inflammatory and cytoprotective agent. Bioorg Med Chem Lett 20:2275–2278

Jeong DW, Kim YH, Kim HH, Ji HY, Yoo SD, Choi WR, Lee SM, Han CK, Lee HS (2007) Dose-linear pharmacokinetics of oleanolic acid after intravenous and oral administration in rats. Biopharm Drug Dispos 28:51–57

Ji HY, Shin BS, Jeong DW, Park EJ, Park ES, Yoo SD, Lee HS (2009) Interspecies scaling of oleanolic acid in mice, rats, rabbits and dogs and prediction of human pharmacokinetics. Arch Pharm Res 32:251–257

Johnson IS, Armstrong JG, Gorman M, Burnett JP Jr (1963) The Vinca alkaloids: a new class of oncolytic agents. Cancer Res 23:1390–1427

Juan ME, Wenzel U, Ruiz-Gutierrez V, Daniel H, Planas JM (2006) Olive fruit extracts inhibit proliferation and induce apoptosis in HT-29 human colon cancer cells. J Nutr 136:2553–2557

Juan ME, Planas JM, Ruiz-Gutierrez V, Daniel H, Wenzel U (2008a) Antiproliferative and apoptosis-inducing effects of maslinic and oleanolic acids, two pentacyclic triterpenes from olives, on HT-29 colon cancer cells. Br J Nutr 26:1–8

Juan ME, Wenzel U, Daniel H, Planas JM (2008b) Erythrodiol, a natural triterpenoid from olives, has antiproliferative and apoptotic activity in HT-29 human adenocarcinoma cells. Mol Nutr Food Res 52:595–599

Khan N, Afaq F, Mukhtar H (2007) Apoptosis by dietary factors: the suicide solution for delaying cancer growth. Carcinogenesis 28:233–239

Kushi L, Giovannucci E (2002) Dietary fat and cancer. Am J Med 113:63S–70S

La Vecchia C (2004) Mediterranean diet and cancer. Public Health Nutr 7:965–968

La Vecchia C (2009) Association between Mediterranean dietary patterns and cancer risk. Nutr Rev 67(S1):S126–S129

La Vecchia C, Negri E, Franceschi S, Decarli A, Giacosa A, Lipworth L (1995) Olive oil, other dietary fats, and the risk of breast cancer (Italy). Cancer Causes Control 6:545–550

Laszczyk MN (2009) Pentacyclic triterpenes of the lupane, oleanane and ursane group as tools in cancer therapy. Planta Med 75:1549–1560

Lee SM, Park JG, Lee YH, Lee CG, Min BS, Kim JH et al (2004) Anti-complementary activity of triterpenoides from fruits of Zizyphus jujuba. Biol Pharm Bull 27:1883–1886

Li J, Guo WJ, Yang QY (2002) Effects of ursolic acid and oleanolic acid on human colon carcinoma cell line HCT15. World J Gastroenterol 8:493–495

Li C, Yang Z, Zhai C, Qiu W, Li D, Yi Z, Wang L, Tang J, Qian M, Luo J, Liu M (2010) Maslinic acid potentiates the anti-tumor activity of tumor necrosis factor alpha by inhibiting NF-kappaB signaling pathway. Mol Cancer 9:73

López-Miranda J, Pérez-Jiménez F, Ros E, De Caterina R, Badimón L, Covas MI, Escrich E, Ordovás JM et al (2010) Olive oil and health: summary of the II international conference on olive oil and health consensus report, Jaén and Córdoba (Spain) 2008. Nutr Metab Cardiovasc Dis 20:284–294

Mantovani A, Allavena P, Sica A, Balkwill F (2008) Cancer-related inflammation. Nature 454:436–444

Marquez-Martin A, De La Puerta R, Fernandez-Arche A, Ruiz-Gutierrez V, Yaqoob P (2006) Modulation of cytokine secretion by pentacyclic triterpenes from olive pomace oil in human mononuclear cells. Cytokine 36:211–217

Marquez-Martín A, De la Puerta R, Fernandez-Arche A, Ruiz-Gutierrez V (2006) Supressive effect of maslinic acid from pomace olive oil on oxidative stress and cytokine production in stimulated murine macrophages. Free Radic Res 40:295–302

Martín R, Carvalho J, Ibeas E, Hernández M, Ruiz-Gutierrez V, Nieto ML (2007) Acidic triterpenes compromise growth and survival of astrocytoma cell lines by regulating reactive oxygen species accumulation. Cancer Res 67:3741–3751

Martín R, Ibeas E, Carvalho-Tavares J, Hernández M, Ruiz-Gutierrez V, Nieto ML (2009) Natural triterpenic diols promote apoptosis in astrocytoma cells through ROS-mediated mitochondrial depolarization and JNK activation. PLoS One 4:e5975

Martínez-González J, Rodríguez-Rodríguez R, González-Díez M, Rodríguez C, Herrera MD, Ruiz-Gutierrez V, Badimon L (2008) Oleanolic acid induces prostacyclin release in human vascular smooth muscle cells through a cyclooxygenase-2-dependent mechanism. J Nutr 138:443–448

Mehta RG, Murillo G, Naithani R, Peng X (2010) Cancer chemoprevention by natural products: how far have we come? Pharm Res 27:950–961

Milner JA (2008) Nutrition and cancer: essential elements for a roadmap. Cancer Lett 269:189–198

Mita AC, Mita MM, Nawrocki ST, Giles FJ (2008) Survivin: key regulator of mitosis and apoptosis and novel target for cancer therapeutics. Clin Cancer Res 14:5000–5005

Mullauer FB, Kessler JH, Medema JP (2010) Betulinic acid, a natural compound with potent anticancer effects. Anticancer Drugs 21:215–227

Newmark HL (1997) Squalene, olive oil, and cancer risk: a review and hypothesis. Cancer Epidemiol Biomarkers Prev 6:1101–1103

Ovesná Z, Vachálková A, Horváthová K, Tóthová D (2004) Pentacyclic triterpenoic acids: new chemoprotective compounds. Neoplasma 51:327–333

Ovesná Z, Kozics K, Slamenová D (2006) Protective effects of ursolic acid and oleanolic acid in leukemic cells. Mutat Res 600:131–137

Owen RW, Haubner R, Würtele G, Hull E, Spiegelhalder B, Bartsch H (2004) Olives and olive oil in cancer prevention. Eur J Cancer Prev 13:319–326

Pérez-Camino MC, Cert A (1999) Quantitative determination of hydroxy pentacyclic triterpene acids in vegetable oils. J Agric Food Chem 47:1558–1562

Reyes FJ, Centelles JJ, Lupiáñez JA, Cascante M (2006) (2Alpha,3beta)-2,3-Dihydroxyolean-12-en-28-oic acid, a new natural triterpene from olea europea, induces caspase dependent apoptosis selectively in colon adenocarcinoma cells. FEBS Lett 580:6302–6310

Reyes-Zurita FJ, Rufino-Palomares EE, Lupiáñez JA, Cascante M (2009) Maslinic acid, a natural triterpene from Olea europaea L., induces apoptosis in HT29 human colon-cancer cells via the mitochondrial apoptotic pathway. Cancer Lett 273:44–54

Rodriguez-Rodriguez R, Ruiz-Gutierrez V (2009) Minor components from olive oil: their most promising biological activities. In: Advances in olive resources. Transworld Research Network, Kerala

Rodriguez-Rodriguez R, Ruiz-Gutierrez V (2010) Functional properties of pentacyclic triterpenes contained in pomace olive oil. In: Olives and olive oil in health and disease prevention. Oxford Academic Press/Elsevier, London

Rodriguez-Rodriguez R, Herrera MD, Perona JS, Ruiz-Gutierrez V (2004) Potential vasorelaxant effects of oleanolic acid and erythrodiol, two triterpenoids contained in 'orujo' olive oil, on rat aorta. Br J Nutr 92:635–642

Rodriguez-Rodriguez R, Perona JS, Herrera MD, Ruiz-Gutierrez V (2006) Triterpenic compounds from "orujo" olive oil elicit vasorelaxation in aorta from Spontaneously Hypertensive rats. J Agric Food Chem 54:2096–2102

Rodriguez-Rodriguez R, Herrera MD, de Sotomayor MA, Ruiz-Gutierrez V (2007) Pomace olive oil improves endothelial function in spontaneously hypertensive rats by increasing endothelial nitric oxide synthase expression. Am J Hypertens 20:728–734

Rodriguez-Rodriguez R, Stankevicius E, Herrera MD, Ostergaard L, Andersen MR, Ruiz-Gutierrez V, Simonsen U (2008) Oleanolic acid induces relaxation and calcium-independent release of endothelium-derived nitric oxide. Br J Pharmacol 155:535–546

Rodriguez-Rodriguez R, Herrera MD, de Sotomayor MA, Ruiz-Gutierrez V (2009) Effects of pomace olive oil-enriched diets on endothelial function of small mesenteric arteries from spontaneously hypertensive rats. Br J Nutr 102:1435–1444

Safayhi H, Sailer ER (1997) Anti-inflammatory actions of pentacyclic triterpenes. Planta Med 63:487–493

Schiff PB, Fant J, Horwitz SB (1979) Promotion of microtubule assembly in vitro by taxol. Nature 277:665–667

Sogno I, Vannini N, Lorusso G, Cammarota R, Noonan DM, Generoso L, Sporn MB, Albini A (2009) Anti-angiogenic activity of a novel class of chemopreventive compounds: oleanic acid terpenoids. Recent Results Cancer Res 181:209–212

Somova LI, Nadar A, Rammanan P, Shode FO (2003) Cardiovascular, antihyperlipidemic and antioxidant effects of oleanolic and ursolic acids in experimental hypertension. Phytomedicine 10:115–121

Song M, Hang TJ, Wang Y, Jiang L, Wu XL, Zhang Z, Shen J, Zhang Y (2006) Determination of oleanolic acid in human plasma and study of its pharmacokinetics in Chinese healthy male volunteers by HPLC tandem mass spectrometry. J Pharm Biomed Anal 40:190–196

Stark AH, Madar Z (2002) Olive oil as a functional food: epidemiology and nutritional approaches. Nutr Rev 60:170–176

Trichopoulou A, Lagiou P, Kuper H, Trichopoulos D (2000) Cancer and Mediterranean dietary traditions. Cancer Epidemiol Biomarkers Prev 9:869–873

Valko M, Leibfritz D, Moncol J, Cronin MT, Mazur M, Telser J (2007) Free radicals and antioxidants in normal physiological functions and human disease. Int J Biochem Cell Biol 39:44–84

Van Waes C (2007) Nuclear factor-kappaB in development, prevention, and therapy of cancer. Clin Cancer Res 13:1076–1082

Willett WC (2001) Diet and breast cancer. J Intern Med 249:395–411

Xi J, Chang Q, Chan CK, Meng ZY, Wang GN, Sun JB, Wang YT, Tong HH, Zheng Y (2009) Formulation development and bioavailability evaluation of a self-nanoemulsified drug delivery system of oleanolic acid. AAPS PharmSciTech 10:172–182

Yamai H, Sawada N, Yoshida T, Seike J, Takizawa H, Kenzaki K, Miyoshi T, Kondo K, Bando Y, Ohnishi Y, Tangoku A (2009) Triterpenes augment the inhibitory effects of anticancer drugs on growth of human esophageal carcinoma cells in vitro and suppress experimental metastasis in vivo. Int J Cancer 125:952–960

Zhang P, Li H, Chen D, Ni J, Kang Y, Wang S (2007) Oleanolic acid induces apoptosis in human leukemia cells through caspase activation and poly(ADP-ribose) polymerase cleavage. Acta Biochim Biophys Sin (Shanghai) 39:803–809

Chapter 19
Dietary Sources of Natural Inducers of Cell Death: Considerations for Cancer Therapy and Prevention

Yvonne Chukwumah

Abstract Programmed cell death (PCD), sometimes referred to as apoptosis, is a natural biological process that plays a key role in tissue maintenance and cellular homeostasis. Although PCD occurs as a normal biological process in multicellular organisms, it is highly regulated by a series of genetic elements which incidentally have also been implicated in carcinogenesis in humans. Thus any anomaly in the expression of the gene will result in the disruption of the highly organized physiological events of PCD resulting in the continuous proliferation and growth of cells, a condition known as carcinogenesis. In fact, most cancer cells exhibit characteristic mutations in the *P53* gene.

While the events of PCD are normally triggered by physiological stimuli, it has been shown that they can also be induced by exogenous factors such as bioactive compounds of plant origin. Some natural plant products have been shown to have anti-tumorigenic properties through the induction of apoptosis. Fruits, vegetables and condiments such as herbs and spices are naturally rich in bioactive compounds which have been shown to exhibit some cytotoxic effect mediated through apoptosis on various tumor cells.

In this chapter, we review pertinent information on dietary sources of natural inducers of cell death and important considerations for cancer prevention and therapy. While studies on their chemopreventive and chemotherapeutic potentials are ongoing, there is a need to consider the effect of processing, gastrointestinal digestion and metabolism on the structural modification of these compounds as well as their bioavailability given their dependency on structure for functionality.

Y. Chukwumah, Ph.D. (✉)
Department of Food and Animal Sciences, Alabama A&M University,
P. O. Box 1628, Normal, AL 35762, USA

M. Diederich and K. Noworyta (eds.), *Natural Compounds as Inducers of Cell Death: Volume 1*, DOI 10.1007/978-94-007-4575-9_19,

19.1 Cancer Development and Natural Cell Death

Cancer is the second leading cause of death in the US accounting for one in every four deaths. Cancer development (carcinogenesis) was first described by Armitage and Doll (1954) as a multi-stage process in which cells transform into tumors due to genetic alterations and become progressively malignant overtime (Armitage and Doll 1954). The first step, generally referred to as the initiation stage, involves the molecular alteration of genetic elements by reactive species leading to DNA mutations. This causes a cell to deviate from activities of a normal cell cycle and proliferate to form clonal cells otherwise called a tumor. Over time, additional genetic alterations occur resulting in the development and growth of clonal cells containing the aberrant genes which causes their inability to respond to cellular signals that control growth resulting in malignancy. This stage is called the tumor promotion stage and it precedes the third and final stage, which is the progression stage. Aberrant malignant cells with the capacity to proliferate rapidly lose their cell adhesion properties which allows them to migrate to other sites in the body were they invade other tissues (metastasis) including the blood and lymphatic system.

Apoptosis is a genetically controlled process for normal development and tissue homeostasis. Characterized by a series of morphological changes such as chromatin condensation, nuclear fragmentation, cell shrinkage and blebbing of cell membrane, it can be activated intrinsically via the mitochondrial pathway or extrinsically by molecular factors. Activation of the mitochondrial pathway occurs through oxidative stress caused by accumulation of reactive oxygen species (ROS) generated by drugs, toxicants, by products of electron transport chain and other oxidizing agents. Oxidative stress results in the reduction of the mitochondrial membrane potential leading to the subsequent release of cyctochrome c, apoptotic protease-activating factor 1 (Apaf-1), endonuclease G and Apoptosis-Inducing Factor (AIF) into the cell cytosol. These compounds form a supramolecular complex with deoxy-ATP and procaspsase-9 that activates capsase-9 by autohydrolysis which initiates a cascade of activation events of caspases that degrades the cell cytoskeleton and activates DNAses.

While intrinsic elicitors of PCD involve stress stimuli such as DNA damage, extrinsic pathway involves the molecular activation of caspases 8 or 10 by cell surface death receptors of certain members of the pro-inflammatory cytokines (TNF, APO-1L, CD95L, CD178 and TNF-related apoptosis-inducing ligand (TRAIL)). Key proteins such as nuclear factor-kappa B (NF-κB), phosphatidylinositol-3-kinase (PI3K), and mitogen-activated protein kinase (MAPKs), related to cellular proliferation and survival transduction pathways are upregulated with the downregulation of the caspases, proapoptotic members of *bcl*-2 family genes (Manson 2003; Surh 2003).

Although apoptosis or lack of it thereof is central to the development of cancer, chronic inflammation induced by the activation of NF-κB which regulates tumor cell development, is a major mediator of the progression of tumor cells (Lu et al. 2006). Ninety percent of all cancer deaths are linked to metastasis of the tumor and thus prevention of chronic inflammation through bioactive dietary components can also reduce the incidence and mortality of cancer.

19.2 Natural Inducers of Cell Death and Their Dietary Sources

Current studies in the area of nutrigenomics have established a link between diet and health (McGinnis and Foege 1993). This has increased awareness among individuals on foods that contain biologically active components that promote health. Epidemiological studies have shown that diet and lifestyle are key environmental factors in the etiology, incidence and prevention of chronic diseases such as cancer (Willett 2002). It is an established fact that 35% of all cancers can be prevented by dietary changes (World Cancer Research Fund and The American Institute for Cancer Research 1997). Also, that the frequent consumption of plant based foods such as fruits, vegetables and nuts rich in bioactive compounds has substantial health benefits especially in the reduction of risk of development of chronic diseases (Block et al. 1992; Benetou et al. 2008; Steinmetz and Potter 1996). Although studies to understand the full extent of their biological activities and mechanisms of action are ongoing, some bioactive compounds have been investigated extensively and their chemopreventive/therapeutic potential evaluated (Kelloff et al. 2000; Khan et al. 2008). Bioactive dietary components have been implicated in the mitigation and chemoprevention of cancers of the gastrointestinal tract, prostate, lungs, breast and skin (Syed et al. 2008; Haseen et al. 2009; Bougnoux et al. 2010; Cranganu and Camporeale 2009; Goralczyk 2009; Bjelakovic et al. 2008). Although a vast number of naturally biologically active exist in the diet, a number of these have been shown to induce cell death as well as inhibit the activation of NF-κB by inflammatory cytokines. Among these are polyphenols, the largest group of phytochemicals (Peterson and Dwyer 1998). They are a diverse group of compounds synthesized by plants of which flavonoids are the largest class (Fig. 19.1).

Polyphenols can affect the overall process of carcinogenesis by several mechanisms. Exogenous polyphenols obtained through a plant-based diet, counteract oxidative stress via their antioxidative and free radical scavenging mechanism thus preventing the onset of tumorigenesis. They also have the added ability to modulate oxidative stress in cancer cells, thereby affecting signal transduction, activation of redox-sensitive transcription factors and expression of specific genes that influence cell proliferation, invasion and apoptosis (Kaefer and Milner 2008). A growing body of evidence indicates that polyphenols can directly interact with specific steps and/or proteins responsible for the regulation of apoptotic process such as the release of cytochrome c with subsequent activation of caspases-9 and caspases-3. Notable compounds among them are the flavanols found in tea and cocoa, isoflavones in legumes and the stilbene resveratrol predominant in grapes. Other compounds implicated in the modulation of carcinogenesis include carotenoids, bioactives from herbs and spices such as cucumin and gingerol (Kaefer and Milner 2008). Table 19.1 provides an inexhaustive list of natural compounds found in various foods with anti-inflammatory, anti-carcinogenic and apoptotic activities. Given their chemical diversity, they target various stages in tumor cell development. Components of green and black tea, such as the flavanol epigallocatechin-3-gallate (EGCG) and

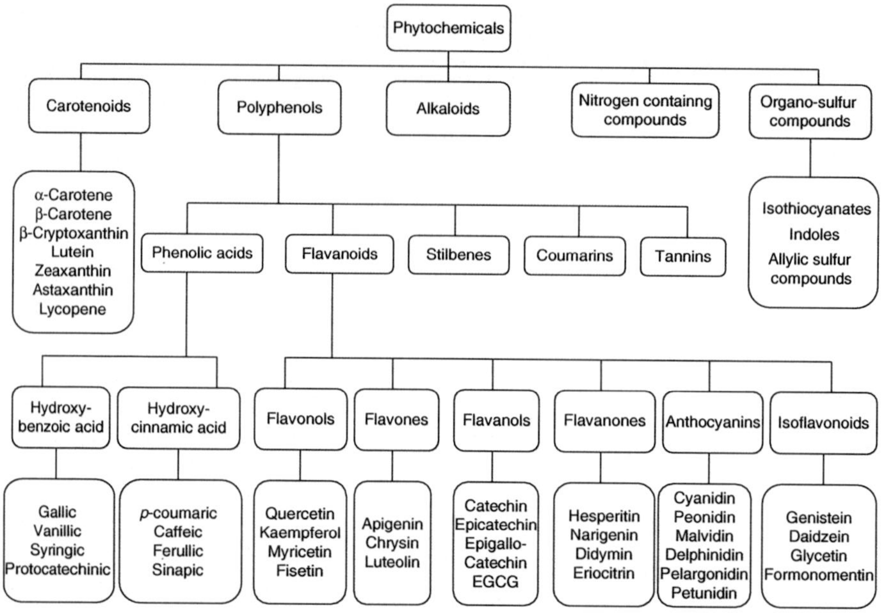

Fig. 19.1 Classification of biologically active compounds found in plant-based foods

theaflavins, induced apoptosis and blocked cell cycle progression in a variety of cancer cells (Mimoto et al. 2000; Chen et al. 2004). EGCG has been shown to inhibit carcinogenesis in a variety of tissues including lung, bladder, skin, small intestine, prostate and breast (Mantena et al. 2005; Stuart et al. 2006; Thangapazham et al. 2007).The apoptotsis induced by EGCG has been shown to be dose dependent and appears to be mediated by the reversible induction of the p57 gene depending on the cell type (Hsu et al. 2001). Another compound found in the diet that has been extensively studied is resveratrol. Naturally occurring in abundance in grapes, studies have shown that it has pro-apoptotic properties in addition to other bioactivities such as antioxidative and anti-inflammatory properties (Goswami and Das 2009). Resveratrol induces apoptosis in cancer cells via cell signaling mechanism. It promotes the phosphorylation of p38 MAP kinase as well as induces the redistribution death receptors in colon cancer cells thereby sensitizing TNF-related apoptosis inducing ligand (Goswami and Das 2009). The isoflavone, genistein, found in soy and other members of the *leguminosae* family, has been shown to inhibit carcinogenesis in animal and human models. It has also been identified as a dietary component that plays a key role in the reduced risk of development and incidence of hormone related cancers such as breast and prostrate cancer in Asian countries were soy is largely consumed (Lampe et al. 2007; Adlercreutz et al. 1993; Mills et al. 1989; Kurahashi et al. 2007; Jacobsen et al. 1998; Peterson and Barnes 1993, 1996).

Studies on the mechanism of action of soy genistein have shown that its anti-carcinogenic properties are effected through the modulation of genes that control

Table 19.1 Some biologically active compounds found in the diet and their dietary sources

Polyphenol	Biological activity	Dietary sources
Flavonols Quercetin Kaempferol	Down-regulation of NF-κB, induce cell cycle arrest, inhibit TNF-α	Onions, chokeberry, elderberry, hot yellow pepper, cilantro
Flavan-3-ols Proanthocyanidins, Catechin, Epicatechin, Epicathechingallate, Epigallocatechingallate (EGCG)	Down-regulation of NF-κB Inhibit IL-1β,TNF-α, and IL-6 production, LOX, COX, iNOS synthase, decreased expression of *Bcl*-2 proteins	Cocoa, cinnamon, apple skin, tea, cranberry, red kidney & pinto beans, sorghum, nuts (almonds, hazelnut, pistachios, pecans)
Isoflavones Genistein	Inhibit IL-2 production, induce apoptosis, inhibit NF-κB transcription	Soy and soy products, legumes (peanuts, clover)
Stilbenes Resveratrol, α-Viniferin	Inhibition of NF-κB activation, TNF-α induced proliferation down-regulation of COX-2, surviving, induce apoptosis, Inhibition of lipid peroxidation	skin of red grapes, red wine, itadori tea, peanut, mulberries
Glucosinolates Indole-3-carbinol Sulphoraphane	Suppress NF-κB activation ⇒ down-regulation of COX-2, LOX and iNOS expression; inhibits TNF- α, interleukin (IL) -1, -2, -6, -8, and −12 production	Cabbage, broccoli and cauliflower
Anthocyanins	Inhibit IL-1β,TNF-α, and IL-6 production	Blackberry, blackcurrant, blueberry, chokeberry, elderberry, red cabbage, black beans, cherries, black plum
Monounsaturated fatty acids (MUFA) *n*-3 Polyunsaturated fatty acids (PUFA)	Inhibition of nuclear factor kappa B (NF-κB) activation via PPARα-dependent pathway	Oily fish (salmon), peanut, olives, tree nuts
Curcumin	Suppress NF-κB activation ⇒ down-regulation of COX-2, LOX and iNOS expression; inhibits TNF-α, interleukin (IL) -1, -2, -6, -8, and −12 production	Tumeric (spice)
Capsaicin	Suppress NF-κB activation ⇒ down-regulation of COX-2, LOX and iNOS expression; inhibits TNF- α, interleukin (IL) -1, -2, -6, -8, and −12 production	Hot Pepper

cell cycle and apoptosis (Spinozzi et al. 1994; Kyle et al. 1997; Moiseeva et al. 2007; Szkudelska and Nogowski 2007; Huang et al. 1992). These mechanisms involve the antagonism of the estrogen- and androgen-mediated signaling pathways that are involved in the processes of carcinogenesis as well as the inhibiting the activation of NF-κB (Li and Sarkar 2002; Takimoto et al. 2003) which maintains the homeostasis of cell cycle and apoptosis. In addition to these, genistein is known to inhibit angiogenesis and metastasis in already developed cancer cells (Krinsky 1989).

Carotenoids with or without provitamin A have also been shown to inhibit nuclear damage at physiological concentrations (Pung et al. 1988; Bendich and Olson 1989). Animal model studies have shown their chemoprotective and chemopreventive effects against UV-induced skin cancer (Hansen and Maret 1988). For chemically induced cancers which occur in tissues not exposed to UV rays, high doses of retinoids seem to be more effective (in rodents) as they block the development of neoplastic lesions in the promotion stage of cancer development (Pung et al. 1988; Bendich and Olson 1989; Ziegler 1989). Carotenoids quench free radicals which otherwise will attack cell membrane lipids causing damage not only to the membrane lipids but ultimately to proteins and nucleic acids. Epidemiological studies have shown an inverse relationship between development of lung cancer in healthy individuals and high serum carotenoid levels as well as consumption of carotenoid-rich fruits and vegetables (Wald et al. 1988; Gey et al. 1987; Ziegler et al. 1986). The presence of other antioxidants present in fruits and vegetables may also play a role in the chemoprevention of cancer development.

While many animal and human (epidemiological, observational and case controlled) studies show the benefits of consuming a plant-based diet due to the presence of bioactive compounds, care must be taken as these compounds especially those with antioxidant properties can be pro-oxidant as high doses as well as act as a mutagen (Li et al. 2008; Skibola and Smith 2000). This must be emphasized as the vitamin supplement and nutraceutical market is currently saturated with purified bioactive compounds.

19.3 Structure-Activity Relationship (SAR)

All flavonoids derive their 15-carbon ring structure the primary plant metabolites, malonyl-CoA and *p*-coumaroyl-CoA Three molecules of malonyl-CoA and one molecule of *p*-coumaroyl-CoA condense to form an intermediate chalcone, which undergoes isomerisation to form flavanone (Harborne and Baxter 1999) Flavanones are 3-ring compounds from which other flavonoid classes are synthesized (Fig. 19.2).

These include their immediate products flavones, isoflavones, flavanols, and dihydroflavanols, together with metabolites of the latter two compounds (Martens and Mithöfer 2005). Further modification occurs at various stages, resulting in alterations in the extent of hydroxylation, methylation, isoprenylation, dimerization and glycosylation (producing O- or C-glycosides). The sugar most commonly involved in

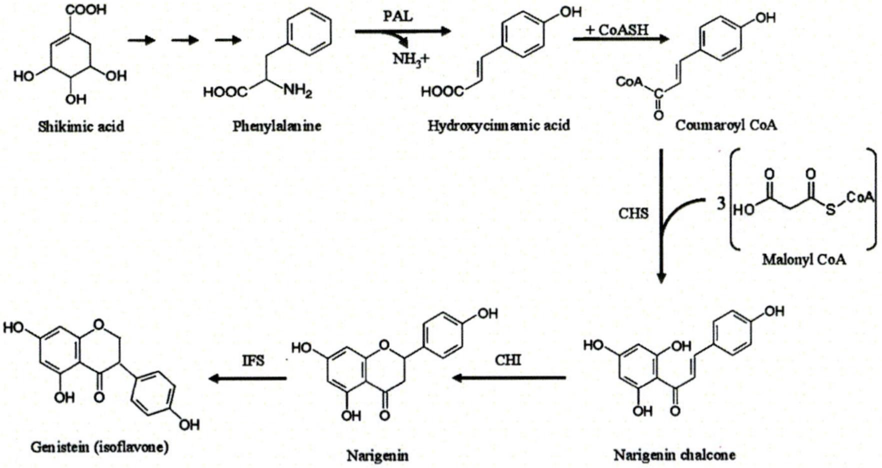

Fig. 19.2 The malonate–shikimate biosynthetic pathway of flavonoids. Phenylalanine lyase (*PAL*), chalcone synthetase (*CHS*), chalcone isomerase (*CHI*), and isoflavone synthetase (*IFS*)

Fig. 19.3 Structures showing backbone of polyphenol rings and pyrogallol

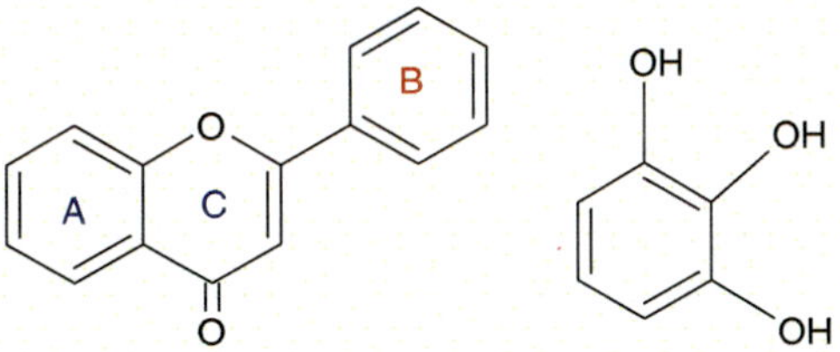

glycoside formation is glucose, although galactose, rhamnose, xylose and arabinose also occur, as well as disaccharides such as rutinose. Most flavonoids exist in nature as glycosides, thus making them more water-soluble and consequently less reactive toward free radicals. Flavonoids can act as antioxidants with mechanisms involving both free radical scavenging and metal chelation due to their structural chemistry. The structural features considered essential for effective radical scavenging activity are the C2, 3 double bond in conjugation with a 4-oxo function in the C-ring. Additionally, the positions of its phenolic hydroxyl groups at positions C-5 and C-7 on the A-ring and C-4′ on the B-ring favor a high antioxidant activity Some flavonoids have been shown to be more effective antioxidants *in-vitro* than vitamins E and C on a molar basis (Rice-Evans and Miller 1996).

In addition to their anti-oxidative activity, many polyphenols have shown cytotoxic activity resulting in apoptosis. One suggested mechanism is DNA-laddering which is common among polyphenols with a pyrogallol-like B ring (Fig. 19.3) enhanced by a gallate moiety attached in a *cis*-conformation at position 3 such as is the case with epigallocatechin (EGC), (–)-epigallocatechin gallate (EGCG) and gallic acid (Mitsuhashi et al. 2008; Saeki et al. 2000).

These compounds are naturally found in tea and reported to induce apoptosis in human ovarian cancer cells (Rao and Pagidas 2010). Other compounds in this category are procyandins found in cocoa cocoa products and grape seeds, *trans*-resveratrol in grapes and quercetin in apples and onions (Kyle et al. 2010).

19.4 Effect of Processing and In-Vivo Metabolism

Given structure activity relationship that exists with most bioactive compounds, it is important that they are chemically stable if they naturally exist in the bioactive conformation and if not, are modified through processing or metabolism to a biologically active form to be effective. Therefore the efficacy of any bioactive compound from dietary sources will depend on their structural conformation at their target sites. An example will be isoflavones in soybeans. These compounds naturally exist as their glycosides which are not biologically active but are water-soluble thus enhancing their solubility in the aqueous microenvironment of the gastrointestinal tract. They have been shown to be sensitive to heat and acidic pH, however the presence of anti-nutritive components such as trypsin inhibitors that can interfere with protein digestion in soy and other legumes requires that soy products be heated to inactivate them (Rostagno et al. 2009; Mathias et al. 2006). Similarly, oxidative enzymes present in vegetable need to be inactivated via blanching to preserve the quality of the vegetables. However, soybean isoflavones are hydrolyzed by intestinal glycosidase to the aglycones, daidzein, genistein and glycitein (Setchell et al. 2001). These can be absorbed or further metabolized. Thus after ingestion of isoflavones-rich foods, the isoflavone glycosides undergoes deglycosylations, resulting in biologically active aglycones that are easily absorbed. Recent studies have also shown that deglycosylation of genistin to genistein begins in the mouth and then continues in the small intestine (Day et al. 1998).

While the phenolic composition and content of foods have reported (Sakakibara et al. 2003) it is also necessary that we determine dietary intake levels and exposure that elicit favorable biological responses that promote health. Key information required to make such determinations lie in the bioavailability of these compounds from foods. This depends on several factors that can be summarized into two main processes, bioaccessibility and absorption. Bioaccessibility is the amount/proportion of nutrients consumed that is made available for absorption into the body. While the amount that is ultimately absorbed, determines the bioavailability of the compound. Factors that can affect bioaccessibility include the food matrix, stability of compounds to digestive process (enzyme activity, pH, presence of other reactive compounds), and solubility in the enterocyte unstirred water layer which facilitates their absorption.

In addition to bioaccessibility, the kinetics of their absorption, effects of hepatic metabolism and excretion have been shown to vary among food sources as well as individuals (Wiseman 1999). Further studies to understand the factors behind this variance are necessary and will be relevant for a chemopreventive approach through dietary bioactives.

19.5 Implications on Effectiveness as Chemopreventive and/or Therapeutic Agent

Thus for any dietary intervention for chemoprevention or cancer therapy to be effective, dietary sources of inducers cell death will need to be individually assessed and evaluated to ensure that these compounds maintain a structural conformation that supports their activity after absorption. Special attention must be paid to the effect of processing on the stability of the compound, the microenvironment, presence of other compounds that may have a synergistic or inhibitory effect and the effect of hepatic metabolism on their structural integrity and concentrations *in-vivo*. This is critical as excessive intake may be detrimental to health. Thus, it is imperative that extensive studies on the bioavailability of the bioactive compounds from each dietary source be evaluated as well as their effective intake level for chemoprevention and anti-carcinogenic properties. This will provide impetus for the development of clear guidelines on dietary sources and intake levels not only for cancer prevention but also for related diseases such as inflammatory diseases

References

Adlercreutz H, Markkanen H, Watanabe S (1993) Plasma concentrations of phyto-oestrogens in Japanese men. Lancet 342:1209–1210

Armitage P, Doll R (1954) The age distribution of cancer and a multi-stage theory of carcinogenesis. Br J Cancer 8:1–12

Bendich A, Olson JA (1989) Biological actions of carotenoids. FASEB J 3(8):1927–1932

Benetou V, Orfanos P, Lagiou P, Trichopoulos D, Boffetta P, Trichopoulou A (2008) Vegetables and fruits in relation to cancer risk: evidence from the Greek EPIC cohort study. Cancer Epidemiol Biomarkers Prev 17:387–392

Bjelakovic G, Nikolova D, Simonetti RG, Gluud C (2008) Antioxidant supplements for preventing gastrointestinal cancers. Cochrane Database Syst Rev (Online) CD004183

Block G, Patterson B, Subar A (1992) Fruit, vegetables, and cancer prevention: a review of the epidemiological evidence. Nutr Cancer 18:1–29

Bougnoux P, Hajjaji N, Maheo K, Couet C, Chevalier S (2010) Fatty acids and breast cancer: sensitization to treatments and prevention of metastatic re-growth. Prog Lipid Res 49:76–86

Chen JJ, Ye ZQ, Koo MW (2004) Growth inhibition and cell cycle arrest effects of epigallocatechin gallate in the NBT-II bladder tumour cell line. BJU Int 93:1082–1086

Cranganu A, Camporeale J (2009) Nutrition aspects of lung cancer. Nutr Clin Pract 24:688–700

Day AJ, DuPont MS, Ridley S, Rhodes M, Rhodes MJ, Morgan MR, Williamson G (1998) Deglycosylation of flavonoid and isoflavonoid glycosides by human small intestine and liver beta-glucosidase activity. FEBS Lett 436(1):71–75

Gey KF, Brubacher GB, Stahelin HB (1987) Plasma levels of antioxidant vitamins in relation to ischemic heart disease and cancer. Am J Clin Nutr 45:1368–1377

Goralczyk R (2009) Beta-carotene and lung cancer in smokers: review of hypotheses and status of research. Nutr Cancer 61:767–774

Goswami SK, Das DK (2009) Resveratrol and chemoprevention. Cancer Lett 284(1):1–6

Hansen S, Maret W (1988) Retinal is not formed in vitro by enzymatic central cleavage of betacarotene. Biochemistry 27:200–206

Harborne JB, Baxter H (1999) The handbook of natural flavonoids, vols 1 and 2. Wiley, Chichester

Haseen F, Cantwell MM, O'Sullivan JM, Murray LJ (2009) Is there a benefit from lycopene supplementation in men with prostate cancer? A systematic review. Prostate Cancer Prostatic Dis 12:325–332

Hsu S, Lewis JB, Borke JL, Singh B, Dickinson DP, Caughman GB, Athar M, Drake L, Aiken AC, Huynh CT, Das BR, Osaki T, Schuster GS (2001) Chemopreventive effects of green tea polyphenols correlate with reversible induction of p57 expression. Anticancer Res 21:3743–3848

Huang J, Nasr M, Kim Y, Matthews HR (1992) Genistein inhibits protein histidine kinase. J Biol Chem 267:15511–15515

Jacobsen BK, Knutsen SF, Fraser GE (1998) Does high soy milk intake reduce prostate cancer incidence? The Adventist Health Study (United States). Cancer Causes Control 9:553–557

Kaefer CM, Milner JA (2008) The role of herbs and spices in cancer prevention. J Nutr Biochem 19(6):347–361

Kelloff GJ, Crowell JA, Steele VE, Lubet RA, Malone WA, Boone CW, Kopelovich L, Hawk ET, Lieberman R, Lawrence JA, Ali I, Viner JL, Sigman CC (2000) Progress in cancer chemoprevention: development of diet-derived chemopreventive agents. J Nutr 130(2S Suppl):467S–471S

Khan N, Afaq F, Mukhtar H (2008) Cancer chemoprevention through dietary antioxidants: progress and promise. Antioxid Redox Signal 10:475–510

Krinsky N (1989) Carotenoids and cancer in animal models. J Nutr 119:123–126

Kurahashi N, Iwasaki M, Sasazuki S, Otani T, Inoue M, Tsugane S (2007) Soy product and isoflavone consumption in relation to prostate cancer in Japanese men. Cancer Epidemiol Biomarkers Prev 16:538–545

Kyle E, Neckers L, Takimoto C, Curt G, Bergan R (1997) Genistein-induced apoptosis of prostate cancer cells is preceded by a specific decrease in focal adhesion kinase activity. Mol Pharmacol 51:193–200

Kyle JA, Sharp L, Little J, Duthie GG, McNeill G (2010) Dietary flavonoid intake and colorectal cancer: a case–control study. Br J Nutr 103(3):429–436

Lampe JW, Nishino Y, Ray RM, Wu C, Li W, Lin MG et al (2007) Plasma isoflavones and fibrocystic breast conditions and breast cancer among women in Shanghai China. Cancer Epidemiol Biomarkers Prev 16:2579–2586

Li Y, Sarkar FH (2002) Inhibition of nuclear factor kappa B activation in PC3 cells by genistein is mediated via Akt signaling pathway. Clin Cancer Res 8:2369–2377

Li N, Liu JH, Zhang J, Yu BY (2008) Comparative evaluation of cytotoxicity and antioxidative activity of 20 flavonoids. J Agric Food Chem 56(10):3876–3883

Lu H, Ouyang W, Huang C (2006) Inflammation, a key event in cancer development. Mol Cancer Res 4:1–13

Manson M (2003) Cancer prevention – the potential for diet tomodulate molecular signaling. Trends Mol Med 9:11–18

Mantena SK, Roy AM, Katiyar SK (2005) Epigallocatechin-3-gallate inhibits photocarcinogenesis through inhibition of angiogenic factors and activation of CD8+ T cells in tumors. Photochem Photobiol 81:1174–1179

Martens S, Mithöfer A (2005) Flavones and flavone synthases. Phytochemistry 66(20): 2399–2407

Mathias K, Ismail B, Corvalan CM, Hayes KD (2006) Heat and pH effects on the conjugated forms of genistin and daidzin isoflavones. J Agric Food Chem 54(20):7495–7502

McGinnis JM, Foege WH (1993) Actual causes of death in the United States. JAMA 270:2207–2212

Mills PK, Beeson WL, Phillips RL, Fraser GE (1989) Cohort study of diet lifestyle and prostate cancer in Adventist men. Cancer 64:598–604

Mimoto J, Kiura K, Matsuo K, Yoshino T, Takata I, Ueoka H, Kataoka M, Harada M (2000) (−) -Epigallocatechin gallate can prevent cisplatin-induced lung tumorigenesis in A/J mice. Carcinogenesis 21:915–919

Mitsuhashi S, Saito A, Nakajima N, Shima H, Ubukata M (2008) Pyrogallol structure in polyphenols is involved in apoptosis-induction on HEK293T and K562 cells. Molecules 13(12):2998–3006

Moiseeva EP, Almeida GM, Jones GD, Manson MM (2007) Extended treatment with physiologic concentrations of dietary phytochemicals results in altered gene expression, reduced growth, and apoptosis of cancer cells. Mol Cancer Ther 6:3071–3079

Peterson G, Barnes S (1993) Genistein and biochanin A inhibit the growth of human prostate cancer cells but not epidermal growth factor receptor tyrosine autophosphorylation. Prostate 22:335–345

Peterson G, Barnes S (1996) Genistein inhibits both estrogen and growth factor-stimulated proliferation of human breast cancer cells. Cell Growth Differ 7:1345–1351

Peterson J, Dwyer J (1998) Flavonoids: dietary occurrence and biochemical activity. Nutr Res 18:1995–2018

Pung A, Rundhaug JE, Yoshizawa CN, Bertram JS (1988) Beta-carotene and canthaxanthin inhibit chemically- and physically-induced neoplastic transformation in 1OTI/2 cells. Carcinogenesis 9:1533–1539

Rao SD, Pagidas K (2010) Epigallocatechin-3-gallate, a natural polyphenol, inhibits cell proliferation and induces apoptosis in human ovarian cancer cells. Anticancer Res 30(7):2519–2523

Rice-Evans CA, Miller NJ (1996) Antioxidant activities of flavonoids as bioactive components of food. Biochem Soc 24(3):790–795

Rostagno MA, Villares A, Guillamón E, García-Lafuente A, Martínez JA (2009) Sample preparation for the analysis of isoflavones from soybeans and soy foods. J Chromatogr A 1216(1): 2–29

Saeki K, Hayakawa S, Isemura M, Miyase T (2000) Importance of a pyrogallol-type structure in catechin compounds for apoptosis-inducing activity. Phytochemistry 53:391–394

Sakakibara H, Honda Y, Nakagawa S, Ashida H, Kanazawa K (2003) Simultaneous determination of all polyphenols in vegetables, fruits, and teas. J Agric Food Chem 51(3):571–581

Setchell KDR, Brown NM, Desai P, Nechemias ZL, Wolfe BE, Brashear WT, Kirscher AS, Cassidy A, Heubi J (2001) Bioavailability of pure isoflavones in healthy humans and analysis of commercial soy isoflavone supplements. J Nutr 131:1362S–1375S

Skibola CF, Smith MT (2000) Potential health impacts of excessive flavonoid intake. Free Radic Biol Med 29(3–4):375–383

Spinozzi F, Pagliacci MC, Migliorati G, Moraca R, Grignani F, Riccardi C et al (1994) The natural tyrosine kinase inhibitor genistein produces cell cycle arrest and apoptosis in Jurkat T-leukemia cells. Leuk Res 18:431–439

Steinmetz KA, Potter JD (1996) Vegetables, fruit, and cancer prevention: a review. J Am Diet Assoc 96:1027–1039

Stuart EC, Scandlyn MJ, Rosengren RJ (2006) Role of epigallocatechin gallate (EGCG) in the treatment of breast and prostate cancer. Life Sci 79:2329–2336

Surh YJ (2003) Cancer chemoprevention with dietary phytochemicals. Nat Rev Cancer 3:768–780

Syed DN, Suh Y, Afaq F, Mukhtar H (2008) Dietary agents for chemoprevention of prostate cancer. Cancer Lett 265:167–176

Szkudelska K, Nogowski L (2007) Genistein – a dietary compound inducing hormonal and metabolic changes. J Steroid Biochem Mol Biol 105:37–45

Takimoto CH, Glover K, Huang X, Hayes SA, Gallot L, Quinn M et al (2003) Phase I pharmacokinetic and pharmacodynamic analysis of unconjugated soy isoflavone administered to individuals with cancer. Cancer Epidemiol Biomarkers Prev 12:1213–1221

Thangapazham RL, Singh AK, Sharma A, Warren J, Gaddipati JP, Maheshwari RK (2007) Green tea polyphenols and its constituent epigallocatechin gallate inhibits proliferation of human breast cancer cells *in vitro* and *in vivo*. Cancer Lett 245:232–241

Wald NJ, Thompson SG, Densem JW, Boreham J, Bailey A (1988) Serum beta-carotene and subsequent risk of cancer: results from the BUPA study. Br J Cancer 49:428–433

Willett WC (2002) Balancing lifestyle and genomics research for disease prevention. Science 296:695–698

Wiseman H (1999) The bioavailability of non-nutrient plant factors: dietary flavonoids and phytooestrogens. Proc Nutr Soc 58:139–146

World Cancer Research Fund, The American Institute for Cancer Research (1997) Food, nutrition and the prevention of cancer: a global perspective. World Cancer Research Fund, The American Institute for Cancer Research, Washington, DC

Ziegler RG (1989) A review of epidemiologic evidence that carotenoids reduce the risk of cancer. J Nutr 119:116–122

Ziegler RG, Mason TJ, Stemhagen A, Hoover R, Schoenberg JB, Gridley G, Virgo PW, Fraumeni JF Jr (1986) Carotenoid intake, vegetables, and the risk of lung cancer among white men in New jersey. Am J Epidemiol 123:1080–1093

Part VII
Phytochemicals in Health and Disease

Chapter 20
Tocotrienols in the Control of Pathological Fibroinflammatory Processes

Eva C. Vaquero and Xavier Molero

Abstract Chronic pancreatitis, liver cirrhosis or inflammatory bowel disease are examples of fibroinflammatory conditions, all of them characterized by a progressive course and poor therapeutic expectations. The signature of these disorders is the perpetual activation of myofibroblasts and the accumulation of redundant fibrotic tissue that progressively replaces the normal parenchyma. Removal of myofibroblast is increasingly recognized as a therapeutic target for the prevention and resolution of fibrosis. Tocotrienols are natural vitamin E compounds with potent anticancer properties. Their antineoplastic credentials are supported by the ability to selectively induce cell death or inhibit proliferation in transformed cells. Recent studies have shown that tocotrienols also strike activated fibroblasts without harming normal cells. This review focus on the current knowledge of the putative role of tocotrienols as antiinflammatory and antifibrogenic agents based on their ability to induce programmed cell death in activated fibroblasts. The review points out to the mitochondria as the main target of tocotrienols to promote apoptosis and autophagy in activated fibroblasts. Most of the available evidence has been gathered using experimental data from pancreatic stellate cells. The overall experimental evidence provides support to consider evaluating clinical trials using tocotrienols to reduce or prevent fibrosis in human fibroinflammatory diseases.

E.C. Vaquero (✉)
Gastrointestinal and Pancreatic Research Group, Hospital Clínic, CIBEREHD, Barcelona, Spain
e-mail: evaquero@comb.es; evaquero@clinic.ub.es

X. Molero
Pancreatic Research Group, Institut de Recerca, Hospital Universitari Vall d'Hebron, Barcelona, Spain

M. Diederich and K. Noworyta (eds.), *Natural Compounds as Inducers of Cell Death: Volume 1*, DOI 10.1007/978-94-007-4575-9_20,

20.1 The Multimolecular Vitamin E

The term vitamin E comprises a group of compounds with similar chemical structures and with biological activity of RRR-α-tocopherol, a naturally occurring vitamin E stereoisomer. A signature that gathers vitamin E compounds is their ability to fully revert all characteristic clinical features that result from vitamin E deficiency. Vitamin E is considered the major lipid-soluble, chain-breaking antioxidant in the body, protecting the integrity of membranes by inhibiting lipid peroxidation. In nature vitamin E is present in plant tissues and vegetable oils as tocopherol and tocotrienol derivatives. These molecules are termed tocochromanols because of their molecular structure consisting in a chroman head with two rings (one phenolic acid and one heterocyclic) and a 15-carbon side chain (Kamal-Eldin and Appelqvist 1996). Both groups differ in the degree of saturation of their side chains. Tocopherols have a saturated phytyl side chain, while tocotrienols possess an unsaturated isoprenoid side chain with three trans double bonds at positions 3′, 7′, and 11′. Both tocotrienols and tocopherols occur in nature as four isomers, designated as α-, β-, γ-, and δ-, which differ from each other by the number and position of methyl groups on the phenol ring.

Most of the vitamin E research has focused on α-tocopherol while all other non-α-tocopherol molecules have been mostly neglected for basic and clinical studies. However, accumulating evidence indicates that tocotrienols display some functionally differences from α-tocopherol and they provide distinctive health benefits, such as neuroprotective, hypocholesterolemic and antitumor effects that are not shared by α-tocopherol (Aggarwal et al. 2010a).

Non-natural vitamin E analogues include a number of synthesized compounds that often display different bioavailability and biological activity than the natural isomers (Birringer et al. 2003). These molecules may differ from the original α-tocopherol in the esther side group, the number and positions of the methyl substitutions on the aromatic ring, or in the aliphatic side chain. Most of these vitamers are redox-silent molecules that have been developed in the search for improved chemical and metabolic stability, water solubility, biopotency or a more selective toxicity towards cancer cells (Behery et al. 2010; Constantinou et al. 2008). Representative examples are α-tocopheryl succinate (α-TOS) and α-tocopheryloxyacetic acid (α-TEA), two semisynthetic derivatives of α-tocopherol with potent antineoplastic effects *in vitro* and *in vivo* (Neuzil 2003; Elson 1992).

20.2 Sources, Absorption and Tissue Distribution of Tocotrienols

Tocotrienols, as tocopherols, are essential components of the human diet. They are synthesized by plants and photosynthetic organisms only. The main sources of tocotrienols are vegetable oils and lipid-rich plants products. Palm oil is one of the most abundant natural sources of tocotrienols (Khosla et al. 2006). They are also found in smaller amounts in monocot seeds such as oat, rice, wheat and barely. However, despite the existence of tocotrienols in natural foods, common dietary sources rarely provide enough amounts of tocotrienols to let their beneficial effects be demonstrated. Therefore, natural supplements might be required to obtain clinical advantages.

Humans absorb all isoforms of vitamin E, but the bioavailability of tocotrienols appears to be much lower than that of tocotrienols. Oral absorption of tocotrienols is limited because its poor water-solubility. Moreover, while α-tocopherol is efficiently transported to tissues by the α-tocopherol transporter protein, it is not yet clear how tocotrienol is delivered to vital organs. Nevertheless, there are convincing data demonstrating that dietary tocotrienols are absorbed by the intestinal epithelium, show measurable plasma levels (Khosla et al. 2006; Yap et al. 2001), and are readily distributed throughout the body, reaching high concentrations in different tissues such as brain, adipose tissue, skin, and mammary glands (Patel et al. 2006). To circumvent the poor oral bioavailability of tocotrienols, emulsifying formulations (Yap and Yuen 2004) and esther modifications of the molecule (Behery et al. 2010) have been developed. Despite the fact that α-tocopherol is the main vitamin E isomer found in plasma and tissues, some studies show that tocotrienols exert higher radical scavenging efficiency in biomembranes than the corresponding tocopherol (Serbinova and Packer 1994; Suzuki et al. 1993). However, this is still a debatable issue as other studies have reported similar antioxidant activities for tocopherols and tocotrienols (Yoshida et al. 2003).

20.3 Tocotrienols as Putative Antineoplastic Agents

There is cumulative evidence to support the notion that tocotrienols have potent antineoplastic effects (Constantinou et al. 2008; Sen et al. 2007; Aggarwal et al. 2010b). *In vitro* studies have demonstrated proapoptotic and antiproliferative activities of tocotrienols in a variety of human cancer cells, such as pancreatic, breast, prostate, liver, colorectal, gastric, and melanoma cells. In animal models, tocotrienols have also been shown to suppress liver, lung, pancreatic, melanoma and breast tumor growth (see the article of Sen et al. ref 16, for a comprehensive analysis of the literature about the *in vitro* and *in vivo* antineoplastic effects of tocotrienols). It is of particular interest the observation that tocotrienols are selectively toxic for cancer cells while sparing normal cell growth and viability (Srivastava and Gupta 2006).

Tocotrienols are potent lipid-soluble antioxidants that incorporate into cellular membranes where they inhibit peroxidation of lipids. But besides their well known antioxidant properties, it is becoming clear that tocotrienols exert important antineoplastic effects beyond their antioxidant function in biological membranes. These redox-silent activities may be attributed to their interaction with various signal transduction pathways (Constantinou et al. 2008), as it will be further discussed below.

20.4 Tocotrienols as Modulators of Chronic Inflammatory Reactions

Inflammation and fibrosis are part of the reparative wound healing response against tissue injury. Inflammation usually precedes and co-exists with fibrosis. Inflammatory cells are recruited to the site of acute injury attracted by TGF-ß, and chemokines such as MCP-1, MIP-1 and MIP-2. The first cells recruited to the site of inflammation are neutrophils and later on macrophages, T and B lymphocytes. The recruited inflammatory cells are a rich source of radical oxygen species, growth factors and mitogenic and fibrogenic cytokines, such as TGFß, PDGF, interleukins, which further activate fibroblasts and engage the fibrogenic process. Although inflammation is a defense response necessary to repair the wounded tissue, uncontrolled inflammation is associated with chronic fibrogenic disorders, such as autoimmune diseases, hepatic cirrhosis, atherosclerosis, cancer, and almost all morbid conditions. Therefore, inflammation appears to be critical for the onset and progression of fibrosis.

Experimental data demonstrate that tocotrienols are potent anti-inflammatory molecules. In murine macrophages (RAW264.7) (Yam et al. 2009) and human monocytic cells (THP-1) (Wu et al. 2008) tocotrienols reduce the proinflammatory response triggered by lipopolysacaride stimulation, as demonstrated by a decrease in a variety of inflammatory molecules, including IL-6, nitric oxide, inducible nitric oxide synthase, TNFα, IL-4, IL-8, prostaglandin E2, cyclooxygenase-1 and –2, and nuclear factor-kB. In human keratinocytes (HaCaT cells) γ-tocotrienol suppresses UVB-induced expression of inflammatory mediators (cyclooxigenase-2, IL-1ß, IL-6, MCP-1) and MAPK activation, while tocopherol cause minimal effects (Shibata et al. 2010). The net result of such anti-inflammatory effect is the prevention of skin photodamage in HR-1 hairless mice treated with oral γ-tocotrienols. Another proof of the anti-inflammatory nature of tocotrienols comes from studies in diabetic rats, in which they reduce levels of serum inflammatory mediators (TNFα, IL-1ß, TGF-ß1), nitrosative and oxidative stress along with the improvement of glycemia and neuropathy (Kuhad and Chopra 2009). Tocotrienols also decrease endothelial expression of adhesion molecules and monocytic cell adherence (Theriault et al. 2002) and is a strong inhibitor of NF-κB, a transcription factor with a central role in inflammation (Kaileh and Sen 2010).

20.5 Tocotrienols as Possible Suppressors of Uncontrolled Fibrogenesis

Fibrosis is a scarring process characterized by extensive and anomalous deposition of extracellular matrix proteins, usually preceded by fibroblast proliferation. It can be considered as the end result of poorly resolved chronic inflammatory reactions promoted by either continuous exposure to injury (such as persistent infections, autoimmune reactions, radiation, mechanical injury, chemical insults, and more) or defective wound healing. The process results in a ceaseless deposition of extracellular matrix that replaces normal parenchymal tissue culminating in structural distortion and organ dysfunction (Wynn 2008).

Organ fibrosis is present in a number of chronic diseases such as liver cirrhosis, chronic pancreatitis, pulmonary fibrosis, interstitial nephritis, keloids, etc. Most of these diseases are progressive and at present there is no treatment that can effectively halt the fibrogenic process. Indeed, there was the conviction that when fibrosis is advanced, reversal to the normal tissue architecture and function is no longer possible. However, current knowledge indicates that fibrosis can be reversible (Ramachandran and Iredale 2009) and one promising way to achieve the resolution of fibrosis is to eliminate the extracellular matrix-producing cells (Elsharkawy et al. 2005; Oakley et al. 2005).

The main cell type responsible for generating the molecular components of the extracellular matrix, such as collagens, fibronectin and laminin, is the myofibroblast. These cells represent a heterogeneous population that are thought to derive from the activation of resident fibroblasts, from epithelial or endothelial cells transdifferentiation (in a process termed epithelial- or endothelial-to- mesenchymal transition), and from circulating fibrocytes originating at the bone marrow (Novo et al. 2009). In some organs myofibroblasts have been well characterized and identified to originate from a specific cell population, like pancreatic stellate cells (Omary et al. 2007) or hepatic stellate cells (Friedman 2008). A great deal of interest has arisen on the elucidation of the biology of these cells since it is now believed that their inactivation by forcing them to return to a quiescent phenotype, to halt proliferation, or to initiate a cell death program would slow, detain or even revert the progression of fibrosis (Elsharkawy et al. 2005). In this setting, and similarly to what occurs in cancer cells, recent data indicate that tocotrienols selectively target activated fibroblasts restraining their proliferating activity or inducing their cell death (Rickmann et al. 2007; Luna et al. 2011; Tappeiner et al. 2010).

Tenon's fibroblasts are just one example (Tappeiner et al. 2010). Failure of glaucoma surgery is mostly due to the formation of a fibrocellular scar generated from the activity of fibroblasts derived from Tenon's capsule. Inhibition of the proliferating activity of these cells by mitomycin C or 5-fluoracil is limited because their toxicity to other ocular cell types and the risk of ocular hypotony. In *in vitro* studies, tocotrienols have been shown to inhibit proliferation, migration and collagen synthesis of human Tenon's fibroblasts and, therefore, tocotrienols may have the potential to function as an anti-scarring agent in glaucoma surgery.

Chronic pancreatitis is an archetypic model of a continuously progressive fibroinflammatory disease. In this condition, pancreatic parenchyma is progressively replaced by scaring and non-functional fibrosis. As a consequence, patients suffering from chronic pancreatitis experience continuous or intermittent abdominal pain, exocrine pancreatic insufficiency and diabetes mellitus. Beyond eliminating predisposing factors, such as alcohol abuse, smoking or duct obstruction, there are no other effective treatments to halt disease progression. However, the recognition of pancreatic stellate cells (PSCs) as one of the main effectors of fibrosis has open new therapeutic approaches (Omary et al. 2007). In the normal pancreas these fibroblast population reside in a quiescent state with no known detrimental activity. Prompted by tissue injury, PSCs transdifferentiate into an activated phenotype to participate very actively in the wound healing process and help to maintain tissue homeostasis. Activated PSCs have the ability to proliferate and generate extracellular matrix components and soluble proinflammatory mediators that attract macrophages and other inflammatory cells that supervise tissue repair. Once the lesion is repaired, activated PSCs may disappear by a self-destroying death program. Otherwise, uncontrolled PSCs proliferation and activity will lead to a ceaseless and unsuccessful reparative process that will overburden the pancreas with redundant matrix load. In this scenario, tocotrienols have been shown to target activated PSCs inducing their own demise by apoptosis and autophagy (Rickmann et al. 2007). Interestingly, the toxic effect of tocotrienols is selectively directed toward activated PSCs, sparing quiescent PSCs and terminal differentiated acinar cells.

Some *in vitro* evidences indicate that tocotrienols activate cell death programs in fibroblasts isolated from human intestinal specimens (Luna et al. 2011). Interestingly, tocotrienols reduce proliferation of intestinal fibroblasts isolated form patients with ulcerative colitis or Crohn disease but not from subjects without inflammatory bowel disease. This observation supports de notion that cell differentiation towards neoplastic or pro-fibrogenic phenotypes endows the cell with survival disadvantages when exposed to tocotrienols.

Beyond the *in vitro* proofs of the antifibrogenic role of tocotrienols, there is so far one *in vivo* study addressing the effect of palm oil in reducing organ fibrosis. This study demonstrates in a rat model of alcoholic liver fibrosis that a diet supplemented with palm oil effectively reverses necrosis, inflammation and fibrosis despite continued alcohol consumption (Nanji et al. 2001).

20.6 Mechanisms of Tocotrienol-Mediated Cell Death

20.6.1 Cancer Cells

The compelling evidence that tocotrienols exert antineoplastic properties without harming normal cells has fostered the search for cellular and molecular targets for tocotrienols in cancer cells. As a result multiple pathways have been found to be modified by tocotrienols in transformed cells that either inhibit proliferation or induce cell death (Yap et al. 2008), but a single molecular interaction that could explain all other cellular events has not yet been identified with accuracy.

Different research groups have shown that some tocotrienol isoforms can induce apoptosis in a wide variety of tumor cells through activation of both the extrinsic and the intrinsic pathways (Sun et al. 2009). Tocotrienol activation of death receptors leading to caspase 8 and caspase 3 activation has been demonstrated in liver and breast cancer cells (Sakai et al. 2006; Park et al. 2010). In gastric and breast cancer cells tocotrienols induce mitochondrial depolarization, release of cytochrome c (in part mediated by upregulation of Bax and/or cleavage of Bid) and activation of caspase 9 upstream to caspase 3 (Sun et al. 2009; Sakai et al. 2006; Takahashi and Loo 2004). In a number of cancer cells including cells from colon, liver, prostate, skin, lung, and breast, tocotrienols have been shown to inhibit survival pathways commonly overexpressed in neoplastic cells: tocotrienols are able to inhibit PKC, p60Src, NF-κB, IKK, GSK-3ß, XIAP, IAP-1, IAP-2, Bcl-2, Bcl-xl, c-FLIP, TRAF-1, survivin, A1, Id proteins and PI3K/AKT (Nanji et al. 2001; Sun et al. 2009; Takahashi and Loo 2004; Agarwal et al. 2004; Ahn et al. 2007). On the side of suppressing cancer cell proliferation rather than inducing cell death, tocotrienols have been found to inhibit HMG-CoA reductase activity and mevalonate synthesis, DNA polymerases, down regulate Rb phosphorylation and repress cyclic-dependent kinases such as cdk2 in breast, colon and pancreatic cancer cells (Hussein and Mo 2009; Wali et al. 2009a; Yang et al. 2010). In addition to mitochondrial destabilization, tocotrienols have been shown to induce apoptosis through ER stress signaling in breast cancer cells (Park et al. 2010; Wali et al. 2009b).

The precise molecular target for tocotrienols that would eventually initiate cell death pathways in cancer cells has not yet been identified. Some investigators believe tocopherol derivatives, either directly or through the generation of metabolites, compete for ubiquinone binding sites at the mitochondria in neoplastic cells. By occupying ubiquinone sites, some of these tocopherol derivatives would disturb the mitochondrial electron transport chain, induce mitochondrial destabilization and accumulation of ROS, promote ATP depletion and mitochondrial membrane permeabilization (Dong et al. 2008) that would ultimately activate enzymatic cascades leading to cell death. Such molecular events appear to affect only transformed cells, not quiescent cells. These particular molecular mechanisms of initiating death in cancer cells, but not in normal cells, have not been described for tocotrienols yet.

20.6.2 Fibroblasts: Lessons from Pancreatic Stellate Cells

We have recently published that tocotrienols induce programmed cell death in activated pancreatic stellate cells (PSCs) and that mitochondria is a key organelle mediating such citotoxic effect (Rickmann et al. 2007). In this *in vitro* model, stellate cells are obtained from rat pancreas and are activated by culturing them on plastic dishes in the presence of growth factors. In active PSCs tocotrienols derived from palm oil switch on a caspase-dependent apoptotic death program and a caspase-independent autophagic death pathway (Fig. 20.1). These two cell death modalities coexist, as concurrent activation of apoptosis and autophagy can be detected. Cells exhibit robust activation of caspase 3, 8, and 9 along with the formation of voluminous acidic vacuoles and expression of lipidated LC3 that indicates a prominent autophagic process. Cell death is found to be associated with a prominent and irreversible destabilization of mitochondria consistent in an early and profound collapse of mitochondrial transmembrane potential, as well as an extensive

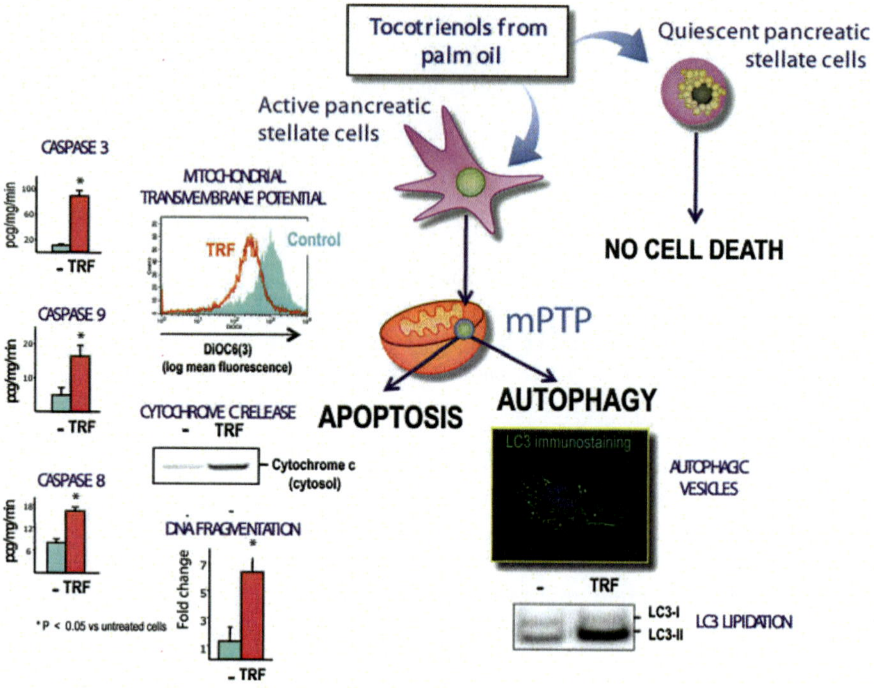

Fig. 20.1 Apoptosis and autophagy are activated in active pancreatic stellate cells. Rat pancreatic stellate cells are cultured for 24 h with TRF, which is abundant in all four tocotrienols isomers (α, β, γ, δ). In the active phenotype, tocotrienols induce a full death program of apoptosis and autophagy mediated by mPTP opening. Apoptosis is characterized by mitochondrial membrane depolarization (flow cytometry), cytochrome c release (western blot) and activation of casapase-3, -8, and -9 (fluorometry). Autophagy is detected by the existence of numerous autophagic vacuoles stained with anti-LC3 and the appearance of a prominent lipidated LC3-II band shown by western blotting. In quiescent PSCs tocotrienols do not elicit any citotoxic effect. *TRF* tocotrienol rich fraction, *mPTP* mitochondrial permeability transition pore

mitochondrial cytochrome c release. Tocotrienols initiate mitochondrial membrane permeabilization through the mitochondrial permeability transition pore (mPTP), as in the presence of the mPTP inhibitor cyclosporin A mitochondrial depolarization and cytochrome c release do no occur. Furthermore, inhibition of mPTP with cyclosporin A blocks both apoptosis and the development of autophagic vacuoles, indicating that tocotrienols interconnect apoptosis and autophagy at an upstream mitochondrial level. However, when caspases are inhibited by the pan-caspase inhibitor zVAD-fmk, cells fail to survive not due to a switch to necrosis, but because autophagy is exacerbated.

Experimental evidence from several cell lines describe tocotrienols as efficacious pro-apoptotic molecules. However, autophagy represents another advantageous cell death type whose analysis in tocotrienol studies has been neglected.

Autophagy is a cell death mechanism distinct from apoptosis, also defined as type II programmed cell death, involving autophagosomic/lysosomal degradation of cellular components (Yang and Klionsky 2010). Also, autophagy represents a homeostatic lysosomal degradative route of cell proteins and organelles. During autophagy, an isolation membrane forms and sequesters cytoplasmic constituents. The edges of the membrane fuse to form a double or multimembranous structure, known as the autophagosome or autophagic vacuole. This fuses with lysosomes where the sequestered material is degraded. Autophagy can be envisioned as an optimized energy saving process that prevents cell collapse and, ultimately, death. It ensures energy during starvation and allows for clearing out damaged and unwanted organelles. At certain undefined point autophagy can still enable cell survival, as long as the conditions that initiated the process subside. If these conditions are maintained or enhanced, autophagy flow can precipitate cell death, as it occurs with some molecules with anti-tumor potential (Turcotte and Giaccia 2010). In this case, induction of autophagy can be advantageous to circumvent mechanisms of apoptosis resistance in transformed cells (Moretti et al. 2007).

Both apoptosis, or type I programmed cell death, and autophagy are characterized for eluding the induction of an inflammatory response in the tissue. During apoptosis there is a breakdown of cytoskeletal elements with preservation of organelles, whereas in autophagy the critical initiating feature is the degradation of organelles without any cytoskeletal damage. In both death modalities cytoplasmic membrane is preserved until late stages, preventing the spill of cytosolic material to the extracellular space and thus achieving a clean cell demise. In contrast, necrosis involves early cytoplasmic membrane disruption with the leak of cellular debris into the extracellular space and the consequent induction of an inflammatory reaction. The ability of tocotrienols to preferentially engage an innocuous death programs in PSCs is of great attractive for their potential use in fibrogenic disorders. Evidence from human intestinal fibroblasts corroborate the capacity of tocotrienols to engage apoptosis and autophagy (Luna et al. 2011).

From observations in fibroblasts (Rickmann et al. 2007; Luna et al. 2011) and from studies in neoplastic cells (Sun et al. 2009; Takahashi and Loo 2004; Agarwal et al. 2004), mitochondria can be considered a key target for tocotrienols to exert citotoxic effects. They induce the mitochondrial permeability pore (mPTP) formation with catastrophic consequences for the cell, since the open pore unleashes pro-apototic molecules, such as cytochrome c, AIF or endonuclease G, promotes energy failure and generation of reactive oxygen species. Although it is accepted that mPTP can precipitate autophagy (Elmore et al. 2001), the mechanisms involved are undetermined. One mechanism that may link mPTP to autophagy postulates that damaged mitochondria engage their own elimination via autophagy (the called mitophagy) and abundant mitophagy precipitates cell death (Kim et al. 2007). Further experiments are needed to clarify this issue.

Induction of mPTP opening by tocotrienols is probably the final consequence of a mitochondrial insult, but how tocotrienols disturb the organelle is still in speculative grounds. Other vitamin E compounds has been shown to target specific sites of the electron mitochondrial chain. This is the case of α-tocopheryl succinate (αTOS), a redox-silent derivative of α-tocopherol in which the hydroxyl group at position C_6 of the chromanol ring (which is responsible for α-tocopherol redox activity) has been substituted by succinic acid (Zhao et al. 2009). αTOS inhibits succinate dehydrogenase activity of mitochondrial complex II by interacting with the ubiquinone binding site (Dong et al. 2008). As a result ubiquinone is displaced from complex II, causing a rapid generation of radical oxygen species responsible to trigger apoptosis. The structural similarities of vitamin E compounds and ubiquinone open the possibility that tocotrienols may be acting as well as an ubiquinone like molecule able to bind to its docking sites in the mitochondrial respiratory complex II. The subsequent mitochondrial electron transport chain disruption would trigger the "eat me" signals of an unhealthy cell. Owing to the fact that activated mitochondria are functionally and structurally different from their normal counterparts (Kroemer and Pouyssegur 2008; Modica-Napolitano and Singh 2004; Gogvadze et al. 2008) it is not risky to think that the selective citotoxic effect of tocotrienols towards cells with a transformed or activated phenotype is dictated by mitochondrial specific traits. This argument would add tocotrienol to the growing list of compounds that selectively target mitochondria of transformed cells (Fulda et al. 2010).

20.7 Perspectives: Possible Therapeutic Roles of Tocotrienols in Chronic Fibroinflammatory Processes

Among the large number of diseases that can affect human beings there is a group of disorders that share in common an unknown or undefined etiopathogenesis, a chronic progressive course, variable degrees of inflammatory cell infiltration, prominent fibrosis accumulation and, ultimately, loss of function of the affected organs. Some of these disorders are conceptually grouped into autoimmune, hyperinflammatory or idiopathic chronic diseases. They tend to be considered as the end result of a wound healing defect, either at the control of the inflammatory cell signaling or at the regulation of extracellular matrix remodeling, or both.

Chronic fibroinflammatory disease can hit any organ in the body, occasionally several organs at a time. Some examples of these conditions may include special forms of chronic bronchitis, chronic renal failure, chronic liver disease, chronic arthritis, inflammatory bowel disease, and chronic pancreatitis. Some of these disorders respond well to steroids or immunosuppressive agents.

Given the fact that tocotrienols seem to be harmless to normal parenchymal cells, may modulate inflammatory reactions and induce apoptosis and autophagy in activated fibroblasts, they may find a role in the therapeutic strategy designed to treat chronic fibroinflammatory diseases. Caution should be taken not to interfere with normal healing processes, otherwise the overall result of tocotrienol treatment may turn to be detrimental. However, all these statements remain largely speculative, since clinical trials are lacking to either prove or discard any of these hypotheses.

References

Agarwal MK, Agarwal ML, Athar M, Gupta S (2004) Tocotrienol-rich fraction of palm oil activates p53, modulates Bax/Bcl2 ratio and induces apoptosis independent of cell cycle association. Cell Cycle 3:205–211

Aggarwal BB, Sundarama C, Prasada S, Kannappana R (2010a) Tocotrienols, the vitamin E of the 21st century: its potential against cancer and other chronic diseases. Biochem Pharmacol 80:1613–1631

Aggarwal BB, Sundaram C, Prasad S, Kannappan R (2010b) Tocotrienols, the vitamin E of the 21st century: its potential against cancer and other chronic diseases. Biochem Pharmacol 80:1613–1631

Ahn KS, Sethi G, Krishnan K, Aggarwal BB (2007) Gamma-tocotrienol inhibits nuclear factor-kappaB signaling pathway through inhibition of receptor-interacting protein and TAK1 leading to suppression of antiapoptotic gene products and potentiation of apoptosis. J Biol Chem 282:809–820

Behery FA, Elnagar AY, Akl MR, Wali VB, Abuasal B, Kaddoumi A, Sylvester PW, El Sayed KA (2010) Redox-silent tocotrienol esters as breast cancer proliferation and migration inhibitors. Bioorg Med Chem 18(22):8066–8075

Birringer M, EyTina JH, Salvatore BA, Neuzil J (2003) Vitamin E analogues as inducers of apoptosis: structure–function relation. Br J Cancer 88:1948–1955

Constantinou C, Papas A, Constantinou AI (2008) Vitamin E and cancer: an insight into the anticancer activities of vitamin E isomers and analogs. Int J Cancer 123:739–752

Dong LF, Low P, Dyason JC, Wang XF, Prochazka L, Witting PK, Freeman R, Swettenham E, Valis K, Liu J, Zobalova R, Turanek J, Spitz DR, Domann FE, Scheffler IE, Ralph SJ, Neuzil J (2008) Alpha-tocopheryl succinate induces apoptosis by targeting ubiquinone-binding sites in mitochondrial respiratory complex II. Oncogene 27:4324–4335

Elmore SP, Qian T, Grissom SF, Lemasters JJ (2001) The mitochondrial permeability transition initiates autophagy in rat hepatocytes. FASEB J 15:2286–2287

Elsharkawy AM, Oakley F, Mann DA (2005) The role and regulation of hepatic stellate cell apoptosis in reversal of liver fibrosis. Apoptosis 5:927–939

Elson CE (1992) Tropical oils: nutritional and scientific issues. Crit Rev Food Sci Nutr 31:79–102

Friedman SL (2008) Hepatic stellate cells: protean, multifunctional, and enigmatic cells of the liver. Physiol Rev 88:125–172

Fulda S, Galluzzi L, Kroemer G (2010) Targeting mitochondria for cancer therapy. Nat Rev Drug Discov 9:447–464

Gogvadze V, Orrenius S, Zhivotovsky B (2008) Mitochondria in cancer cells: what is so special about them? Trends Cell Biol 18:165–173

Hussein D, Mo H (2009) d-Dlta-tocotrienol-mediated suppression of the proliferation of human PANC-1, MIA PaCa-2, and BxPC-3 pancreatic carcinoma cells. Pancreas 38:124–136

Kaileh M, Sen R (2010) Role of NF-kappaB in the anti-inflammatory effects of tocotrienols. J Am Coll Nutr 29(3 Suppl):334S–339S

Kamal-Eldin A, Appelqvist LA (1996) The chemistry and antioxidant properties of tocopherols and tocotrienols. Lipids 31:671–701

Khosla P, Patel V, Whinter JM, Khanna S, Rakhkovskaya M, Roy S, Sen CK (2006) Postprandial levels of the natural vitamin E tocotrienol in human circulation. Antioxid Redox Signal 8:1059–1068

Kim EH, Sohn S, Kwon HJ, Kim SU, Kim MJ, Lee SJ, Choi KS (2007) Sodium selenite induces superoxide-mediated mitochondrial damage and subsequent autophagic cell death in malignant glioma cells. Cancer Res 67:6314–6324

Kroemer G, Pouyssegur J (2008) Tumor cell metabolism: cancer's Achilles' heel. Cancer Cell 13:472–482

Kuhad A, Chopra K (2009) Tocotrienol attenuates oxidative-nitrosative stress and inflammatory cascade in experimental model of diabetic neuropathy. Neuropharmacology 57:456–462

Luna J, Masamunt MC, Rickmann M, Mora R, España C, Delgado S, Llach J, Vaquero E, Sans M (2011) Tocotrienols have potent antifibrogenic effects in human intestinal fibroblasts. Inflamm Bowel Dis 17(3):732–741

Modica-Napolitano JS, Singh KK (2004) Mitochondrial dysfunction in cancer. Mitochondrion 4:755–762

Moretti L, Yang ES, Kim KW, Lu B (2007) Autophagy signaling in cancer and its potential as novel target to improve anticancer therapy. Drug Resist Updat 10:135–143

Nanji AA, Jokelainen K, Tipoe GL, Rahemtulla A, Dannenberg AJ (2001) Dietary saturated fatty acids reverse inflammatory and fibrotic changes in rat liver despite continued ethanol administration. J Pharmacol Exp Ther 299:638–644

Neuzil J (2003) Vitamin E succinate and cancer treatment: a vitamin E prototype for selective antitumour activity. Br J Cancer 89:1822–1826

Novo E, di Bonzo LV, Cannito S, Colombatto S, Parola M (2009) Hepatic myofibroblasts: a heterogeneous population of multifunctional cells in liver fibrogenesis. Int J Biochem Cell Biol 41:2089–2093

Oakley F, Meso M, Iredale JP, Green K, Marek CJ, Zhou X, May MJ, Millward-Sadler H, Wright MC, Mann DA (2005) Inhibition of inhibitor of kappaB kinases stimulates hepatic stellate cell apoptosis and accelerated recovery from rat liver fibrosis. Gastroenterology 128:108–120

Omary MB, Lugea A, Lowe AW, Pandol SJ (2007) The pancreatic stellate cell: a star on the rise in pancreatic diseases. J Clin Invest 117:50–59

Park SK, Sanders BG, Kline K (2010) Tocotrienols induce apoptosis in breast cancer cell lines via an endoplasmic reticulum stress-dependent increase in extrinsic death receptor signaling. Breast Cancer Res Treat 124:361–375

Patel V, Khanna S, Roy S, Ezziddin O, Sen CK (2006) Natural vitamin E alpha-tocotrienol: retention in vital organs in response to long-term oral supplementation and withdrawal. Free Radic Res 40:763–771

Ramachandran P, Iredale JP (2009) Reversibility of liver fibrosis. Ann Hepatol 8:283–291

Rickmann M, Vaquero EC, Malagelada JR, Molero X (2007) Tocotrienols induce apoptosis and autophagy in rat pancreatic stellate cells through the mitochondrial death pathway. Gastroenterology 132:2518–2532

Sakai M, Okabe M, Tachibana H, Yamada K (2006) Apoptosis induction by gamma-tocotrienol in human hepatoma Hep3B cells. J Nutr Biochem 7:672–676

Sen CK, Khanna S, Rink C, Roy S (2007) Tocotrienols: the emerging face of natural vitamin E. Vitam Horm 76:203–261

Serbinova EA, Packer L (1994) Antioxidant properties of alpha-tocopherol and alpha-tocotrienol. Methods Enzymol 234:354–366

Shibata A, Nakagawa K, Kawakami Y, Tsuzuki T, Miyazawa T (2010) Suppression of gamma-tocotrienol on UVB induced inflammation in HaCaT keratinocytes and HR-1 hairless mice via inflammatory mediators multiple signaling. J Agric Food Chem 58:7013–7020

Srivastava JK, Gupta S (2006) Tocotrienol-rich fraction of palm oil induces cell cycle arrest and apoptosis selectively in human prostate cancer cells. Biochem Biophys Res Commun 346:447–453

Sun W, Xu W, Liu H, Liu J, Wang Q, Zhou J, Dong F, Chen B (2009) Gamma-tocotrienol induces mitochondria-mediated apoptosis in human gastric adenocarcinoma SGC-7901 cells. J Nutr Biochem 20:276–284

Suzuki YJ, Tsuchiya M, Wassall SR, Choo YM, Govil G, Kagan VE, Packer L (1993) Structural and dynamic membrane properties of alpha-tocopherol and alpha-tocotrienol: implication to the molecular mechanism of their antioxidant potency. Biochemistry 32:10692–10699

Takahashi K, Loo G (2004) Disruption of mitochondria during tocotrienol-induced apoptosis in MDA-MB-231 human breast cancer cells. Biochem Pharmacol 67:315–324

Tappeiner C, Meyenberg A, Goldblum D, Mojon D, Zingg JM, Nesaretnam K, Kilchenmann M, Frueh BE (2010) Antifibrotic effects of tocotrienols on human Tenon's fibroblasts. Graefes Arch Clin Exp Ophthalmol 248:65–71

Theriault A, Chao JT, Gapor A (2002) Tocotrienol is the most effective vitamin E for reducing endothelial expression of adhesion molecules and adhesion to monocytes. Atherosclerosis 160:21–30

Turcotte S, Giaccia AJ (2010) Targeting cancer cells through autophagy for anticancer therapy. Curr Opin Cell Biol 22:246–251

Wali VB, Bachawal SV, Sylvester PW (2009a) Combined treatment of gamma-tocotrienol with statins induce mammary tumor cell cycle arrest in G1. Exp Biol Med 234:639–650

Wali VB, Bachawal SV, Sylvester PW (2009b) Endoplasmic reticulum stress mediates gamma-tocotrienol-induced apoptosis in mammary tumor cells. Apoptosis 14:1366–1377

Wu SJ, Liu PL, Ng LT (2008) Tocotrienol-rich fraction of palm oil exhibits anti-inflammatory property by suppressing the expression of inflammatory mediators in human monocytic cells. Mol Nutr Food Res 52:921–929

Wynn TA (2008) Cellular and molecular mechanisms of fibrosis. J Pathol 214:199–210

Yam ML, Abdul Hafid SR, Cheng HM, Nesaretnam K (2009) Tocotrienols suppress proinflammatory markers and cyclooxygenase-2 expression in RAW264.7 Macrophages. Lipids 44:787–797

Yang Z, Klionsky DJ (2010) Eaten alive: a history of macroautophagy. Nat Cell Biol 12:814–822

Yang Z, Xiao H, Jin H, Koo PT, Tsang DJ, Yang CS (2010) Synergistic actions of atorvastatin with gamma-tocotrienol and celecoxib against human colon cancer HT29 and HCT116 cells. Int J Cancer 126:852–863

Yap SP, Yuen KH (2004) Influence of lipolysis and droplet size on tocotrienol absorption from self-emulsifying formulations. Int J Pharm 281:67–78

Yap SP, Yuen KH, Wong JW (2001) Pharmacokinetics and bioavailability of α-, γ- and δ-tocotrienols under different food status. J Pharm Pharmacol 53:67–71

Yap WN, Chang PN, Han HY, Lee DT, Ling MT, Wong YC, Yap YL (2008) Gamma-tocotrienol suppresses prostate cancer cell proliferation and invasion through multiple-signalling pathways. Br J Cancer 99:1832–1841

Yoshida Y, Niki E, Noguchi N (2003) Comparative study on the action of tocopherols and tocotrienols as antioxidant: chemical and physical effects. Chem Phys Lipids 123:63–75

Zhao Y, Neuzil J, Wu K (2009) Vitamin E analogues as mitochondria-targeting compounds: from the bench to the bedside? Mol Nutr Food Res 53:129–139

Chapter 21
Anthocyanins: Janus Nutraceuticals Displaying Chemotherapeutic and Neuroprotective Properties

Erika K. Ross, Natalie A. Kelsey, and Daniel A. Linseman

Abstract Anthocyanins are natural polyphenolic compounds widely distributed as pigments in many fruits and vegetables. In addition to displaying antioxidant properties, these nutraceuticals exhibit anti-inflammatory, anti-proliferative, and pro-apoptotic activities suggesting their potential as novel chemotherapeutic agents. Through cell cycle down-regulation, and context-specific pro-oxidant activity, anthocyanins induce cytotoxicity in cancer cells *in vitro* and *in vivo*. Specifically, via regulation of the Bcl-2 protein family and induction of caspase-dependent or caspase-independent apoptotic pathways, anthocyanins inhibit the growth of cancers by inducing cell death. Moreover, by modulating the activities of specific kinases and proteases, including (but not limited to) cyclin-dependent kinases, mitogen-activated protein kinases, matrix metalloproteases, and urokinase-type plasminogen activators, anthocyanins induce apoptosis, inhibit motility, and suppress invasion of cancer cells. In marked contrast to their effects in cancer cells, we have found that anthocyanins display significant *anti-apoptotic* activity in neurons. Antioxidant properties of these nutraceuticals, particularly at the level of the mitochondria, appear to underlie their neuroprotective effects. The opposing effects of anthocyanins on cancer cells and neurons suggest that these nutraceuticals are promising candidates for development

E.K. Ross • N.A. Kelsey
Department of Biological Sciences and Eleanor Roosevelt Institute,
University of Denver, Denver, CO, USA

D.A. Linseman (✉)
Department of Biological Sciences and Eleanor Roosevelt Institute,
University of Denver, Denver, CO, USA

Research Service, Veterans Affairs Medical Center, Denver, CO, USA

Division of Clinical Pharmacology and Toxicology, Department of Medicine,
University of Colorado Denver, Aurora, CO, USA

Department of Biological Sciences, University of Denver,
2199 S. University Blvd, Denver, CO 80208, USA
e-mail: daniel.linseman@du.edu

M. Diederich and K. Noworyta (eds.), *Natural Compounds as Inducers of Cell Death: Volume 1*, DOI 10.1007/978-94-007-4575-9_21,

as either chemotherapeutic agents or novel neuroprotective compounds for the treatment of cancers or neurodegenerative diseases, respectively.

Keywords Anthocyanin • Apoptosis • Antioxidant • Chemotherapy • Neurodegeneration • Neuroprotection • Nutraceutical

21.1 Introduction

Anthocyanins are a major sub-class of the extensive flavonoid family, and they are responsible for the distinctive red, blue, and purple pigments in many fruits and vegetables. Found in widely consumed foods, including berries, purple sweet potatoes, red rice, and grapes, they exist in relatively high concentrations compared to other dietary polyphenolic compounds (Del Rio et al. 2010). Anthocyanins display a number of potential health benefits that warrant their investigation as potential clinical treatments for several human disorders. Due to their anti-inflammatory and antioxidant properties, these novel nutraceuticals have proven effective in both *in vitro* and *in vivo* models of various chronic human conditions, including cardiovascular disease, obesity, atherosclerosis, ophthalmologic disorders, and type II diabetes (Boucher and Martin 2008; Seymour et al. 2009; Kalt et al. 2010; Mauray et al. 2010; Basu et al. 2010).

The polyphenolic and cationic attributes of anthocyanins and their metabolites activate a variety of cellular responses. Anthocyanins consist of an aglycon component, or anthocyanidin, and a sugar moiety (glucose, galactose, or arabinose). This anthocyanin structure is more stable than its aglycon alone, specifically in acidic environments such as the stomach. The polyphenolic nature of anthocyanins is principally responsible for their strong antioxidant and free radical scavenging activities, and their overall metabolic benefits. There are many known anthocyanins varying in the anthocyanidin skeleton and the complexity of the attached glycoside (Fig. 21.1), necessitating multiple pathways for absorption (Prior and Wu 2006).

Recent bioavailability studies suggest that anthocyanins are absorbed rapidly from the stomach and small intestine, and they are highly metabolized resulting in very low to undetectable concentrations of the parent compound being observed in plasma within only a few hours of consumption (Azzini et al. 2010; Woodward et al. 2009). The low concentrations of parent anthocyanins are seemingly paradoxical to the beneficial role displayed by anthocyanins *in vivo*. This issue has drawn interest to their specific mechanism of action, in particular which metabolites of anthocyanins produce their positive health effects (Milbury and Kalt 2010; Tsuda et al. 2006). Studies have shown that anthocyanins are absorbed and metabolized through two prominent mechanisms. The first mechanism involves the rapid absorption of the intact, parent anthocyanin. These nutraceuticals are detected as either whole glycosides on their corresponding aglycons or glucoronide metabolites in plasma of rats following oral administration, indicative of rapid adsorption across the gastric mucosa (ElMoheson et al. 2006; He et al. 2006). This method of absorption is unique to

Fig. 21.1 Structure of common anthocyanins

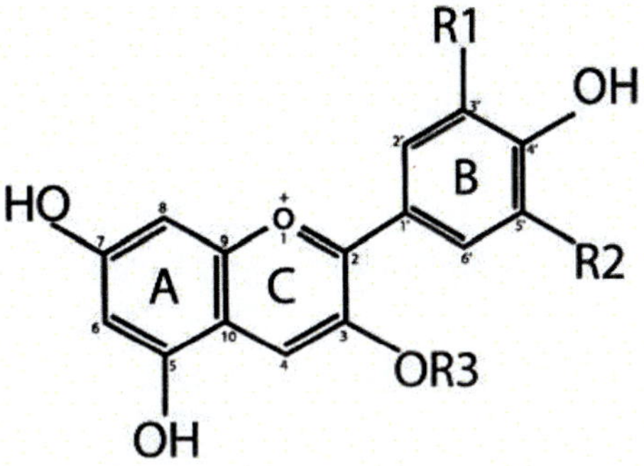

	R_1	R_2
Cyanidin	OH	H
Peonidin	OCH_3	H
Delphinidin	OH	OH
Malvidin	OCH_3	OCH_3
Pelargonidin	H	H

R_3= Glucose, galactose or arabinose

anthocyanins, and it appears that this mechanism involves the hepatic membrane transporter bilitranslocase in the small intestine as well as in vascular endothelium and kidney (Prior et al. 2010; Harada et al. 2004; Arts et al. 2004; Passamonti et al. 2003; Karawajczyk et al. 2007; Maestro et al. 2010; Vanzo et al. 2008). Possibly working in concert with the first mechanism, the second method of absorption relies on metabolism of anthocyanins by gut microflora through deglycosylation and anthocyanidin heterocyclic ring, yielding specific phenolic acids and phenolic aldehydes (Aura et al. 2005; Keppler and Humpf 2005). Which of the above anthocyanin metabolites contribute most to the beneficial health effects of these novel nutraceuticals is currently unclear.

After they are absorbed and metabolized, anthocyanins and their active metabolites produce effects on many normal cellular processes, resulting in diverse actions including enhanced free radical scavenging, reduction of inflammation, decreased cell proliferation, diminished angiogenesis, as well as the induction of apoptosis. Generally, anthocyanins drive the cellular activities by modulating expression of the associated genes (Wang and Stoner 2008). The etiology and pathophysiology of many chronic human conditions are correlated with cellular oxidative stress, including most cancers and neurodegenerative diseases. With limited systemic toxicity, anthocyanins appear to alter biochemical mechanisms associated with damage caused by oxidative stress, which suggests that these novel nutraceuticals may be potentially useful in combating these types of chronic conditions. Anthocyanins have demonstrated a variety of strong anti-cancer effects on highly metastatic cells (Ding et al. 2006). They have also recently proven to be neuroprotective in a model of oxidative stress induced secondary to psychological stress (Rahman et al. 2008), as well as in a mouse model of Alzheimer's disease (Hartman et al. 2006).

Their effectiveness against cancer cells, protective effects in neurons, and limited toxicity to healthy cells, emphasizes the potential of developing anthocyanins as both chemotherapeutic and neuroprotective agents.

21.2 Chemical Properties of Anthocyanins

21.2.1 Antioxidant Activity

Mammalian cells are constantly exposed to toxic reactive intermediates and many types of free radicals, including, but not limited to, reactive oxygen species (ROS). The source of these free radicals may be extrinsic (i.e. from the extracellular environment) or intrinsic, (i.e. from within the cell). In particular, the mitochondria are both a prominent source and target of ROS. The aberrant accumulation of ROS and other free radicals causes damage to essential sub cellular processes. These cellular oxidative stressors contribute to the pathogenesis of many chronic human disorders and are important therapeutic targets for these diseases. Oxidative stress typically causes damage to key macromolecules including DNA, proteins, and lipids, ultimately triggering activation of additional cellular processes, such as apoptosis, or mutagenesis (Ames and Gold 1991). As a result, oxidative stress is associated with many degenerative diseases and arguably contributes to aging (Ames et al. 1993).

Anthocyanin fractions of various fruits and vegetables display significant antioxidant activity and appear to be beneficial in degenerative disorders such as cardiovascular disease (Cote et al. 2010; Ruel and Couillard 2007; Heinonen 2007; Dulebohn et al. 2008; Zhu et al. 2010). There are two suggested mechanisms through which anthocyanins act as antioxidants. The first involves anthocyanins acting as direct scavengers of ROS, thus reducing the concentration of these free radicals before they are able to cause intracellular damage. The second mechanism involves *indirect facilitation* of endogenous antioxidant defenses, which enhances the capacity of the cell to subdue free radicals (Ruel and Couillard 2007; Heinonen 2007; Dulebohn et al. 2008; Zhu et al. 2010). This induction of endogenous antioxidant activity occurs principally through the induction of specific enzyme function. Anthocyanins are documented as activating phase II enzymes in cultured cells (Dulebohn et al. 2008). Phase II enzymes, including glutathione reductase (GR) and glutathione peroxidase (GPx), are responsible for the endogenous production and utilization of glutathione (GSH), respectively. The association between anthocyanin treatment and phase II enzyme activation yielded similar results with different anthocyanin compounds. Antioxidant/detoxifying gene expression regulates the levels of antioxidant activity and intracellular ROS. Studies suggest that anthocyanins regulate these phase II enzymes through the antioxidant response element (ARE). The ARE is present in the promoter region of many genes that code for endogenous antioxidant enzymes (Yu and Kensler 2005). Multiple *in vitro* studies provide evidence that anthocyanin activation of the many cytoprotective and antioxidant genes occurs via the redox-sensitive transcription factor Nrf2 (Vari et al. 2011; Shih et al. 2007; Dai et al. 2009). Specific anthocyanin metabolites have demonstrated protective effects in cellular oxidative stress models. Protocatechuic acid (PCA) is a recognized metabolite of anthocyanins, which is especially noted for its antioxidant properties in such models (Vari et al. 2011; Kay et al. 2004; Tsuda et al. 1999; Nguyen et al. 2009). In accord with whole anthocyanin treatment, PCA seemingly affects cellular oxidative stress by modulating enzymatic phase II antioxidants, and up-regulating cellular antioxidant capacity (Renis et al. 2008).

21.2.2 Anti-inflammatory Activity

Inflammation plays a significant pathological role in various degenerative diseases, including the promotion of many cancers (Kwon et al. 2007; Coussens and Werb 2002). ROS accumulation and the activation of specific signaling cascades are known inducers of cellular inflammation. The mitogen-activated protein kinase (MAPK) signaling cascade is one of the more important pathways in the inflammatory response (Arbabi and Maier 2002). Anthocyanins inhibit the phosphorylation and activation of extracellular signal-related kinase 1 (ERK-1) and ERK-2 by suppression of the upstream kinase, MAPK kinase 1 (MEK1) activation. This inhibitory activation of anthocyanins has a potent modulatory effect on the expression of specific genes and proteins involved in the inflammatory response. In particular, this inhibitory effect of anthocyanins on MEK/ERK signaling limits the expression of certain pro-inflammatory cytokines, such as cyclooxygenase-2 (COX 2) and interleukin-6 (IL-6) in *in vitro* models of inflammation (Rasheed et al. 2009; Bae et al. 2009).

Downstream of MAPK in the pro-inflammatory cascade are nuclear factor kappa B (NF-κB) and activating protein (AP) -1, both of which are also inhibited by anthocyanins. NF-κB and AP-1 are typically hyper activated in many types of cancer (Bae et al. 2009; Hsu et al. 2007). NF-κB and AP-1 are transcription factors involved in many critical physiological responses, including apoptosis, cell differentiation, cell proliferation, oxidative stress, and tumor metastasis. Most pertinent to the latter processes are the roles these transcription factors play in the expression of many pro-inflammatory molecules and tumor metastasis (Bahassi et al. 2004). Due to the effects of its inhibitory protein, IκBα, NF-κB is generally sequestered in the cytosol. Upon exposure to various extracellular stimuli, IκBα is degraded resulting in the release of NF-κB from its inhibited state. Upon its release, NF-κB translocates into the nucleus where it modulates the expression of many pro-inflammatory genes (Collart et al. 1990). It is mainly through the suppression of NF-κB activation that anthocyanins are able to down regulate these inflammatory responses. For example, anthocyanins have been shown to decrease production of monocyte chemo attractant protein 1 (MCP-1), a chemokine responsible for stimulating the recruitment of macrophages to sites of inflammation (Garcia-Alonso et al. 2004). Pro-inflammatory chemokines strongly promote the induction of COX-2. In turn, elevated COX-2 stimulates the production of prostoglandin E_2 (PGE_2) and inducible nitric oxide synthase (iNOS) (Bahassi et al. 2004; Collart et al. 1990; Aggarwal and Shishodia 2004; Kim et al. 2008). Primarily by decreasing the affinity for DNA binding by NF-κB, and facilitating IκBα activity, the anthocyanins are capable of suppressing the expression of critical pro-inflammatory target genes like COX-2, MCP-1, PGE_2, and iNOS (Hafeez et al. 2008; Saric et al. 2009; Cuevas-Rodriguez et al. 2010; Cardile et al. 2010; Zhang et al. 2009; Mulabagal et al. 2009; Zdarilova et al. 2010).

21.2.3 Anti-proliferative Activity

Many treatment modalities for chronic human degenerative disorders target abnormal cell proliferation as an important process in pathogenesis. As mammalian cell growth and proliferation are largely mediated through cell cycle progression, defects in the cell cycle are one of the most common features of cancerous cells (Fridrich et al. 2008). Anthocyanins have been shown to mediate defects in cell cycle progression and proliferation (Marko et al. 2004). Specific anthocyanin metabolites have also shown inhibitory effects on cell proliferation in colon cancer cells, though the mechanism remains unclear, and may contribute to the overall anti-proliferative benefit of anthocyanins (Shih et al. 2005; Forester and Waterhouse 2010). By significantly down-regulating cyclin dependent kinase (CDK) -1, CDK-2, cyclin B1, and cyclin D1, anthocyanins have proven to modulate unchecked cell proliferation in human breast carcinoma, gastric adenocarcinoma cells, and prostate cancer cells, resulting in G2/M arrest (Reddivari et al. 2010; Chen et al. 2005). Cell cycle transition from G2 to M phase is regulated by the complex formation of dephosphorylated CDK-1 with cyclin-B1, and cell cycle arrest occurs at this juncture when these protein and kinase levels are depleted. This mechanism of control has a strong inhibitory effect on cell growth and proliferation, and is extremely interesting for the potential development of this nutraceutical.

21.2.4 Pro-apoptotic Activity

Apoptosis, or programmed cell death, is a critical endogenous mechanism for the disposal of cells harboring DNA damage that could otherwise lead to tumor formation if allowed to survive and proliferate. Anthocyanins derived from a variety of sources appear to induce apoptosis of cancer cells via several different pathways (Shih et al. 2005; Chen et al. 2005; Seeram et al. 2006; Chang et al. 2005; Katsube et al. 2003). The first apoptotic signaling pathway is the extrinsic pathway, which involves activation of a member of the death receptor family, such as Fas. In this pathway, Fas ligand (FasL) will activate Fas by binding to its receptor and recruiting a Fas-associated death domain (FADD) adapter protein and pro-caspase-8. This will cause the activation of pro-caspase-8 to caspase-8, which is required for cell death (Alnemri 1997). Active caspase-8 then cleaves and activates the executioner, caspase-3, which plays a central role in apoptosis, and a point of convergence for many pro-apoptotic signaling cascades, including those stimulated by chemotherapeutic agents and ionizing radiation (Pauwels et al. 2010). The second pathway is the intrinsic, or mitochondrial pathway, which involves members of the Bcl-2 family, such as anti-apoptotic Bcl-2 and Bcl-X_L, and pro-apoptotic Bax and Bid proteins. Bcl-2 is a potent suppressor of apoptosis and will form a heterodimer with Bax to neutralize its pro-apoptotic activity. The ratio of Bcl-2 to Bax is an important gauge of cellular apoptosis. Bid cleavage by caspase-8, a means by which the extrinsic pathway interacts with the intrinsic cascade, forms truncated Bid (tBid) which induces conformational activation of Bax at the mitochondria which results in the release of cytochrome c, and downstream activation of caspase-9 and -3 (Luo et al. 1998). The activation of caspase-3 also results in the cleavage of poly (ADP ribose) polymerase (PARP), activation of caspase-activated DNAses (CADs), and DNA fragmentation.

Anthocyanins seemingly affect both of these caspase-dependent pathways. These nutraceuticals have been shown to activate either the intrinsic or extrinsic apoptotic cascade in several different cellular models. Anthocyanin treatment results in the activation of caspase-3, -8, and -9 and induces PARP cleavage in multiple cellular models (Coussens and Werb 2002; Shih et al. 2005; Chen et al. 2005; Chang et al. 2005; Shin et al. 2009). Anthocyanins also appear to have an affect on the regulation of Bcl-2 and Bax, as the ratio of Bcl-2 to Bax is altered in favor of apoptosis in cancer cells, suggesting that anthocyanins up-regulate Bax and down-regulate Bcl-2 in transformed cells (Yeh and Yen 2005; Malik et al. 2005). In addition, anthocyanins are demonstrated to be key regulators of FasL expression and tBid cleavage (Lo et al. 2007).

There are many important signaling pathways that influence cell survival, including the ERK, JNK, and p38 MAPK cascades. In addition to the key involvement of MAPK cascades in the inflammatory and proliferative responses, the kinases are also intimately associated with apoptosis. The activities of several proteins in the MAPK pathway are altered in cells with the addition of anthocyanin extracts (Lee et al. 2009a; Liu et al. 2008). The mechanism involved in this alteration is theorized to involve p53 protein and p38-MAPK, by outwardly triggering upstream caspase activation. Anthocyanins also appear to attenuate the phosphorylation of JNK, which is an essential process in apoptosis signaling (Liu et al. 2008). Anthocyanins appear to be potent inducers of cancer cell apoptosis through both the mitochondrial and death receptor pathways.

21.2.5 Additional Activity

Anthocyanins display a wide array of additional activities in different cell models, though many of these properties are not well understood. In addition to their more

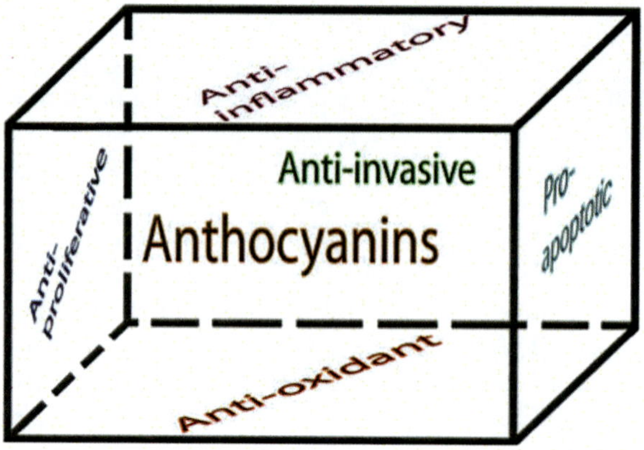

Fig. 21.2 Summary of anthocyanin properties

thoroughly recognized chemotherapeutic attributes, the potential utility of these nutraceuticals in other chronic human diseases has recently become a point of interest. Anthocyanins have been studied *in vivo* in a model of obesogenic high fat diet-fed mice, where they lowered fat levels to the equivalent of a low fat diet-fed animal. It is suggested that the mechanism of their lipid-lowering effect involves β-cell function and serum leptin, however the specific signaling pathway remains to be investigated (Seymour et al. 2009).

Anthocyanins display cardioprotective properties, partially due to their antioxidant and anti-inflammatory activities, but these compounds also regulate specific genes associated with heart disease. These genes include those coding for the cholesterol transporter ABCA-1, the scavenger receptor CD36, and the vasoconstrictor endothelin-1, which are expressed in human macrophages or endothelial cells (Kao et al. 2009; Lazze et al. 2006). Moreover, anthocyanins modulate genes coding for adhesion molecules and those that have been implicated in the regulation of angiogenesis, such as JAM-A and VEGF. Cell-cell adhesion is affected as well, through the regulation of genes such as CRB3, CLDN14, or CDH4, which are associated with this process (Mauray et al. 2010).

Importantly, anthocyanins have also been shown to reduce the expression of matrix metalloproteinase (MMP)-9 and urokinase-type plasminogen activator (u-PA), which are both associated with cell invasion (Chen et al. 2006). These enzymes promote degradation of the ECM, giving rise to cell invasion and enhanced cancer cell motility (Westermarck and Kahari 1999). The anthocyanin-induced decrease in enzymatic activity is predicted to diminish cell invasion and motility, which would significantly decrease the metastatic potential of cancer cells. The major chemical properties of anthocyanins described above are summarized in Fig. 21.2.

21.3 Chemotherapeutic Potential of Anthocyanins

21.3.1 Mechanisms of Cancer Cell Death

21.3.1.1 Anthocyanin-Induced Cell Cycle Down Regulation

Unchecked cell proliferation is a hallmark of tumorogenesis. Cancer cells typically possess elevated levels of CDK-1 and -2 (Chen et al. 2005). The ability of anthocyanins to down regulate these cell cycle proteins in cancer is a key point of interest. As anthocyanins are potent suppressors of CDK-1 and -2, cyclin B1, and cyclin D1, they are able to blunt unchecked cell proliferation in many highly metastatic cancer cell models (Chen et al. 2005). The down regulation of cyclins and their associated kinases has been shown to cause an accumulation of cells in the pre-G1 phase in malignant Caco-2 and Hep-G2, and nonmalignant 3T3-L1 cells, though the mechanism of the arrest at this point in the cell cycle is still unclear (Liu et al. 2010). In addition, anthocyanins appear to have direct effects on microtubules, resulting in the accumulation of cancer cells in G2/M (Nguyen et al. 2010). An additional and likely more significant mechanism behind the G2/M arrest of cancer cells is attributed to the depletion of CDK-1 and -2, as well as cyclin B1 and D1, induced by anthocyanins. Significantly, the activity of anthocyanins to cause cell cycle arrest often precedes induction of apoptosis in cancer cells (Chen et al. 2005; Malik et al. 2005; Nguyen et al. 2010).

21.3.1.2 Context-Specific Pro-oxidant Activity

One of the most interesting and counterintuitive aspects of anthocyanins is their ability to act as antioxidants in some systems and as pro-oxidants in other cellular models. The data supporting this activity are limited and necessitate further investigation, but it would appear that anthocyanins exhibit this activity uniquely in select types of cancer cells. For instance, anthocyanins induce DNA fragmentation in human colon cancer cells in a concentration-dependent manner. This effect is more dramatic when anthocyanin metabolites are introduced, as opposed to the parent anthocyanin, arguing for the efficacy of anthocyanin metabolites in chemotherapy (Vari et al. 2011). Cyanidin-3-rutinoside is proven to induce the accumulation of peroxides in human HL-60 promyelocytic leukemia cells, which results in cellular apoptosis (Feng et al. 2007). Significantly, this anthocyanin did not induce ROS accumulation of apoptosis in normal tumor peripheral blood mononuclear cells, indicating a cancer cell-specific pro-oxidant effect. Anthocyanins also cause accumulation of hydrogen peroxide and cause DNA strand breaks in cancer cells, resulting in reduced proliferation (Lee et al. 2005). These activities are quite remarkable and unique to anthocyanins, and their context-specific pro-oxidant effects may indeed play a key role in their anticancer activity.

21.3.1.3 Modulation of Bcl-2 Family

Mitochondrial function and intrinsic apoptosis are controlled by several factors, but none are more critical than the pro- and anti-apoptotic, and intrinsic apoptosis members of the Bcl-2 family. Studies suggest that the addition of anthocyanin fractions to cancer cells alters the expression and/or formation of multiple members of the Bcl-2 family. Specifically, Bcl-2, Bax, and Bid appear to be affected by the addition of anthocyanins *in vitro*. After treatment with hibiscus anthocyanins, human promyelocytic leukemia cells responded with an increase in the truncated form of Bid, tBid, as well as increased levels of cytochrome c in the cytosol, a marker for induction of the mitochondrial apoptosis pathway (Chang et al. 2005). The authors of this study concluded that activation by anthocyanins of the p38 MAPK, downstream of Fas stimulation, induces apoptosis in HL-60 cells. Additional studies argue for mitochondrial dysfunction in cancer cells induced by anthocyanin treatment. Anthocyanin-induced increases in Bax and decreases in Bcl-2 results in mitochondrial depolarization, cytochrome c release, and subsequent activation of caspase-9, causing apoptotic cell death in human leukemia cells (Lee et al. 2009b). Two additional groups investigating the involvement of Bcl-2 family members in anthocyanin-induced apoptosis similarly found a decrease in Bcl-2 protein levels post-anthocyanin treatment. The studies also demonstrated an increase in the Bax/Bcl-2 ratio after the introduction of anthocyanins in human hepatoma cells (Yeh and Yen 2005). These data provide more evidence towards anthocyanin fractions inducing apoptosis, at least in part, through the mediation of Bcl-2 family proteins. Moreover, these data indicate that anthocyanins induce apoptosis of cancer cells through the intrinsic, as well as the extrinsic apoptotic pathway.

21.3.1.4 Caspase-Dependent and Caspase-Independent Pathways

Apoptotic cell death can occur via caspase-dependent or caspase-independent apoptotic pathways. Cancer cells typically have a defect in programmed cell death, making caspase-dependent and caspase-independent apoptotic pathways potential targets for chemotherapy. Anthocyanins have cell-specific effects in terms of the mechanisms of cell death they induce, targeting alternative apoptotic cascades in different cell models. Anthocyanins may activate a caspase-dependent cascade in one cancer cell line and a caspase-independent pathway in another. For example, in prostate cancer models, anthocyanins are cytotoxic to androgen-dependent cells through both caspase-dependent and caspase-independent pathways, whereas anthocyanins solely caused apoptosis through a caspase-independent mechanism in androgen-independent tumor cells (Reddivari et al. 2007). Apoptosis inducing factor (AIF) and endonuclease G (Endo G) are classical markers for caspase-independent apoptosis. Levels of each of these factors increased in both androgen dependent and androgen independent prostate cancer cells after treatment with anthocyanin fractions from potato extracts (Reddivari et al. 2007). Caspase-dependent apoptosis is typically measured by the cleavage of caspases and PARP. Increased levels of anthocyanin fraction *in vitro* resulted in elevated levels of cleaved caspase-3, caspase-9, and PARP, exclusively in the androgen-dependent prostate cancer cells (Reddivari et al. 2007). Though most data suggest that anthocyanins cause apoptosis predominantly through caspase-dependent pathways, studies demonstrate that they may also cause apoptosis via caspase-independent mechanisms.

21.3.2 Suppression of Cancer Cell Motility and Invasion

The degradation and invasion of basement membrane collagen is a decisive event in determining the metastatic potential of a given cancer. Tumor cells typically secrete proteolytic enzymes to facilitate successful invasion of extracellular matrix barriers. MMPs and plasminogen activators regulate ECM degradation. One mechanism by which anthocyanins inhibit cancer cell invasion is through decreasing levels of MMP and u-Pa. In addition, anthocyanins also appear to increase levels of tissue inhibitors of MMP-2, as well as inhibitors of plasminogen activator (Chen et al. 2006; Brandstetter et al. 2001; Lamy et al. 2007). In SKHep-1 cells, a highly invasive hepatoma cell line, anthocyanin fractions increased levels of these endogenous MMP and u-Pa inhibitors. Black rice anthocyanin fractions, including cyanidin-3-glucoside and peonidin-3-glucoside reduced the invasion and motility of these highly invasive cells *in vitro* (Chen et al. 2006). This anti-metastatic activity was not only observed in SKHep-1 cells, but also Huh-7, HeLa, and SCC-4 cells, drawing the conclusion that these results are more universal for cancer cells than initially assumed (Chen et al. 2006). AP-1 is a transcription factor responsible for the expression of ECM degrading proteases. Anthocyanin treatment decreased AP-1 binding activity in the hepatoma cells as well (Chen et al. 2006).

The molecular mechanism by which anthocyanins down regulate or inhibit invasion and motility has been investigated in H1229 Lewis lung carcinoma cells (Ho et al. 2010). These studies suggest that anthocyanin derivatives inhibit MMP and u-Pa expression through the inactivation of ERK and AP-1-dependent transcriptional events. The decreased AP-1 DNA binding activity, coupled with inhibition of MEK and ERK 1/2 activity, results in the down regulation of MMP-2, MMP-9, and u-Pa expression. This study strongly argues that peonidin-3-glucoside inhibits the metastasis of Lewis lung carcinoma, at least in part, by decreasing cell invasion and motility (Ho et al. 2010). Another study aimed at investigating the relationship between anthocyanins and their anti-invasive activity in human colon cancer cells suggests a different mechanism for the decreased expression of MMP-2 and MMP-9 (Yun et al. 2010). This study found that anthocyanins decrease MMP-2 and MMP-9 expression in HT-29 colon cancer cells via suppression of NFκB-dependent gene transcription (Yun et al. 2010). Thus, anthocyanins decrease the invasive capacity of cancer cells by diminishing the expression of key ECM-degrading enzymes. The mechanism underlying this down regulation appears to involve anthocyanin inhibition of specific transcription factors that normally promote ECM enzyme expression. The main chemotherapeutic pathways utilized by anthocyanins are shown in Fig. 21.3.

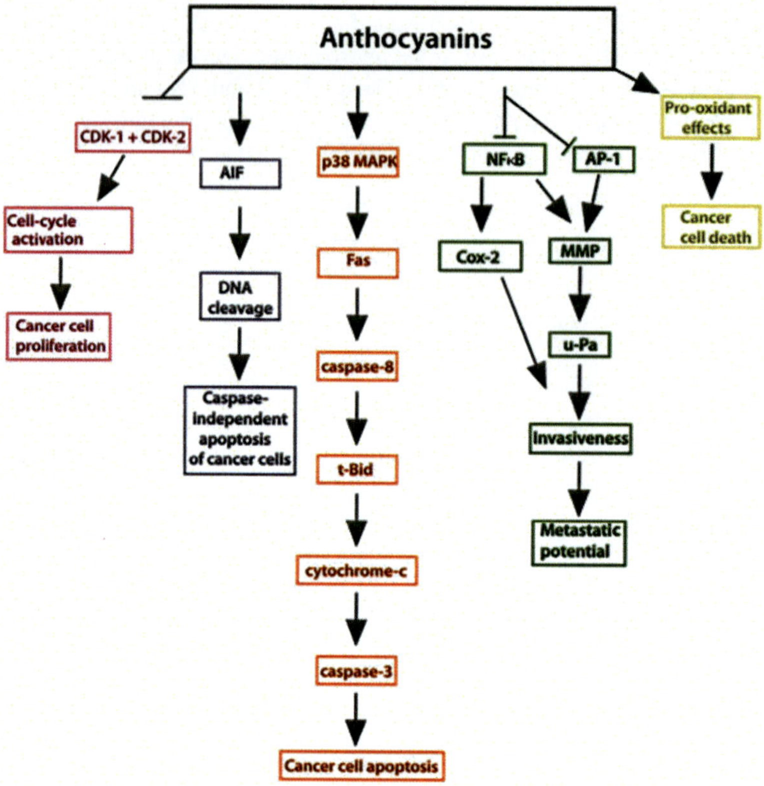

Fig. 21.3 Main pathways for anthocyanin-induced cancer cell death

21.3.3 Other Mechanisms of Anthocyanin Anti-cancer Effects

In addition to the well-documented anti-cancer properties discussed above, anthocyanins are noted for their anti-angiogenic capacity. These nutraceuticals inhibited the expression of vascular endothelial growth factor (VEGF), a key regulator of tumor angiogenesis *in vitro* (Bagchi et al. 2004). Anthocyanins also diminished expression of monocyte chemoattractant protein-1 (MCP-1), whose expression is positively correlated with angiogenic activity (Bagchi et al. 2004). The anti-angiogenic effects of anthocyanins have been confirmed in several additional studies (Roy et al. 2002; Garcia-Alonso et al. 2009). This anti-angiogenic property further supports a key role for anthocyanins in chemoprevention and chemotherapy.

Another novel property of anthocyanins is their ability to regulate cancer cells through the induction of differentiation. This is an especially unique tool for chemotherapy, as it is less toxic than many pharmaceuticals targeting alternative mechanisms for prevention and treatment. Studies suggest that anthocyanin-treatment of leukemic cells results in induction of apoptosis through a variety of stress mechanisms (Del Pozo-Insfran et al. 2006). In a similar manner, anthocyanin extracts induce

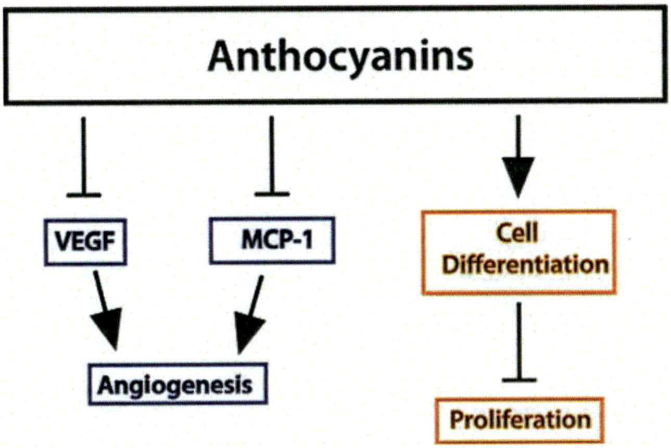

Fig. 21.4 A summary schematic of other chemotherapeutic contributory anthocyanin pathways

terminal differentiation of squamous cell carcinoma cells (Rodrigo et al. 2006). This activity was accompanied by decreased cell proliferation, activation of transglutamate enzymes involved in keratin production, an indication of their ability to induce cell differentiation (Rodrigo et al. 2006). The anti-angiogenic and pro-differentiation effects of anthocyanins are summarized in Fig. 21.4.

21.4 Effects of Anthocyanins in Animal Models of Cancer

Anthocyanins display significant chemotherapeutic activity in animals harboring cancerous genetic mutations and in carcinogen-treated animals. In the Apc^{min} mouse model of intestinal tumor development, anthocyanins inhibited growth and development if cecal adenomas but had no effect on colonic tumor growth (Kang et al. 2003). In a similar study, Apc^{min} mice fed anthocyanin-rich extract showed a 74% decrease in cecal tumors compared to mice on a control diet (Wang and Stoner 2008). Anthocyanins have also been demonstrated to reduce the promotion of colon tumors caused by 2-amino-1-methyl-6-phenylimidazo[4,5-*b*]pyridine in a rat model of colorectal carcinogenesis (Hagiwara et al. 2001).

Anthocyanins also appear to be effective chemotherapeutic agents in esophageal cancer models *in vivo*. In one study, rats were treated with *N*-nitrosomethylbenzylamine (NMBA), a known inducer of squamous cell carcinoma. The results indicate that animals treated with anthocyanin fractions from freeze-dried strawberries had a 42–47% reduction in tumor numbers, a significant improvement over the control animals (Stoner et al. 2007).

In SKHep-1 xenograft nude mice, anthocyanin feeding resulted in a significant reduction of tumor volume compared to control animals. Interestingly, this occurred after only 40 days of oral administration, a brief time-course for administration of chemotherapy (Chen et al. 2006). In A549 lung cancer xenograft nude mice, anthocyanin treatment resulted in an approximate 50% size reduction compared to control mice (Ding et al. 2006). Macroscopic and microscopic examination of these anthocyanin-fed mice also revealed a substantial decrease in tumor involvement in the abdominal wall and cavity compared to positive control mice, indicating a strong anti-metastatic effect of the anthocyanins. In similar studies involving either prostate carcinoma or glioma tumor xenograft mice, anthocyanin treatment resulted in a substantial delay in tumor growth, a difference of about 20 days for the tumor to reach maximum volume, and in some cases, tumor regression (Malik et al. 2005; Jeong et al. 2010). Collectively, these results suggest that anthocyanin treatment not only inhibits growth of a primary tumor, but likely inhibits cancer migration and invasion *in vivo.*

In a more mechanistic study investigating the antioxidant and anti-inflammatory effects of anthocyanins derived from sour cherry juice, the results demonstrated concentration-dependent effects of anthocyanins *in vivo*. Anthocyanin treatment increased GSH peroxidase and superoxide dismutase activity, and exhibited strong antioxidant effects. Interestingly, this study also revealed an inhibition of COX-2 activity in mice (Saric et al. 2009). These findings confirm that the antioxidant and anti-inflammatory activity exhibited by anthocyanins *in vitro* carries over to the *in vivo* situation.

21.5 Neuroprotective Effects of Anthocyanins

In marked contrast the their ability to kill cancer cells, anthocyanins significantly protect neurons in several *in vitro* models of neurotoxicity and *in vivo* models of neurodegeneration. Current consensus agrees that anthocyanin-mediated neuroprotection is largely due to their antioxidant and anti-inflammatory activities. These properties are important for agents targeting neurodegenerative disease, as the mechanisms that underlie these conditions often involve the accumulation of ROS and other free radicals. As anthocyanins display overt cytotoxicity in cancer cell models, it is perhaps unexpected that they would promote survival in neuronal cultures. However, they appear to have strong antioxidant and anti-apoptotic effects in non-cancerous cells, including neurons (Solomon et al. 2010). Anthocyanins derived from mulberry fruit displayed protection of dopaminergic cells *in vitro* (Kim et al. 2010). After treatment with either 6-hydroxydopamine (6-OHDA) or 1-methyl-4-phenylpyridinium (MPP+), *in vitro* models of Parkinson's disease (PD), cells pre-treated with anthocyanins showed less apoptosis and a significant decrease in indices of oxidative stress. Anthocyanins and their metabolites demonstrate protective effects in other *in vitro* models of neuronal injury. For example, in SH-SY5Y cells, anthocyanins and their metabolites inhibit H_2O_2-induced oxidative stress, ROS accumulation, and apoptosis (Tarozzi et al. 2007). Anthocyanins from purple sweet potatoes have also been shown to protect rat pheochromocytoma PC-12 cells from Aβ-induced oxidative stress and lipid peroxidation (Ye et al. 2010).

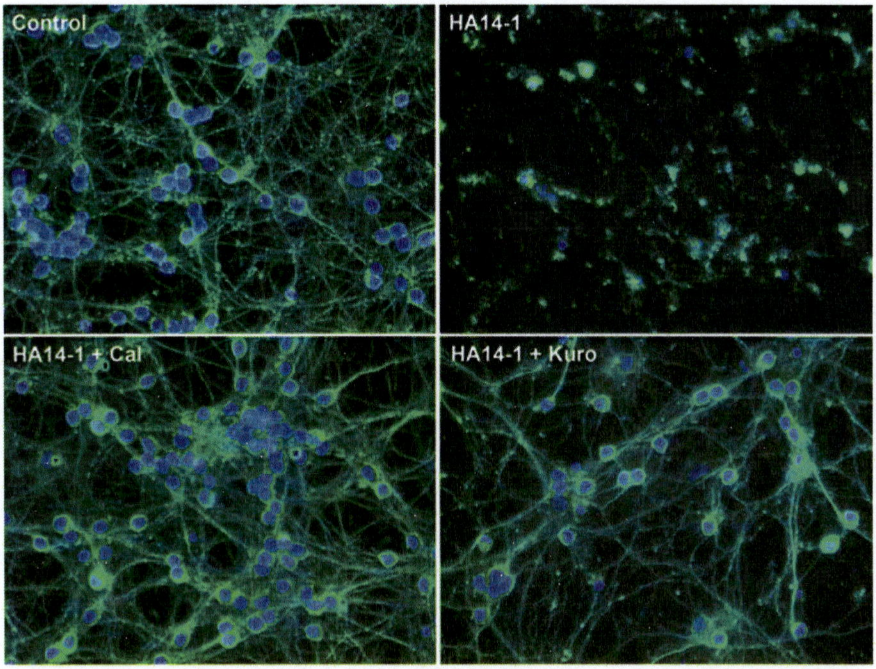

Fig. 21.5 CGNs treated with HA14-1 after pre-treatment with either 213 μM Callistephin or 103 μM Kuromanin

Although most results point to direct ROS scavenging and phase II enzyme activation, preliminary studies suggest secretory phospholipase A_2 ($sPLA_2$) as an additional target for anthocyanins and their metabolites. Specifically, group V $sPLA_2$ seems to be inhibited by anthocyanins, this may be important since $sPLA_2$s take part in regulating inflammatory responses associated with neurodegeneration (Dreiseitel et al. 2009).

Exposure of cultured rat cerebellar granule neurons (CGNs) to the Bcl-2 inhibitor, HA14-1, induces GSH-sensitive mitochondrial oxidative stress and intrinsic apoptosis. (Zimmerman et al. 2007). Inspired by the many suggested benefits of anthocyanin treatment, we have recently examined several anthocyanins that had yet to be tested in a neuronal model of oxidative stress-induced apoptosis. We found that callistephin (pelargonidin-3-*O*-glucoside) and kuromanin (cyanidin-3-*O*-glucoside) displayed significant protection in this neuronal model, as shown in Fig. 21.5. Anthocyanin-mediated neuroprotection was due at least in part, to preservation of mitochondrial GSH and decreased oxidation of the mitochondrial lipid, cardiolipin. Collectively, the above data demonstrate that anthocyanins provide significant protection from oxidative stress in cultured neurons.

Recently, several *in vivo* studies have exhibited exciting results, suggesting that these novel nutraceuticals could be beneficial in a clinical setting for neurodegenerative diseases. A central aim of these studies was to examine the therapeutic potential of anthocyanins in the treatment of specific neurodegenerative diseases, specifically using animal models of PD. In the MPTP mouse, a neurotoxin model widely used to test potential therapeutic options for PD, anthocyanin treatment preserved dopamine neurons in the substantia nigra pars compacta and dopaminergic innervation of the striatum (Kim et al. 2010). Anthocyanins have also exhibited neuroprotection in rats subjected to unilateral striatal lesioning with 6-OHDA, reinforcing their potential in this particular neurodegenerative disease (Roghani et al. 2010). Anthocyanins have also been shown to have neuroprotective effects in *in vivo* models of acute neuronal injury such as middle cerebral artery occlusion and reperfusion in rats (Shin et al. 2006).

Anthocyanins have also been examined in models of aging, as research suggests that oxidative stress plays a large role in the etiology of aging. Recent studies investigating anthocyanins have reveled other potential benefits of these nutraceuticals. Anthocyanins appear to diminish age-related oxidative stress (Lu et al. 2010; Krikorian et al. 2010). Treatment with anthocyanins significantly attenuated cytosolic cytochrome c release, and promoted neuronal survival in a model of D-galactose-induced brain aging in old mice (Lu et al. 2010). Finally, in a recent clinical study, consumption of wild blueberry juice for 12 weeks enhanced memory performance in older adults with early symptoms of dementia (Krikorian et al. 2010). These data are suggestive of a possible therapeutic role for anthocyanins in age-associated cognitive impairment.

21.6 Conclusions

An important element of anthocyanin treatment is the cell specific effects of these compounds exhibited both *in vitro* and *in vivo*. As they act in a pro-apoptotic fashion in cancer cells, and as anti-apoptotic agents in neurons, it is clear that their effects on cell physiology are complex. Anthocyanins also exhibit this specificity between cancer cells and other non-cancer cells of the same or surrounding tissue. For example, they are shown to have pro-apoptotic effects against both estrogen receptor positive breast cancer cells, as well as triple negative breast cancer cells. However, in the same study, they exhibited anti-apoptotic effects in normal breast cells (Li et al. 2009).

Anthocyanins affect many different signaling pathways in different cell systems. They exhibit anti-proliferative, anti-inflammatory, and pro-apoptotic effects in cancer cells, supportive of their use as chemotherapeutic agents. They also exhibit strong antioxidant and anti-apoptotic effects in neuronal injury models, which provides evidence toward the potential of anthocyanins as a novel treatment for neurodegeneration. *In vivo* studies in animal models of carcinogenesis or neurodegeneration involving anthocyanins have delivered promising results that may lean towards their clinical development for both neurodegenerative diseases and chemotherapy. Studies in human subjects are limited, but are also promising for both treatment modalities. In preliminary clinical studies, anthocyanins have exhibited very positive data regarding their use for colorectal cancer intervention and in oral intraepithelial neoplasia. These studies both suggest the further evaluation of anthocyanin use in chemoprevention (Thomasset et al. 2009; Shumway et al. 2008).

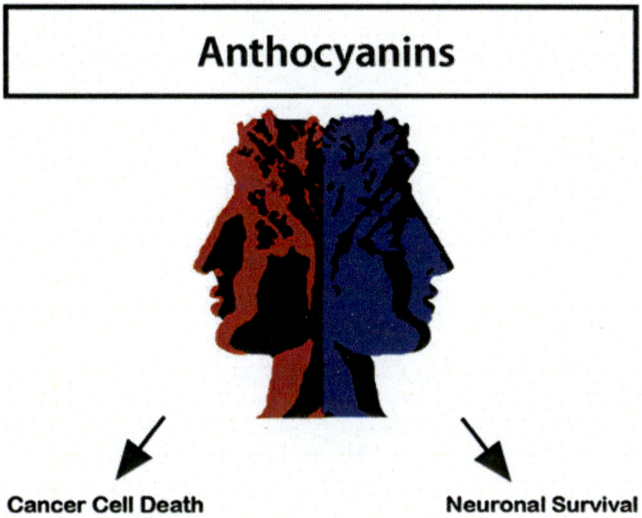

Fig. 21.6 The Janus effects of anthocyanins

These novel nutraceuticals have also displayed promising effects in preliminary clinical studies of memory impairment in older adults, again suggesting the potential benefit of developing anthocyanins for the treatment of neurodegenerative diseases (Krikorian et al. 2010). Though the data in human models is limited and preliminary, they provide a basis for more comprehensive human trials of anthocyanins, both as chemotherapeutic and neuroprotective agents. Seeing the clinical potential of anthocyanins, recent studies are directed towards delivery methods of these anthocyanins *in vivo*, even looking toward slow anthocyanin-releasing implants for sustained, long-term delivery of these nutraceuticals (Desai et al. 2010).

The Janus character of anthocyanins is evidenced by their contrasting anti-apoptotic effects in neurons and pro-apoptotic effects in cancer cells (Fig. 21.6). The unique properties of anthocyanins may be extremely beneficial for the clinical treatment of chronic human diseases, as diverse as cancer and neurodegeneration. Future development of these nutraceuticals as chemopreventative, chemotherapeutic, and neuroprotective agents will one day hopefully lead to their use in a clinical setting for the treatment of neurodegenerative diseases as well as highly invasive cancers.

Acknowledgements Funding was provided by a VA merit review grant and R01NS062766 from NINDS.

References

Aggarwal BB, Shishodia S (2004) Suppression of the nuclear factor-kappaB activation pathway by spice-derived phytochemicals: reasoning for seasoning. Ann N Y Acad Sci 1030:434–441

Alnemri ES (1997) Mammalian cell death proteases: a family of highly conserved aspartate specific cysteine proteases. J Cell Biochem 64:33–42

Ames BN, Gold LS (1991) Endogenous mutagens and the causes of aging and cancer. Mutat Res 250:3–16

Ames BN, Shigenaga MK, Hagen TM (1993) Oxidants, antioxidants, and the degenerative diseases of aging. Proc Natl Acad Sci USA 90:7915–7922

Arbabi S, Maier RV (2002) Mitogen-activated protein kinases. Crit Care Med 30:S74–S79

Arts IC, Sesink AL, Faassen-Peters M, Hollman PC (2004) The type of sugar moiety is a major determinant of the small intestinal uptake and subsequent biliary excretion of dietary quercetin glycosides. Br J Nutr 91:841–847

Aura AM, Martin-Lopez P, O'Leary KA, Williamson G, Oksman-Caldentey KM, Poutanen K, Santos-Buelga C (2005) In vitro metabolism of anthocyanins by human gut microflora. Eur J Nutr 44:133–142

Azzini E, Vitaglione P, Intorre F, Napolitano A, Durazzo A, Foddai MS, Fumagalli A, Catasta G, Rossi L, Venneria E, Raguzzini A, Palomba L, Fogliano V, Maiani G (2010) Bioavailability of strawberry antioxidants in human subjects. Br J Nutr 104:1–9

Bae JY, Lim SS, Kim SJ, Choi JS, Park J, Ju SM, Han SJ, Kang IJ, Kang YH (2009) Bog blueberry anthocyanins alleviate photoaging in ultraviolet-B irradiation-induced human dermal fibroblasts. Mol Nutr Food Res 53:726–738

Bagchi D, Sen CK, Bagchi M, Atalay M (2004) Anti-angiogenic antioxidant and anti-carcinogenic properties of a novel anthocyanin-rich berry extract formula. Biochemistry (Mosc) 69:75–80, 71ppreceding75

Bahassi ELM, Karyala S, Tomlinson CR, Sartor MA, Medvedovic M, Hennigan RF (2004) Critical regulation of genes for tumor cell migration by AP-1. Clin Exp Metastasis 21:293–304

Basu A, Rhone M, Lyons TJ (2010) Berries: emerging impact on cardiovascular health. Nutr Rev 68:168–177

Boucher F, Martin C (2008) Chronic dietary intake of plant-derived anthocyanins protects the rat heart against ischemia-reperfusion injury. J Nutr 138:747–752

Brandstetter H, Grams F, Glitz D, Lang A, Huber R, Bode W, Krell HW, Engh RA (2001) The 1.8-A crystal structure of a matrix metalloproteinase 8-barbiturate inhibitor complex reveals a previously unobserved mechanism for collagenase substrate recognition. J Biol Chem 276:17405–17412

Cardile V, Frasca G, Rizza L, Rapisarda P, Bonina F (2010) Antiinflammatory effects of a red orange extract in human keratinocytes treated with interferon-gamma and histamine. Phytother Res 24:414–418

Chang YC, Huang HP, Hsu JD, Yang SF, Wang CJ (2005) Hibiscus anthocyanins rich extract-induced apoptotic cell death in human promyelocytic leukemia cells. Toxicol Appl Pharmacol 205:201–212

Chen PN, Chu SC, Chiou HL, Chiang CL, Yang SF, Hsieh YS (2005) Cyanidin 3-glucoside and peonidin 3-glucoside inhibit tumor cell growth and induce apoptosis in vitro and suppress tumor growth in vivo. Nutr Cancer 53:232–243

Chen PN, Kuo WH, Chiang CL, Chiou HL, Hsieh YS, Chu SC (2006) Black rice anthocyanins inhibit cancer cells invasion via repressions of MMPs and u-PA expression. Chem Biol Interact 163:218–229

Collart MA, Baeuerle P, Vassalli P (1990) Regulation of tumor necrosis factor alpha transcription in macrophages: involvement of four kappa B-like motifs and of constitutive and inducible forms of NF-kappa B. Mol Cell Biol 10:1498–1506

Cote J, Caillet S, Doyon G, Sylvain JF, Lacroix M (2010) Bioactive compounds in cranberries and their biological properties. Crit Rev Food Sci Nutr 50:666–679

Coussens LM, Werb Z (2002) Inflammation and cancer. Nature 420:860–867

Cuevas-Rodriguez EO, Dia VP, Yousef GG, Garcia-Saucedo PA, Lopez-Medina J, Paredes-Lopez O, Gonzalez de Mejia E, Lila MA (2010) Inhibition of pro-inflammatory responses and antioxidant capacity of Mexican blackberry (Rubus spp.) extracts. J Agric Food Chem 58:9542–9548

Dai J, Gupte A, Gates L, Mumper RJ (2009) A comprehensive study of anthocyanin-containing extracts from selected blackberry cultivars: extraction methods, stability, anticancer properties and mechanisms. Food Chem Toxicol 47(4):837–847

Del Pozo-Insfran D, Percival SS, Talcott ST (2006) Acai (Euterpe oleracea Mart.) polyphenolics in their glycoside and aglycone forms induce apoptosis of HL-60 leukemia cells. J Agric Food Chem 54:1222–1229

Del Rio D, Borges G, Crozier A (2010) Berry flavonoids and phenolics: bioavailability and evidence of protective effects. Br J Nutr 104(Suppl 3):S67–S90

Desai KG, Olsen KF, Mallery SR, Stoner GD, Schwendeman SP (2010) Formulation and in vitro-in vivo evaluation of black raspberry extract-loaded PLGA/PLA injectable millicylindrical implants for sustained delivery of chemopreventive anthocyanins. Pharm Res 27:628–643

Ding M, Feng R, Wang SY, Bowman L, Lu Y, Qian Y, Castranova V, Jiang BH, Shi X (2006) Cyanidin-3-glucoside, a natural product derived from blackberry, exhibits chemopreventive and chemotherapeutic activity. J Biol Chem 281:17359–17368

Dreiseitel A, Korte G, Schreier P, Oehme A, Locher S, Hajak G, Sand PG (2009) SPhospholipase A(2) is inhibited by anthocyanidins. J Neural Transm 116:1071–1077

Dulebohn RV, Yi W, Srivastava A, Akoh CC, Krewer G, Fischer JG (2008) Effects of blueberry (Vaccinium ashei) on DNA damage, lipid peroxidation, and phase II enzyme activities in rats. J Agric Food Chem 56:11700–11706

ElMoheson MA, Marks J, Kuhnle G, Moore K, Debnam E, Kaila Srai S, Rice-Evans C, Spencer JP (2006) Absorption, tissue distribution and excretion of pelargonidin and its metabolites following oral administration to rats. Br J Nutr 95:51–58

Feng R, Ni HM, Wang SY, Tourkova IL, Shurin MR, Harada H, Yin XM (2007) Cyanidin-3-rutinoside, a natural polyphenol antioxidant, selectively kills leukemic cells by induction of oxidative stress. J Biol Chem 282:13468–13476

Forester SC, Waterhouse AL (2010) Gut metabolites of anthocyanins, Gallic acid, 3-O-methylgallic acid, and 2,4,6-trihydroxybenzaldehyde, inhibit cell proliferation of caco-2 cells. J Agric Food Chem 58:5320–5327

Fridrich D, Teller N, Esselen M, Pahlke G, Marko D (2008) Comparison of delphinidin, quercetin and (−)-epigallocatechin-3-gallate as inhibitors of the EGFR and the ErbB2 receptor phosphorylation. Mol Nutr Food Res 52:815–822

Garcia-Alonso M, Rimbach G, Rivas-Gonzalo JC, De Pascual-Teresa S (2004) Antioxidant and cellular activities of anthocyanins and their corresponding vitisins a–studies in platelets, monocytes, and human endothelial cells. J Agric Food Chem 52:3378–3384

Garcia-Alonso M, Minihane AM, Rimbach G, Rivas-Gonzalo JC, de Pascual-Teresa S (2009) Red wine anthocyanins are rapidly absorbed in humans and affect monocyte chemoattractant protein 1 levels and antioxidant capacity of plasma. J Nutr Biochem 20:521–529

Hafeez BB, Siddiqui IA, Asim M, Malik A, Afaq F, Adhami VM, Saleem M, Din M, Mukhtar H (2008) A dietary anthocyanidin delphinidin induces apoptosis of human prostate cancer PC3 cells in vitro and in vivo: involvement of nuclear factor-kappaB signaling. Cancer Res 68:8564–8572

Hagiwara A, Miyashita K, Nakanishi T, Sano M, Tamano S, Kadota T, Koda T, Nakamura M, Imaida K, Ito N, Shirai T (2001) Pronounced inhibition by a natural anthocyanin, purple corn color, of 2-amino-1-methyl-6-phenylimidazo[4,5-b]pyridine (PhIP)-associated colorectal carcinogenesis in male F344 rats pretreated with 1,2-dimethylhydrazine. Cancer Lett 171:17–25

Harada K, Kano M, Takayanagi T, Yamakawa O, Ishikawa F (2004) Absorption of acylated anthocyanins in rats and humans after ingesting an extract of ipomoea batatas purple sweet potato tuber. Biosci Biotechnol Biochem 68:1500–1507

Hartman RE, Shah A, Fagan AM, Schwetye KE, Parsadanian M, Schulman RN, Finn MB, Holtzman DM (2006) Pomegranate juice decreases amyloid load and improves behavior in a mouse model of Alzheimer's disease. Neurobiol Dis 24:506–515

He J, Magnuson BA, Lala G, Tian Q, Schwartz SJ, Giusti MM (2006) Intact anthocyanins and metabolites in rat urine and plasma after 3 months of anthocyanin supplementation. Nutr Cancer 54:3–12

Heinonen M (2007) Antioxidant activity and antimicrobial effect of berry phenolics–a finnish perspective. Mol Nutr Food Res 51:684–691

Ho ML, Chen PN, Chu SC, Kuo DY, Kuo WH, Chen JY, Hsieh YS (2010) Peonidin 3-glucoside inhibits lung cancer metastasis by downregulation of proteinases activities and MAPK pathway. Nutr Cancer 62:505–516

Hsu YL, Kuo PL, Cho CY, Ni WC, Tzeng TF, Ng LT, Kuo YH, Lin CC (2007) Antrodia cinnamomea fruiting bodies extract suppresses the invasive potential of human liver cancer cell line PLC/PRF/5 through inhibition of nuclear factor kappaB pathway. Food Chem Toxicol 45:1249–1257

Jeong JC, Jang SW, Kim TH, Kwon CH, Kim YK (2010) Mulberry fruit (moris fructus) extracts induce human glioma cell death in vitro through ROS-dependent mitochondrial pathway and inhibits glioma tumor growth in vivo. Nutr Cancer 62:402–412

Kalt W, Hanneken A, Milbury P, Tremblay F (2010) Recent research on polyphenolics in vision and eye health. J Agric Food Chem 58:4001–4007

Kang SY, Seeram NP, Nair MG, Bourquin LD (2003) Tart cherry anthocyanins inhibit tumor development in Apc(Min) mice and reduce proliferation of human colon cancer cells. Cancer Lett 194:13–19

Kao ES, Tseng TH, Lee HJ, Chan KC, Wang CJ (2009) Anthocyanin extracted from hibiscus attenuate oxidized LDL-mediated foam cell formation involving regulation of CD36 gene. Chem Biol Interact 179:212–218

Karawajczyk A, Drgan V, Medic N, Oboh G, Passamonti S, Novic M (2007) Properties of flavonoids influencing the binding to bilitranslocase investigated by neural network modelling. Biochem Pharmacol 73:308–320

Katsube N, Iwashita K, Tsushida T, Yamaki K, Kobori M (2003) Induction of apoptosis in cancer cells by bilberry (vaccinium myrtillus) and the anthocyanins. J Agric Food Chem 51:68–75

Kay CD, Mazza G, Holub BJ, Wang J (2004) Anthocyanin metabolites in human urine and serum. Br J Nutr 91:933–942

Keppler K, Humpf HU (2005) Metabolism of anthocyanins and their phenolic degradation products by the intestinal microflora. Bioorg Med Chem 13:5195–5205

Kim JM, Kim JS, Yoo H, Choung MG, Sung MK (2008) Effects of black soybean [Glycine max (L.) Merr.] seed coats and its anthocyanidins on colonic inflammation and cell proliferation in vitro and in vivo. J Agric Food Chem 56:8427–8433

Kim HG, Ju MS, Shim JS, Kim MC, Lee SH, Huh Y, Kim SY, Oh MS (2010) Mulberry fruit protects dopaminergic neurons in toxin-induced Parkinson's disease models. Br J Nutr 104:8–16

Krikorian R, Shidler MD, Nash TA, Kalt W, Vinqvist-Tymchuk MR, Shukitt-Hale B, Joseph JA (2010) Blueberry supplementation improves memory in older adults. J Agric Food Chem 58:3996–4000

Kwon JY, Lee KW, Hur HJ, Lee HJ (2007) Peonidin inhibits phorbol-ester-induced COX-2 expression and transformation in JB6 P+cells by blocking phosphorylation of ERK-1 and –2. Ann N Y Acad Sci 1095:513–520

Lamy S, Lafleur R, Bedard V, Moghrabi A, Barrette S, Gingras D, Beliveau R (2007) Anthocyanidins inhibit migration of glioblastoma cells: structure-activity relationship and involvement of the plasminolytic system. J Cell Biochem 100:100–111

Lazze MC, Pizzala R, Perucca P, Cazzalini O, Savio M, Forti L, Vannini V, Bianchi L (2006) Anthocyanidins decrease endothelin-1 production and increase endothelial nitric oxide synthase in human endothelial cells. Mol Nutr Food Res 50:44–51

Lee KW, Hur HJ, Lee HJ, Lee CY (2005) Antiproliferative effects of dietary phenolic substances and hydrogen peroxide. J Agric Food Chem 53:1990–1995

Lee JH, Lee YH, Lee HJ, Lee HJ, Lee EO, Ahn KS, Shim BS, Bae H, Choi SH, Ahn KS, Baek NI, Kim DK, Kim SH (2009a) Caspase and mitogen activated protein kinase pathways are involved in solanum lyratum herba induced apoptosis. J Ethnopharmacol 123:121–127

Lee SH, Park SM, Park SM, Park JH, Shin DY, Kim GY, Ryu CH, Shin SC, Jung JM, Kang HS, Lee WS, Choi YH (2009b) Induction of apoptosis in human leukemia U937 cells by anthocyanins through down-regulation of Bcl-2 and activation of caspases. Int J Oncol 34:1077–1083

Li L, Adams LS, Chen S, Killian C, Ahmed A, Seeram NP (2009) Eugenia jambolana Lam. Berry extract inhibits growth and induces apoptosis of human breast cancer but not non-tumorigenic breast cells. J Agric Food Chem 57:826–831

Liu B, Chen Y, St Clair DK (2008) ROS and p53: a versatile partnership. Free Radic Biol Med 44:1529–1535

Liu J, Zhang W, Jing H, Popovich DG (2010) Bog bilberry (Vaccinium uliginosum L.) extract reduces cultured Hep-G2, Caco-2, and 3 T3-L1 cell viability, affects cell cycle progression, and has variable effects on membrane permeability. J Food Sci 75:H103–H107

Lo CW, Huang HP, Lin HM, Chien CT, Wang CJ (2007) Effect of hibiscus anthocyanins-rich extract induces apoptosis of proliferating smooth muscle cell via activation of P38 MAPK and p53 pathway. Mol Nutr Food Res 51:1452–1460

Lu J, Wu DM, Zheng YL, Hu B, Zhang ZF (2010) Purple sweet potato color alleviates D-galactose-induced brain aging in old mice by promoting survival of neurons via PI3K pathway and inhibiting cytochrome C-mediated apoptosis. Brain Pathol 20:598–612

Luo X, Budihardjo I, Zou H, Slaughter C, Wang X (1998) Bid, a Bcl2 interacting protein, mediates cytochrome c release from mitochondria in response to activation of cell surface death receptors. Cell 94:481–490

Maestro A, Terdoslavich M, Vanzo A, Kuku A, Tramer F, Nicolin V, Micali F, Decorti G, Passamonti S (2010) Expression of bilitranslocase in the vascular endothelium and its function as a flavonoid transporter. Cardiovasc Res 85:175–183

Malik A, Afaq F, Sarfaraz S, Adhami VM, Syed DN, Mukhtar H (2005) Pomegranate fruit juice for chemoprevention and chemotherapy of prostate cancer. Proc Natl Acad Sci U S A 102:14813–14818

Marko D, Puppel N, Tjaden Z, Jakobs S, Pahlke G (2004) The substitution pattern of anthocyanidins affects different cellular signaling cascades regulating cell proliferation. Mol Nutr Food Res 48:318–325

Mauray A, Felgines C, Morand C, Mazur A, Scalbert A, Milenkovic D (2010) Bilberry anthocyanin-rich extract alters expression of genes related to atherosclerosis development in aorta of apo E-deficient mice. Nutr Metab Cardiovasc Dis 22:72–80

Milbury PE, Kalt W (2010) Xenobiotic metabolism and berry flavonoid transport across the blood–brain barrier. J Agric Food Chem 58:3950–3956

Mulabagal V, Lang GA, DeWitt DL, Dalavoy SS, Nair MG (2009) Anthocyanin content, lipid peroxidation and cyclooxygenase enzyme inhibitory activities of sweet and sour cherries. J Agric Food Chem 57:1239–1246

Nguyen T, Nioi P, Pickett CB (2009) The Nrf2-antioxidant response element signaling pathway and its activation by oxidative stress. J Biol Chem 284:13291–13295

Nguyen V, Tang J, Oroudjev E, Lee CJ, Marasigan C, Wilson L, Ayoub G (2010) Cytotoxic effects of bilberry extract on MCF7-GFP-tubulin breast cancer cells. J Med Food 13:278–285

Passamonti S, Vrhovsek U, Vanzo A, Mattivi F (2003) The stomach as a site for anthocyanins absorption from food. FEBS Lett 544:210–213

Pauwels B, Wouters A, Peeters M, Vermorken JB, Lardon F (2010) Role of cell cycle perturbations in the combination therapy of chemotherapeutic agents and radiation. Future Oncol 6:1485–1496

Prior RL, Wu X (2006) Anthocyanins: structural characteristics that result in unique metabolic patterns and biological activities. Free Radic Res 40:1014–1028

Prior RL, Wilkes SE, Rogers TR, Khanal RC, Wu X, Howard LR (2010) Purified blueberry anthocyanins and blueberry juice alter development of obesity in mice fed an obesogenic high-fat diet. J Agric Food Chem 58:3970–3976

Rahman MM, Ichiyanagi T, Komiyama T, Sato S, Konishi T (2008) Effects of anthocyanins on psychological stress-induced oxidative stress and neurotransmitter status. J Agric Food Chem 56:7545–7550

Rasheed Z, Akhtar N, Anbazhagan AN, Ramamurthy S, Shukla M, Haqqi TM (2009) Polyphenol-rich pomegranate fruit extract (POMx) suppresses PMACI-induced expression of pro-inflammatory cytokines by inhibiting the activation of MAP Kinases and NF-kappaB in human KU812 cells. J Inflamm (Lond) 6:1–2

Reddivari L, Vanamala J, Chintharlapalli S, Safe SH, Miller JC Jr (2007) Anthocyanin fraction from potato extracts is cytotoxic to prostate cancer cells through activation of caspase-dependent and caspase-independent pathways. Carcinogenesis 28:2227–2235

Reddivari L, Vanamala J, Safe SH, Miller JC Jr (2010) The bioactive compounds alpha-chaconine and gallic acid in potato extracts decrease survival and induce apoptosis in LNCaP and PC3 prostate cancer cells. Nutr Cancer 62:601–610

Renis M, Calandra L, Scifo C, Tomasello B, Cardile V, Vanella L, Bei R, La Fauci L, Galvano F (2008) Response of cell cycle/stress-related protein expression and DNA damage upon treatment of CaCo2 cells with anthocyanins. Br J Nutr 100:27–35

Rodrigo KA, Rawal Y, Renner RJ, Schwartz SJ, Tian Q, Larsen PE, Mallery SR (2006) Suppression of the tumorigenic phenotype in human oral squamous cell carcinoma cells by an ethanol extract derived from freeze-dried black raspberries. Nutr Cancer 54:58–68

Roghani M, Niknam A, Jalali-Nadoushan MR, Kiasalari Z, Khalili M, Baluchnejadmojarad T (2010) Oral pelargonidin exerts dose-dependent neuroprotection in 6-hydroxydopamine rat model of hemi-parkinsonism. Brain Res Bull 82:279–283

Roy S, Khanna S, Alessio HM, Vider J, Bagchi D, Bagchi M, Sen CK (2002) Anti-angiogenic property of edible berries. Free Radic Res 36:1023–1031

Ruel G, Couillard C (2007) Evidences of the cardioprotective potential of fruits: the case of cranberries. Mol Nutr Food Res 51:692–701

Saric A, Sobocanec S, Balog T, Kusic B, Sverko V, Dragovic-Uzelac V, Levaj B, Cosic Z, Macak SZ, Marotti T (2009) Improved antioxidant and anti-inflammatory potential in mice consuming sour cherry juice (Prunus Cerasus cv. Maraska). Plant Foods Hum Nutr 64:231–237

Seeram NP, Adams LS, Zhang Y, Lee R, Sand D, Scheuller HS, Heber D (2006) Blackberry, black raspberry, blueberry, cranberry, red raspberry, and strawberry extracts inhibit growth and stimulate apoptosis of human cancer cells in vitro. J Agric Food Chem 54:9329–9339

Seymour EM, Lewis SK, Urcuyo-Llanes DE, Tanone II, Kirakosyan A, Kaufman PB, Bolling SF (2009) Regular tart cherry intake alters abdominal adiposity, adipose gene transcription, and inflammation in obesity-prone rats fed a high fat diet. J Med Food 12:935–942

Shih PH, Yeh CT, Yen GC (2005) Effects of anthocyanidin on the inhibition of proliferation and induction of apoptosis in human gastric adenocarcinoma cells. Food Chem Toxicol 43:1557–1566

Shih PH, Yeh CT, Yen GC (2007) Anthocyanins induce the activation of phase II enzymes through the antioxidant response element pathway against oxidative stress-induced apoptosis. J Agric Food Chem 55:9427–9435

Shin WH, Park SJ, Kim EJ (2006) Protective effect of anthocyanins in middle cerebral artery occlusion and reperfusion model of cerebral ischemia in rats. Life Sci 79:130–137

Shin DY, Lee WS, Lu JN, Kang MH, Ryu CH, Kim GY, Kang HS, Shin SC, Choi YH (2009) Induction of apoptosis in human colon cancer HCT-116 cells by anthocyanins through suppression of Akt and activation of p38-MAPK. Int J Oncol 35:1499–1504

Shumway BS, Kresty LA, Larsen PE, Zwick JC, Lu B, Fields HW, Mumper RJ, Stoner GD, Mallery SR (2008) Effects of a topically applied bioadhesive berry gel on loss of heterozygosity indices in premalignant oral lesions. Clin Cancer Res 14:2421–2430

Solomon A, Golubowicz S, Yablowicz Z, Bergman M, Grossman S, Altman A, Kerem Z, Flaishman MA (2010) Protection of fibroblasts (NIH-3 T3) against oxidative damage by cyanidin-3-rhamnoglucoside isolated from fig fruits (Ficus carica L.). J Agric Food Chem 58:6660–6665

Stoner GD, Wang LS, Chen T (2007) Chemoprevention of esophageal squamous cell carcinoma. Toxicol Appl Pharmacol 224:337–349

Tarozzi A, Morroni F, Hrelia S, Angeloni C, Marchesi A, Cantelli-Forti G, Hrelia P (2007) Neuroprotective effects of anthocyanins and their in vivo metabolites in SH-SY5Y cells. Neurosci Lett 424:36–40

Thomasset S, Berry DP, Cai H, West K, Marczylo TH, Marsden D, Brown K, Dennison A, Garcea G, Miller A, Hemingway D, Steward WP, Gescher AJ (2009) Pilot study of oral anthocyanins for colorectal cancer chemoprevention. Cancer Prev Res (Phila) 2:625–633

Tsuda T, Horio F, Osawa T (1999) Absorption and metabolism of cyanidin 3-O-beta-D-glucoside in rats. FEBS Lett 449:179–182

Tsuda T, Ueno Y, Yoshikawa T, Kojo H, Osawa T (2006) Microarray profiling of gene expression in human adipocytes in response to anthocyanins. Biochem Pharmacol 71:1184–1197

Vanzo A, Terdoslavich M, Brandoni A, Torres AM, Vrhovsek U, Passamonti S (2008) Uptake of grape anthocyanins into the rat kidney and the involvement of bilitranslocase. Mol Nutr Food Res 52:1106–1116
Vari R, D'Archivio M, Filesi C, Carotenuto S, Scazzocchio B, Santangelo C, Giovannini C, Masella R (2011) Protocatechuic acid induces antioxidant/detoxifying enzyme expression through JNK-mediated Nrf2 activation in murine macrophages. J Nutr Biochem 22(5):409–417
Wang LS, Stoner GD (2008) Anthocyanins and their role in cancer prevention. Cancer Lett 269:281–290
Westermarck J, Kahari VM (1999) Regulation of matrix metalloproteinase expression in tumor invasion. FASEB J 13:781–792
Woodward G, Kroon P, Cassidy A, Kay C (2009) Anthocyanin stability and recovery: implications for the analysis of clinical and experimental samples. J Agric Food Chem 57:5271–5278
Ye J, Meng X, Yan C, Wang C (2010) Effect of purple sweet potato anthocyanins on beta-amyloid-mediated PC-12 cells death by inhibition of oxidative stress. Neurochem Res 35:357–365
Yeh CT, Yen GC (2005) Induction of apoptosis by the Anthocyanidins through regulation of Bcl-2 gene and activation of c-Jun N-terminal kinase cascade in hepatoma cells. J Agric Food Chem 53:1740–1749
Yu X, Kensler T (2005) Nrf2 as a target for cancer chemoprevention. Mutat Res 591:93–102
Yun JW, Lee WS, Kim MJ, Lu JN, Kang MH, Kim HG, Kim DC, Choi EJ, Choi JY, Kim HG, Lee YK, Ryu CH, Kim G, Choi YH, Park OJ, Shin SC (2010) Characterization of a profile of the anthocyanins isolated from Vitis coignetiae Pulliat and their anti-invasive activity on HT-29 human colon cancer cells. Food Chem Toxicol 48:903–909
Zdarilova A, Rajnochova SA, Chytilova K, Simanek V, Ulrichova J (2010) Polyphenolic fraction of Lonicera caerulea L. Fruits reduces oxidative stress and inflammatory markers induced by lipopolysaccharide in gingival fibroblasts. Food Chem Toxicol 48:1555–1561
Zhang ZF, Fan SH, Zheng YL, Lu J, Wu DM, Shan Q, Hu B (2009) Purple sweet potato color attenuates oxidative stress and inflammatory response induced by d-galactose in mouse liver. Food Chem Toxicol 47:496–501
Zhu F, Cai YZ, Yang X, Ke J, Corke H (2010) Anthocyanins, hydroxycinnamic acid derivatives, and antioxidant activity in roots of different Chinese purple-fleshed sweetpotato genotypes. J Agric Food Chem 58:7588–7596
Zimmerman MC, Oberley LW, Flanagan SW (2007) Mutant SOD1-induced neuronal toxicity is mediated by increased mitochondrial superoxide levels. J Neurochem 102:609–618

Index

M. Diederich and K. Noworyta (eds.), *Natural Compounds as Inducers of Cell Death: Volume 1*, DOI 10.1007/978-94-007-4575-9,